DATE DUE

NOV 1 1 2000	
APR OCT 3 1 2000 APR 1 9 2000	
APR 2 5 2001	
MAY - 7 2003 MAY - 6 2003	
FEB 2 0 2006	
APR 1 0 2006	
MAY 1 2006	
MAY - 1 2006	
MAY 2 2007 MAY - 2 2007 OCT 2 1 2009	
NOV 1 3 2009	

GAYLORD   PRINTED IN U.S.A.

REHABILITATIVE AUDIOLOGY:
CHILDREN AND ADULTS

THIRD EDITION

REHABILITATIVE AUDIOLOGY:
CHILDREN AND ADULTS

THIRD EDITION

EDITORS

Jerome G. Alpiner, Ph.D.
Jerome G. Alpiner, Ph.D. & Associates
Littleton, Colorado

Patricia A. McCarthy, Ph.D.
Professor
Department of Communication Disorders and Sciences
Rush University
Rush-Presbyterian-St. Luke's Medical Center
Chicago, Illinois

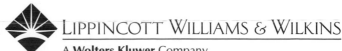
LIPPINCOTT WILLIAMS & WILKINS
A **Wolters Kluwer** Company
Philadelphia • Baltimore • New York • London
Buenos Aires • Hong Kong • Sydney • Tokyo

Editor: John P. Butler
Managing Editor: Matthew J. Hauber
Marketing Manager: Anne Smith
Project Editor: Paula C. Williams
Back cover graphic designed by Randy Hansen

Printed in the United States of America

First Edition, 1987
Second Edition, 1993

Library of Congress Cataloging-in-Publication Data

Rehabilitative audiology: children and adults/editors, Jerome G. Alpiner, Patricia A. McCarthy.—3rd. ed.
   p.   cm.
   Includes bibliographical references and index.
   ISBN 0–683–30652–9
   1. Hearing impaired—Rehabilitation. 2. Deaf—Rehabilitation. 3. Audiology. I. Alpiner, Jerome G., 1932– II. McCarthy, Patricia A.
   RF297 .R44 2000
   617.8′9—dc21   99–32657
                                                              CIP

To purchase additional copies of this book, call our customer service department at **(800) 638-3030** or fax orders to **(301) 824-7390.** International customers should call **(301) 714-2324.**

99 00 01 02 03
1 2 3 4 5 6 7 8 9 10

To my wife, Victoria, and our family: Steven, Susan, Sharon, David, Bill, Carol, Dan, Benjamin, Rachel, Shayna, Anna, and Charley, who have supported me with their love and encouragement. This book is also dedicated to my students, colleagues, and other family members, who have meant so much to me and have provided continuing inspiration for the things I accomplish. And to the memory of Judy.

J.G.A.

To my husband and my son, Richard and Kevin Peach, who anchor me with their unconditional love and consistent support. And to my parents, Joanne and Dan McCarthy, who have given me a lifetime of encouragement, inspiration, and total approval.

P.A.M.

PREFACE

More than 20 years have passed since the publication of the first edition of *Handbook of Adult Rehabilitative Audiology* in 1978. In the preface to that edition, we noted that "the book attempts to fill a void in the literature for those who have any contact with hearing-impaired adults." A second edition followed in 1982, and in 1987 the first edition of the expanded *Rehabilitative Audiology: Children and Adults* was introduced. The years since 1978 have seen numerous and significant changes in the field of audiology. Whereas early texts on the subject could be perused quickly and without intensive concentration, the body of knowledge in "Audiologic Rehabilitation" today has expanded considerably for both children and adults. Gone are the days when aural rehabilitation was primarily confined to lipreading and auditory training.

Today, a greater number of professional audiologists and other health care providers have become involved in various aspects of rehabilitation. Many areas of audiologic rehabilitation have emerged, and there are more options for clients in need of professional assistance for loss of hearing. Audiology students of two decades ago would likely be amazed at a contemporary course outline for audiologic rehabilitation. Chapter 19 on Future Directions is intended to alert readers to the recent advances in audiologic rehabilitation and to emphasize the need for study in additional areas as we begin the 21st century.

This third edition of *Rehabilitative Audiology: Children and Adults* is organized in five sections: Philosophy and Service Provision; Audiologic Rehabilitation: Children; Audiologic Rehabilitation: Adults; Technology in Audiologic Rehabilitation; and Future Directions. Chapter 18 on Outcome Measures makes its debut—all other chapters have been updated. A new feature in this edition is the attachment section at the end of the text. This section includes all Self-Assessment Tools for Audiologic Rehabilitation which appear in the book. Current information covers audiologic rehabilitation in various types of practices, cochlear implants, assistive technology, computer applications, needs of the geriatric population, aspects of audiologic rehabilitation for children, and research needs.

The contributors of this edition represent a variety of audiology work settings: universities, hospitals, schools, hearing aid dispensing practices, private practices, and industry. These authors, nationally recognized, bring many years of experience and hands-on treatment with clients and provide a comprehensive view of audiologic rehabilitation in the United States. We are fortunate to have so many authorities represented, complemented by the comprehensive references provided to other experts in the profession.

We hope that audiologic rehabilitation becomes a regular and challenging part of your day-to-day professional work life. Come and experience the fascinating and changing field of *audiologic rehabilitation.* Work with us in benefiting the children and adults of today and tomorrow "who don't hear very well."

Welcome to the new millennium!

J.G.A.
P.A.M.

Alpiner, Jerome G., Ph.D., Jerome G. Alpiner, Ph.D. & Associates, Littleton, Colorado

Beiter, Anne L., M.S., Director of Education and Training, Cochlear Corporation, Englewood, Colorado

Bentler, Ruth A., Ph.D., Associate Professor, Department of Speech Pathology & Audiology, University of Iowa, Iowa City, Iowa

Brimacombe, Judith A., M.A., Senior Director of Customer and Clinical Services, Advanced Bionics Corporation, Sylmar, California

Compton, Cynthia L., Ph.D., Assistant Professor of Audiology, Department of Audiology & Speech Language Pathology, Gallaudet University, Washington, DC

Erler, Susan F., Ph.D., Project Coordinator, Northwestern University, Evanston, Illinois

Erdman, Sue Ann, M.A., Research Associate, Hearing Rehabilitation Laboratory, Department of Psychology, University of Maryland Baltimore County, Baltimore, Maryland

Garstecki, Dean C., Ph.D., Professor and Chairman, Communication Sciences and Disorders Department, Northwestern University, Evanston, Illinois

Gottermeier, Linda, M.A., Rochester Institute of Technology, National Technical Institute for the Deaf

Hansen, Elaine M., M.ed., Audiological Consultants, Inc., Denver, Colorado

Hasenstab, Suzanne M., Ph.D., Department of Audiology, Medical College of Virginia-Virginia Commonwealth University, Richmond, Virginia

Houston, K. Todd, Ph.D., Clinical Assistant Professor, Department of Speech-Language Pathology and Audiology, University of South Carolina, Columbia, South Carolina

Johnson, Cheryl DeConde, Ed.D., Senior Consultant, Deaf/Hard of Hearing Disabilities and Audiology Services, The Colorado Department of Education & Educational Audiologist, Special Education Unit, Greeley, Colorado

Kaufman, Kristen J., M.S., ENT Associates, Sioux Falls, South Dakota

Kricos, Patricia B., Ph.D., Professor of Audiology, Department of Communication Sciences and Disorders, University of Florida, Gainesville, Florida

Laughton, Joan, Ph.D., Director of Deaf/Hard of Hearing, Communication Sciences & Disorders, University of Georgia, Athens, Georgia

Madell, Jane R., Ph.D., Director, Communicative Disorders, Long Island College Hospital, Professor, Clinical Otolaryngology, State University of New York, Brooklyn, New York

McCarthy, Patricia A., Ph.D., Professor, Department of Communication Disorders and Sciences, Rush University, Rush-Presbyterian-St. Luke's Medical Center, Chicago, Illinois

Meyer, Dianne H., Ph.D., Chairperson, Department of Communication Disorders and Sciences, Rush University, Rush-Presbyterian-St. Luke's Medical Center, Chicago, Illinois

Montano, Joseph, Ed.D., Associate Professor of Education, Department of Speech and Hearing, Long Island University, C.W. Post Campus, Brookville, New York

Montgomery, Allen A., Ph.D., Research Professor, Department of Speech-Language Pathology, University of South Carolina, Columbia, South Carolina

Mueller, H. Gustav, Ph.D., Associate Adjunct Professor, Vanderbilt University; Senior Consultant in Audiology, Siemens Hearing Instruments, Castle Rock, Colorado

Palmer, Catherine V., Ph.D., Assistant Professor, University of Pittsburgh, Pittsburgh, Pennsylvania; Director of Audiology, Eye and Ear Institute, University of Pittsburgh Medical Center, Pittsburgh, Pennsylvania

Sapp, Julie Vesper, Ph.D., Audiologist, Northeast Georgia RESA, Winterville, Georgia

Schow, Ronald L., Ph.D., Professor, Department of Speech Pathology and Audiology, Idaho State University, Pocatello, Idaho

Sims, Donald G., Ph.D., Associate Professor, National Institute for the Deaf, Rochester Institute of Technology, Rochester, New York

Tye-Murray, Nancy, Ph.D., Professor and Director of Research, Central Institute for the Deaf, St. Louis, Missouri

Weinstein, Barbara E., Ph.D., Professor and Program Director, Lehman College, CUNY, Bronx, New York

Yoshinaga-Itano, Christine, Ph.D., Chairperson, Department of Speech, Language, and Hearing Sciences, University of Colorado, Boulder, Colorado

CONTENTS

S E C T I O N **III**
AUDIOLOGIC REHABILITATION: ADULTS

S E C T I O N **IV**
TECHNOLOGY IN AUDIOLOGIC REHABILITATION

S E C T I O N **V**
FUTURE DIRECTIONS

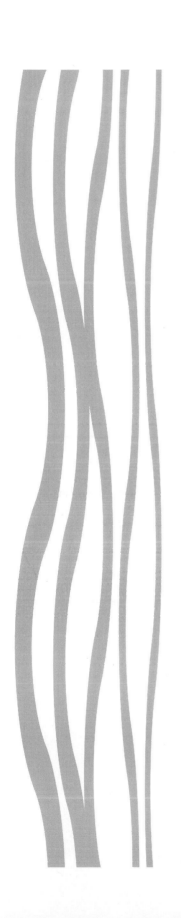

PHILOSOPHY AND SERVICE PROVISION

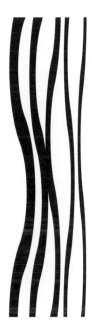

Transition: Rehabilitative Audiology Into the New Millennium

Jerome G. Alpiner, Ph.D., Elaine M. Hansen, M.Ed., and
Kristen J. Kaufman, M.S.

Aural rehabilitation emerged as a result of World War II. It began out of a need to help thousands of soldiers who became hearing-impaired due to the war. In contemporary terminology, "rehabilitative audiology" developed as a remediation process to lessen the consequences of hearing loss on an individual's everyday life. As we enter the new millennium, it is important to sequence the transition of aural rehabilitation in the beginning to rehabilitative audiology now.

The emphasis during the early days was primarily on lipreading (speechreading) and auditory training. Hearing aids existed, were very helpful, but were primitive by today's technology. Visualize the commonplace "body type aids"—large batteries and dangling cords resting in shirt pockets or undergarments. Hearing aids were dispensed only by hearing aid dealers until the 1970s. Audiologists were not permitted to sell hearing aids to clients; the Code of Ethics of the American Speech-Language-Hearing Association (ASHA) prohibited the sale of products. This situation changed in the 1970s and appeared to alter the profession of audiology. Previously, audiologists performed hearing aid evaluations and then referred clients to hearing aid dealers. Usually there was little rehabilitative follow-up. The change af-

forded the audiologist the opportunity to assume full responsibility for rehabilitative audiology from evaluation through dispensing to preremediation and postremediation follow-up. Hearing aid dispensing became a major aspect of rehabilitation.

Audiology As a Profession

The past decade found many audiologists on a roller coaster ride in defense of their profession. Criticisms from the Food and Drug Administration (FDA) about unsubstantiated claims of hearing aid performance put skepticism into the minds of many consumers. Most audiologists and hearing aid dispensers do operate in a professional and ethical manner. When consumers read certain advertisements in newspapers, however, they become confused. Why does this situation exist? Recent advertisements, for example, in the *Denver Rocky Mountain News* newspaper expound the following: hearing aid, $129; free pack of batteries, free video otoscopic picture of your ears; free hearing test; free 1-year warranty. The client is confused! How can one sell that "wonderful" hearing aid for $129, when an audiologist the client has visited quoted a price of $750 for the aid and $75 for the hearing test (1999)?

As we promote ourselves and our services, we find some obstacles along the way. We are not the only providers of hearing aids; credentialed hearing aid dispensers sell hearing aids and some physicians sell hearing aids (without the services of an audiologist). In addition, managed care may affect the way we do business.

Nevertheless, we continue with our desire to become more autonomous. Through the efforts of many audiologists, ASHA has taken a more intensive look at autonomy for audiology. ASHA has tried to show its support for the profession by adding a Vice-President for Audiology on its Executive Board. Still, a large number of audiologists felt the need to establish their own association, the American Academy of Audiology (AAA), in 1988. There has been concern at the national level about the relationship and mission of ASHA and AAA with regard to audiology and the credentials necessary to be a practicing audiologist. Consequently, the same struggles of ASHA and AAA became mirrored on a state level. Some audiologists have formed their own state academies of audiology; some state associations attempted to upgrade audiologists through licensure and/or registration.

As consumers become more sophisticated and inquisitive, many audiologists find themselves taking different tactics when dealing with their clients. Rehabilitative audiology, which sometimes comprised a very little to an almost nonexistent part of the dispensing process in the past, is becoming an integral part of service to clients. High-technology hearing aids have led to high expectations from consumers. Even manufacturers have become cognizant of the benefit of rehabilitative audiology, which in turn reduces hearing aid return rates. Some manufacturers of hearing aids now provide rehabilitation programs for use by audiologists for their clients.

Northern (1998) described one audiological rehabilitation program offered by HEARx in which the rate of hearing aid returns was reduced through a patient education program. Records were reviewed from a large sample of patients (n = 9868) who ordered hearing aids between January and June 1997. Approximately one-third of the patients (n = 3306) elected to attend a free series of audiological rehabilitation classes. Rehabilitation participants showed a 3.5% hearing aid return rate compared with a 12% return/cancellation rate in those patients who did not attend the classes. Northern states that these results should satisfy audiologists who often question the necessity of aural rehabilitation in hearing aid programs.

Electone, Inc. (Harford PR, Aural Rehabilitation [Program by Electone, Inc.], Longwood, FL, 1994) developed an aural rehabilitation protocol. The purpose of the protocol is to support the dispenser's efforts to improve the quality of life of those individuals with hearing loss. It is recommended that aural rehabilitation be integrated into the current system of hearing care. The protocol states that a patient has a better opportunity for success with amplification if a regimented rehabilitation program is followed. The Electone program cites three reasons for aural rehabilitation as part of a hearing aid program:

1. It educates the patient and the patient's significant other on the subject of hearing loss and sets realistic expectations for the ability of hearing instruments to assist in better communication.
2. It outlines the patient's responsibilities in the use of hearing instruments and the adjustment to hearing instruments in a variety of environments.
3. It adds value to the dispensing practice, which leaves the patient with a lasting, favorable impression, thereby increasing referrals.

There are several components to this program. A confidential patient case history is taken that includes a hearing aid assessment screening tool. An otoscopic examination is performed, and medical aspects are considered regarding any necessary physician referral. Both pure tone and speech testing are accomplished. A review of the findings are explained to the patient, including the effect on understanding speech. Amplification recommendations are discussed, including hearing aid options. Counseling is provided both before and after the hearing aid fitting. A hearing adjustment program is outlined for the patient and includes several goals. Some of the patient topics include (a) performing selective listening, (b) involving others with better hearing, (c) becoming accustomed to his or her own voice, (d) becoming positively assertive, (e) modifying communication behavior, (f) listening for ideas, (g) improving communication using visual clues, (h) improving communication in competing noise, (i) participating in small group conversation, (j) accepting realistic expectations from hearing instrument use, and (k) listening in various environments.

We participated in a hearing aid study for an electronics manufacturer. One of the purposes of the project was to determine the reactions of first-time wearers to hearing aids. One phase of the evaluation aspect was to present an expectation questionnaire before and after hearing aid use (Chapter Appendices 1.1 and 1.2). There are numerous assessment tools available for pretesting and posttesting of communication performance and hearing aid benefit. The expectation questionnaire provided an additional dimension to consider, that is, what does the patient expect? Did the hearing aid fulfill those expectations? We believe that this kind of information offers an informative way for audiologists to plan rehabilitation for their clients and also serves as a quality check on counseling.

Definitions

A variety of definitions have been used to describe audiology and the remediation process for persons with hearing loss. In this text, we use rehabilitative audiology, habilitative audiology, and aural rehabilitation interchangeably. We prefer rehabilitative audiology because it has been defined as a more comprehensive terminology in working with the whole person, regardless of onset of hearing loss or modality of communi-

cation. It is helpful to refer to Preferred Practice Patterns for audiologists which have been suggested by ASHA (1997):

1. Audiologic rehabilitation assessment
   a. Clinical indications—individuals of all ages are assessed on the basis of results of audiologic assessment; hearing aid or assistive system/device assessment, fitting, or orientation; sensory aid assessment; and communication needs or preferences.
   b. Clinical process—(a) assessment includes evaluation of reception, comprehension, and production of language in oral, signed, or written modalities; speech and voice production; perception of speech and non-speech stimuli in multiple modalities; listening skills; speechreading; and communication strategies; (b) performance in both clinical and natural environments is considered; and (c) audiologic (aural) rehabilitation assessment may be part of an intradisciplinary and interdisciplinary process.
2. Audiologic rehabilitation
   a. Clinical indications—audiologic (aural) rehabilitation is provided to persons of all ages who have any degree or type of hearing loss on the basis of the results of an audiologic (aural) rehabilitation assessment.
   b. Clinical process (highlights) treatment that focuses on reception, comprehension, and production of language; speech and voice production; auditory training; speechreading; visual; auditory-visual; tactile training; communication strategies; education and counseling; family/caregiver participation; discharge planning; follow-up service; interdisciplinary involvement; and quality assurance.

From these practice patterns, it appears that the role of the audiologist in rehabilitation has greatly expanded and is considerably more substantive than even 10 to 15 years ago. These patterns also include aspects that guide the audiologist in providing help to oral-aural, total, and manual clients.

From an applied viewpoint, Ross (1997) has indicated that the rehabilitation needs of most clients can be met within the hearing aid dispensing process. He proposes a group hearing aid orientation program (HAO) for both previous and new hearing aid users. Ross further provides a rationale for an orientation program:

1. The incidence of hearing aid returns is likely to be much less for persons who attend such programs than for those who do not.
2. An HAO program is going to translate into more satisfied and loyal clients.
3. More satisfied users mean more word-of-mouth referrals.
4. During the course of the program, some monaural users will opt for a binaural fitting.
5. The program provides sufficient time to display, demonstrate, and dispense other types of hearing assistance technologies.
6. Although a group HAO program should supplement and not supplant individual orientation programs, it is likely that the group meetings may eliminate the necessity of some individual sessions.
7. The inclusion of family members multiplies the number of contacts and future referral sources.
8. The additional time available for instructions on trouble-shooting should translate into less returns for problems such as those due to excessive cerumen.
9. The program provides a logical opportunity to sign people up for a "battery club."

We believe that HAO programs are appropriate and necessary. This type of program helps to move rehabilitative audiology into a total assistance program, with amplification serving as the anchor for the process. However, it is often not possible to engage in group programs for several reasons. We have found it difficult to establish set times for all participants, resulting in a number of "no-shows." Continuity of the

program, therefore, was not able to be followed. Many clients had varying degrees of hearing loss, from mild to profound, causing interference in the flow of the program. Differences in the types of hearing aids worn caused difficulties in orientation and resulted in frustration. We did have some success with "captive" audiences, such as Veterans Administration (VA) programs at which attendance was required, although the problems mentioned above still occurred on occasion. We do endorse both individual and group HAO programs and recommend either depending on the compatibility of the individuals.

Incidence

Standing at the threshold of the new millennium, we can appreciate the progress made in increasing the awareness of hearing and hearing loss. Hearing impairment among individuals such as President Clinton, former Miss America Heather Whitestone, and General Norman Schwarzkopf has spurred this campaign. Despite these great strides, hearing professionals, the hearing industry, and related hearing groups must continue their efforts to inform society about hearing and hearing loss.

Currently, there are millions of children and adults in the United States who have varying degrees of hearing loss that may affect performance in everyday living environments. Hearing impairment is often a very handicapping condition that may go unnoticed if a hearing aid is not visible to others or if one does not hear the speech of a congenitally deaf youngster. The 1996 edition of AHSA *Communication Facts* provides the latest estimates available of hearing loss in the United States. Approximately 28 million individuals have hearing loss (Adams and Marano, 1995). The most common causes of hearing loss for adults are presbycusis and noise exposure. Figure 1.1 indicates the percentage of people with hearing loss by age (National Center for Health Statistics, 1996). Presbycusic trends are demonstrated with 13.7% of the 45- to

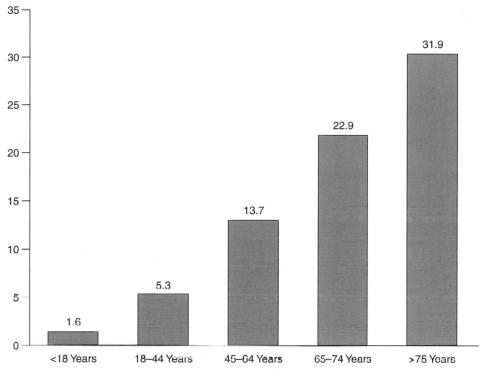

Figure 1.1. Percentage of persons with hearing loss by age (1994) (National Center for Health Statistics).

64-year-old group having hearing loss, increasing to 22.9% of the 65- to 74-year-old group, and to 31.9% of those older than 75. The ASHA fact sheet (1998) presents other information of interest: (1) of individuals younger than 45 years of age with hearing loss, 58.8% were males and 41.2% were females; (2) the greatest disparity between males and females was reported in the 45 to 64 year age group—67.2% were males and 32.8% were females; (3) African-Americans are underrepresented in the population reporting hearing loss compared with the general population, with only 6.8% reporting hearing loss; (4) 10 million persons are affected by noise-induced hearing loss; (5) approximately 17 million people have sensorineural hearing loss; and (6) bothersome tinnitus affects from 6 to 20% of the U.S. population (Axelsson and Ringdahl, 1989).

The most common causes of hearing loss in children are genetic/hereditary factors and middle ear pathology. Otitis media has become the most common treatable illness for which children visit their physicians (ASHA, 1995). Approximately 50% of childhood hearing loss is genetically based. Surprising to some, hearing loss ranks third, only behind arthritis and hypertension, as a health concern expressed by adults 65 years and older (Brechtelsbauer, 1990). In view of these demographics, the audiologist is faced with a myriad of rehabilitative schemes to consider to serve their pediatric through geriatric clientele successfully.

With regard to incidence, Dickenson (1998) discusses the "Doomed Boomer Generation." It is not a startling event to hear members of the "boom box generation" driving around, defiantly contending that loud noises will not harm them, indeed nothing will harm them. What are the facts? One of 12 30-year-olds is already hearing-impaired. From 1971 to 1991, the number of Americans with hearing loss increased by 53%. What about the 40-year-olds? Because of the baby-boom bulge, more 40-year-olds than 50-year-olds suffer from hearing loss.

At age 50, 1 in 8 will be hearing-impaired. Typically, the 50-year-old will spend 7 years in denial before submitting to a hearing aid. No matter how intense our denial of hearing loss, it will happen to a certain number of individuals and a considerable amount of time will be spent in a denial or a lack of awareness response before reality emerges.

Myths About Rehabilitative Audiology

The early days of aural rehabilitation focused on speechreading and auditory training. These strategies were recommended to improve communication ability regardless of whether hearing aids were worn. Academic training programs were the primary providers of these therapies to expose students to clinical practice. Speechreading and auditory training became synonymous with aural rehabilitation, and that belief still lingers for some. These strategies, however, are only smaller components of a more comprehensive approach to the rehabilitation process. The Preferred Practice Patterns designated by ASHA exemplify this broader concept.

Whether good or bad, there is an ever-increasing need for the "quick fix." We live in the age of the World Wide Web, fast food, fax transmissions, overnight express delivery, and microwaveable everything. This mentality is demonstrated in all aspects of our lives: social, vocational, financial, spiritual, technological, and health. The hearing health care profession is not immune from this way of thinking, that is, the myth that we can provide an immediate "fix" for the ears.

Time is our invaluable commodity. Think about it. Time management consultants/seminars are a booming industry. Why? The "need for speed" requires constant evaluation of time. Both consumers and professionals define parameters and expectations relative to the time and energy they are willing to expend on a task or project. This results in giving tangible and immediate solutions priority, thus the quick fix.

Not to be forgotten in this quick-fix generation is the prerequisite that quality not be compromised. Today's consumers are more sophisticated as they seek ways to optimize their hearing and quality of life in general. So as the consumer demands immediate yet quality solutions for hearing impairment, the goal of the hearing professional must be to maintain the balance between a comprehensive hearing health care plan that can be individualized for each client, yet not imposing on the time constraints of themselves or the client. A comprehensive plan by front line professionals (Tye-Murray et al., 1994) offers options such as home training programs, client libraries, children or family centers, and assistive technology centers for consideration of one or all for the busy clinical setting.

Essential to this balancing act is the acknowledgment that instrumentation is not the "cure all." There is no disputing that technology is dramatically improving the habilitative/rehabilitative process. Digital and programmable instrumentation allow finger-tip flexibility and individualized customization. However, we agree with Rihs (1997) that the hearing instrument myth that states "audiologically based solutions such as compression, the number of channels and the use of signal processing algorithms present the solution to *all* of the communication needs of hearing-impaired users" must be dismissed.

For time's sake, some of the first elements of the hearing evaluation/treatment process to be eliminated or abbreviated are the case history, prefitting inventory/questionnaire, appropriate counseling on realistic expectations, or an assistive listening devices (ALD) needs assessment (Fuller, 1998). When we eliminate these valuable measures, we potentially miss medical information that would reveal confounding medical factors (Ulrich, 1998), unrealistic expectations regarding what treatment can provide, and identification of day-to-day needs related to communication that exist for the client. Evaluation of the client's expectations and specific communication needs before initiating the element of instrumentation may actually improve the end result of customer satisfaction.

With the pediatric client, we seem to have a broader approach to treatment. We would never consider ignoring the need for other ALDs (i.e., FM system for academic setting), nor should we do this for the adult or geriatric client. More and more professionals are acknowledging the need for some form of ALD components. Morris (1998) suggests that professionals consider one of three packages when including an ALD component in their services. First, an outsourcing package in which a professional resource is provided without committing to selling/training/support time. Second, a referrals package which includes assessment is initiated and a communication assessment report, with a technology plan, is received. The professional can be in the loop without becoming involved in inventory and billing processes. Third, a full-service package in which ALDs are directly dispensed and a technical support is set up, with a flexible inventory control and on-site consulting/technical training of staff.

Another myth is that individuals do not buy hearing aids because they cost too much money. Although money may be a factor for some, Ross (1992) presents several reasons why only approximately 20 to 25% of persons who need aids obtain them. He states that there is no single reason for rejection of amplification.

Association with age is one factor. Our society is bombarded with advertisements that emphasize youth through use of pictures and physical activity. It is not uncommon to hear our older clients insist that hearing aids will make them look and feel old, even with completely in the canal (CIC) instruments.

Association with disability is another factor for consideration. It is not necessarily only the hearing loss that is troublesome, but that problem coupled with others such as heart disease, dementia, and so forth. These difficulties may cause feelings of frustration that one is different from other "normal" persons.

Association with high cost can be a consideration for many persons. Hearing aid costs may range from $800 to $3000 for one instrument depending on technology, options, and other factors. Binaural amplification will double the cost. However, we cannot ignore the fact that quality of life may be improved significantly with amplification in a society that demands expressive and receptive communication. There is no easy answer regarding this issue. Compounding this matter is the fact that there are approximately 2.5 million low-income children and adults in the United States who need hearing help but cannot afford hearing aids (U.S. Department of Commerce, 1995; Hoffman, 1996).

Assistance for Low-Income Children and Adults

The issue of children and adults who want and need hearing aids and cochlear implants but do not have the financial resources needs to be addressed further. Although this population goes largely unrecognized, various service clubs, churches, and community groups are available to help low-income persons obtain hearing aids and cochlear implants, usually at the local level. In addition, one major national nonprofit organization, HEAR NOW, provides assistance for low-income individuals in all U.S. states and territories. HEAR NOW was founded in 1988 and, projected through 1999, 17,000 hearing aids were provided to low-income children and adults. In 1998, assistance was provided for 20 cochlear implants.

HEAR NOW is like the March of Dimes for hearing. Interested persons contact HEAR NOW, complete application procedures to verify that they meet financial criteria, and find an audiologist or hearing aid dispenser who volunteers to order and fit the hearing aids provided by HEAR NOW. More than 2500 audiologists and hearing aid dispensers volunteer their time to assist these individuals. HEAR NOW is a community service supported by foundations, corporations, individual donors, special events, and a hearing aid recycling program.

HEAR NOW engages in providing quality assurance and surveying providers and recipients about the help received from hearing aids. Standardized procedures such as the *Abbreviated Profile of Hearing Aid Benefit* (Cox, 1995) are used before and after the hearing aid fitting. An additional tool is used as well, the *Expectation Questionnaire* (Alpiner and Hansen, 1996), which was previously used in a hearing aid study for an electronics manufacturer. It is especially helpful to know what clients expect from a hearing aid before they wear it and, after a certain period of use, to determine if expectations are fulfilled.

Low-income clients are evaluated in the same way as "paying" clients. It is HEAR NOW's goal to enable these children and adults to hear so that they may become productive members of society. People who want to hear should not be denied that critical connection to society due to a lack of financial resources. Additional information can be obtained by calling HEAR NOW at 1-800-648-HEAR.

Quality of Life and Consumer Expectations

Does the hearing aid do it all now? Is the end of hearing loss in reach? Digital sound processing (DSP) technology is now readily available and implemented in many practices. Advances in hearing aid technology continue to change, much like personal computers. Software upgrades for programming instruments continue to improve. With all these advances in technology, testing and fitting techniques, and the ability to customize or program the hearing instrument, is it possible to meet the satisfaction of the consumer? The MarkeTrak satisfaction survey found satisfaction rates of 75% or more for advanced hearing aids compared with the MarkeTrak average of 64% for conventional instruments (Kochkin, 1997).

There is an increase in the satisfaction with hearing aids and service. There is also improved technology due to CIC hearing aids, programmable devices, cochlear implants, and other implantable devices. The needs have been met for the entire range of hearing loss from mild to the most profound impairment. Hearing aid sales increased 7.5% in 1997 primarily due to high-performance hearing aid devices (Kirkwood, 1998b). The universal NOAH software system has given the dispenser a more affordable means of providing digitally programmable and DSP programmable instruments for clients. Although the stigma of hearing aids is still an issue, they are beginning to be viewed more favorably. The return rate of hearing aids, however, still remains the same or slightly increased at 17.8%. The return rate for CIC instruments is the highest at 25.2% (Kirkwood, 1998a). We can surmise that perfection has not yet been achieved even with today's advanced hearing instruments.

There is a tendency for consumers to look for simple answers to complex hearing problems. There are a variety of dimensions to hearing loss that need to be addressed. Therefore, follow-up service is important. It is an ongoing service, a relationship that is developed between the professional audiologist and the client. Extensive rehabilitative audiology usually is not on the mind of hearing aid consumers. Even cochlear implant clients rarely stay in rehabilitation for lengthy periods. We tell our clients that patience is a virtue with regard to achieving the most benefit from their hearing instruments.

The relationship between quality of life and rehabilitative audiology has long been recognized by hearing professionals. However, effective measurement tools (specific to hearing impairment) are in their early stages of development. Different terms are used—life satisfaction, quality of life, and functional health status—all referring to the level of an individual's social, physical, and emotional well-being. Crandell (1998) states that hearing impairment decreases psychosocial and physical health, specifically shown by an increased incidence of health-related difficulties with sensorineural hearing loss. Current research is more clearly defining the association between quality of life and sensory impairment, as well as demonstrating improved functional health status with hearing instrument utilization (Crandell, 1996). One study, reported by Radcliffe (1998), revealed that "Sensory aids are effective in counteracting the negative effect of sensory dysfunction on quality of life. Subjects using sensory aids showed a higher mood level, richer social relationships and better performance in the activities of daily living than subjects with non-corrected sensory impairments".

We hope this surge will document for the medical field and the general public what hearing professionals have known for quite some time. We specify the medical field due to the ever-increasing demand for health care accountability. More and more, managed care is demanding assurances and/or additional documentation to substantiate that audiologic services are cost-effective and of proven value. In response to this increased demand, ASHA in 1995 developed a Functional Assessment of Communication Skills, known as the ASHA FACS. This was formed as an outcome measure of communication disability specific to speech, language, hearing, or cognition deficits as they affect performance of daily activities. Another benefit to this outcome measure movement might be the possibility, albeit somewhat far-reaching, that amplification may be viewed as a necessary rather than an elective component of health care (Bridges and Bentler, 1998).

In addition to solutions to communication difficulties, consumers also expect their service providers to be ethical and follow professional standards. The general public expects a higher level of conduct from those in health and health-related professions (Metz, 1997).

In a survey by Age Wave Health Services (1997), it was found that senior citizens were more concerned with the qualifications of hearing aid dispensers (48%) than any other factor, including the cost of the instruments. Good client rapport is essential in the rehabilitation process; first impressions can set the stage for continuing dialogue. It is this rapport that offers promise for a willingness on the part of clients to pursue a total rehabilitation program and, it is hoped, to dispel the notion of the quick fix.

Matkin and Estrada (1997) (Table 1.1) bring together the client, the client's support person, and the clinician with regard to advocacy as part of the total adult aural rehabilitation process. Their goal is to enhance the communication effectiveness of the individual who has a hearing loss. Quality of life may be enhanced by addressing these different perspectives of the client, the significant other, and the audiologist.

A Communication Model

Many authorities recognize that there is a direct relationship between effective communication and quality of life. Effective communication is a dynamic process of exchanging ideas with both expressive and receptive characteristics. Audiologists are concerned primarily with the receptive aspects of communication behavior. Alpiner and Meline (1989) developed a communication model (Fig. 1.2) that emphasizes the receptive process. This model attempts to illustrate factors that are pertinent to the quality of life of persons with hearing loss by exemplifying the multifaceted issues that an audiologist must address in clinical service delivery. Any breakdown in the communication process will interfere with quality of life. As stated so well by Toubbeh (1973) "Human communication is action; it is culture; it is the history of man; it is the fabric of all societies; its absence negates man's existence."

There are four levels of concern in this model:

- Level 1 is message expression. A communication event is transmitted through sound, touch, and movement. It must transcend environmental barriers to reach the receiver. These barriers to reception may include telephone lines that have static or a room with a high level of background noise.
- Level 2 deals with message encoding. The individual must have the ability to receive

Table 1.1
Perspectives of those involved in a hearing rehabilitation plan

Client	Support Person	Clinician
Accept your hearing loss	Accept the hearing loss of your significant other	Accept your limitations as a clinician
Determine a course of action	Determine your role in the rehabilitation plan	Determine a course of action
Value your clinician's input	Value your significant other	Value your client
Overcome your fear of the hearing loss	Overcome your fear of the hearing loss	Overcome fear of counseling
Communicate with your clinician and support person	Communicate with your significant other and clinician	Communicate with the client and support person
Assert yourself in communication efforts	Assert yourself	Adapt to your client
Teach others about your hearing loss	Teach other family members and friends about hearing loss	Teach your client and support person about the hearing loss
Educate yourself	Educate yourself	Educate yourself

the communication. The integrity of the receiver's auditory, tactile, and visual systems must be intact to receive whatever message is being sent.

- Level 3 involves message decoding. Once the message has reached the receiver, it must be interpreted. These interpretations are often determined by internal cognitive factors and by the social, vocational, and emotional needs of the individual.
- Level 4 is message perception. The receiver of the communication internalizes the message, may ask for clarification, may observe the speaker's feedback, and may repair the perceived meaning of the message before formulating a response.

In essence, this model demonstrates that the message is sent to a person who is a listener; is encoded by the auditory-visual and tactile systems; is related to the environment of the individual as a social, vocational, or emotional need; and is perceived by the receiver.

Effects of Managed Care

An increasing number of corporations are using managed care health insurance plans.

Managed care programs have forced health clinics, private practices, hospitals, and other facilities to become providers with designated fee schedules. Services are required to be under the direction of a physician or by referral. Many managed care or health maintenance organizations (HMOs) use the primary care physician (PCP) as the gatekeeper. If a specialist needs to be included in patient care, it usually requires the approval of the PCP. It is important for the patient to maintain good rapport with the PCP. The MarkeTrak IV survey found that the majority of patients (45%) who did not use amplification would discuss hearing loss with family physicians, compared with 40% with ENT (ear, nose, and throat) physicians, 35% with audiologists, and 14% with hearing instrument specialists (Kochkin, 1998). These figures demonstrate a need for increased communication, education, and rapport between audiologists and PCPs. Health care providers, including audiologists, do not automatically become an authorized HMO provider.

Update: Rapid Changes in Hearing Care (Practice Builder Association, 1998) provides significant information regarding managed care not previously considered by most audiologists. Initial exposure to this re-

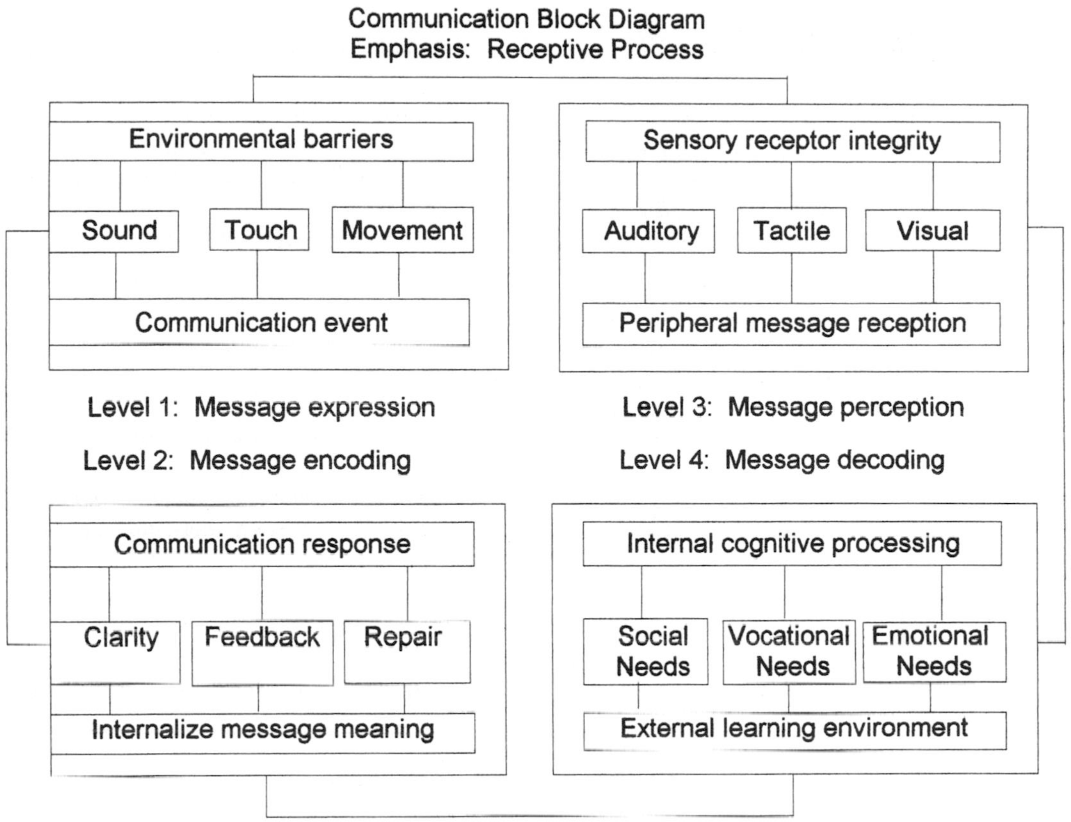

Communication Block Diagram
Emphasis: Receptive Process

Environmental barriers		
Sound	Touch	Movement
Communication event		

Sensory receptor integrity		
Auditory	Tactile	Visual
Peripheral message reception		

Level 1: Message expression

Level 2: Message encoding

Level 3: Message perception

Level 4: Message decoding

Communication response		
Clarity	Feedback	Repair
Internalize message meaning		

Internal cognitive processing		
Social Needs	Vocational Needs	Emotional Needs
External learning environment		

Figure 1.2. Communication model.

port may cause real concern to some audiologists, whereas others will consider health care changes as an opportunity for change. This report states that these rapid changes will devastate 60% of audiology and hearing instrument practices, with the remaining 40% gaining market share and major profits. Because hearing aids represent the anchor of rehabilitative audiology, we present *Updates*'s eight major factors (1998):

1. Projected to last until 2030, explosive growth is coming to the financial fortunes of hearing care providers. This will be caused by Baby Boomer demographics and impressive advances in hearing aid technology that will overcome perceived cosmetic and acoustic shortcomings.
2. Well-funded *Wall Street* corporations have discovered a way to own private hearing care practices. Therefore, the lion's share of these new profits will go to *Wall Street*'s practice management companies.
3. Most, if not all, of *Wall Street*'s practice management companies will market heavily. They will cut prices to gain crucial managed care contracts. This will encourage price-cutting across the profession and cause great stress for some private practitioners.
4. Practice management companies have already grown from 0 to 4% of the hearing care market from 1995 to 1998. They will consume 15% from 1999 to 2002 and 33% in the next 36 months. Even the smallest local audiology and hearing instrument specialty practice across the continent will be affected within the next 1 to 3 years (anticipated from 1999 through 2001).
5. There will be winners and losers in private practice. The losing practices will

soon begin to feel the impact. Within five years, "losing" hearing care practitioners will see revenues fall an average of 36%.

6. Within 10 years, trend line projections indicate that almost 60% of all hearing care practitioners will become employees of large corporations before a leveling-off occurs. After this majority of private practitioners have lost to their competition, closed their offices, or been bought, they will become salaried employees. However, salaries will be lower than what many practitioners expect.

7. The remaining 40% of hearing care practitioners in private practice will be bigger, better, and quite well off. They will be the winners. All will have achieved a minimum of $1,000,000 gross annually; most will be more than $5,000,000, and some will be more than $10,000,000.

8. Unfortunately, some private practitioners will deny changes are taking place. In the coming years, these are the practitioners who will economically suffer the most.

Kirkwood (1997a) states that managed care is a fact of life. He indicates that there are concerns about its possible effect on hearing care and that hearing health care providers will need to make it work for themselves and their patients.

Degrees and Credentials

DEGREES

In the previous edition of this book, we discussed the educational directions for audiology. The major emphasis of that discussion was for the Doctor of Audiology (Au.D.) degree. A major proponent of the Au.D., Goldstein (1989) stated that audiology programs did not allow students to earn a "professional degree"; programs were mainly academic rather than oriented toward service delivery. We also indicated in the previous edition that it appeared that new programs would begin soon.

As of this writing, we can state that philosophical differences continue to exist on how the Au.D. is earned but that several programs now offer the degree. This is a significant event for students currently in training because varying options are available. As of June 1998, *Audiology Express* (June, 1998) listed the following Au.D. programs:

1. Accepting current practitioners with a Master's degree by distance learning technology:
   a. Central Michigan University, Mt. Pleasant, Michigan/Vanderbilt University, Nashville, Tennessee
   b. Nova Southeastern University, Ft. Lauderdale, Florida
2. Accepting applicants holding a Bachelor's degree for a resident 4-year Au.D. degree:
   a. Ball State University, Muncie, Indiana
   b. Central Michigan University, Mt. Pleasant, Michigan
   c. Gallaudet University, Washington, DC
   d. University of Florida, Gainesville, Florida
   e. University of Louisville, Louisville, Kentucky

The universities listed above offer the degree in the traditional sense: a "university *earned* degree." The other major option is earning the Au.D. through earned entitlement (EE). This Au.D. does not represent an earned university degree, but rather the audiologist (usually a Master's degree audiologist) files an application through an organization that evaluates credentials. If the audiologist meets the required experience, the Au.D. designation is awarded. Proponents of the EE are not opposed to an earned degree but rather wish to upgrade the profession more quickly to enhance the status of the professional audiologist. A variety of arguments have been presented either way. A major consideration is whether state regulatory agencies will permit the use of an unearned Au.D degree. Some audiologists believe that one should be able to practice without obtaining an Au.D. The issue remains controversial. The AAA surveyed its members in 1998. The survey was sent to

1942 randomly selected members, and 1248 responses received. The survey found the following:

1. Audiology should move to a doctoral level degree.
2. The transition will not have a positive or negative effect on respondents personally—most are neutral.
3. The transition will have a positive effect on the profession of audiology.
4. The Au.D. is a degree designation rather than a credential.
5. Most respondents are not considering obtaining an Au.D. degree.
6. Features important to Au.D. degree programs include the following: distance learning (very important), credit for experience, traditional classroom instruction, and traditional clinic setting (less or not important).
7. Those wishing to use the Au.D. degree should earn it.
8. Use of the term Doctor of Audiology by those who have not earned a degree from a regionally accredited university is confusing and misleading to the public.
9. The lack of an earned degree damages the reputation of the profession with consumers and other professionals.
10. Only degrees from accredited institutions should be used in statements regarding professional services.

The issue of why the majority are neutral may be related to the following questions: (1) will the degree increase my knowledge, (2) will I provide better care, and (3) will it improve my compensation status?

Kirkwood (1998b) regards the long struggle to convert audiology to a doctoral discipline as the outstanding professional development of the 1990s. We can speculate that the Au.D., in one form or another, will continue and grow in the new millennium. We further hope that rehabilitative audiology will also gain similar momentum. As reported by Sykes et al. (1997), there appears to be a lack of training in audiologic rehabilitation for graduate-level students in au-diology. They indicate that these same students receive considerable training in areas such as pathology and diagnostics, for example, but do not always receive hands-on experience in the rehabilitation of these patients. The concern is for students who graduate, take positions in audiology, and lack the necessary ability to treat patients appropriately. Special mention is made of the proper rehabilitation experience to work with cochlear implant recipients, patients with vestibular disorders, and patients with central auditory processing disorders.

Martin et al. (1998) report on the seventh survey of audiometric practices in the United States. They sent questionnaires to 500 audiologists who were randomly selected from the AAA directory. Audiologists were asked what they were doing clinically and how they did it. Although it was indicated that 70% of those audiologists dispensing hearing aids engaged in hearing aid orientation with their patients, little mention was made about how they did it compared with the more lengthy statements regarding diagnostic procedures. Regarding counseling, it was noted that performing this task in a physician's office may be more controversial. It was indicated, however, that audiologists are the primary counselors of their patients.

CREDENTIALS

Another contemporary matter deals with credentialing of audiologists to provide service to clients. Since the inception of the credential for audiology, ASHA has been the organization providing certification for audiologists. Certification attests to the individual's competence to provide audiology services. The student will have completed a specified program of training, completed a clinical fellowship year, and successfully passed a national examination. ASHA claims that the value, respect, and credibility of the Certificate of Clinical Competence—Audiology (CCC-A) represents years of careful and meticulous deliberations. ASHA contends that the CCC-A is widely regarded within the profession, by consumers, health insurance payers, employers, legislators, educators, and consumers.

The AAA has developed its plan for certification of audiologists. A major impetus for AAA to establish its own certification plan, independent of membership, has been a desire of audiologists to have their own organization dealing with hearing. Some audiologists perceived that ASHA focused more on speech-language pathology than on audiology. There are far more speech-language pathologists than audiologists, approximately an 8:1 ratio.

In an effort to seek a solution, representatives from ASHA and AAA continue to engage in joint meetings. AAA has suggested an independent certification program that includes mandatory continuing education (ASHA does not currently do so), the requirement that the Au.D. become the entry level for audiology in the future, and the elimination of the tie between certification and accreditation. The last report on this issue was that there should not be duplicative certification programs. There will be certification in the 21st century; we do not yet know what it will be.

States also have their own individual licensure or registration programs for audiologists. Some states have patterned their programs after ASHA; others use different models. It appears that there may be individual decisions to be made by students and practitioners related to national certification, state licensure/registration, and the pursuit or upgrade of an academic degree. Our profession continues to grow, and issues and decisions will need to be addressed in the new millennium.

A Service Delivery Model

We present a service delivery model (Fig. 1.3) that may help in the establishment of an effective program. The complexities of the rehabilitation process can be narrowed by use of this model, which permits us to develop and use the philosophies with which we are most comfortable. This model also enables us to determine expectations for outcome measures.

The first phase in the model is the identification of the child or the adult. Children in school programs usually are screened on a periodic basis and identified in this manner. Infants may be identified in hospital newborn screening programs; certain states now mandate newborn screening. Adults with hearing loss have less chance of being identified early because there are no mandatory adult testing programs. Adults usually have to take the initiative to have their hearing tested. Many communities have annual health fairs that include hearing screening, providing an opportunity for adults to be tested. Many adults, however, are not terribly interested in knowing about their hearing, probably because hearing loss for most is gradual and not obvious to them. Many general and family practice physicians do not screen hearing as part of physical examinations.

Whatever the identification program, the audiologist needs to make some clinical judgments when hearing loss exists:

1. Is rehabilitative audiology necessary after completion of the audiologic evaluation?
2. Should a hearing aid evaluation be administered to determine if the hearing impairment can be minimized with amplification? Will assistive devices be helpful? Is the client a candidate for a cochlear implant?
3. Is rehabilitation indicated after the completion of the hearing aid evaluation and/or possible hearing aid fitting? Here and in item 1, remediation is not recommended if on the basis of the audiologist's information and judgment, the client is able to communicate effectively without assistance. Conversely, on the same basis, remediation is recommended when the client needs assistance to improve communication ability or to minimize any concomitant problems resulting from hearing loss. Is remediation recommended after a cochlear implant?
4. What are the client's communication

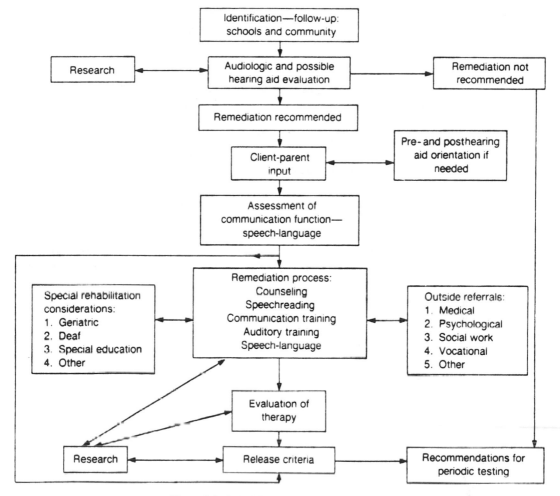

Figure 1.3. Rehabilitative audiology process.

needs? In the initial stages of rehabilitation, client and parent input help to provide significant information regarding communication status. Preorientation and postorientation may be necessary if amplification is considered.

5. Should therapy be terminated? An assessment of communication function, and speech/language (for a child) goals are considered in the process to determine the need for additional rehabilitation or termination of therapy. When treatment is terminated, recommendations may be made for periodic follow-up. We recommend follow-up once a year or sooner if a change occurs in the client's communication ability.

6. Which rehabilitative audiology procedures should be recommended? Procedures may include counseling, hearing aid orientation, auditory training, repair strategies, and so forth.

7. Should referrals be made? The child's or adult's situation may require referral to other professionals such as psychologists, family counselors, pediatricians, and otologists. Professionals in other disciplines should refer back to the audiologist with a report and recommendations.

8. Are special treatment considerations appropriate? Additional procedures may be indicated when dealing with profoundly deaf children, geriatric clients in extended care facilities, persons with multiple

handicaps, and clients with strokes and other disorders. It is also desirable to include family members in audiologic rehabilitation; hearing loss is a "family affair."

9. Has therapy been successful? During the course of therapy, periodic assessment needs to be made with regard to both success and termination as related to outcome measures.

10. How can research serve this process? Research in the total rehabilitative process is recommended for more meaningful and valid approaches. Research applications are usually accomplished in university settings.

General Effects of Hearing Loss on Children and Adults

As later chapters will explore in-depth, the effects of hearing impairment can be devastating at any age. Hearing loss, whether mild or profound, has certain fundamental psychosocial implications. There are social and emotional aspects of hearing loss that affect not only the hearing-impaired individual, but their family members and anyone interacting with them on a daily basis. Wayner and Abrahamson (1998) (Fig. 1.4) provide a useful summary of the issues for positions on communicative interaction. Other considerations that must be made, regardless of age, are the factors of anatomy/

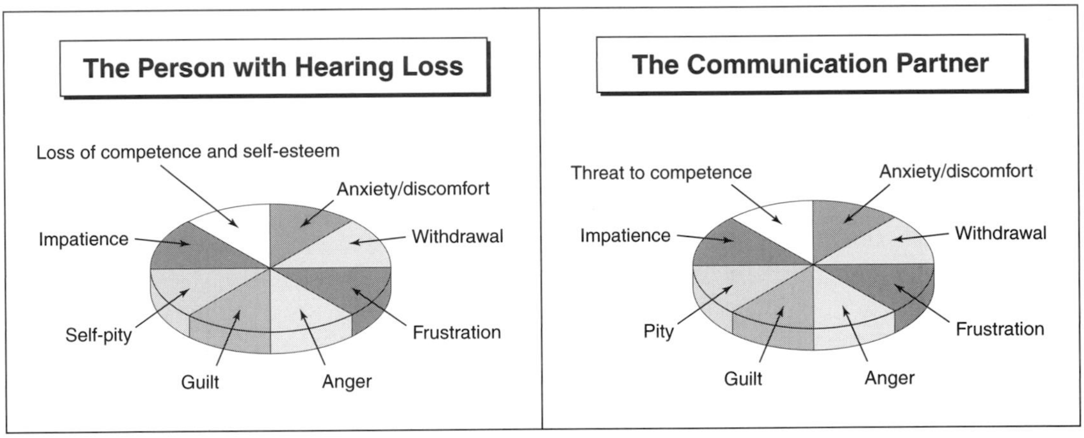

- Frustration: Can't understand
- Anxiety/discomfort: "Will I again not understand and appear confused?"
- Impatience with others for not taking time to speak clearly, face me, speak slowly, one at a time, or with a cigarette in their mouth or a hand in front of their face.
- Anger: At others for not trying harder, not being included in a conversation, and for "forgetting" (when, in fact, they never heard properly). Additionally, anger can be directed at self.
- Feeling of loss of competence and diminished self-esteem: More intense if person is already struggling with other changes/losses such as retirement, reduction in income, decline in health, etc.
- Self-pity: "Poor me. It's not worth trying."
- Guilt for making demands or for being a "burden."
- Withdrawal: "It's better not to get involved than to have so much trouble understanding."

- Frustration: Can't make self understood.
- Anxiety/discomfort: Not knowing what to do or feeling awkward in certain situations.
- Impatience for not being understood and/or for constantly having to repeat things. Frustration from the hearing-impaired person's unwillingness to try other means and feeling it's not worth the time.
- Anger at person with hearing loss for complaining, making demands, or for being angry. A feeling of wanting to say, "What do you expect from me?"
- Threat to competence: Because of uncertainty of dealing with hearing loss. May view other person as losing competence or mental abilities.
- Pity: For the person with hearing loss, but also for not being understood.
- Guilt: For not knowing what to do and for being impatient. Particularly important for spouses.
- Withdrawal: Poor communication may be misperceived as a lack of interest in the relationship.

Figure 1.4. Communication interaction. (First published in *The Hearing Review* 1998;5 . Reprinted courtesy of *The Hearing Review* and Fladmark Publishing Co. All rights reserved.)

sensory capabilities, prelinguistic or postlinguistic onset, and motivation (whether intrinsic or extrinsic).

A 40-year-old working individual may find a mild hearing loss to be a significant handicap in his or her rigorous work environment and interactions. A 65-year-old retired individual who resides alone may not express concern over his or her moderately severe hearing loss. For both of these adults, the normal aging process may actually increase or compound the effect of their hearing loss. In Chapter 13 of this text, McCarthy and Sapp outline sensory changes that occur with aging, both structural and functional. The hearing professional must maintain a broad view of these other sensory modalities. The rehabilitative audiologic plan can change dramatically, as in the case of a client who has had a cerebrovascular accident (CVA) and has hemiparesis and diminished range of vision. Although binaural amplification may be most appropriate, monaural may need to be instituted if the client is to be independent.

The onset of hearing loss is a primary factor in the direction of the rehabilitation/habilitation of a hearing-impaired individual. Prelinguistic versus postlinguistic onset affects the fundamental components of the comprehensive plan. The habilitation process for a congenitally deafened child throughout his or her lifetime may present the largest "cost" due to the obvious length of therapy time. Early intervention is the key element to an improved outcome in the habilitation of a newborn with congenital hearing loss. The issues related to and the development of speech and language for hearing-impaired infants are a major focus and require a cooperative team approach. Numerous professionals (audiologists, speech language pathologists, teachers for the hearing impaired, psychologists, social workers, and so forth) will be necessary to treat the prelingual hearing-impaired patient effectively.

Chartrand (1990) identifies possible psychological effects related to degree of loss: (a) mild loss may bring mild defensiveness, loss of selective hearing, and increased stress; (b) moderate loss brings added frustration, depression, antisocial tendencies,

and increased resistance to seek help for the problem; and (c) severe loss brings increased isolation, severe depression, resentfulness, and acute psychological barriers against seeking help. Motivation is also a key element. An individual (or parent in the case of a child) must acknowledge the hearing problem, accept its existence, and be motivated to pursue assistance. If this is missing, the success of any rehabilitation/habilitation plan is in jeopardy.

In the previous edition of this book, we emphasized numeric classifications. For example, a person with a hearing loss between 26 and 40 dB will only have difficulty with faint speech, or a person with a hearing loss between 71 and 90 dB will understand only shouted or amplified speech. Numeric classification systems have been used for medical/legal purposes. For example, the amount of compensation paid to a service-connected veteran is based, in part, on a numeric classification, as is the case for a construction worker under Workers' Compensation. The concept of a numeric classification is presented by Northern and Downs (1991) (Table 1.2). The level of hearing loss, however, and the handicap caused by that loss is another matter.

To address this issue better, the Joint Committee of the ASHA and the Council on Education of the Deaf (CED) developed a position statement to consider for adoption (ASHA, 1998). The statement attempts to delineate a continuum of communication function to describe persons with hearing loss. Terms, for example, that have general acceptance by some individuals who have hearing loss include hard of hearing, hearing-impaired, late deafened, Deaf, and deaf. In addition, persons with hearing loss may communicate using signed, spoken, or written languages; other methods; or combinations of methods. The statement also indicates that the description of hearing loss should reflect the personal preferences of the individuals involved as well as facilitate eligibility of entitlement and access to various services. The Joint Committee of ASHA and the CED (1998) based its position on the following assumptions:

Table 1.2
Numeric classification of hearing loss[a]

Average Threshold Level at 500–2000 Hz (ANSI)	Description	Common Causes	What Can Be Heard Without Amplification	Degree of Handicap (If not Treated in First Year of Life)	Probable Needs
0–15 dB	Normal range		All speech sounds	None	None
16–25 dB	Slight hearing loss	Serious otitis, perforation monomeric membrane, sensoineural loss, tympansclerosis	Vowel sounds heard clearly, may miss unvoiced consonant sounds	Possible mild or transitory auditory dysfunction Difficulty in perceiving some speech sounds	Consideration of need for hearing aid, lip reading, auditory training, speech therapy, preferential seating, appropriate surgery
26–40 dB	Mild hearing loss	Serious otitis, perforation, tympanosclerosis, monomeric membrane, sensorineural loss	Hears only some of speech sounds—the more loudly voiced sounds	Auditory learning dysfunction, mild language retardation, mild speech problems, inattention	Hearing aid, lipreading, auditory training, speech therapy, appropriate surgery
41–65 dB	Moderate hearing loss	Chronic otitis, middle ear anomaly, sensorineural loss	Misses most speech sounds at normal conversational level	Speech problems, language retardation, learning dysfunction, inattention	All of the above plus consideration of special classroom situation
		Sensorineural loss or mixed loss due to sensorineural loss plus middle ear disease	Hears no speech sound of normal conversations	Severe speech problems, language retardation, learning dysfunction, inattention	All of the above; probable assignment to special classes
96+ dB	Profound hearing loss	Sensorineural loss or mixed	Hears no speech or other sounds	Severe speech problems, language retardation, learning dysfunction, inattention	All of the above; probable assignment to special classes

Reprinted with permission from Northern JL, Downs MP. Hearing in children. 4th ed. Baltimore: Williams & Wilkins, 1991:99.

[a]Classification of hearing handicap as a function of average hearing threshold level of the better ear.

1. Individuals who are deaf or hard of hearing constitute a heterogeneous population.
2. The relationship that exists between an individual's hearing level and that individual's ability to develop a language or languages in one or more communication modalities varies among individuals.
3. A variety of factors affect the communication function of individuals with hearing loss. These include, but are not limited to, the presence of concomitant disabilities related to vision, fine and gross motor function, and/or cognitive functioning.
4. Communication choices are influenced by such factors as the age of the individual when the hearing loss occurred, when the hearing loss was identified, the type of intervention/educational services available, and when those services were initiated.
5. Family, cultural values, and community support of individuals with hearing loss can have a strong effect on the individual. This can include, but is not limited to, access to language, communication approaches, and use of residual hearing and spoken or signed languages.
6. Individuals with hearing loss often interact differently depending on their work, education, community, and social environment. Communication is influenced by the presence or absence of access to interpreters, appropriate technology, and communication partners.

Ultimately, the Joint Committee notes the complexity of the communication interchange and the need to facilitate opportunities for personal, educational, social, and vocational development. We believe the statement emphasizes the need for clinicians to be cognizant of the total audiologic rehabilitation process.

Areas of Rehabilitative Audiology

We have covered a variety of topics in the overview of rehabilitative audiology, some areas in which change is continuing to taking place. These topics are covered in depth in this book. We consider five major areas of study: (1) philosophy and service provision, (2) rehabilitative audiology for children, (3) rehabilitative audiology for adults, (4) technology in rehabilitative audiology, and (5) future directions.

In the philosophy and service provision section, trends in rehabilitative audiology since its inception are presented. Traditional and nontraditional relationships between hearing care providers and individuals with impaired hearing are covered; these relationships can also include diagnosticians, rehabilitationists, counselors, advocates, policy-makers, researchers, educators, technologists/inventors, and other health care providers. Gone are the days when the audiologist was an all-inclusive expert who "did everything" for the client. There are also professional practice issues related to federal and state legislation, scope of practice guidelines, insurance constraints, and managed care. Also gone are the days when most audiology was done in the comfortable confines of the university environment. Audiology is now accomplished in hospital settings, schools, community clinics, private practice, governmental agencies, long-term care facilities, and university clinics. We now need to think about marketing, overhead costs, business taxes, and increased competition from chains. Audiologists and students in training programs have more choices to make, including the type of work environment. For example, do you want to work for yourself or for someone else? Are jobs available in the area in which you wish to work?

It is feasible for audiologists to be well trained so that they may be able to emphasize or specialize in diagnostics, rehabilitation, or both. Economics is a factor not to be ignored in terms of salaries and benefits. Audiologists often encounter clients who are interested in our services but quickly reject rehabilitation when they learn that insurance does not cover the service. Diagnostic audiology procedures are usually reimbursed, but adult rehabilitative services are not unless bundled into the cost of evaluation or hearing aids. We need to be aware of this issue so that we can involve ourselves in legislation that one day will lead to reimbursement for rehabilitation.

The section on hearing-impaired children focuses on identification, evaluation, and impact of hearing loss in children; amplification for children; assessment and intervention with infants, preschoolers, and school-age children; and the counseling process for both children and parents. In addition, newborn hearing screening programs are emerging across the United States. Reports about increasing high-frequency hearing loss among young people continue to appear in both lay and professional publications. Although many children and teenagers believe their ears are immune to hearing loss, noise exposure takes its toll. Hearing health care providers will continue to be busy in the 21st century.

One of the goals of rehabilitation for adults is to provide support therapy. While we address different approaches to rehabilitation, we also must address other issues that relate to the treatment process for adults. Assessing the effect of hearing loss on the individual is a good starting point. Assessment tools allow us to determine how hearing loss affects the emotional, social, and vocational aspects of everyday living. Other assessment type procedures can help to define hearing aid benefits; still others may help us to evaluate quality of life issues. These various instruments may, in many cases, be used before and after rehabilitation to define improvement from initial baseline levels. Amplification is often the anchor of the rehabilitative audiology process. Many audiologists think that hearing aids represent the major aspect of our service. This may be true to a certain degree, particularly in view of the fact that hearing aid technology has permitted the provision of much better products than in the past. We need to remember, however, that hearing aids still are not the same as new ears, that 20 to 25% of hearing aids are returned by unsatisfied

users, and that only 20 to 25% of those in need of hearing aids obtain them. These statements are not intended in any way to discredit hearing aids, but rather to emphasize that rehabilitation is very much an essential ingredient for audiologists.

There are other areas of rehabilitative audiology that continue to develop and refine themselves as a result of technologic developments. Cochlear implants have been of significant help to both children and adults. Only a few years ago, there was little (if anything) that could be done for the profoundly or severely deaf person, short of limited amplification and some form of manual or total communication. Audiologists and speech-language pathologists are challenged to assimilate the vast amounts of information and techniques being made available in the implant field today. Assistive devices for the hearing-impaired are increasing in significance and use. This interest is positive, because our clients may benefit further by participating in everyday communication activities. Such devices include special alarm clocks, light indicators, television/radio listening systems, closed caption television, FM systems, and so forth. Many hearing aid practices now include ancillary assistive device options to offer clients ways for more effective communication. We continue to be more aware, if only by media sources, of the Internet, interactive communication, and computer programs. This new technology is feared by some who have never been exposed to it and ignored by others who feel intimidated. School children are now teaching their parents about new technologies. The new millennium belongs, in part, to those who are willing to learn about and use things like the new technologic hardware and software. New technologies and computers are discussed in Chapters 16 and 17.

The concluding section of this book includes research and development needs in rehabilitative audiology and a new chapter on outcome measures. The procedures that interface with the clinician's goals and the results obtained by clients help to provide indications of success or failure of the rehabilitation process. Quality of care is considered. Domains of function to be considered in the audiologic rehabilitation process are impairment, disability, and handicap measures. In this ever-changing era of health care, we have been challenged to demonstrate that our services are effective; outcome measures can help us to quantify audiologic rehabilitation. The final chapter, which deals with research, focuses on conversation and communication therapy, speech recognition testing, sensory aids, and speech perception training. The research aspects are related to both children and adults. This chapter emphasizes our need for continuing research so that clinicians may better fulfill the mission of rehabilitative audiology.

Finally, mention should be made about the various contributors to this book. The information is presented in a format that allows them to use their individual styles. Readers will have the opportunity to realize that different philosophies, definitions, and beliefs exist in the profession; there is not always just one way to do things. We believe that this will give us a greater appreciation and understanding of rehabilitative audiology as we enter the 21st century.

REFERENCES

Adams PF, Marano MA, National Center for Health Statistics. (Cited in Prevalence of hearing loss in the United States. In: Communication facts. Rockville, MD: American Speech-Language-Hearing Association, 1995.)

Age Wave Health Services for the American Academy of Audiology. 1997 AAA marketing study. Audiol Today 1998;10:10–14.

Alpiner JG, Hansen, EM. Project CIC/FT, Hear Now Denver, CO, (1996), Appendices I, II.

Alpiner JG, Meline NC. A communication model. Paper presented at the annual convention of the Alabama Speech and Hearing Association, Birmingham, Alabama, 1989.

American Academy of Audiology. Opinion survey of doctor of audiology. Audiol Express 1998;4.

American Speech-Language-Hearing Association. *Communication Facts.* (1995).

American Speech-Language-Hearing Association. Preferred practice patterns for the profession of audiology. Rockville, MD: American Speech-Language-Hearing Association, 1997;November:43–46.

ASHA. Hearing loss: terminology and classification. ASHA Suppl 1998;40(Suppl 18):22–23.

Axelsson A, Ringdahl A. Tinnitus—A study of its prevalence and characteristics. Br J Audiol 1989;23:53–62.

Brechtelsbauer DA. Adult hearing loss. Prim Care 1990;17:249–266.

Bridges JA, Bentler RA. Relating hearing aid use to well-being among older adults. Hear J 1998;51:39–44.

Chartrand MS. Working with the psychology of the hearing impaired. Hear Instruments 1990;41:22–24.

Cox R, Alexander G. The abbreviated profile of hearing aid benefit. Ear Hear 1992;16:176–186.

Crandell CC. Effects of hearing instruments on psychosocial and functional health. Hear Rev 1996;3:38, 40, 66.

Crandell CC. Hearing aids: their effects on functional health status. Hear J 1998;51:22–30.

Denver Rocky Mountain News, July 28, 1999, 14A, 33A.

Dickenson B. Listen up-while you still can. Hear Rev 1998;5:67.

Fuller D. Assistive devices and client safety: a responsibility issue. Hear Rev 1998;5:46–47.

Goldstein D. The doctoring degree in audiology. ASHA 1989;31:33–35.

Hoffman H. National Institute on Deafness and Other Communication Disorders. (Cited in Prevalence of hearing loss in the United States. In: Communication facts. Rockville, MD: American Speech-Language-Hearing Association, 1996.)

Kirkwood DH. Managed care: it's a fact of life. Hear J 1997a;50:23.

Kirkwood DH. 1988–1997: rise of technology. Hear J 1997b;50:32–38.

Kirkwood DH. Hearing aid sales increase 7.5% in 1997: expansion expected to continue. Hear J 1998a;51:21–28.

Kirkwood DH. One giant leap for audiology. Hear J 1998b; 51:4.

Kochkin S. Customer satisfaction & subjective benefit with high performance hearing aids. Hear Rev 1997;2(High Performance Hearing Solutions Suppl):4–10.

Kochkin S. MarkeTrak IV: correlates of hearing aid purchase intent. Hear J 1998;51:30–41.

Martin FN, Champlin CA, Chambers J. Seventh survey of audiometric practices in the United States. J Am Acad Audiol 1998;9:95–104.

Matkin N, Estrada C. Audiology Today 1997;9(5):11.

Metz MJ. Ethical, legal, or moral? "If it feels good . . . " Hear J 1997;50:10–16.

Morris R. Hearing instruments + ALDs = a winning combination. Hear J 1998;51:59–66.

National Institute on Deafness and Other Communication Disorders. (Cited in Prevalence of communication disorders among children in the United States. In: Communication facts. Rockville, MD: American Speech-Language-Hearing Association, 1996.)

Northern JL. Reducing hearing aid returns patient education. Paper presented at the Academy of Rehabilitative Audiology Summer Institute, Lake Geneva, Wisconsin, June 12, 1998.

Northern JL, Downs MP. Hearing in children. 4th ed. Baltimore: Williams & Wilkins, 1991.

Practice Builder Association. Update: rapid changes in hearing care. Hearing care research report no. 98–229. Irvine, CA: Market Research Division, 1998:1–12.

Radcliffe D. The high cost of hearing lost: what our publics need to know. Hear J 1998;51:21–30.

Rihs A. Perspective: is the hearing industry on the right track? Hear Rev 1997;2(Suppl):47–49.

Ross M. Why people won't wear hearing aids. Hear Rehab Quart 1992;17.

Ross M. A retrospective look at the future of aural rehabilitation. J Acad Rehab Audiol 1997;30:11–28.

Sykes S, Tucker D, Herr D. Aural rehabilitation and graduate audiology programs. J Am Acad Audiol 1997;8: 314–321.

Toubbeh J. Human communication disorders. *Rehabilitation Record,* 1973:1–4.

Tye-Murray N, Witt S, Schum L, et al. Feasible aural rehabilitation services for busy clinical settings. Am J Audiol 1994;3:33–45.

Ulrich ML. Remember, ears are body parts. Hear J 1998; 51:78–79.

U.S. Department of Commerce, U.S. Bureau of the Census, Income Statistics Branch/HHES Division. Poverty 1995. Persons and families in poverty by selected characteristics. Washington, DC, 1995.

Wayner DS, Abrahamson JE. Social & emotional aspects of hearing loss. Hear Rev 1998;5:26, 28, 76.

APPENDIX
1.1 *Expectations Questionnaire*

Answer true or false to each question

When I am using my hearing aids . . .

_____   1.   Conversation over the telephone will be easy to understand.

_____   2.   Watching people's lips and faces will always be a major part of my communication.

_____   3.   In background noise, I will be able to understand speech.

_____   4.   Most television programs will be easy to understand with hearing alone.

_____   5.   It will be possible for me to separate one word from another when listening to normal conversation.

_____   6.   I will be able to understand all speech when using my hearing aids.

_____   7.   I will be able to understand speech when at a theater, church, etc.

_____   8.   It will be possible to hear my own voice.

_____   9.   I may have better job opportunities by using my hearing aids.

_____   10.   I will be able to hear and appreciate music with the hearing aids.

_____   11.   Others will not know that I have a hearing disability.

_____   12.   Speech will sound natural to me.

APPENDIX
1.2 *Fulfillment of Expectations*

Answer true of false to each question

When I am using my hearing aids . . .

_____ 1.   Conversation over the telephone is easy to understand.

_____ 2.   Watching people's lips and faces is a major part of my communication.

_____ 3.   In background noise, I understand speech.

_____ 4.   Most television programs are easy to understand with hearing alone.

_____ 5.   It is possible for me to separate one word from another when listening to normal conversation.

_____ 6.   I understand all speech.

_____ 7.   I understand speech when at a theater, church, etc.

_____ 8.   I hear my own voice.

_____ 9.   I have better job opportunities by using my hearing aids.

_____ 10. I hear and appreciate music with the hearing aids.

_____ 11. Others do not know that I have a hearing disability.

_____ 12. Speech sounds natural to me.

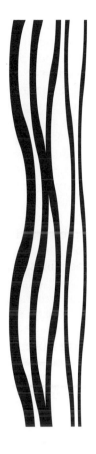

Hearing Care Providers and Individuals With Impaired Hearing: Continuing and New Relationships in the New Millennium

Dean C. Garstecki, Ph.D., and Susan F. Erler, Ph.D.

When hearing loss presents a permanent and continuing predicament, affecting communication and learning, independence, and quality of life, a cadre of audiologists, otologists, speech-language pathologists, educators of the hearing-impaired, counselors, social workers, support group members, family members, and others may be involved in providing hearing care. Each has a unique and important contribution to make to the hearing loss management process. None can do all that needs to be done alone. Each depends on others and, in the process, continuing and new professional and personal relationships are established. Some relationships thrive during critical periods then dissipate, others continue throughout a lifetime.

This chapter focuses on factors that will cause continuing hearing care relationships to be stretched and challenged and new relationships to be created in the new millennium. Hearing care in the future will be different from what it is today. It will be delivered in a variety of settings and under changing service delivery systems by individuals with professional backgrounds including and extending beyond those listed above. Overall philosophy toward hearing care will change from diagnosis and treatment to an emphasis on wellness and prevention of hearing loss and hearing handicap. There will be increasing linkage between treatment progress and third-party reimbursement. Changing demographics will favor treatment of greater numbers of older adults and individuals from diverse cultural backgrounds more in the future than any time in the past. Clinical practice will be enhanced by advanced computer technology, increased use of information on the World Wide Web, and dependence on telehealth procedures. Hearing care providers and recipients will benefit from vast amounts of readily available information.

To begin preparing for these changes, hearing care provider relationships, population trends, clinical service delivery, personal-professional relationships, and ethical challenges are reviewed.

Hearing Care: Continuing and New Relationships

Hearing care is defined as care provided to individuals seeking relief from the effects of permanent hearing loss, that is, hearing loss that is medically/surgically irreversible (Bratt et al., 1996). Relationships are established and maintained among individuals with impaired hearing, their families, significant others, and the professionals who provide services to them in the course of hearing care (Table 2.1). Concerns related to any hearing loss, regardless of permanency, are often first addressed by a physician. The child's pediatrician, a family physician, or gerontologist may be the first professional to be consulted. Referrals then may be made to an ear specialist or otologist. This practice may be necessitated because resolving a hearing problem medically or surgically may obviate the need for further intervention. A medical case history will be recorded and a physical examination conducted. After all diagnostic data are obtained, the otologist will explain the findings to the individual with impaired hearing and, in the

case of a child, to his or her parents. Children with impaired hearing may require medical/surgical treatment and/or hearing aids. Middle ear problems are the most common cause of hearing loss in children and are typically medically treated. Longer-standing and/or significant hearing loss may require the services of a speech-language pathologist, modification in educational placement, and medical follow-up (Clark and Terry, 1991). Adults typically require hearing aids and periodic medical follow-up. They also will benefit from participation in an audiologic rehabilitation program. In the case of permanent hearing loss, the otologist and audiologist will become long-term providers of hearing care.

The audiologist plays an integral role on the hearing care team. The audiologist's rehabilitation responsibilities are defined by scope of practice guidelines issued by the American Speech-Language-Hearing Association (ASHA, 1996). Current practice in audiology includes rehabilitative services relating to:

1. Development of communication competence;
2. Psychosocial adjustment to hearing loss;
3. Selection, evaluation, fitting, and use of hearing aids, assistive hearing devices, and other sensory aids;
4. Adjustment to use of a cochlear implant;
5. Selection of and instruction in the use of alerting systems, telecommunication systems, and captioning devices;
6. Management of hearing loss in educational settings; and
7. Communication access.

Audiologists rely on otologists for cerumen management, and otologists rely on audiologists when making decisions concerning candidacy for cochlear implantation. The otologist-audiologist relationship is likely to be the longest-term working relationship among members of the hearing care team. The frequency of medical care for any individual with impaired hearing is likely to diminish over time, with less need as an adult.

Table 2.1
Members of the hearing care team

Principal members
  Audiologist
  Family physician
  Otologist
  Speech-language pathologist
Additional members
  Educators of children with hearing
    impairment
  Mental health counselors
  Psychologists
  "Regular" educators
  Sensory device manufacturers and
    distributors
  Social workers
  Telecommunication and captioning service
    providers
  Vocational counselors

Because hearing loss potentially affects communication and learning and, in turn, personal adjustment, the audiologist is likely to maintain a working relationship with several professionals. They include speech-language pathologists; school personnel, particularly educators of children with impaired hearing; counselors concerned with mental health, family, or occupational matters; and social workers dealing with pragmatic solutions to problems associated with hearing loss. Working relationships also may need to be established with psychologists, mental health counselors, hearing device manufacturers and distributors, cochlear implant manufacturers and distributors, telecommunication and captioning service representatives, educators, and vocational counselors (as appropriate and necessary) in addition to core team members. Drawing on the insight, expertise, and experience of the individual with impaired hearing, family members and friends, and professionals will enhance the success of audiologic rehabilitation.

Population Trends

Rehabilitative audiologists in the new millennium will serve an older, larger, more ethnically diverse population than in previous decades. Several trends are of particular importance. First, the number of older adults (65 years and older) is increasing dramatically (Figs. 2.1 and 2.2). Second, the incidence of hearing impairment is increasing. Finally, the proportion of children and adults requiring hearing care who come from culturally diverse backgrounds is increasing. Each of these factors will affect the demand for service and shape service delivery to meet the disparate needs of these older adults, children, and their families.

OLDER ADULTS

The majority of growth in the older adult population is expected to occur between 2010 and 2030 when Baby Boomers begin to reach age 65. Who are the aging Baby Boomers? Born during the years following World War

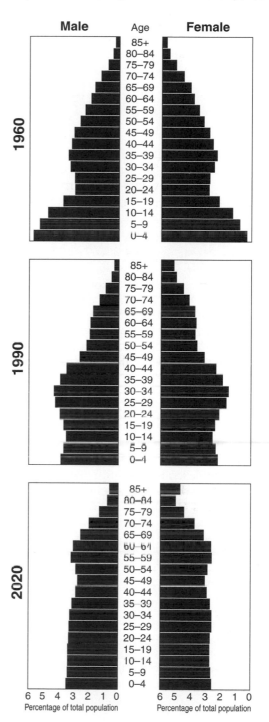

Figure 2.1. Population age structure: 1960 to 2020. (From US Bureau of the Census.)

II through the early 1960s, these adults will be the trend-setters and predominant consumers of audiologic rehabilitation services in the years to come. Although there is great

Elderly

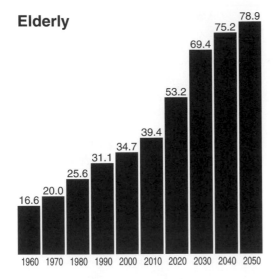

Oldest Old

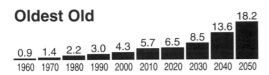

Figure 2.2. Population 1960 to 2050 (in millions). (From US Bureau of the Census.)

variability within this group, on average they have been described as well-educated, technologically savvy, and reaching retirement with more disposable income than previous generations. Women in this group are likely to spend a significant portion of their adult life in the work force. The older adults of the new millennium who have impaired hearing are expected to approach audiologic rehabilitation as consumers demanding the latest technological advances and treatment technologies available. The audiologists who serve them will need expertise in these technologies and must be well-versed in adult development. Specialization as "geri-audiologists" will become more common.

HEARING IMPAIRMENT

It is estimated that between 20 and 28 million Americans have impaired hearing (ASHA, 1995) (see Chapter 1 for further information about the incidence of impaired hearing).

Presbycusis refers to the gradual decline in hearing associated with aging. However, hearing loss acquired during adulthood may stem from a variety of etiologies, with incidence varying by gender. Although men are more likely to report hearing loss due to noise exposure and trauma, women more often experience hearing impairment due to Meniere's disease, otosclerosis, ear surgery, and exposure to ototoxic drugs (Moscicki et al., 1985). As social mores and safety standards evolve, etiology, incidence, and severity of hearing impairment may also change. For example, jobs that involve exposure to noise are no longer exclusively filled by men, increasing the incidence of noise-induced hearing loss in women. In contrast, safety and health standards will reduce exposure to environmental and medical threats to hearing (Garstecki and Erler, 1998a).

Hearing aids are the rehabilitative tool of choice for most adults with impaired hearing. In 1997, 5.6 million persons reported using a hearing aid (Kochkin, 1997). This represents less than 20% of the population with impaired hearing. The vast majority of hearing aid users (72%) are older than 65 years of age, with hearing aid use increasing with the severity of the hearing impairment. Hearing aid consumer behavior is most often linked to issues of cost, technological limitations, stigma, and perceived benefit (Kochkin, 1993). Recent findings suggest that psychological control beliefs and problem-solving behaviors differ between hearing aid users and nonusers as well as between women and men (Garstecki and Erler, 1998b). Further, availability of satisfactory social support also influences adherence to professional recommendations to obtain hearing aids. Clearly, numerous instrumental and psychological barriers to hearing aid use remain, representing a challenge to rehabilitative audiologists, particularly in their roles as educators and counselors.

Although most hearing loss is associated with aging, 5.6% of those with impaired hearing experience their loss before the age of 3 years and 21% before the age of 19 years (ASHA, 1995). It is estimated that 1 of every 1000 children is born with severe to profound sensorineural hearing loss, with 2.1% of children younger than 18 years of age experiencing hearing loss of any degree (National Institutes of Health, 1993). The incidence is somewhat higher among children enrolled in special education programs.

The most common cause of impaired hearing in children is middle ear infection. By the age of 6 years, 90% of children have had at least one bout of otitis media (ASHA, 1994a), accounting for 24 million physician visits per year. Even with good medical follow-up, 10% of preschoolers continue to have chronic episodes of otitis media (Downs, 1995). Although most hearing impairment related to otitis media is temporary, children who experience frequent bouts may demonstrate problems in acquisition and development of speech and language as well as long-term problems associated with academic achievement. Large-scale studies are currently underway to examine the efficacy of a vaccine to protect against several strains of pneumococcus, the cause of approximately 30 to 50% of all cases of acute otitis media (Rennels et al., 1998). Although medical advances should reduce the number of cases of pneumococcal otitis media in the future, hearing care providers will continue to play an essential role in providing information to parents, educators, and physicians about the long-term sequelae of middle ear problems.

A number of demographic changes among young children with permanent hearing impairment have been noted during the past two decades (Holden-Pitt and Diaz, 1998). These include recent increases in the number of children with impaired hearing who are younger than 3 years of age, children with mild to moderate hearing impairment (i.e., average thresholds <70 dB HL), and children with impaired hearing who are from diverse ethnic backgrounds. The Gallaudet Research Institute Annual Survey of Deaf and Hard-of-Hearing Children and Youth, now in its 30th year, represents the largest database of information about children with impaired hearing in the United States (Holden-Pitt and

Diaz, 1998). Annual Gallaudet surveys report data related to incidence, etiology, and degree of hearing impairment as well as information about educational setting, communication method for instruction, and presence of other disabilities.

Although some factors, such as the ratio of males to females with impaired hearing, have remained consistent over the years, others have changed significantly (Table 2.2). First, the number of cases (i.e., children with hearing impairment reported to the Gallaudet Survey) has increased during the past decade, although current numbers are not as high as recorded in 1977. Higher incidence 20 years ago was due predominantly to the number of children and adolescents who were part of the so-called rubella bulge that began in the 1960s. Although 21% of the reported cases were due to maternal rubella in 1977, today only 1% of cases report this etiology. When compared with children in other age groups, the proportion of children with impaired hearing who are younger than 5 years of age remains small, indicative of limitations of services for very young children and delays in identification. Changes in the degree of hearing loss are also of interest. In general, more children with milder hearing loss and fewer with severe to profound hearing loss were reported in 1997 than in 1977. This change is attributed not only to fewer cases of hearing loss due to maternal rubella, but to improved identification of milder impairments. The ethnic background of children reported in the Gallaudet Survey has changed significantly, reflecting similar changes within the United States at large. In 1977, 71% of the cases reported were identified as White/non-Hispanic. Today, the proportion is 58%. In contrast, only 9% of cases were identified in 1977 as Hispanic compared with 18% in 1997. Changes in the survey itself parallel evolutions that are seen in audiologic rehabilitation. For example, informants now are questioned about the degree to which additional handicapping conditions limit the child's function in their educational setting, rather than merely assigning a categoric

Table 2.2
Responses to the Gallaudet Research Institute annual survey of deaf and hard-of-hearing youth, 1977–1997

	1977–1978	1987–1988	1996–1997
Gender	N = 53,954	N = 46,885	N = 50, 404
Male	54%	54%	54%
Female	46%	46%	46%
Age (as of 12/31 in year of survey) (in years)	N = 53,681	N = 46,227	N = 49,748
<3	1%	3%	2%
3–5	8%	11%	10%
6–9	21%	25%	24%
10–13	36%	25%	28%
14–17	22%	25%	26%
18 +	11%	11%	9%
Degree of hearing loss (better ear average)	N = 51,268	N = 45,844	N = 46,097
<27 dB HL	4%	7%	12%
Mild	5%	9%	11%
Moderate	9%	12%	13%
Moderately severe	13%	13%	12%
Severe	25%	19%	17%
Profound	44%	41%	35%
Racial/ethnic background	N = 50,566	N = 46,174	N = 49,115
White/Non-Hispanic	71%	65%	58%
Black/Non-Hispanic	17%	17%	17%
Hispanic	9%	13%	18%
Asian/Pacific Islander	1%	3%	4%
American Indian	<1%	1%	1%
School type	N = 48,866	N = 38,158	N = 43,267
Residential	36%	25%	20%
Day (full-time hearing impaired)	15%	9%	8%
Regular/local	46%	61%	69%
Academic integration with hearing children	N = 36,808	N = 39,313	N = 42,629
Not integrated	66%	46%	38%
Part-time integrated	26%	21%	22%
Full-time integrated	18%	32%	40%

Adapted from Holden-Pitt L, Diaz JA. Thirty years of the Annual Survey of Deaf and Hard-of-Hearing Children and Youth: a glance over the decades. *Am Ann Deaf* 1998;142:72–76.

label (e.g., visually impaired). Other items relate to sociocultural changes. For example, included among etiologic choices is deafness resulting from maternal drug abuse.

Despite the proven effectiveness of early intervention programs, the average age at identification of hearing impairment in chil-dren is 3 years (National Institutes of Health, 1993), a delay that threatens language acquisition during a critical period of development. This is far later than ASHA's recommendation that children with impaired hearing be identified before the age of 6 months (ASHA, 1994a). Further, significant delays continue to occur between the time hearing loss is suspected and diagnosed and again until the time intervention is initiated (Stein et al., 1990; Harrison and Roush, 1996). As neonatal screening becomes universal and hearing professionals provide adequate information and guidance about risk factors associated with impaired hearing to parents and professionals, the timing of identification and intervention can be expected to improve.

DIVERSITY

Perhaps one of the greatest changes in continuing and new relationships that is likely to occur within the practice of audiologic rehabilitation will be an appreciation of diversity, as reflected by gender, socioeconomic status, ethnicity, and social support resources.

Gender

Among children with impaired hearing, 54% are boys and 46% are girls; this ratio of boys to girls is somewhat greater among children attending residential programs for children with impaired hearing (Walker-Vann, 1998). An abundance of information exists underscoring gender-related differences in behavior, academic achievement, and learning styles among children with normal hearing. Schildroth and Hotto (1993) report that boys with impaired hearing have more behavioral problems and learning disabilities. In contrast, girls with impaired hearing may experience lower self-esteem and greater anxiety (Loeb and Sarigiani, 1986).

Among adults of any age with impaired hearing, slightly more than half (57%) are men. However, older women outlive older men. Sixty percent of the population older than age 65 is female, increasing to 70% by age 85 (U.S. Bureau of the Census, 1995). As women age, they are more likely to experience chronic health problems than men (Rodin and Ickovics, 1990), which may affect the importance they assign to seeking professional intervention for hearing impairment. Pure-tone threshold gender reversals are frequently reported (e.g., Garstecki and Erler, 1998a,b), with women demon-

strating poorer low-frequency hearing and men poorer high-frequency hearing. Configurations of hearing thresholds, combined with word recognition and central auditory processing abilities that vary by gender, may influence the perceived need for audiologic rehabilitation as well as benefit from such intervention. Women also demonstrate an advantage for nonverbal communication that may influence communication strategy preference and proficiency. To increase accountability, hearing professionals will need to design service programs that reflect gender-related diversity and needs. Relationships with female clients, whether children or adults, will vary from those with male clients, taking into account physical and emotional differences and learning styles.

Socioeconomic Factors

More education is associated with better health and higher financial status. Both may influence attitudes toward and accessibility of audiologic rehabilitation. Among today's older adults, only 64% have completed high school, compared with 85% of those 35 to 64 years of age, a group that includes Baby Boomers (U.S. Bureau of the Census, 1995). It is expected that by 2015, 20% of older adults will have a Bachelor's degree. Today, only 13% of older adults have completed college. In general, the financial status of older adults has improved during the past 20 years. The number of older adults living in poverty has declined from 15% in 1975 to 11% in 1995 (U.S. Bureau of the Census, 1995). However, poverty rates vary by age, gender, and ethnicity. Poverty rates are higher among those who are 75 and older (13% compared with 9% of those 65 to 75 years of age), female (14% compared with 6% of elderly men), and Black or Hispanic (25% and 24%, respectively, compared with 9% of Whites). Among children living in single-parent homes, 39% live at the poverty level (U.S. Bureau of the Census, 1993). At present, third-party reimbursement for audiologic services is limited. Until payment for hearing services (including costs associated with hearing aids and audiologic rehabilitation) through public or private insurance is routine, financial resources will be of concern. Relationships among audiologists, health service delivery systems, and policy-makers will be critical to maintaining the availability of audiologic rehabilitation services for children and adults.

Diversity

Some of the greatest changes to come in the new millennium will be related to ethnic diversity. Indeed, in some geographic areas there are ethnic groups that were once considered the minority and are now the majority. In 1994, 10% of the older adult U.S. population was non-White. That proportion will double within the next 50 years, with the greatest increases in the Hispanic population. Similar increases in the number of children with impaired hearing who are from ethnic minorities are also noted (Schildroth et al., 1989). The term Hispanic refers to a heterogeneous population, arriving in the United States from various countries. Children who are both Hispanic and have impaired hearing are more likely to have parents who are undereducated, underemployed, and limited in their English-speaking ability than children with impaired hearing from other ethnic and cultural backgrounds. These children may find themselves exposed to a bilingual, and in some cases trilingual, environment incorporating spoken Spanish at home and spoken and/or signed English at school (MacNeil, 1990). Currently, non-White children who are deaf demonstrate lower academic achievement and are less likely to be mainstreamed (Kluwin, 1994). Hearing care providers must accommodate cultural values and traditions as well as language needs. Specifically, culture may influence acceptance of hearing loss and its treatment, interaction with government agencies, adherence to traditional medical regimens, and nonverbal and verbal communication styles (Yacobacci-Tam, 1987).

Social Support

The composition of the American family has changed significantly and will continue to do so. No longer is a two-parent family the norm, nor is it usual practice for older parents to live with and be cared for by their adult children. Today, 25% of children live in single-parent homes; that proportion is higher for African-American (50%) and Hispanic (33%) families (Roush and McWilliam, 1994). Such family structures may affect financial status and the amount of time mothers and fathers are able to devote to the treatment of their child's hearing impairment. Further, a parent's ability to cope with the emotional impact of having a child with impaired hearing may be influenced by restricted social support resources. When compared with mothers of children with normal hearing, mothers of preschool children with severe to profound hearing loss report significantly greater parenting stress, smaller support networks, and less frequent contact with support sources (Quittner et al., 1990). Similar barriers to satisfactory social support are noted among aging adults, especially older women. Seventy-five percent of older men and 36% of older women are married (Williams, 1992). One-third of women aged 65 to 74 years live alone. Among the oldest-old, 81% live alone. Limited social support is associated with poorer health and psychological adjustment. The role of significant others in adjustment to chronic conditions, including impaired hearing, is considerable, yet older adults are likely to experience declines in hearing sensitivity at the same time their sources of support diminish.

The obligation of the audiologist is to help clients compensate for barriers to rehabilitative success that may be associated with gender, socioeconomic status, ethnicity, and sources of social support. This will be accomplished through strong relationships with clients and their families and significant others.

Clinical Service Delivery

Professional associations, licensing agencies, and funding sources increasingly are insistent that the benefit of services must be verifiable. Audiologists and other service providers will need to develop and implement assessment and treatment protocols that meet the individual needs of children and adults with impaired hearing.

INTERNATIONAL CLASSIFICATION OF IMPAIRMENT, DISABILITY, AND HANDICAP-2

Recognizing the need for a more meaningful system of classification that focuses on the individual, the World Health Organization (WHO) recently developed a revised *International Classification of Impairment, Disability, and Handicap-2* (ICIDH-2) (World Health Organization, 1997). The previous system consisted of classifications by (1) disease or disorder, (2) impairment, (3) disability, and (4) handicap (World Health Organization, 1980). That format has been criticized for focusing more on the condition/situation than on the individual with a particular health condition. WHO has attempted to revise its classifications to recognize the need for a common global language in the field of health (Fig. 2.3).

Impairment, activities, and participation represent function at the level of the body, person, and society, respectively. Impairment refers to a loss or abnormality of psychological, physiological, or anatomic structure or function. In the context of hearing, impairment would be demonstrated by deviations from normal pure-tone thresholds.

Activities refer to the nature and extent of deviations in normal function at the level of the individual. Changes in the essential characteristics of the activity, including its duration and quality, may occur. In other words, based on what is normal for the person, what difficulty do they experience in performing daily activities, such as problems communicating in specific environments or maintaining satisfactory employment?

Participation refers to the nature and extent of a person's ability to be involved in one's normal roles and must consider the effects of the hearing impairment on the individual, significant others, and the community. Encompassed within this category are nonauditory effects of hearing loss such as restricted socialization.

Impinging on the categories of impairment, activities, and participation are the disease/disorder condition itself and environmental and personal contextual factors unique to the individual. Etiology, onset, and progression of hearing loss may vary and affect the degree of impairment and restrictions to activity and participation. For example, prelinguistic onset of hearing loss in a young child is likely to affect the ability to acquire language (i.e., activity) and educational placement (i.e., participation). The effect of postlinguistic hearing loss may be quite different. Similarly, a young, employed adult with sudden-onset hearing loss due to Meniere's disease is likely to experience vastly different effects on activities and participation than an older, retired adult with presbycusis.

Perhaps of even greater importance is the role of the context in which a disease or disorder is experienced. Environmental factors include such tangible variables as architectural characteristics as well as social attitudes and structures. Personal characteristics that interact with impairment, activities, and participation may include demographic

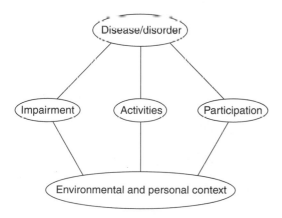

Figure 2.3. World Health Organization Classifications. Adapted from World Health Organization. International classification of impairments, disabilities and handicaps-2: a manual of dimensions of disablement and functioning (beta-1 draft for field trials). Geneva: World Health Organization, 1997.

variables (e.g., age, gender, education), profession, experience, and coping style. Individual functioning, therefore, is a synthesis of physical or mental conditions as well as social and physical environment. Restrictions to activities and participation will require individualized treatment plans, including use of assistive devices, environmental modifications, and communication training. Professionals may also be involved in prevention efforts to negate or limit restrictions. Preventive activities may include providing public education about hearing loss, advocating for accessibility of services and employment, and developing public policies to promote hearing health and hearing loss management.

The revised WHO classification system serves several purposes. First, it provides a means for standardization of assessment and interpretation of data. Second, it serves as a framework for evaluating hearing health care. Finally, an agreed-on classification system may be used to introduce and amend legislation and other social policies.

HEARING CARE COST, SERVICE DELIVERY PRACTICE, AND TREATMENT OUTCOMES ISSUES

Practical issues in service delivery relate to cost, delivery practice, treatment outcome and efficacy, and reimbursement issues. As costs for hearing care rise, there will be increasing dependence on third-party reimbursement and innovative service delivery programs. Demand for closer accounting of treatment outcomes will increase. Reimbursement for services will depend on treatment outcome data. While costs rise, technological advances will bring new benefits, particularly in regard to information access and communication. Shifting demographics will cause a change in the types of services that are made available and in how they are delivered. The scope of practice in audiology will change to accommodate new needs and approaches to treatment. Finally, each change potentially challenges professional standards of ethical practice.

Costs

Health care costs spiraled from the late 1960s to the mid-1990s at a rate that, if left unchecked, would consume 100% of the gross national product by 2050 (Banja, 1994). Public concern over escalating health care costs reached a crescendo in 1994, culminating in a major effort to reform health care at the federal level that eventually failed. Subsequent attempts also failed, suggesting that success in the future is likely to depend on political alignment between the majority party in Congress and the presidency (Pietranton, 1998). Because little reimbursement for hearing care in general, and audiologic rehabilitation in particular, is available though public or private sources, new efforts to support hearing care may be dependent on convincing key legislators and members of Congress of its importance. The future of audiologic rehabilitation may be tied to the success of such efforts and the relationships established by hearing care providers in the political arena.

Cost factors also will dictate where services are provided. For example, there will be fewer hospitals in the future, but the ones that exist will be large, for-profit, multipurpose medical centers (Kiplinger, 1986). These "super-meds" will incorporate a full range of hospital and insurance services and include health maintenance organizations/preferred provider organizations (HMOs/PPOs), walk-in clinics, pharmacies, and facilities for dental care and mental illness treatment. They may offer "plug-in" home computer services to monitor vital health signs and to provide self-help instruction. Audiologic rehabilitation in such an environment is likely to involve establishing relationships with a broad spectrum of health care providers functioning as a comprehensive health service team. Other hospitals will close, merge, or convert to alternate types of health care facilities (e.g., extended care or nursing facilities). Hearing care in the future may also be provided in the homes of individuals with impaired hearing.

Hearing care costs will continue to rise for an indefinite period, then level off. This, coupled with increasing numbers of the largest health-care–consuming segment of the population (e.g., older adults), bodes well for the future of audiology as a rehabilitation-emphasis profession. Health care costs will be held in check, at least minimally, by a shift in population interest toward wellness, prevention, and self-help approaches to health care management. Thus, the scope of practice in audiology is likely to incorporate greater emphasis on public education in understanding hearing loss and its ramifications, as well as on development and implementation of distance treatment and self-instruction programs in hearing loss management. Rehabilitation audiologists may find it beneficial to establish working relationships with educational program developers.

Service Delivery Practices

Hearing care in a fee-for-service system is provider-driven. The provider sets the fees, determines the types and levels of service needed, delivers the service, and is reimbursed directly from the individual served or a third party. Payment typically is provided on a per-visit basis. Provider income increases with increased numbers of individuals treated and/or treatment procedures provided. The payor prefers minimal service to control costs. The provider delivers as much service as can be justified clinically. The relationship between the provider and consumer is one in which the audiologist is motivated to provide comprehensive, extended care. This will not be the most common service delivery paradigm in the future.

In the new millennium, managed care will essentially control clinical service delivery. The number of individuals enrolled in HMOs grew to 46 million in 1993 (Pietranton, 1998). In 1996, 70% of all health insurance in the United States was under managed care. Unlike in the traditional fee-for-service system, under managed care hearing care is payor-driven. The payor determines a capitated (per head) rate for a covered population. The provider's interest is in controlling cost and increasing the profit margin by providing minimal service. The financial risk is shifted from the payor to the provider through capitated contractual agreements. A fee is negotiated for each potential recipient of a specified service in advance of the service being provided. The fee is multiplied by the number of eligible individuals or enrollees in a given managed care plan and paid to the provider in advance of the service being rendered. If service costs exceed the capitated amount of reimbursement received, the provider absorbs the excess cost as a loss. If the cost is less, the provider realizes a profit (Pietranton, 1998).

Under managed care, the provider and consumer continue to have a working relationship, however, the audiologist/provider will be motivated by profit to provide minimal care. This suggests that in the future the hearing care consumer will want to establish a relationship with a hearing care provider whose services are reimbursable by a more flexible and generous managed care plan. Whatever payment procedure is applied, reimbursement is likely to be contingent on demonstrated treatment outcome data.

Treatment Outcome Measures

Treatment outcome measures demonstrate the relationship between service costs and benefits. Outcome measures are needed to justify reimbursement and therefore need to be multidimensional, addressing a range of clinical management issues that include the following (Pietranton, 1998):

1. Clinical status: the hearing condition, other sensory deficits, and other physical or mental factors that influence the potential to self-manage hearing loss independently should be demonstrated.
2. Functional status: communication ability, psychosocial adjustment to hearing loss, and personal performance in social, academic, and vocational settings should be noted.
3. Well-being: the status of pertinent physical and mental health conditions should be reported.
4. Satisfaction with care: a report of personal reaction to clinical service should be obtained from the hearing care recipient.
5. Cost: a report of costs associated with clinical service delivery to the recipient

and the health care system should be maintained.

This multidimensional approach to measuring treatment outcome attempts to balance the perspectives of all involved in the hearing care process. A detailed examination of outcome measures can be found in Chapter 18.

In addition to services related to audiologic assessment and sensory device selection and fitting, the current scope of practice in audiology includes the following rehabilitative services expected by hearing care consumers (ASHA, 1996):

1. Counseling to understand and adjust to hearing loss and its effects.
2. Counseling in regard to selection and potential benefit from use of sensory aids, assistive devices, and large area amplification systems.
3. Improvement of communication competence;
4. Development of individualized education programs (IEPs) for school-age children.
5. Development of individualized family service plans (IFSPs) for children from birth to 36 months.

Hearing care providers will be responsible for developing and using appropriate outcome measures for each service provided. Treatment outcome data have many uses including prediction of treatment duration and progress milestones, determination (in advance) of likely benefit from treatment, and establishment of guidelines for the average number of visits needed to effect change in behavior or function (Task Force on Treatment Outcomes and Cost Effectiveness, 1997).

Treatment Efficacy

How can hearing care professionals demonstrate that the services they provide are diminishing the impairment and restrictions of activities and participation of the client? Treatment efficacy, as it relates to audiologic rehabilitation, refers to the likelihood that a person with impaired hearing in a spe-cific diagnostic category will benefit from an intervention (Montgomery, 1994). Further, such intervention will be assessed by performance at or above a specified criterion using valid, reliable outcome measures. In a recent review of treatment efficacy related to children with impaired hearing, Carney and Moeller (1998) identified several problems with existing efficacy research. They suggest that variations within and between research populations, assessment tools, and interventions limit our ability to draw reliable conclusions. The same can be said for research related to adults with impaired hearing. Because audiologic rehabilitation is concerned primarily with improving receptive and expressive communication, developing valid, reliable outcome measures is a complex process. Hearing care providers will be challenged to improve outcome measures to assure treatment benefit.

The service provider's assessment protocol must be tailored to the individual client. Assessment should vary based on disease/disorder condition and environmental and personal context, determining outcomes relevant to impairment, activities, and participation. Traditionally, assessments have reflected a medical model, relying on audiometric measures of the degree of hearing loss, middle ear function, and word recognition. Objective measures of hearing aid benefit are routinely administered. Audiometric measures provide accurate assessment of peripheral and central auditory function under ideal conditions (i.e., hearing impairment). Audiometric protocols focus on the individual's capability to perform tasks, such as responding to sound and recognizing speech. Glass (1998) refers to this as experimental function. These measures relate to the individual's clinical status.

To augment audiometric data, numerous self-report and self-assessment tools exist. Recent ASHA (1998) guidelines related to hearing aid fitting have been expanded to encompass self-assessment inventories. Self-assessments provide information about communication performance and personal adjustment to hearing loss (i.e., activity and/or participation) and rely on the perceptions of the individual with impaired hearing and/or significant others. These measures may provide information about the individual's perception of their functional status. Numerous self-report instruments are available for adults with impaired hearing, including those designed to determine hearing aid benefit (e.g., the Abbreviated Profile of Hearing Aid Benefit; Cox and Alexander, 1995), communication performance and personal adjustment (e.g., the Communication Profile for the Hearing Impaired; Demorest and Erdman, 1987), and hearing handicap in specific populations (e.g., Hearing Handicap Inventory for the Elderly; Ventry and Weinstein, 1982). These self-report instruments are discussed further in Chapters 10, 11, and 13, and can be found in the attachments at the end of this book. No similar standardized instruments are available for use with children and their families.

TECHNOLOGICAL ADVANCES

Another aspect of service delivery relates to changes in technology. Advances in sensory device design and medical technology will greatly affect audiologic rehabilitation. These topics are explored in-depth elsewhere in this text. Clinical service will increasingly depend on computer technology and information available on the Internet. Although Chapter 17 specifically examines the role of computer technology in aural rehabilitation, the following briefly addresses issues related to hearing care relationships.

Computers

Expert systems that compress and then provide knowledge on a given topic are becoming available for hearing care. Such a system should enable individuals with impaired hearing to gather considerable information concerning hearing loss and treatment options in advance of visiting an otologist, audiologist, or any other health care provider. Provider-consumer relationships may be set at a higher shared knowledge level than in the past. Expert systems provide reference sources for tutors, planners and designers,

managers, and coaches. They will be of benefit in any instance in which a body of knowledge can be reduced to an "If this, then what?" system of rules and methods.

Use of expert systems will be enhanced by voice-activated computers. Individuals will speak to the computer and the computer will present a response. For universal application, advances will first need to be made in voice input-output systems for the computer to recognize more than a few thousand words spoken by a single speaker. A computer that responds to any voice should become a reality in the future, although special challenges will lay ahead for individuals whose hearing condition has influenced their speech intelligibility. Speech-language pathologists may have a new reason for improving articulation skills among individuals with impaired hearing. Although computers will be programmed to respond to spoken questions, it is unlikely that they will reach the stage of emulating such human brain processes as reasoning by analogy. The ultimate goal would be for a computer to solve a problem with only the instruction to do so.

Other uses of computer technology relate to academics and communication training. For example, using computer-assisted note-taking, a note-taker types information into a computer and the student with impaired hearing reads from a television monitor. Although the success of this approach depends on the skills of the note-taker, it reduces the student's need to attend to auditory-visual cues while they write (Youdelman and Messerly, 1996). Others are developing computer-based drills for auditory-visual speech recognition (Lansing and Bienvenue, 1994). This method allows for individualization of lessons while greatly reducing clinician time commitments. Although one cannot imagine what the computer will become to providers and recipients of hearing care, it is certain that it is likely to compete with the hearing aid as the critical tool in the rehabilitation process.

Web-Based Learning

In 1994, few people knew about the World Wide Web. During a 3-month period 2 years later, 24 million people accessed the Web at least once. By the beginning of the new millennium, 14 million people will have access to the Web in their place of employment (Tsantis and Keefe, 1996). Today, the Web is the most important force in communication and will profoundly influence society for many years to come. The Web simplifies access to information to build a learning environment beyond traditional boundaries. It accomplishes this by creating synthetic environments that simulate real-world settings. Knowledge webs complement existing sources of information, and virtual communities provide interaction capabilities that complement face-to-face relationships (e.g., mentoring, peer coaching, teleapprenticeships) (Tsantis and Keefe, 1996).

By creating synthetic environments (e.g., chat rooms) the Web has become the great equalizer in that hearing and speaking disabilities are no longer impediments to interpersonal communication. Chat room relationships may create an important opportunity for catharsis, lessening (unfortunately) the need for support group participation (Tsantis and Keefe, 1996).

Knowledge webs containing archival resources include images, audio files, and video segments that are accessed through search engines (e.g., Alta Vista, Yahoo, InfoSeek). In time, virtual communities will be established, providing opportunities for replacement of face-to-face meetings, counseling sessions, and treatment with on-line meetings. For individuals with impaired hearing, seeing as well as hearing a communication partner and making use of speechreading, facial expression, and body language cues add significantly to communication success. Virtual communities can beget virtual relationships without the limitations of physical distance. In the new millennium, access—not knowledge—will be power (Tsantis and Keefe, 1996).

Personal-Professional Relationships

Ultimately, accommodations made for serving targeted populations, new delivery practices, and new demands for service benefit verification will succeed only when working relationships are established among providers and with families. The nature and importance of these relationships are discussed below.

A DEVELOPMENTAL VIEW OF RELATIONSHIPS

From birth to death, relationships are established to nurture, guide, direct, build autonomy, and engender a high quality of life. By understanding normal development throughout the life course, appropriate relationships within the context of audiologic rehabilitation can be established.

Erikson (1963) describes eight stages in the life cycle, which when examined within the framework of impaired hearing suggest different types of relationships that may develop. These serve as guideposts to understanding how relationships are formed and cultivated and how early relationships prepare for new relationships.

In the first stage, trust versus mistrust, most infants discover that the world is a safe place. The positive and predictable relationship developed between a baby and its parents or caregivers helps accomplish this task. Cry and mother appears like clockwork! Development of trust is threatened when an infant has impaired hearing. The child may only be soothed by physical contact, rather than the sound of the parent's voice. Parents of a newly diagnosed hearing-impaired child may feel uncertain about their parenting abilities. If the child's condition is not yet diagnosed, parents may be caught in the "medical funnel," unsure of which professionals to consult and waiting for answers and referrals.

During the next stage, autonomy versus shame and doubt, children begin to establish control over physical and mental activities. During this stage, the child begins to communicate his or her wants and learns the power of "No." The child with impaired hearing is likely to experience delays in the ability to communicate effectively through spoken language. Failure to be understood frequently results in frustration for both the child and the caregiver. For children with more severely impaired hearing, relationships will be established with hearing care providers, physicians, and speech-language pathologists. For children with lesser degrees of hearing loss, delays in the acquisition of speech and language may generate confusion and doubt among parents, ultimately leading them to seek professional assistance.

As the number of communication partners increases, new connections are made. Soon the young child realizes his or her potential for establishing new relationships with the adult world. Initiative versus guilt is the stage in which children demonstrate inordinate curiosity, activity, and at times aggression. Impaired hearing may limit the child's ability to interact effectively with other children and adults. In turn, parents find themselves torn between encouraging and limiting exploration because of concerns about their child's safety. Relationships with professionals are likely to extend to early intervention specialists and other school personnel.

Armed with knowledge well beyond the home environment, the child progresses to the next stage, industry versus inferiority. In this stage, the child is ready for formal learning. School relationships are waiting to be conquered and, ideally, bring positive reinforcement, personal satisfaction, pride, and pleasure. The degree of the child's hearing impairment may affect the amount of integration with hearing peers, resulting in recognition of differences and, in the worst case, feelings of inferiority.

The following stage, identity versus role confusion, encompasses the adolescent experience. Strong connections are established through social relationships with age peers. Adolescence is an inherently difficult stage, and its challenges may be exacerbated by the presence of impaired hearing. For example, teenagers may resist wearing sensory devices, particularly those that are more visible. An adult-like identity is acquired largely through relationships made outside the home and family environment.

The next stage, intimacy versus isolation, is a time of mature relationship-building.

The focus is on establishing new primary social relationships (adult friends) and an occupation. Energy is directed toward establishing a satisfying means of independent social and economic survival. Interpersonal relationships acquire high intensity and importance. For an adult with impaired hearing, there may be concerns about maintaining the types of social and work relationships necessary to capitalize on opportunities to make new acquaintances or to advance in a job.

Generativity versus stagnation is the next stage. This is a time when relationships are established by adults with younger individuals with the intention of preparing them for the future. It is also a time of formal and informal teaching, either as parents or experts. Adults who acquire a hearing loss may feel limited in their ability to achieve personal and professional goals. They will establish relationships with hearing professionals, physicians, and counselors to obtain appropriate treatment and guidance.

The final stage, ego integrity versus despair, is the stage of wisdom. Younger generations reach out to their elders for lessons on life. Sense of control and coping style will influence attitudes toward disability, as will experiences and life history. Some older adults with impaired hearing will become isolated, whereas others will feel little handicapping effect. Relationships with family members, friends, and professionals will reflect these attitudes, reinforcing either feelings of helplessness or independence. Some older adults may have little motivation to develop new social relationships; however, this seems to be more true for older men than for older women. Results of a study by Garstecki and Erler (1998b) revealed that effective social communication was more important for older women than older men. In an earlier study, Garstecki and Erler (1996) found that social communication was of less importance to older than younger adults, but grew in importance as communication settings became more intimate or confined. Although the relationship between perceived effectiveness and communication importance requires further study, inability to communicate effectively in social situations obviously impedes relationship-building.

Relationships develop throughout the life course. The roles of family members, friends, and professionals vary with time and circumstance. Having considered the developmental nature of relationships among individuals regardless of hearing ability and challenges that may be encountered, the next section addresses relationships within families and with hearing care providers.

FAMILY AND HEARING CARE PROVIDER RELATIONSHIPS

Given the pervasive nature of hearing loss, hearing care affects the involved individual within the context of a family environment. What affects one family member will affect other family members in various ways. Family members intimately know the individual with impaired hearing, interacting on a daily basis. Hearing care providers must establish effective relationships with family members. To do so, they must understand how families function, their resources, and interaction style (DeConde-Johnson et al., 1997).

Today, a family is best self-defined. Each child or adults' family may vary in structure, role, culture, language, socioeconomic status, and belief system. A family may consist entirely of blood relatives. Children enrolled in audiologic habilitation may come from families in which there is only one parent or one in which a grandparent assumes responsibility for making decisions. Older adults may rely on adult children or close friends for support and assistance or they may prefer to make decisions independently.

The concept of family continues to evolve. For example, today 17 million couples in the United States are divorced, and only 58% of all children live with their biological parents. Seventy-five percent of divorced men spend less than 2 days a month with their children when they are young, even less when their children are older.

Even among more traditional families, parents spend on average only 17 hours per week with their children (Cleminshaw, 1996).

Adults are increasingly likely to live alone, and this is especially true for women as they age. Only 6% of women younger than 45 years of age live alone, compared with 40% of women 65 to 74 years of age and 53% of those 75 years and older (U.S. Bureau of the Census, 1995). In contrast, only 17% of men aged 65 to 74 years and 23% of those 75 years and older live alone. Clearly, reliance on support from friends and professionals becomes increasingly important.

According to Turnbull and Turnbull (1986), the family, whatever its composition, exists as a system of interrelated components including resources (e.g., socioeconomic status), interactions (e.g., frequency of contact), functions (e.g., activities of each member), and lifestyle (e.g., roles). Within each component, change affecting one individual influences others. For example, the cost of hearing care for one family member limits funds available for others. Time spent with a child with special needs affects parents' time with other children.

The family system can be sabotaged in a variety of ways. Luterman (1991) studied family members, noting factors that potentially complicate relationship-building with health care providers. First, consider spouses. Marriage implies contractual expectations for each partner. Although marriage partners pledge "for better or for worse," neither partner plans for spousal disability (e.g., permanent hearing loss). When disability occurs, some consider the contract violated. Some spouses become angry, whereas others grieve the loss of a partner with whom they planned to share their life and in whom they confide. Hearing loss may draw spouses together or may act as a divisive factor. New marriages survive when young couples are aware of a disability or its potential in advance. Other marriages crumble because partners lack experience in coping with the stress related to hearing impairment (Luterman, 1991). When such a situation is encountered in the process of establishing a hearing care relationship, it may be important for professionals to attend to the needs of the unimpaired spouse for there to be a long-term, positive effect on the spouse with the disability.

Next, consider parents and children. Under ideal conditions, parenting is an extremely difficult task. There is always conflict, not only with children, but among parents themselves over their nurturing or control-guiding functions. When parents are close emotionally and a child with a disability is born, the parents are likely to fulfill their child-raising responsibilities successfully. Those who do not equally share parenting responsibilities or who have dissimilar expectations will have more difficulty coping with the demands of a child with impaired hearing (Luterman, 1991). This may first become apparent to the hearing care provider at the time the child enters a preschool program if one parent is less involved. This suggests that hearing care providers may need to focus on optimizing the parent-child relationship.

Other important family members are grandparents. They function as caretakers, mediators, role models, and historians. They may also introduce stress in the home (Luterman, 1991). Grandparents are generally slower in their acceptance of disability than parents. Disability may occur at a time they are least prepared to cope with emotional emergencies. Grandparents often lack current information about a disorder and know far less than their children in regard to how to deal with it. Parents may then be forced to parent their own parents. Ideally, grandparents will become a source of emotional support. Some may also provide financial assistance (Atkins, 1994). Depending on existing relationships and the manner in which such assistance is given, financial support may enhance positive bonds or may increase feelings of resentment and lack of control. Parents and grandparents may need assistance from the hearing care provider to help bridge the gap. Professionals can provide much-needed information and can also facilitate communication between grandparents and their grandchildren.

Finally, there are siblings. The sibling relationship generally is a long-term relationship. The sibling system teaches children to negotiate, cooperate, compete, and be supportive. Siblings are almost always affected when a brother or sister has a disability. Positive outcomes include a greater understanding of individuals with disabilities, compassion, and sensitivity to prejudice. Alternately, siblings may feel cheated out of their own childhood, neglected by their parents, even shameful (Luterman, 1991). Atkins (1994) points out that some siblings feel pressure to be high-achieving students, in a sense compensating for limitations their brother or sister may have. Again, hearing care providers need to provide age-appropriate information and support to parents and siblings, and parents may need assistance in balancing the needs of each of their children.

A MODEL FOR RELATIONSHIP BUILDING

Traditional approaches to rehabilitation in the past relied on a professional-centered model in which hearing was assessed and treatment regimens prescribed by a hearing care professional. The professional identified problems related to hearing loss, prioritized needs, developed a plan of treatment, and provided services in locations and at times convenient to the hearing care provider. In essence, the client was acted upon. Two shifts in this approach have occurred since the 1970s. First, legislative actions, primarily related to special education, have focused on the importance of family-centered and client-centered intervention. Second, there is a growing recognition of the benefits of collaboration among clients and professionals (e.g., Matkin, 1994).

Beginning in 1975 with the Education of All Handicapped Act (PL94–142), the federal government not only guaranteed that all children had the right to a free and appropriate education, it mandated the development of IEPs for each child receiving special education services, including those with impaired hearing. The IEP process emphasizes bringing together parents and professionals to share information (including the results of formal assessments), identify current levels of function, discuss needs, and cooperatively develop appropriate goals and objectives. More recent enactment of PL 99-457 (1986), the Individuals with Disabilities Education Act and amended by PL105-17 (1997), introduced the concept of an IFSP, which stresses the concept that intervention for young children must be family-centered. The IFSP must be developed by a multidisciplinary team, including the child's family. It takes into consideration not only the child's functional levels and needs, but includes the family's self-assessed needs and priorities. Goals are then developed to meet both child and family concerns.

To some extent, the Americans with Disabilities Act of 1990 (ADA) (United States Architectural and Transportation Barriers Compliance Board, 1991) focuses attention on the individual needs and rights of adults with impaired hearing. The ADA protects individuals from workplace discrimination, mandating appropriate accommodations to allow satisfactory employment and advancement. Other aspects of the ADA address issues of accessibility in public places and includes accessibility to telecommunications.

Although one of the primary outcomes of these legislative acts has been to focus intervention on the individual, secondarily it has underscored the need for collaboration. Collaboration has been described as a process that brings individuals with diverse expertise together to develop solutions to mutually agreed-on problems (Idol et al., 1986). Ideally, collaboration produces outcomes that are superior to those resulting from the efforts of any single team member.

Collaborative teams may be multidisciplinary, interdisciplinary, or transdisciplinary. Multidisciplinary team members function independently. That is, assessment and goal development are discipline-specific. Information may or may not be shared formally. In this scenario, an individual might receive services from a physician (e.g., treatment of a middle ear problem), an audiologist (e.g., assessment of hearing loss and recommendation to purchase hearing aids), and a speech-language pathologist (e.g., communication training) with little or no interaction among team members.

In an interdisciplinary team format, professionals again maintain roles related to their specific areas of expertise. However, results of assessments and observations are shared formally, and team members (including clients and family members) make decisions as a group. Intervention is carried out by specific team members according to their area of expertise, with periodic reviews of progress.

In a transdisciplinary approach, team members share expertise. Professionals, family members, and clients may participate in assessments and goal development that transcend their specific area of expertise. Intervention roles are integrated. For example, a speech-language pathologist may work full-time in a classroom for children with impaired hearing, providing on-going communication skill-building and participating in and leading a variety of classroom activities. Some professionals may be reluctant to agree to therapeutic priorities that do not recognize their discipline as most important. Others may have difficulty assuming roles that extend well beyond their formal training. Parents and clients may feel hesitant or incapable to assume a major role in developing goals. Professionals, families, and clients are likely to feel more comfortable functioning within a specific team model, and individual circumstances will dictate which model is most appropriate.

Rehabilitative relationships that are family-centered and client-centered increase problem ownership and decrease feelings of helplessness. The family or client is the constant, whereas hearing care professionals may be involved episodically (Winton and Bailey, 1994). The professional's first priority is to help families and clients feel empowered and supported (Bowe, 1995). Empowerment is a process that helps people feel a sense of control. For example, the purpose and nature of assessments should be explained in advance to alleviate fears and create reasonable expectations (Blosser, 1996). Results of assessments should be reported thoroughly and interpretations justified. A parent or spouse should not feel like a surrogate service provider. Rather, the family and client's opinions, observations, experience, knowledge, and feelings should be respected and valued.

In addition to fostering a sense of empowerment, successful relationships prioritize goals based on the family's or client's assessment of a problem. The Client Oriented Scale of Improvement (COSI) (Dillon et al., 1997) is an excellent example of client-guided assessment and rehabilitation. Other self-assessment tools and observations allow the client to personalize treatment. Family-centered and client-centered rehabilitation is provided at times and in places that are convenient for the individual, not the professional. Many clinical programs now offer extended weekday hours and Saturday appointments. Early intervention programs may incorporate parent-child activities on weekends to accommodate working parents.

Families that are successful in coping with impaired hearing are characterized by clear and direct communication among family members, clearly defined roles, acceptance of limitations, intimacy and equity among members, and stability (Luterman, 1991). Successful family members are high in self-esteem, philosophical about their lives, and feel their burdens are shared. In addition, they are committed to each other and demonstrate common beliefs and values (Cleminshaw, 1996). Successful professional members of the team demonstrate flexibility and respectfulness. They are open-minded and tolerant of values, beliefs, and traditions that are different from their own. Hearing care providers must be knowledgeable, adept at gathering information, and able to effectively communicate with others.

Parents of children with impaired hearing identified several professional characteristics and actions they find most helpful (Roush, 1994). Most of their "advice" is equally applicable to professionals who work with adults. Although facts and information are critical, families appreciate a caring attitude. Parents (and adults) want to be guided to make decisions, not simply told what to choose. If an educational or therapeutic choice is no longer appropriate, families want to be able to change their minds. Families appreciate praise for their abilities, not judgment of their limitations. Likewise, professionals are encouraged to see the abilities of the person with impaired hearing, not their disabilities. Families want the opportunity to share ideas, support, and experiences with other families and adults coping with hearing loss. Families appreciate professionals who recognize and involve all members of their support network. To develop satisfying rehabilitative relationships, family members, clients, and professionals must view their partnership as a dynamic one, changing with time and circumstance.

Providing services and maintaining relationships must occur within a framework of accepted ethical conduct. The final section of this chapter addresses issues related to professional ethics.

Professional Ethics

Unlike nonprofessional members of the rehabilitative team, hearing care providers must function within guidelines that assure adherence to professional and legal standards. Individuals who encounter ear disease, ear disorders, or head and ear injuries may experience physical pain, mental anguish, personal frustration, and inconvenience in addition to hearing loss. Because of these effects, individuals with impaired hearing may be vulnerable to exploitation. Also, bad decisions by hearing care providers can have dire consequences. Finally, it is commonly recognized that "turf battles" occur among hearing care team members. These conditions and others, alone and in tandem, create a situation that mandates adherence to ethical standards to assure high-quality, professional care.

Professional codes of ethics serve multiple purposes. They may be directive in that they provide guidance for the behavior of members of a profession. They protect the rights of all involved in hearing care: providers, recipients, significant and concerned others, and the public at large. Codes of ethics address potential problems, issues, and dilemmas of concern to a profession. They are enforceable and enforced (Scott, 1998). The ASHA Code of Ethics (ASHA, 1994b) and the American Academy of Audiology Code of Ethics (American Academy of Audiology, 1998–1999) are included in Appendices 2.1 and 2.2.

MORALS, ETHICS, AND THE LAW

Ethical practices are based in morality and blended with law to form standards of professional conduct. Morals are formed by personal beliefs regarding what is right and what is wrong. Moral beliefs are grounded in religion or secular philosophic theory. They are culture-based, culture-driven, time-dependent, and intrapersonal in nature. Universal morals, for example, prohibit murder, rape, and incest. Although one is not compelled to abide by another person's morals, ethical and legal mandates of a community and society at large must be observed (Scott, 1998).

Ethics relate to personal and professional conduct. Rules of ethics are grounded in moral theory. Ethical problems often are direct, temporary, and resolvable (e.g., whether to carry out a treatment plan that calls for less than optimal intervention). Ethical issues involve debate or controversy and are normally resolved through compromise (e.g., whether to seek legal redress in regard to encroachment on professional practice by another professional). Ethical dilemmas involve making decisions between equally favorable or unfavorable choices (e.g., whether to accept or challenge a physician's application of therapeutic privilege). Every ethical problem, issue, or dilemma has three fundamental components: an agent, conduct (action or nonac-

tion), and an effect associated with the agent's conduct (Scott, 1998). Under the systems approach to hearing care, resolution of professional ethical issues involves consideration of sociocultural factors, legal implications, ethical imperatives, economic impact, and political ramifications (Scott, 1998). Each ethical issue has its own unique set of considerations.

Finally, hearing care provider practices are governed by law. Every provider is obliged to comply with existing administrative, civil, and criminal laws. These include constitutional law authority (e.g., Health Care Financing Administration [HCFA]), statutory law authority (e.g., state statutes regulating licensure of health care providers), case law authority (i.e., common law), and administrative law (i.e., regulatory agencies at the local, state, and federal levels). In addition, a secondary legal authority includes professional association ethical practice standards (e.g., Joint Commission on Accreditation of Healthcare Organizations [JCAHO]) (Scott, 1998). It is the consideration of morals, ethics, and laws that ensure control and provide order in health care delivery.

ETHICAL CHALLENGES IN THE NEW MILLENNIUM

In the new millennium, ethical issues related to hearing care provider and recipient relationships will continue. They are likely to be exacerbated by higher health care costs, tightened competition for health service contracts, changes in the scope of service delivery, and technological advances. They also will be affected by behaviors of individual team members, growing tendencies to treat professionals with less authority and respect, increased suspicion in regard to quality of care under managed care delivery systems, and increased amounts of damages awarded by jurors in health service delivery complaints (Pannbacker et al., 1996). By virtue of built-in incentives to hold costs at a minimum, providers may feel compelled to "do more with less" and not disclose treatment data to care recipients.

Managed Care

One area in which professional ethics may be challenged is managed care. Managed care is an organized system of health care service that links financial and clinical service matters. The term managed care refers to HMOs, PPOs, and managed care service delivery techniques. Potential care recipients are directed to specific providers by a physician "gatekeeper," usually a primary care physician (PCP) who specializes in family medicine, internal medicine, obstetrics/gynecology, or pediatrics. Services are offered by a specified group of providers to a covered population under contractual terms. Providers are paid a salary or contractual amount by the managed care plan, rather than a fee for service. Information systems are applied to monitor costs, appropriateness of and access to care, and treatment efficiency and effectiveness (ASHA Governmental and Social Policies Coordinating Committee, 1996).

Ideally, providers of hearing care, including audiologic rehabilitation, are expected to help individuals with impaired hearing develop their full potential. Progress toward this end must be demonstrated by documented indications of functional improvement, not merely changed performance on a select battery of tests. Treatment outcomes must represent real, demonstrable improvement such as renewed ability to converse over the telephone or conduct conversations in noisy settings. In addition, the provider must demonstrate that the services provided are the least costly means of achieving the desired outcome. Under managed care, the emphasis in audiologic service delivery shifts from concern over minimizing the impairment to minimizing the hearing disability or handicap. Less time will be spent in attempting to resolve the impairment than in compensating for its effects.

One risk to ethical practice in the future relates to reimbursement (ASHA Council on Professional Ethics, 1993). Whenever reimbursement for clinical service is guaranteed by contractual agreement, there may be the temptation to schedule services to fill the authorized period of reimbursement. As a result, services may be provided when no further benefit can be realized. This constitutes ethical dishonesty. Services for which reimbursement is approved may not represent actual services rendered. A provider cannot bill for a covered service (i.e., audiologic assessment) when another legitimate service (e.g., speechreading training) is provided to help a person cover the cost of a needed service. Indicating that an individual was referred by a named physician when, in fact, that person did not authorize referral is misrepresentation. Changing dates of service to match dates of insurance coverage is misrepresentation and ethically dishonest. Providing service when no reasonable benefit can be realized is ethically dishonest. Service provision beyond the point of maximum benefit cannot be rationalized on the basis that no harm is done in continuing. Providing support unrelated to treatment does not justify billing for treatment, and progress reports cannot be exaggerated to obtain, continue, or discontinue treatment. In every instance, it is unethical to bill solely to increase the amount of reimbursement. Requests for reimbursement must be accurate and consistent with treatment rendered (see Appendix 2.1: ASHA Code of Ethics, Principle of Ethics I [Rules E and J], Principle of Ethics III [Rule C], and Principle of Ethics IV [Rule B]).

Another ethical consideration is conflict of professional interest (ASHA Council on Professional Ethics, 1993). Professional judgment should be rendered without primary emphasis on personal gain. Gifts and economic benefits may be accepted if they benefit the individual served professionally. Situations involving, or appearing to involve, self-dealing should be avoided. If they are unavoidable, timely disclosure should be made of relevant information. Voluntary and full disclosure demonstrates good faith on the part of the provider and may be an influential factor in determining whether a conflict of interest exists. Conflicts of interest erode trust in the professional and the profession. Professional practices that include or suggest conflicts of interest are unethical (see Appendix 2.1: ASHA Code of Ethics, Principle of Ethics I, Principle of Ethics III [Rule B], and Principle of Ethics IV).

A third ethical concern relates to prescription (ASHA Council on Professional Ethics, 1993). Comprehensive hearing care incorporates input from and involvement of a team of professionals. The clinical process often involves collective decision-making. It is possible that recommendations regarding content, frequency, and duration of hearing care may be developed by collaboration, rather than by the hearing care provider alone. The overall plan is intended to be in the best interests of the individual with impaired hearing. Thus, the hearing care provider has an obligation to consider implementation of the plan. In all circumstances, however, it is incumbent on the provider to determine when to accept limitations on professional responsibility. As long as independence in professional judgment and the prerogative to provide appropriate services and accept responsibility for their outcomes are maintained, there is no violation of the ASHA Code of Ethics.

Ethical issues related to support personnel must be considered (ASHA Council on Professional Ethics, 1993). As health care service costs rise and the number of potential recipients increases, greater use may be made of support personnel in service delivery. Support services may be delegated to individuals who are neither clinically certified nor in the certification process. In such cases, support personnel cannot independently evaluate, treat, or advise hearing care recipients. They must be supervised by certified clinicians. Improper delegation of clinical responsibility is inconsistent with the ASHA Code of Ethics. Support personnel must avoid situations of possible misrepresentation, and supervisors must avoid situations of only cursory supervision or situations in which the welfare of persons served is compromised.

Butler (1996) noted that the ethical challenges created by managed care would be minimized significantly by separating funding issues from clinical service decisions. This would reduce the likelihood of someone conducting procedures outside the designated scope of practice, or providing services within the scope of practice but outside one's level of training and experience. There would be less likelihood of services being provided to individuals who are not likely to benefit from them. In sum, a number of ethical problems, issues, and dilemmas could be avoided.

To ensure that clinical practice is ethical and legal, the following suggestions are offered by Roberts and Cornett (1994). First, the practitioner must know the scope of practice in his or her profession. State licensure statues contain this information. The practitioner should know the ASHA Code of Ethics, the American Academy of Audiology Code of Ethics, and that of any other organization representing audiologists and other members of the hearing care provider team (Appendix 2.2). The practitioner should also know the established mechanisms of managed care plan appeals, minimize the risk of liability by remaining alert to possible conflicts of interest, be an advocate for individuals to whom service is provided, and insist on the right to exercise independent clinical judgment in the best interest of the patient.

Ethics and the Internet

In the new millennium it is possible that, because of physical distance, the best resource for hearing care may be available via the Internet. E-mail will enable long-distance communication, including reference to information on the Internet. Hearing care providers may need to be responsible for knowing about Internet information sources and relaying information to care recipients. Is this treating by correspondence an ethical practice?

In the opinions of the American Psychological Association's Ethics Committee, E-mail is not a confidential form of communication and, therefore, is an inappropriate medium for providing professional care. Concerns relate to confidentiality of "discussions" of clinical information on paid subscription "listservs," confidentiality of clinical or case information presented on Web sites, and confidentiality of clinical case information presented without informed consent. Journal articles and textbooks may be presented on the Web without peer review or professional endorsement. Users of such information will need to depend on their own critical evaluation and verification skills (Kuster, 1997).

Telehealth

Telehealth, a federal priority, is the use of telecommunication technology to deliver health services. It is of particular interest in delivering home health services and serving rural or remote communities. It is considered applicable to noninstrumental evaluation of speech, language, hearing, and swallowing problems. It may be used for long-distance consultations, including those involving hearing aid modification. Its use will become widespread as computers, video systems, long-distance costs, Internet, and Web rates become lower in cost and face-to-face health care costs increase. Telehealth practices may be as simple as using a telephone or looking up a health reference source on the Web. It ensures access regardless of distance or ability to pay (Goldberg, 1997).

Unfortunately, technical standards and clinical and ethical practice guidelines for telehealth practices are nonexistent. Some of the "bugs" relate to state licensure laws that prohibit interstate practice and reimbursement policies that do not compensate for services delivered by telehealth systems. Malpractice liability is also an issue. For example, if a complaint is filed by a hearing care recipient living in California for services provided in Illinois, which state's rules and regulations apply? Concerns about confidentiality of information create ethical practice dilemmas. Standards are slow to develop when cost-effectiveness data are lacking and infrastructure (i.e., equipment comparability, communication system charges) planning is uncoordinated (Gold-

berg, 1997). However, changes are on the way.

The Universal Service Provision of the 1996 Telecommunication Act ensures information access to rural/remote and underserved consumers. The Federal Communications Commission recently backed this interest with allocation of $400 million per year to rural health care providers and $2.25 billion to schools and libraries. Other progress includes the creation of the 1995 Joint Working Group on Telemedicine to develop telehealth policy recommendations, a 1997 Balanced Budget Act provision to broaden the term "telemedicine" to "telehealth," support in the amount of $646 million dedicated to federal telehealth projects from 1994 to 1996, and the HCFA's Telemedicine Demonstration Program that allows Medicare reimbursement for teleconsulting services.

Federal and state legal and policy issues need to be addressed. The federal government has the responsibility to guarantee free interstate commerce. States have the right to protect the health and well-being of their residents. If states do not accommodate telehealth practice, the federal government will, and state licensure boards may find themselves out of business.

Telehealth systems have been in place for the past 25 years but failed when federal support was withdrawn. What is required is a needs assessment to determine what might be improved in the current system. There also should be some determination of whether the technology exists to support clinical application. In addition, there is the question of how subsystems might function. For example, where does one refer a patient who happens to have a prominent skin lesion for a hearing evaluation? Finally, there is the question of whether electronic consultation is as effective as person-to-person contact (Peters and Peters, 1998).

Summary

This chapter examined factors that will influence continuing and new relationships among hearing care providers and individuals who receive professional services in the new millennium. Otologists, audiologists, speech-language pathologists, educators of the hearing-impaired, counselors, and social workers will continue to play important roles in the hearing loss management process. In addition, increasing dependence may be placed on psychologists, mental health counselors, hearing device distributors, cochlear implant manufacturers and distributors, telecommunication and captioning service representatives, "regular" educators, and vocational counselors. Much of the expansion of the potential provider pool is due to a predicted change in philosophy from diagnosis and treatment to wellness, prevention, and self-help. This change in philosophy will reflect the interests of increasing numbers of older adults (including the Baby Boom cohort). Most importantly, diversity in gender, socioeconomic, ethnic, and social support status will be better recognized.

To be efficient and efficacious, hearing care service programs will need to accommodate such differences in the future. Family composition will change in the new millennium, and family member responsibilities in the audiologic rehabilitation process will be better defined as family dynamics and life course development are better understood and appreciated by hearing care providers. In rehabilitative treatment, there will be greater emphasis on functional outcome measures, not only for determining degree of disability and handicap, but to justify third-party reimbursement. Managed care programs already in existence will become pervasive in the new millennium in an effort to contain health care costs. Advancements in computer and information technology will bring new resources to the hearing care provider and consumer for general educational and self-help purposes as well as to facilitate rehabilitative service delivery (e.g., telehealth).

Suggestions for relationship-building were provided, emphasizing the partnership among professionals, individuals with impaired hearing, and family members. Fi-

nally, reference was made to the importance of professional ethics in all professional relationships, now and in the future. Particular emphasis was directed toward ethical challenges in the new millennium, challenges created by the changes that are noted above.

Hearing care will be different in the new millennium. In some ways it may be better. Ultimately, its value and importance will depend on the quality of relationships established among hearing care providers and with individuals with impaired hearing and their families. By collaboratively dedicating their interest and efforts to alleviating the negative effects of impaired hearing, they will ensure that the new millennium will bring hope for those who navigate through life with less than optimal hearing ability.

REFERENCES

American Academy of Audiology. Code of ethics. American Academy of Audiology Membership Directory 1998–1999:230–232.

ASHA (American Speech-Language-Hearing Association) Council on Professional Ethics. Ethics: resources for professional preparation and practice. Rockville, MD: American Speech-Language-Hearing Association, 1993.

ASHA. Prevalence of hearing loss in the United States. Communication facts. Rockville, MD: American Speech-Language-Hearing Association. 1994a.

ASHA. Code of ethics. ASHA 1994b;36(Suppl 13):1–2.

ASHA. Hearing loss and hearing aid use in the United States: highlights of the National Center for Health Statistics' report prevalence and characteristics of persons with hearing trouble: United States, 1990–1991. Communication facts. Rockville, MD: American Speech-Language-Hearing Association, 1995.

ASHA. Scope of practice in audiology. ASHA 1996;38 (Suppl 16):12–15.

ASHA. Guidelines for hearing aid fitting for adults. Am J Audiol (in press).

ASHA Ad Hoc Committee on Hearing Aid Selection and Fitting. Guidelines for hearing aid fitting for adults. American Journal of Audiology. 1998;7:1, 5–13.

ASHA Governmental and Social Policies Coordinating Committee. Curriculum guide to managed care. Rockville, MD: American Speech-Language-Hearing Association, 1996.

Atkins DV. Counseling children with hearing loss and their families. In: Clark JG, Martin FN, eds. Effective counseling in audiology: perspectives and practice. Englewood Cliffs, NJ: Prentice-Hall, 1994:116–146.

Banja JD. Ethics, outcomes, and reimbursement. Rehab Manage 1994;7:61–65, 136.

Blosser J. Working with families. ASHA 1996;38:34–35.

Bowe F. Birth to five: early childhood special education. New York: Delmar, 1995.

Bratt G, Freeman B, Hall JW, et al. The audiologist as an entry point to healthcare: models and perspectives. In: Zapal D, Mendel LL, eds. Hearing care service delivery: essays and articles. Semin Hear 1996;17:227–235.

Butler K. Managed care: emerging issues in clinical ethics. ASHA 1996;38:7.

Carney AE, Moeller MP. Treatment efficacy: hearing loss in children. J Speech Lang Hear Res 1998;41(Suppl):61–84.

Clark KA, Terry DL. A collaborative framework for intervention. In: Roeser RJ, Downs MP, eds. Auditory disorders in school children: the law, identification, remediation. 3rd ed. New York: Thieme 1991:169–187.

Cleminshaw H. The American family. ASHA 1996; 38:36–37.

Cox RM, Alexander GC. The abbreviated profile of hearing aid benefit (APHAB). Ear Hear 1995;16:176–186.

DeConde-Johnson C, Benson PV, Seaton JB. Educational audiology handbook. San Diego: Singular Publishing Group, 1997.

Demorest ME, Erdman SA. Development of the communication profile for the hearing impaired. J Speech Hear Res 1987;52:129–143.

Dillon H, James A, Ginis J. Client oriented scale of improvement (COSI) and its relationship to several other measures of benefit and satisfaction provided by hearing aids. J Am Acad Audiol 1997;8:27–43.

Downs MP. Contribution of mild hearing loss to auditory language learning problems. In: Roeser RJ, Downs MP, eds. Auditory disorders in school children: the law, identification, remediation. 3rd ed. New York: Thieme, 1995:188–200.

Education of handicapped children, PL94–142 regulations. Fed. Reg. 1977;42:163.

Erikson E. Childhood and society. 2nd ed. New York: Norton, 1963.

Garstecki DC, Erler SF. Older adult performance on the communication profile for the hearing impaired. J Speech Hear Res 1996;39:28–42.

Garstecki DC, Erler SF. Hearing and aging. Topics Gerontol Rehab 1998a;14:1–17.

Garstecki DC, Erler SF. Hearing loss, control, and demographic factors influencing hearing aid use among older adults. J Speech Lang Hear Res 1998b;41:527–537.

Glass TA. Conjugating the "tenses" of function: discordance among hypothetical, experimental, and enacted function in older adults. Gerontologist 1998;38:101–112.

Goldberg B. Linking up with telehealth. ASHA 1997; 39:26–31.

Harrison M, Roush J. Age of suspicion, identification, and intervention for infants and young children with hearing loss: a national study. Ear Hear 1996;17:55–62.

Holden-Pitt L, Diaz JA. Thirty years of the annual survey of deaf and hard-of-hearing children and youth: a glance over the decades. Am Ann Deaf 1998;142:72–76.

Idol L, Paolucci-Whitcomb P, Nevin A. Collaborative consultation. Austin, TX: Pro-Ed, 1986.

Kiplinger Washington Letter Staff. Kiplinger forecasts: the new American boom. Washington, DC: The Kiplinger Washington Editors, 1986.

Kluwin T. The interaction of race, gender and social class effects in the education of deaf students. Am Ann Deaf 1994;139:465–471.

Kochkin S. MarkeTrak III: Why 20 million in U.S. don't use hearing aids for their hearing loss. Hear J 1993;46:26, 8–31.

Kochkin S. MarkeTrak IV: What is the viable market for hearing aids? Hear J 1997;50:31–39.

Kuster JM. Ethics and the Internet. ASHA 1997;39:33.

Lansing CR, Bienvenue LA. Intelligent computer-based systems to document the effectiveness of consonant recognition training. Volta Rev 1994;96:41–49.

Loeb R, Sarigiani P. The impact of hearing impairment on self-perceptions of children. Volta Rev 1986;88:89–100.

Luterman DM. Counseling the communicatively disordered and their families. 2nd ed. Austin, TX: Pro-Ed, 1991.

MacNeil B. Educational needs for multicultural hearing-impaired students in the public school system. Am Ann Deaf 1990;135:75–82.

Matkin ND. Strategies for enhancing interdisciplinary collaboration. In: Roush J, Matkin ND, eds. Infants and toddlers with hearing loss: family-centered assessment and intervention. Baltimore: York Press, 1994:83–97.

Montgomery AA. Treatment efficacy in adult audiological rehabilitation. In: Gagne J P, Tye-Murray N, eds. Research in audiological rehabilitation: current trends and future directions. J Acad Rehab Audiol Monogr Suppl 1994;27:317–336.

Moscicki EK, Elkins EF, Baum HM, et al. Hearing loss in the elderly: an epidemiologic study of the Framingham heart study cohort. Ear Hear 1985;6:184–190.

National Institutes of Health. Early identification of hearing impairment in infants and young children. Program and abstracts from the NIH Consensus Development Conference. Bethesda, MD: NIH, 1993.

Pannbacker M, Middleton GF, Vekovius GT. Ethical practices in speech-language pathology and audiology: case studies. San Diego: Singular Publishing Group, 1996.

Peters LJ, Peters DP. Telehealth part II: a total system approach. ASHA 1998;40:31–33.

Pietranton A. Clinical service delivery reform. In Johnson AF, Jacobson BH, eds. Medical speech-language pathology: a practitioner's guide. New York: Thieme, 1998: 669–684.

Quittner AL, Gluekauf RL, Jackson DN. Chronic effects of parenting stress: moderating versus mediating effects of social support. J Pers Soc Psychol 1990;59:1266–1278.

Rennels MB, Edwards KM, Keyserling IIL, et al. Safety and immunogenicity of heptavalent pneumococcal vaccine conjugated to CRM197 in United States infants. Pediatrics 1998;101:604–611.

Roberts KB, Cornett BS. Professional ethics in a managed care environment. In: Managing managed care: a practical guide for audiologists and speech-language pathologists. Rockville Pike, MD: American Speech-Language-Hearing Association, 1994:29–31.

Rodin J, Ickovics JR. Women's health: review and research agenda as we approach the twenty-first century. Am Psychol 1990;45:1018–1034.

Roush J. Strengthening family-professional relations: Advice from parents. In: Roush J, Matkin ND, eds. Infants and toddlers with hearing loss: family-centered assessment and intervention. Baltimore: York Press, 1994:337–351.

Roush J, McWilliam RA. Family-centered early intervention: historical, philosophical, and legislative issues. In Roush J, Matkin ND, eds. Infants and toddlers with hearing loss: family-centered assessment and intervention. Baltimore: York Press, 1994:3–21.

Schildroth AN, Hotto SA. Annual survey of hearing-impaired children and youth: 1991–92 school year. Am Ann Deaf 1993;138:163–171.

Schildroth AN, Rawlings BW, Allen TE. Hearing-impaired children under age 6: a demographic analysis. Am Ann Deaf 1989;133:63–69.

Scott R. Professional ethics: a guide for rehabilitation professionals. St. Louis: Mosby, 1998.

Stein L, Jabeley T, Spitz R, et al. The hearing-impaired infant: patterns of identification and rehabilitation revisited. Ear Hear 1990;11:201–205.

Task Force on Treatment Outcomes and Cost Effectiveness. Treatment outcomes data for adults in health care environments. ASHA 1997;39:26–31.

Tsantis L, Keefe D. Reinventing education. ASHA 1996; 38:38–41.

Turnbull A, Turnbull H. Families, professionals, and exceptionality: a special partnership. Columbus, OH: Merrill Publishing, 1986.

United States Architectural and Transportation Barriers Compliance Board. Americans with Disabilities Act (ADA): accessibility guidelines for buildings and facilities. Fed Reg 1991; 56, 144, 35455–35542.

U.S. Bureau of the Census. Poverty in the United States: 1992. Current population reports no. p60–185. Washington, DC: U.S. Bureau of the Census, 1993.

U.S. Bureau of the Census. Population projections of the United States by age, sex, race, and Hispanic origin: 1995–2050. Current population reports no. P25–1130. Washington, DC: U.S. Bureau of the Census, 1995.

Ventry IM, Weinstein BE. The hearing handicap inventory for the elderly: a new tool. Ear Hear 1982;3:128–134.

Walker-Vann C. Profiling Hispanic deaf students: a first step toward solving the greater problems. Am Ann Deaf 1998;143:46–54.

Williams TF. Demographics of aging. Cardiovasc Clin 1992; 22:2, 3–7.

Winton PJ, Bailey DB. Becoming family centered: strategies for self-examination. In Roush J, Matkin ND, eds. Infants and toddlers with hearing loss: family-centered assessment and intervention. Baltimore: York Press, 1994: 23–39.

World Health Organization. International classification of impairments, disabilities and handicaps: a manual of classification relating to the consequence of disease. Geneva: World Health Organization, 1980.

World Health Organization. International classification of impairments, disabilities and handicaps-2: a manual of dimensions of disablement and functioning (beta-1 draft for field trials). Geneva: World Health Organization, 1997.

Yacobacci-Tam P. Interacting with the culturally different family. Volta Rev 1987;89:46–58.

Youdelman K, Messerly C. Computer-assisted notetaking for mainstreamed hearing impaired students. Volta Rev 1996;98:191–199.

APPENDIX 2.1 *American Speech-Language-Hearing Association Code of Ethics, Revised January 1, 1994*

Preamble

The preservation of the highest standards of integrity and ethical principles is vital to the responsible discharge of obligations in the professions of speech-language pathology and audiology. This Code of Ethics sets forth the fundamental principles and rules considered essential to this purpose.

Every individual who is (a) a member of the American Speech-Language-Hearing Association, whether certified or not, (b) a nonmember holding the Certificate of Clinical Competence from the Association, (c) an applicant for membership or certification or (d) a Clinical Fellow seeking to fulfill standards for certification shall abide by this Code of Ethics.

Any action that violates the spirit and purpose of this Code shall be considered unethical. Failure to specify any particular responsibility or practice in this Code of Ethics shall not be construed as denial of the existence of such responsibilities or practices.

The fundamentals of ethical conduct are described by Principles of Ethics and by Rules of Ethics as they relate to responsibility to persons served, to the public and to the professions of speech-language pathology and audiology.

Principles of Ethics, aspirational and inspirational in nature, form the underlying moral basis for the Code of Ethics. Individuals shall observe these principles as affirmative obligations under all conditions of professional activity.

Rules of Ethics are specific statements of minimally acceptable professional conduct or of prohibitions and are applicable to all individuals.

PRINCIPLE OF ETHICS I

Individuals shall honor their responsibility to hold paramount the welfare of persons they serve professionally.

Rules of Ethics

A. Individuals shall provide all services competently.
B. Individuals shall use every resource, including referral when appropriate, to ensure that high-quality service is provided.
C. Individuals shall not discriminate in the delivery of professional services on the basis of race or ethnicity, gender, age, religion, national origin, sexual orientation, or disability.
D. Individuals shall fully inform the persons they serve of the nature and possible effects of services rendered and products dispensed.
E. Individuals shall evaluate the effectiveness of services rendered and of products dispensed and shall provide services or dispense products only when benefit can reasonably be expected.
F. Individuals shall not guarantee the results of any treatment or procedure, directly or by implication; however, they may make a reasonable statement of prognosis.
G. Individuals shall not evaluate or treat speech, language, or hearing disorders solely by correspondence.

H. Individuals shall maintain adequate records of professional services rendered and products dispensed and shall allow access to these records when appropriately authorized.
I. Individuals shall not reveal, without authorization, any professional or personal information about the person served professionally, unless required by law to do so, or unless doing so is necessary to protect the welfare of the person or of the community.
J. Individuals shall not charge for services not rendered, nor shall they misrepresent,[1] in any fashion, services rendered or products dispensed.
K. Individuals shall use persons in research or as subjects of teaching demonstrations only with their informed consent.
L. Individuals whose professional services are adversely affected by substance abuse or other health-related conditions shall seek professional assistance and, where appropriate, withdraw from the elected areas of practice.

PRINCIPLE OF ETHICS II

Individuals shall honor their responsibility to achieve and maintain the highest level of professional competence.

Rules of Ethics

A. Individuals shall engage in the provision of clinical services only when they hold the appropriate Certificate of Clinical Competence or when they are in the certification process and are supervised by an individual who holds the appropriate Certificate of Clinical Competence.
B. Individuals shall engage in only those aspects of the professions that are within the scope of their competence, considering their level of education, training, and experience.
C. Individuals shall continue their professional development throughout their careers.
D. Individuals shall delegate the provision of clinical services only to persons who are certified or to persons in the education or certification process who are appropriately supervised. The provision of support services may be delegated to persons who are neither certified nor in the certification process only when a certificate holder provides appropriate supervision.
E. Individuals shall prohibit any of their professional staff from providing services that exceed the staff member's competence, considering the staff member's level of education, training, and experience.
F. Individuals shall ensure that all equipment used in the provision of services is in proper working order and is properly calibrated.

PRINCIPLE OF ETHICS III

Individuals shall honor their responsibility to the public by promoting public understanding of the professions, by supporting the development of services designed to fulfill the unmet needs of the public, and by providing accurate information in all communications involving any aspect of the professions.

Rules of Ethics

A. Individuals shall not misrepresent their credentials, competence, education, training, or experience.
B. Individuals shall not participate in professional activities that constitute a conflict of interest.
C. Individuals shall not misrepresent diagnostic information, services rendered, or products

---

[1]For purposes of this Code of Ethics, misrepresentation includes any untrue statements or statements that are likely to mislead. Misrepresentation also includes the failure to state any information that is material and that ought, in fairness, to be considered.

dispensed or engage in any scheme or artifice to defraud in connection with obtaining payment or reimbursement for such services or products.

D. Individuals' statements to the public shall provide accurate information about the nature and management of communication disorders, about the professions, and about professional services.

E. Individuals' statements to the public—advertising, announcing, and marketing their professional services, reporting research results, and promoting products—shall adhere to prevailing professional standards and shall not contain misrepresentations.

PRINCIPLE OF ETHICS IV

Individuals shall honor their responsibilities to the professions and their relationships with colleagues, students, and members of allied professions. Individuals shall uphold the dignity and autonomy of the professions, maintain harmonious interprofessional and intraprofessional relationships, and accept the professions' self-imposed standards.

Rules of Ethics

A. Individuals shall prohibit anyone under their supervision from engaging in any practice that violates the Code of Ethics.

B. Individuals shall not engage in dishonesty, fraud, deceit, misrepresentation, or any form of conduct that adversely reflects on the professions or on the individual's fitness to serve persons professionally.

C. Individuals shall assign credit only to those who have contributed to a publication, presentation, or product. Credit shall be assigned in proportion to the contribution and only with the contributor's consent.

D. Individuals' statements to colleagues about professional services, research results, and products shall adhere to prevailing professional standards and shall contain no misrepresentations.

E. Individuals shall not provide professional services without exercising independent professional judgment, regardless of referral source or prescription.

F. Individuals shall not discriminate in their relationships with colleagues, students, and members of allied professions on the basis of race or ethnicity, gender, age, religion, national origin, sexual orientation, or disability.

G. Individuals who have reason to believe that the Code of Ethics has been violated shall inform the Ethical Practice Board.

H. Individuals shall cooperate fully with the Ethical Practice Board in its investigation and adjudication of matters related to this Code of Ethics.

Reprinted with permission from American Speech-Language-Hearing Association. Code of ethics. ASHA 1994b;36(Suppl 13):1–2

APPENDIX 2.2 *American Academy of Audiology Code of Ethics*

Preamble

The Code of Ethics of the American Academy of Audiology specifies professional standards that allow for the proper discharge of audiologists responsibilities to those served, and that protect the integrity of the profession. The Code of Ethics consists of two parts. The first part, the Statement of Principles and Rules, presents precepts that members of the Academy agree to uphold. The second part, the Procedures, provides the process which enables enforcement of the Principles and Rules.

Part I.
Statement of Principles and Rules

PRINCIPLE 1: Members shall provide professional services with honesty and compassion, and shall respect the dignity, worth, and rights of those served.
Rule 1a: Individuals shall not limit the delivery of professional services on any basis that is unjustifiable or irrelevant to the need for the potential benefit from such services.

PRINCIPLE 2: Members shall maintain high standards of professional competence in rendering services, providing only those professional services for which they are qualified by education and experience.
Rule 2a: Individuals shall use available resources, including referrals to other specialists, and shall not accept benefits or items of personal value for receiving or making referrals.
Rule 2b: Individuals shall exercise all reasonable precautions to avoid injury to persons in the delivery of professional services.
Rule 2c: Individuals shall not provide services except in a professional relationship, and shall not discriminate in the provision of services to individuals on the basis of sex, race, religion, national origin, sexual orientation, or general health.
Rule 2d: Individuals shall provide appropriate supervision and assume full responsibility for services delegated to supportive personnel. Individuals shall not delegate any service requiring professional competence to unqualified persons.
Rule 2e: Individuals shall not permit personnel to engage in any practice that is a violation of the Code of Ethics.
Rule 2f: Individuals shall maintain professional competence, including participation in continuing education.

PRINCIPLE 3: Members shall maintain the confidentiality of the information and records of those receiving services.
Rule 3a: Individuals shall not reveal to unauthorized persons any professional or personal information obtained from the person served professionally, unless required by law.

PRINCIPLE 4: Members shall provide only services and products that are in the best interest of those served.
Rule 4a: Individuals shall not exploit persons in the delivery of professional services.
Rule 4b: Individuals shall not charge for services not rendered.
Rule 4c: Individuals shall not participate in activities that constitute a conflict of professional interest.

Rule 4d: Individuals shall not accept compensation for supervision or sponsorship beyond reimbursement of expenses.

PRINCIPLE 5: Members shall provide accurate information about the nature and management of communicative disorders and about the services and products offered.
Rule 5a: Individuals shall provide persons served with the information a reasonable person would want to know about the nature and possible effects of services rendered, or products provided.
Rule 5b: Individuals may make a statement of prognosis, but shall not guarantee results, mislead, or misinform persons served.
Rule 5c: Individuals shall not carry out teaching or research activities in a manner that constitutes an invasion of privacy, or that fails to inform persons fully about the nature and possible effects of these activities, affording all persons informed free choice of participation.
Rule 5d: Individuals shall maintain documentation of professional services rendered.

PRINCIPLE 6: Members shall comply with the ethical standards of the Academy with regard to public statements.
Rule 6a: Individuals shall not misrepresent their educational degrees, training, credentials, or competence. Only degrees earned from regionally accredited institutions in which training was obtained in audiology, or a directly related discipline, may be used in public statements concerning professional services.
Rule 6b: Individuals' public statements about professional services and products shall not contain representations or claims that are false, misleading, or deceptive.

PRINCIPLE 7: Members shall honor their responsibilities to the public and to professional colleagues.
Rule 7a: Individuals shall not use professional or commercial affiliations in any way that would mislead or limit services to persons served professionally.
Rule 7b: Individuals shall inform colleagues and the public in a manner consistent with the highest professional standards about products and services they have developed.

PRINCIPLE 8: Members shall uphold the dignity of the profession and freely accept the Academy's self-imposed standards.
Rule 8a: Individuals shall not violate these Principles and Rules, nor attempt to circumvent them.
Rule 8b: Individuals shall not engage in dishonesty or illegal conduct that adversely reflects on the profession.
Rule 8c: Individuals shall inform the Ethical Practice Board when there are reasons to believe that a member of the Academy may have violated the Code of Ethics.
Rule 8d: Individuals shall cooperate with the Ethical Practice Board in any matter related to the Code of Ethics.

Part II.
Procedures for the Management of Alleged Violations

INTRODUCTION

Members of the American Academy of Audiology are obligated to uphold the Code of Ethics of the Academy in their personal conduct and in the performance of their professional duties.

To this end it is the responsibility of each Academy member to inform the Ethical Practice Board of possible Ethics Code violations. The processing of alleged violations of the Code of Ethics will follow the procedures specified below in an expeditious manner to ensure that violations of ethical conduct by members of the Academy are halted in the shortest time possible.

PROCEDURES

1. Suspected violations of the Code of Ethics should be reported in letter format giving documentation sufficient to support the alleged violation. Letters must be signed and addressed to: Chair, Ethical Practice Board
   American Academy of Audiology
   8201 Greensboro Drive, Suite 300
   McLean, VA 22102
2. Following receipt of the alleged violation the Board will request from the complainant a signed Waiver of Confidentiality indicating that the complainant will allow the Ethical Practice Board to disclose his/her name should this become necessary during investigation of the allegation. The Board may, under special circumstances, act in the absence of a signed Waiver of Confidentiality.
3. On receipt of the Waiver of Confidentiality signed by the complainant, or on the decision of the Board to assume the role of active complainant, the member(s) implicated will be notified by the Chair that an alleged violation of the Code of Ethics has been reported. Circumstances of the alleged violation will be described and the member(s) will be asked to respond fully to the allegation.
4. The Chair may communicate with other individuals, agencies, and/or programs, for additional information as may be required for Board review. The accumulation of information will be accomplished as expeditiously as possible to minimize the time between initial notification of possible Code violation and final determination by the Ethical Practice Board.
5. All information pertaining to the allegation will be reviewed by members of the Ethical Practice Board and a finding reached regarding infractions of the Code. In cases of Code violation, the section(s) of the Code violated will be cited, and a sanction specified when the Ethical Practice Board decision is disseminated.
6. Members found to be in violation of the Code may appeal the decision of the Ethical Practice Board. The route of Appeal is by letter format through the Ethical Practice Board to the Executive Committee of the Academy. Requests for Appeal must:
   a. be received by the Chair, Ethical Practice Board, within 30 days of the Ethical Practice Board notification of violation.
   b. state the basis for the appeal, and the reason(s) that the Ethical Practice Board decision should be changed.
   c. not offer new documentation.

The decision of the Executive Committee regarding Appeals will be considered final.

SANCTIONS

1. Reprimand. The minimum level of punishment for a violation consists of a reprimand. Notification of the violation and the sanction is restricted to the member and the complainant.
2. Cease and Desist Order. Violator(s) may be required to sign a Cease and Desist Order which specifies the non-compliant behavior and the terms of the Order. Notification of

the violation and the sanction is made to the member and the complainant, and may on two-thirds vote of the Ethical Practice Board be reported in an official publication.

3. Suspension of Membership. Suspension of membership may range from a minimum of six (6) months to a maximum of twelve (12) months. During the period of suspension the violator may not participate in official Academy functions. Notification of the violation and the sanction is made to the member and the complainant and is reported in official publications of the Academy. Notification of the violation and the sanction may be extended to others as determined by the Ethical Practice Board. No refund of dues or assessments shall accrue to the member.

4. Revocation of Membership. Revocation of membership will be considered as the maximum punishment for a violation of the Code. Individuals whose membership is revoked are not entitled to a refund of dues or fees. One year following the date of membership revocation the individual may reapply for, but is not guaranteed, membership through normal channels and must meet the membership qualifications in effect at the time of application. Notification of the violation and the sanction is made to the member and the complainant and is reported in official publications of the Academy for at least three (3) separate issues during the period of revocation. Special notification, as determined by the Ethical Practice Board, may be required in certain situations.

RECORDS

1. A Central Record Depository shall be maintained by the Ethical Practice Board which will be kept confidential and maintained with restricted access.
2. Complete records shall be maintained for a period of five years and then destroyed.
3. Confidentiality shall be maintained in all Ethical Practice Board discussion, correspondence, communication, deliberation, and records pertaining to members reviewed by the Ethical Practice Board.
4. No Ethical Practice Board member shall give access to records, act or speak independently, or on behalf of the Board, without the expressed permission of the Board members then active, to impose the sanction of the Board, or to interpret the findings of the Board in any manner which may place members of the Board, collectively or singly, at financial, professional, or personal risk.
5. A Book of Precedents shall be maintained by the Ethical Practice Board which shall form the basis for future findings of the Board.

Reprinted with permission from American Academy of Audiology. Code of ethics. American Academy of Audiology Membership Directory. 1998–1999:230–232.

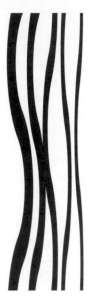

Audiologic Rehabilitation in Different Employment Settings

Jane R. Madell, Ph.D., and Joseph Montano, Ed.D.

Need for Rehabilitative Audiology in All Aspects of Audiology

REHABILITATION AND THE PRACTICE OF AUDIOLOGY

Audiology has a long history. It is frequently thought of as beginning during World War II as the need developed to provide aural rehabilitation to veterans with service-connected hearing losses. In fact, the rehabilitative component of the profession began much earlier. When we look at the history of audiology, we find community centers, guilds, or leagues for the hard of hearing (such as the New York League for the Hard of Hearing, the Boston Guild for the Hard of Hearing, the Chicago Hearing Society, and the Bay Area Hearing Society) that provided lipreading training and vocational assistance for persons with impaired hearing as early as 1910. In addition to providing lipreading training to adults, many of the programs also provided lipreading training to children in schools. Before the first degree was conferred in audiology, several schools offered degrees to teachers of lipreading. Some were offered at institutions such as Columbia University's Teacher's College, and others were in independent schools such as the Nitchie and Mueller-

Walle Schools that trained teachers of lipreading to provide lipreading training, support, and counseling to hearing-impaired children and adults.

The early practice of the profession had a very strong rehabilitative direction, with technology having only a minor role. Certainly this was, in large part, because the technology available was very limited. The hearing aids that were available were large, had limited battery life, limited gain, and poor acoustic quality. As a result, they were used primarily for clients who had only conductive hearing loss. If people with hearing impairment were going to be a part of the mainstream, developing good lipreading skills would be critical. As technology improved, it began to "take over" audiology, with rehabilitation frequently taking a back seat. The march away from rehabilitation increased as audiology services began to be provided primarily in medical settings in which rehabilitation was less valued. This direction is an unfortunate one for clients and professionals alike. It deprives persons with hearing loss of the ability to learn significant skills and limits audiologists to the technical roles of diagnosis and evaluating and dispensing amplification.

Audiologists provide service in a variety of settings. Their perception of rehabilitation may differ, and many may consider themselves solely diagnostic clinicians. Although audiologists profess the importance of audiologic rehabilitation, they frequently do not consider themselves "therapists." Schow et al. (1993) reported that only 68% of audiologists surveyed (n = 169) described aural rehabilitation in their general clinical duties.

Malinoff et al. (1990) surveyed more than 900 hearing aid dispensers—including private dispensing audiologists, otolaryngologists, hearing instrument specialists, and hospital-based dispensing audiologists—on treatment practices. When queried regarding the factors perceived as being most important in providing better service to patients with hearing impairment, less than 10% of respondents identified aural rehabilitation.

Clearly, rehabilitative service is not thought to be the primary role of many practicing audiologists. The American Speech-Language-Hearing Association Special Interest Division 7 (ASHA SID 7) (Aural Rehabilitation and Its Instrumentation) stated that "audiologic rehabilitation is Audiology" (ASHA, 1992). They went on to describe the process of audiologic rehabilitation as multifaceted, involving assessment and the impact of hearing loss on the "individual, the family and society." Having the broadest view of the field of audiology opens up vast possibilities for clinician and client alike. By looking more closely at all aspects of what we do, audiologists should be able to develop rehabilitation programs in every type of audiology facility. Rehabilitation does not mean simply providing speechreading. It encompasses interviewing, counseling, performing many aspects of diagnosis (especially those related to assessing auditory function), and providing treatment. Treatment services viewed broadly from the prospective of rehabilitation include selection of amplification, assistive living devices, hearing aid counseling, family counseling, and support groups for patients and families in addition to speechreading, auditory training, speech-language training, communication strategies training, and school and vocational support.

Basic Assumptions

Let us begin with some basic assumptions.

- *Habilitative and rehabilitative audiology is a basic part of the practice of audiology.* The diagnostic and technical components of audiology are certainly critical, and in most cases the necessary first step, but they cannot operate in isolation. At the very least, every audiology practice should provide counseling, descriptions of rehabilitation options, and referral. Any practice that evaluates amplification should include information and, if possible, demonstration of assistive living and assistive listening devices. Any practice that dispenses amplification should provide hearing aid adjustment counseling. All practices should include information about therapy options such as speechreading, auditory training, and hearing aid orientation and speech-language training for children. If support and self-help groups are not available within the practice, referrals should be available for groups in the community. In other words, there is no audiology practice that should not provide rehabilitative audiology as a necessary component unless the audiologist is working as a technician and another professional is providing the rehabilitation.
- *Every hearing-impaired patient and his or her family will benefit from a habilitative/rehabilitative program.* Any hearing loss that is not short term (lasting only a few weeks) is going to affect the person with impaired hearing and his or her family. It will interfere with communication and increase family stress. Therefore, it is critical that rehabilitation be included in the care of every person with impaired hearing. Whereas hearing aids will reduce many problems associated with hearing loss, they will not eliminate all hearing problems. Adults will still have difficulty hearing in any situation in which the signal is degraded (i.e., over distance, when there is noise, when speaking to persons with accents). Children will have language-learning and academic difficulties. Family members will need assistance in

understanding that hearing aids do not "solve the problem" and in developing realistic expectations and techniques for improving communication.

• *Having a habilitative/rehabilitative component will improve the quality of almost every diagnostic program.* By including a habilitative/rehabilitative component as part of the diagnostic program, the probability that the patient will accept the diagnosis and take responsibility for planning treatment is increased. A major role in rehabilitation is to provide education. This is truly a case of "an educated consumer is the best customer." The more the consumer knows, the more likely it is that he or she will accept the results of the diagnostic testing and move on to rehabilitation to improve communication functioning.

• *The addition of a habilitative/rehabilitative component will increase work satisfaction for everyone involved in the program.* Audiologists who work in technician roles in which they perform evaluations that are discussed with the patient by others and those who have jobs limited to describing test results to patients frequently find that they are unhappy with their jobs. There are only so many times that masking can be exciting, and only so many auditory brainstem responses (ABRs) that are unusual and interesting. There needs to be some

other aspect of the job that makes it interesting. Dealing with people is never boring. It is always interesting and always changing. As our skills improve, we learn to understand our clients better and to find better ways to help them accept what they need. It is the problem-solving aspect of audiology that keeps people excited and involved. As a result, programs that have rehabilitative components are likely to have more satisfied staff with less staff turnover.

The idea of a diagnostic audiologist cannot be realized if we are to accept either the above assumptions or the description provided by ASHA SID 7. Our concept of the diagnostician is more fully embedded into the medical model of service delivery, whereas the ASHA SID 7 description of audiologic rehabilitation fits into the rehabilitative model.

Reviewing the Characteristics of Delivery Models in Audiology

Erdman et al. (1994) described the characteristics of service delivery models frequently seen in audiology (Table 3.1). The models are categorized as medical and rehabilitative. The medical model is thought of as the traditional method of service delivery. It focuses on the identification of the hearing

Table 3.1
Characteristics of service delivery models

Medical Model	Rehabilitation Model
Top down communication	Horizontal communication
Authoritarian	Interactive, facilitative
Clinician determines diagnosis and treatment of clients' conditions	Clinician helps clients identify and resolve clients' problems
Clinician does something "to" clients	Clinician does something "with" clients
Appropriate and necessary in acute emergency situations	Ideal for chronic conditions and preventive measures requiring adherence to treatment regimen
Assumes clinician knows what's right and best for clients	Assumes clients' perceptions and needs will decide treatment goals and strategies
Oriented toward disease and pathology	Oriented toward self-actualization, adjustment, and well-being.

From Erdman SA, Wark DJ, Montano JJ. Implications of service delivery models in audiology. *J Acad Rehab Audiol* 1994;27:45–60.

impairment and the prescribed method of treatment. Under this model, the individual with a hearing impairment is primarily a passive participant in treatment. The audiologist will perform the diagnostic evaluation and report the findings. The focus of this model is on the identification of pathology. Recommendations will be made based on the information obtained on the audiogram. Further evaluation, medical referral, or amplification decisions are directed by the audiologist with little responsibility placed on the patient.

The rehabilitative model emphasizes patient/audiologist interaction. The individual with a hearing impairment is an active participant in the care. The patient is viewed as being directly responsible for the resolution of the problem. The focus is on disability rather than on pathology. Treatment goals are directed by the patient's perceptions and needs. It is believed that compliance with treatment recommendations will improve when the patient is motivated to participate in the process. Participation begins immediately, at the identification of hearing loss, and continues throughout its management.

Aspects of audiologic rehabilitation* are present wherever an audiologist practices. What needs to occur is a shift in focus and approach. To maximize the effectiveness of our rehabilitation programs, we need to evaluate our service delivery model and the underlying goals of our practice. The philosophies of the rehabilitative model can help guide us in our quest to further develop and implement inclusive rehabilitation programming.

Our attempts at preventing or reducing the handicapping effects of hearing loss may be fostered through the use of an ecologic approach to audiologic rehabilitation. An ecologic approach to treatment is client-

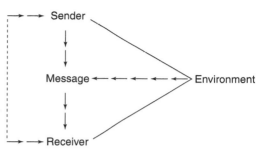

Figure 3.1. Components of an ecologic approach to audiologic rehabilitation for analyzing and remediating communication handicap. (From Jennings MB, Head BG. Development of an ecological audiologic rehabilitation program in a home-for-the- aged. J Acad Rehab Audiol 1994;27:73–88.)

centered. It stresses the inclusion of the patient and his or her communication partners within the context of their environment and real life situations. (Jennings and Head, 1994; Noble and Hetu, 1994; Gagne et al., 1995). Gagne et al. (1995) reported that "a client's hearing problem can only be defined by that person." The definition of the problem will be directly influenced by the patient's perception of the problem and the context in which it occurs.

Jennings and Head (1994) described the components of an ecologic approach to audiologic rehabilitation (Fig. 3.1). The components highlight the direct interaction between the sender and receiver within a dynamic environment. To achieve effective communication, both the patient and the communication partner play distinct roles. Treatment will need to include an emphasis on education and assessment with perhaps modification of the barriers within the communication environment.

Samples of communication partners and various environments are shown in Table 3.2. A young adult may have a multitude of communication partners including spouse, significant others, children, parents, coworkers, and friends. His or her communication environments and life situations will be varied and may include home, office, automobile, soccer field with children, or relatives' homes. The audiologist working with adults will need to invite them into the treatment

---

* The terms "aural rehabilitation" and "audiologic rehabilitation" are frequently used interchangeably in the professional literature. We have chosen to use audiologic rehabilitation as our preferred terminology, because it more closely identifies with the service provision described in this chapter. The term aural rehabilitation is used only in reference to citations by other authors.

Table 3.2
Communication partners and communication environments

Subject	Environment	Communication Partners	Communication Needs
Child with hearing impairment	Home	Parents, siblings, grandparents, extended family, friends	Interpersonal, telephone, TV signal alerting, recreational
	School	Teachers, visitors, classmates	Classroom, schoolyard, public speaking, extracurricular activities
	Community	Merchants, public service providers, health care workers	Interpersonal emergencies, assistance, recreational
Adult with hearing impairment	Home	Spouse, children, parents, extended family, neighbors	Interpersonal, intimacy, recreational, telephone, TV, music
	Work	Coworkers, superiors, clients, visitors	Meetings, telephone, lunchroom, interpersonal
	Community	Merchants, public service providers, health care workers	Interpersonal, emergencies, assistance, recreational, religious activities
Elderly person with hearing impairment	Home	Spouse, children, grandchildren, extended family, neighbors, friends, friends with hearing impairments	Interpersonal, intimacy, recreational, telephone, TV
	Community	Merchants, health care providers, service providers	Interpersonal, emergencies, assistance recreational, religious activities
	Long-term Care	Family, nurses, physicians, nurse assistants, therapists, residents, residents with hearing impairments	Interpersonal, assistance, therapy, dining room, recreational, telephone, auditorium

regimen and make them active participants in rehabilitation. Each patient comes into the audiologic assessment with his or her own personalized communication portfolio. The audiologist must thoroughly review it to establish appropriate priorities.

Any assessment and identification of hearing impairment must include the identification of the needs of all communicatively related parties. Noble and Hetu (1994) reported that the program design needs to address the following areas:

1. Identification of the hearing handicap as it relates to the situational conditions of the individual with the impairment.

2. Assessment of the need for psychosocial support.

3. Evaluation of the possible ways to reduce the disability associated with the hearing impairment; this would include not only the hearing aid, but the need for assistive listening devices, signal alerting technology, and communication strategies.

4. Implementation of achievable goals to help reduce the disability and identification of the need for supportive intervention for those who interact with the individual with hearing impairment.

The development of rehabilitation programs can include a variety of traditional components. It is the manner in which the audiologist chooses to implement the program that will affect the program design and its success. The following are some areas for consideration in the creation of a rehabilitation program. These components can be incorporated into an ecologic therapeutic approach by focusing on the client, the environment, and the communication partners.

Developing an Audiologic Rehabilitative Program

EVALUATING THE POSSIBLE COMPONENTS OF A HABILITATIVE/REHABILITATIVE PROGRAM

The first step in developing a program is to evaluate all the components of a rehabilitation program (Table 3.3). Almost all audiology programs should provide many of these services. If the services are not provided, they should be available by referral. Even programs that are primarily diagnostic (providing presurgery and postsurgery evaluations) should include some determination of whether rehabilitation services may be needed by patients so they can be appropriately referred.

- *Communication history*—A communication history assesses how the person and/or family believes he or she communicates.

Table 3.3
Components of a habilitative/rehabilitative program

Communication history
Communication assessment
    Auditory function
    Speechreading
    Conversation skills
    Self-assessment scales for patient and family
      members
Assessment of hearing impairment/handicap
Amplification selection
Dispensing of amplification systems
Hearing aid orientation/training
Communications training
    Speechreading
    Auditory training
    Conversational skills training
Counseling
Peer support groups

What situations cause problems? What is the person able to hear well? What has the family discovered that will improve communication? How has auditory function changed over time? How do the hearing-impaired person and family view the problem? Why have they come for evaluation?

- *Communication assessment*—The communication assessment evaluates a variety of different communication skills. It begins with audiologic assessment of degree of hearing loss and assessment of word recognition skills at comfortably loud levels (31 to 40 dB, re: SRT). More information will be gained about daily listening skills by testing at normal (50 dB) and soft (35 dB) conversational levels in quiet and with competing noise. The communication assessment then proceeds with assessment of speechreading, other auditory skills, and conversational communication skills. For children, it includes assessment of speech and language skills.

- *Assessment of auditory processing skills*—Assessing auditory processing skills is part of the assessment of auditory function. Assessments may be limited to testing at soft conversational levels in quiet and in competing noise or may include standardized tests of auditory processing.

- *Assessment of hearing impairment/ handicap*—In assessing impairment/handicap, an attempt is made to determine how an individual's hearing loss affects functioning. The same hearing loss will affect different people differently. A mild hearing loss can be devastating for a child in school, difficult for a business person who has many meetings in which listening is critical, and no problem at all for an older adult who lives alone and does not socialize. Self-assessment scales are very useful in assessing hearing impairment/handicap.

- *Amplification evaluation and dispensing*—Amplification is at the base of audiologic rehabilitation. The first treatment procedure is to reduce hearing loss to the greatest extent possible. After any appropriate medical treatment is completed, the next step is usually the selecting and fitting of amplification systems.

- *Hearing aid orientation/training*—Hearing aid orientation and training consists of basic training in caring for amplification, directions for using amplification including how to adjust to it, and techniques for optimizing function in difficult listening situations. It also includes training in being assertive about listening needs, including reduction of noise when possible and seat selection. Group hearing aid orientation provides support from others with similar problems with regards to learning to accept amplification and in developing communication strategies.

- *Assistive listening and assistive living systems*—Assessment of auditory difficulties that are not being solved by amplification is the first step. This is followed by provision of information about and demonstration of assistive devices to improve communication and reduce the stress of daily living.

- *Communication training*—Communication training includes training in speechreading, auditory training, conversational skills strategies, assertiveness training, and for children speech and language therapy.

- *School support*—School support includes providing information to classroom personnel to maximize communication, including use of FM systems, preferential seating, communication strategies for assuring that the child receives all the information, teaching strategies, and information about modifying the acoustic conditions in the classroom.

- *Employment counseling*—Employment counseling has two components: improving the current workplace environment and selecting new employment opportunities that best meet the communication needs of the person with impaired hearing. Improving the current workplace environment involves assisting a hearing-impaired employee and his or her employer in adapting the work environment to maximize the functioning of the employee by using both technology and communication skills. An audiologist and/or a vocational rehabilitation counselor may do this. Assistance in selecting a new employment situation due to a hearing loss is not usually accomplished by an audiologist, but by a vocational counselor who is experienced with hearing-impaired people and is working in conjunction with an audiologist.

- *Peer support groups*—No amount of experience working with patients who have hearing loss and their families can make audiologists understand what it is like to experience a hearing loss. Peer groups provide support, validation about emotions, and suggestions for problem-solving that are not available in any other format. A hearing-impaired teen is more likely to be able to get another teen to wear a hearing aid than are parents or audiologists. Adults who are embarrassed about asking for assistance or about wearing a visible hearing aid are more likely to be convinced by peers. Parents of young children with hearing loss and spouses of adults with hearing loss will appreciate having the opportunity to express feelings to each other in an environment that is accepting. Possible groups include those for parents, teens, young adults, middle-aged adults, older adults who are living independently, older adults living in group homes, spouses, and children and other family members.

- *Counseling*—There are two types of counseling in rehabilitative audiology: information counseling and support counseling. Information counseling includes providing a description of the degree and type of hearing loss, types of amplification, types of assistive devices, and available therapies. Support counseling deals with feelings, expectations, and disappointment related to the hearing loss.

THE PLACE OF THE PRODUCT IN AN AUDIOLOGIC REHABILITATION PROGRAM

All too often, the hearing aid is seen as the goal of the rehabilitation program. Adults with hearing loss frequently request amplification assuming that once it arrives, all communication problems will be resolved.

Parents often assume that once hearing aids are dispensed, their hearing-impaired children will talk. Sometimes, as audiologists, we contribute to this view by the way we describe the expected benefit that amplification will provide and by our failure to discuss the other components of audiologic rehabilitation. Sometimes we do this because we fear that if we tell clients that hearing aids have limitations, they will not wish to purchase them; sometimes it is because we are not comfortable talking about or providing rehabilitation. When we do this we deprive our patients of the benefit of other components of rehabilitation and limit the practice of audiology. By remembering that the practice of audiology is vast, we enrich our lives and those of our patients.

EVALUATING THE EXISTING PROGRAM

The initial step in developing a new program is to evaluate the current program carefully. By reviewing all activities, it will be possible to determine what current activities can easily be expanded and what new activities can be added. This begins by reviewing the services that are currently provided and considering how each one can be expanded to meet increased rehabilitation needs.

Virtually every audiologist obtains a patient history as part of most evaluations. The initial step in evaluating the program is to review what is included in the history. Is it limited to medical information related to etiology and time of onset? If so, the history can be expanded to include communication history. Topics should include specific descriptions of situations in which the hearing-impaired person has difficulty hearing or understanding (Table 3.4). The routine use of self-assessment scales for hearing-impaired patients and their families should be considered; these scales can assist the audiologist in understanding how hearing-impaired persons and their families see the problem. Repeating these scales after treatment can help to understand if the person feels that function has changed and can help the audiologist to see what is needed next (see Chapter 10). Better understanding of how the person

Table 3.4
Components of a communication history

Onset of hearing loss
Progression of hearing loss
Situations in which hearing is difficult
    Individual conversational
    Group conversation—2, 4, 6 or more people
    Quiet versus noise
    Distance
    Knowledge of conversation topic
    Specific difficult listening situations
      TV
      Movies
      Lecture
      Temple/church
      Classroom
      Street
      Dinner table
      Other
Strategies that you have found to make
    listening easier
Are communication problems the same at all
    times or do they change (e.g., time of day,
    tiredness, weather, etc.)

views the problem will assist in planning rehabilitation and counseling.

All programs do some form of communication assessment. For some programs this may only consist of the pure tone audiogram and word recognition testing under earphones at comfortably loud levels. Although this is important information, it does not provide information about everyday communication. This can only be obtained by assessing auditory function in conditions in which the person functions every day, such as word recognition testing at normal (50 dB HL) and soft (35 dB HL) conversational levels in quiet and with competing noise. Although the audiologist may be able to estimate from previous experience what kinds of problems a person with a 40-dB or 60-dB hearing loss may have, it cannot be known how this hearing loss will affect a particular patient unless measurable results can be demonstrated. This information also provides a good counseling tool. A patient who does not think he or she has a serious problem because family members raise their voices when talking will learn a great deal by seeing functional communication testing. Family members will also be able to understand why communication has been so difficult. Performing the specific testing permits the audiologist to demonstrate to the patient and family exactly how the hearing loss is affecting daily functioning.

Other aspects of communication assessment include assessing speechreading and auditory training skills as well as measuring auditory processing skills (see Chapters 10 and 12). Programs that do not provide therapy may not want to provide the diagnostic testing. On the other hand, providing the testing is likely to help the audiologist to understand more about the patient's function and assist in counseling as well as to understand problems with amplification and assist in making appropriate referrals. Programs in which amplification is dispensed or in which cochlear implant surgery is performed may need to consider strongly the provision of a complete communication assessment and therapy or an association with a nearby center that can provide these services.

Dispensing amplification, cochlear implants, or assistive devices opens the door for many rehabilitation services. During the program review, it would be helpful to determine what the current patients think about the services offered by the program. What kind of patients are being drawn to the dispensing practice? Where do referrals come from? Do patients return for follow-up? For additional hearing aids? Are dispensing referrals received from other programs? How is the selection of hearing aids and assistive devices determined? Is there a wide variety meeting different audiologic and financial needs? Are there are a large number of hearing aid returns? Are hearing aids in stock or must they be ordered for each evaluation? A financial review is essential to determine if stock aids are practical. Consideration should be given to how many evaluations are done monthly, how many aids are dispensed, and how many patients will choose to go to other facilities if they need to wait. If group hearing aid orientation is not being offered, it may be useful to consider beginning a program. Madell

(1973), Wayner (1990), and others have reported that clients who attend hearing aid orientation are better hearing aid users, have more realistic expectations about amplification, and have fewer hearing aid returns.

Therapy services including speech-language therapy, speechreading, and auditory training require staff members with expertise and interest. A well-trained audiologist may be able to provide these services, but they are most frequently provided by speech-language pathologists. If staff members are already in the program they can learn the necessary skills. If not, they will need to be recruited. Having therapy programs at your facility makes it very attractive to families who can have "one stop shopping." If the program is not sufficiently large to make it worthwhile to have a clinician on staff who does therapy, a relationship needs to be developed with clinicians or clinics in the community where these services are available.

Only very large programs will realistically be able to afford a vocational counselor, but all programs can arrange for services to be available at the local rehabilitation agency or at another community facility. If the vocational counselor does not know a great deal about hearing loss, the audiologist will need to take responsibility for assisting the counselor in understanding what effect the hearing loss will have on work. Suggestions for modifying the work environment, desk placement, and acoustic treatment should be considered as well as assistive listening systems such as FM systems and amplified telephones. The use of a sign or oral interpreter during training should be considered.

School consultation can be offered by an audiologist, speech-language-pathologist, or teacher of hearing-impaired children who has experience in the educational setting. Table 3.4 provides information about what to look for when doing a school visit. An outside consultant, such as an audiologist from a hospital or clinic, can sometimes be very helpful in reviewing the services that a school is providing and providing an outside view. This is especially useful for children who are mainstreamed and who may not be receiving services at school from clinicians who are experienced with hearing loss.

Peer support groups can be formed easily by monitoring the patient flow. If scheduling and volume permits, classes can be scheduled in advance and people referred to them as needed. If the patient population is small, it may be more reasonable to wait until there are a sufficient number of patients and then schedule the sessions. A staff member will need to be available to keep the group on target and to allow all group members to speak. A psychologist or social worker experienced in working with hearing-impaired children is likely to be the best group leader, although audiologists and speech-language pathologists can develop the necessary skills.

Counseling is a critical part of every audiology program, whether or not staff members consider the program to be rehabilitative. All audiology programs provide informational counseling; however, an insufficient number provide support counseling. This can be provided individually or in peer groups. Most audiologists feel comfortable with informational counseling, but many are not comfortable dealing with supportive counseling. Crandell (1997) reviewed counseling training in graduate programs in audiology. He reported that less than half of audiology programs offered a counseling course, and only 27% required a counseling course. Of those that offered counseling courses, most were taught by audiologists and not by persons with degrees in counseling. Therefore, it is not surprising that many audiologists do not feel comfortable providing supportive counseling. Support counseling, however, is a critical part of audiology. If patients or family members cannot accept their hearing losses, they are not likely to be able to make maximum use of rehabilitation measures, including the acceptance of amplification. If the program is large enough, it may be possible to hire a counselor or social worker to provide some of these services. A part-time person from another program may be able to provide services at the facility to help round out the program.

WHAT PATIENTS WILL BE SERVED?

When considering the development of a rehabilitation program, one should begin by determining what population is currently served by the center and what services are provided to each population served. For example, adult services may be provided in great depth but services to children may be limited. Knowing this helps to evaluate the program better. A decision needs to be made as to where the services are going to be directed. If the center is currently providing services mostly to adults, it would seem reasonable to begin there. If there is a large pediatric population, it may be reasonable to begin with children. Consideration should be given to staff preferences. If there is a particular group that the staff wants to serve, this is a good place to begin. Information will also be gained by finding out what services patients and referral sources would like to have added. Another consideration is to look at what services are available in the community and to make an effort to serve a population that is unserved or underserved.

STAFF REQUIREMENTS

A review of the current staff is necessary to determine what skills are available within the program. Training and academic preparation are critical, as are interest, attitude, and experience. Some clinicians are not interested in doing rehabilitation. The time and effort involved is not the way they wish to spend their time. If the majority of the staff feel that way, it will be very difficult to get a rehabilitation program started. However, if there are members of the staff who are interested in rehabilitation, others may develop an interest as the program develops.

WHO IS ON THE TEAM?

The team that is currently available may influence what services are initially available. An adult program would need to have audiologists who have skills in diagnostic audiology and in amplification selection at a minimum. Someone should be available to provide therapy and counseling services or to arrange for referrals. Peer groups are relatively easy to organize and should be available in most settings. This means that the team will consist of one or two audiologists, a speech-language pathologist or rehabilitative audiologist, a social worker or psychologist, and a physician. The team for any individual patient also includes the patient and family. Not all staff members need be full time.

A pediatric program will benefit greatly by having rehabilitation services and parent counseling available. School support will also be critical to maximize functioning. The staff will include one or more audiologists, a speech-language pathologist, a rehabilitative audiologist and/or teacher of hearing-impaired children, an educational audiologist for school support, a social worker or psychologist, and a physician. Again, the child and family are critical members of the team, as are the classroom teacher and other school personnel.

HOW IS THE TEAM COORDINATED?

In some settings it will be obvious who should be on an individual patient's team and who should coordinate team activities. In some cases, the parents or adult patient will be the best team managers. In other cases, it may be the audiologist who is managing the amplification; in others it may be the clinician who is responsible for therapy or the classroom teacher. If services are provided in a number of different settings, it will be important that someone be responsible for working out how the services will be coordinated and assuring that everyone knows what is going on at the other facilities.

Special Considerations for Providing Rehabilitation in Different Settings

HOSPITALS

Audiologic rehabilitation can be provided in a hospital setting on either outpatient or inpatient bases. Hospital audiology departments vary in the scope of the programs available. Many are valued as providers of diagnostic information with little emphasis on the rehabilitation of patients with hearing impairment. Audiology programs may be housed in departments of otolaryngology, rehabilitation medicine, or neurology and at times can be free-standing. Even programs focusing on diagnostic audiology can include many components that will emphasize the rehabilitative nature of the service provided.

Inpatient stays at hospitals have decreased significantly over the years due to changes in hospital regulations and insurance reimbursement. For patients with hearing impairment, hospitalization can be particularly stressful when limited rehabilitation services are available within the facility. Many patients with hearing impairment enter the hospital environment without the audiology department being aware of their presence. Communication breakdowns between patients and hospital personnel (including nurses, physicians, and technicians) are common occurrences. Assistive listening devices for the telephone and television as well as one-to-one communication devices are often unavailable or underutilized.

Assessing the context of need and the environment of care, the importance of inservicing, and personnel training is apparent. Hospital staff members need to be aware of the effect of hearing impairment on communication and how to deal with the resultant problems. At the minimum, personnel need to be aware of the presence of audiology services in the hospital and the assistance that is available. Trouble-shooting amplification, utilization of assistive technology, and basic communication strategies are all important components of an inpatient audiologic rehabilitation program. A system of communication needs to be developed to ensure that the audiologist is aware of a patient who reports a history of hearing impairment or wears amplification.

Audiologists need to take a more active role in maximizing communication efforts for the hearing-impaired hospital inpatient. Community and consumer organizations, such as SHHH (Self-Help for Hard of Hearing) and the League for the Hard of Hearing, have taken leadership positions in identifying the need for education of hospital personnel. Advocates for Better Communication, a consumer-driven group affiliated with the League for the Hard of Hearing, have produced and widely distributed a series of education materials addressing the concerns of meeting the needs of inpatients with hearing impairment. This program consists of videotape information, educational pamphlets, and stickers to identify those individuals with hearing loss in the hospital. (Additional information on Advocates for Better Communication is available through the League for the Hard of Hearing, 71 West 23 Street, New York, NY 10010.)

Outpatient hospital audiology programs have tended to focus on the diagnostic procedures of patient management. Hospital dispensing of rehabilitation technology has increased over the years, and the role of the hospital-based audiologist has begun to expand. Audiologic rehabilitation services have now expanded beyond the audiogram or electrophysiologic evaluation and have begun to encompass all aspects of communication.

The hearing aid fitting is considered by many to be the primary component of the audiologic rehabilitation program. The amplification system cannot, by itself, solve all the communication problems experienced by hearing-impaired listeners. Amplification must be part of an individualized program that attempts to identify the self-assessed needs of the patient, the significant others (including family, coworkers, and friends), and the environments of communication. There are numerous options to consider in amplification selection. An important part of the rehabilitation program would be choosing the device(s) that would best serve the needs of the patient within his or her environment and the people with whom he or she communicates.

The processes of fitting an earmold, programming an instrument, or replacing a battery are only parts of audiologic service delivery. It is not only the physical mechanics that need to be mastered, but the interactive services of counseling and hearing aid orientation that need to become primary components of the program. Kochkin (1998) reported on the importance of counseling in the hearing aid process. He identified an increase in hearing aid satisfaction as a result of counseling and hearing aid orientation. It would seem that this aspect of amplification fitting is crucial to client success.

SCHOOLS

Educational audiology programs received their mandate in the Code of Federal Regulations on Education, Title 34, Section 300.13 (1986) (Flexer, 1989). According to the law, audiology includes the following.

1. Identifying children with hearing loss;
2. Determining the range, nature, and degree of hearing loss, including referral for medical or other professional attention for the habilitation of hearing;
3. Providing habilitative activities such as language habilitation, auditory training, speechreading, hearing evaluation, and speech conservation;
4. Creating and administrating programs for prevention of hearing loss;
5. Providing counseling and guidance of pupils, parents, and teachers regarding hearing loss; and
6. Determining the child's needs for group and individual amplification, selecting and fitting an appropriate aid, and evaluating the effectiveness of amplification.

By law, all children with permanent or fluctuating hearing losses are entitled to these services, yet the majority of school systems are not providing them. If schools were able to provide these services, hearing-impaired children would have better options.

School programs have the advantage of not having to search for patients. All children who are in the school district are candidates for services. The very best school programs, and there are many, develop programs very much like those in hospitals and community clinics and include all services mandated in Title 34. They see their role as directly providing all the necessary services that the children in their program need, without referrals to other facilities. Many provide all of the evaluation and treatment services discussed above. Some do not dispense hearing aids and rely on community agencies for those services. Even those programs that do not dispense hearing aids should have audiologists who can check amplification daily to be certain that the amplification is working maximally and dispense and monitor FM systems for classroom use. The educational audiologist will also work with teachers and other school staff members to be certain that amplification systems are being used optimally and to monitor classroom noise.

The fact that the audiologist is in the school on a regular basis is a significant advantage, because he or she is able to develop a good long-term working relationship with teachers and other staff members providing ongoing in-service training about hearing and amplification. The educational staff can also provide in-service training to the audiologist about the educational needs of the hearing-impaired child. The fact that all staff members are working together on a regular basis allows them to develop good teamwork. If the school has a sufficiently large number of hearing-impaired children, it may provide a vocational counselor to assist in planning secondary education, training, or job placement. If the school does not have a vocational counselor, it may be possible to arrange for vocational counseling at the school through the local rehabilitation agency.

If there are services that cannot be met by the school, someone in the school program should be assigned the responsibility of coordinating services with outside programs. Part of the coordination of services must include assuring family participation. When families take their children for services at outside facilities, they have the opportunity to talk with audiologists and therapists about what is happening in treatment and can get information for follow-through at home. School programs must make a concerted effort to include parents in team meetings, to provide them with information about educational and therapeutic activities, and to discuss activities parents can work on at home. Parent support and education groups should be offered. If children are receiving all services in school, the parents may not have an opportunity to meet other parents of hearing-impaired children. They still need support from other parents, and group meetings offer the best opportunity for this. Educational activities may be needed for some groups of parents. This is particularly important for families of children who are using sign language or cued speech in school.

Schools do not usually charge for services. Providing all the necessary services can be a problem for some school systems because it may require significant additional staff. Some school systems develop clinics outside the school buildings which provide the required services but can bill for them. Others bill insurance companies or state physically handicapped programs for providing the necessary services. As more children continue to be mainstreamed and as private and public funding for therapy services become more limited, school systems will need to develop cost-effective and efficient ways to meet the needs of children with hearing impairments.

UNIVERSITIES

University training programs do not only educate graduate students in becoming practicing audiologists and speech-language pathologists, they also provide an active clinical program for patients with hearing impairment. Recent changes by the ASHA Council of Academic Accreditation have reduced the number of audiologic rehabilitation practicum hours needed by speech-language pathology graduate students to meet certification requirements. Before this change (which became effective in September 1998), speech-language pathology students needed a total of 35 practicum hours in audiology that were split between diagnostic and rehabilitation experiences. The new standard calls for a total of only 20 practicum hours in any combination of diagnostic or rehabilitation audiology. In other words, it is now possible for a speech-language pathologist to meet certification requirements without having ever experienced audiologic rehabilitation. This becomes further disheartening because aural rehabilitation is identified as being within the scope of practice for a certified speech-language pathologist.

The university clinic offers many opportunities for audiologic rehabilitation, and services do not need to be limited to speechreading or auditory training. There should be a rehabilitative component to any diagnostic audiologic procedure. With the increase in amplification dispensing within the university setting, hearing aid orientation, fitting procedures, and counseling should be readily available.

The patient population in a university-based speech and hearing center will be varied depending on location of the clinic within the community. Generally there is a mix of both children and adults, with many clinics accepting referrals from various outside sources such as hospitals, schools, and industry and health centers. Services provided to meet the needs of the community can encompass more than just a diagnostic audiologic evaluation. The use of self-assessment inventories, such as the Communication Profile for the Hearing Impaired (Demorest and Erdman, 1987) and the Hearing Handicap Inventory for the Elderly (Ventry and Weinstein, 1982), are tools that can help the clinician identify the issues related to hearing handicap and disability and can help educate the student in the underlying effects of hearing impairment on psychosocial functioning and communication. Self-assessment tools can be important to the counseling process and instrumental in determining treatment goals.

Counseling before and after the audiologic assessment can help determine issues of greatest importance for patients with hearing impairment and their families. Understanding their communication situations can aid the clinician in providing the necessary treatment to increase communication accessibility.

There are many university programs that offer advanced degrees only in speech-language pathology and not audiology. They may provide audiologic services on a limited basis or place their students in external sites to fulfill their audiology practicum requirements. A visit to these external placement sites is necessary to determine process and protocol of audiologic procedures. This would enable the university faculty to help the student distinguish the rehabilitation components of the program and discuss them in lecture and seminar sessions.

LONG-TERM CARE FACILITIES

The long-term care facility presents a unique challenge to the audiologist. As the older adult population demographics change with increased life expectancy, chronic rather than acute conditions will be one of the most prevalent health issues facing the elderly (Weinstein and Clark, 1989), with hearing impairment being among the most common chronic conditions in this population (National Center for Health Statistics [NCHS], 1987). Although the majority of older adults reside in their own homes or with their families, an increasing number are seeking or requiring alternative levels of care ranging from assistive living facilities, subacute care, and skilled nursing facilities.

Audiologic services are primarily available to older adults through outpatient facilities, community agencies, hospitals, and universities. When an audiologist is affiliated with long-term care (either a subacute or skilled nursing facility), availability of positions may vary from full or part-time employment, to limited consultation, to an outside referral source only. Many long-term care facilities have no affiliation at all with an audiologist, and the care for the residents with hearing impairment is left to nursing personnel or, if available, the speech-language pathologist.

Rehabilitation of older adults with hearing impairment depends largely on the cooperative efforts of the audiologist, patient, family, and caregivers. For those providing services within the long-term care facility, the communication partners and environmental conditions play pivotal roles in success. Lubinski (1981) identified the long-term care environment as deficient for effective communication. A communication-impaired environment (Lubinski et al., 1981) was described as a setting in which little opportunity exists for successful and meaningful communication. Many long-term care facilities meet this definition when residents are placed in large day rooms facing walls or are placed in front of televisions, giving little chance for any effective conversation with other residents or staff members.

Communication partners within the long-term care facility include caregivers (consisting primarily of nurses and nurse assistants), other residents, and visiting family and friends. Because the nursing personnel frequently have the most opportunity for communication with the residents, their role in audiologic rehabilitation is extremely important. Montano (1993) stated that nursing personnel in long-term care facilities demonstrated deficiency in the information necessary to care for their residents with hearing impairment. He identified the need for further in-service education on topics such as identification of characteristics and behaviors of individuals with hearing impairment, hearing aid management skills, and strategies necessary for successful communication. Education was recommended as a critical component of any audiologic rehabilitation program within the long-term care environment.

The relevance of the ecologic approach to audiologic rehabilitation described earlier in this chapter is apparent when one views the environmental issues related to communication in long-term care facilities. Jennings and Head (1994) described the development and implementation of an ecologic audiologic rehabilitation program in a home for the aged, noting that standard clinical approaches were insufficient for long-term care. Their program consisted of various audiologic services including assessment, provision and maintenance of rehabilitation technology, environmental modifications, staff education, self-help groups, and an audiology drop-in clinic. Audiologic rehabilitation services involved the residents, their communication partners, and in particular the staff involved in daily care. Hearing aids and assistive listening devices were used to help maximize environmental accessibility. Participation in resident case conferences helped increase the knowledge the audiologists had regarding their patients' communication activity and allowed for the opportunity to educate other service providers. In-service and staff development were critical components of the program. A series of four 30-minute programs were developed that highlighted areas such as hearing loss and aging, the effects of hearing loss on communication, hearing aids, assistive listening devices, and environmental coping and problem-solving.

There are numerous problems inherent in providing audiologic rehabilitation services in long-term care. Certainly, the physical and mental deterioration of many residents who require skilled nursing care would make the provision of audiologic rehabilitation challenging. Traditional hearing aid fittings and dispensing are the exceptions to the rule, and amplification systems frequently require modifications to allow independent use or lengthy therapy for training and education. Many residents are incapable of acquiring independent functioning with their amplification, and staff education is the only way to achieve successful remediation. Limited staffing levels and multiple job responsibilities make attendance at in-service programs difficult for all facility personnel, particularly nurses and nurse assistants. In addition, the need for training staff members on all work shifts is necessary for continuity of care.

COMMUNITY AGENCIES

Community agencies were among the first to provide rehabilitation services and continue to be significant providers of these services in many communities. These programs vary in size and services provided. Some provide speech and hearing services only, and others provide a variety of rehabilitation services. Some, like the various Leagues and Guilds for the Hard of Hearing, only provide services to persons with hearing loss; others provide more expanded services to children and adults with a variety of speech, hearing, and physical disorders. Some restrict their services to one age group (children or adults), and others provide services to everyone in need. Frequently, community agencies meet needs that are not being met by other programs in the community. Because most hospital programs do not provide rehabilitative services, this job falls to the community agencies.

Years ago, services at community agencies were frequently provided at little or no cost. This can no longer be afforded, and community agencies need to charge for services like any other program. Because of the way they are organized, community agencies can usually raise funds directly from the community and corporations to meet some of the costs of running the service. As fund-raising becomes more difficult and as health insurance pays for fewer rehabilitation services, community agencies may experience a more difficult time funding their operations.

PRIVATE PRACTICE

Unlike hospitals, schools, and community agencies who can raise funds and may have endowments, private practices rely entirely on fees to run their programs. This forces staff to develop an efficient use of time and resources. Private practitioners need to analyze carefully the needs of the community and the demand for services (just as all other programs do) and determine what the market wants. Many restrict their rehabilitative activities to the dispensing of hearing aids. Others have found that providing other services can increase the number of referrals for hearing aids. Hearing aid orientation classes are frequently cost-effective for many practices because the more a consumer knows, the happier he or she is likely

to be with amplification and the fewer will be the postfitting visits required. This results in fewer hearing aid returns and better word-of-mouth referrals. Some programs have found it useful to offer a discount on hearing aid purchase or free batteries to encourage attendance at hearing aid orientation classes. Offering other rehabilitative services, especially those not offered in the community, will draw attention to the practice and increase the referral base. Other clinicians in the community may be willing to offer services at the private practice office and share expenses and income from the services which will benefit both parties and their hearing-impaired clients.

Tye-Murray et al. (1994) acknowledge the influence of hectic workday schedules in a busy clinical setting such as a private practice. They recommend the implementation of a variety of programs that can be incorporated into most practices. Services described include home training programs, a client lending library, a family center (a room designed for counseling and demonstrating real-life speech perception situations), and an assistive listening device center.

COORDINATING SERVICES BETWEEN SETTINGS

When services are provided at more than one center to a child or adult with a hearing loss, it is critical that the programs work together if they are going to provide optimal services. In some cases the adult client or spouse, or the parent of a hearing-impaired child, can provide this activity. However, this is not always optimal. It frequently works best if services are coordinated by one clinician. This is usually best done by a person who sees the client frequently. If the client is in therapy and seen weekly, that clinician might be the best person to coordinate services. If the child is receiving most services in a school, someone from the school staff may be the ideal coordinator. Sometimes the audiologist who sees the child only occasionally will be a good coordinator because of his or her ability to summarize and organize things with an outsider's view.

The responsibilities of the team coordinator include being certain that all clinicians know what other clinicians are doing and assuring that they have the same goals and are not working at cross-purposes. This can best be accomplished by periodic team meetings. If the same team is working with a large group of clients (as is frequently the case in schools and community agencies), cases can be reviewed at weekly team meetings. Although every client may not be discussed each week, the opportunity is available to discuss problems as they arise. At the very least, team meetings should occur quarterly, and more often for any clients who are having difficulties.

The coordinator is also responsible for arranging for periodic evaluations to measure progress. Reports of all specialists should be shared, and the team, client, and family should determine if things are moving along as expected or if changes need to be made in the program.

Team coordination is ideally carried out in person but can be done by conference call or by sharing reports. However, unless the team gets the opportunity to discuss things with each other in person or by telephone (not just by paper), they will not be able to truly discuss problems and work out solutions.

Legislative Issues

Audiologic rehabilitation should be viewed as a growing component of our profession. Improvements in technology, consumer advocacy, and legislative efforts lead to an optimistic view for the future (Binnie, 1994). There have been a number of recent public laws that have a direct effect on the provision of audiologic rehabilitation services, in particular the Individuals with Disabilities Education Act (IDEA) and the Americans with Disabilities Act (ADA). These laws support the services necessary to enhance the communication abilities of children and adults in schools, the workplace, and society.

The IDEA, as amended in 1997, was designed to "ensure that all children with disabilities have available to them a free appropriate public education that emphasizes special education and related services designed to meet their unique needs and prepare them for employment and independent living" (1997). Included within the definition of related services are the supportive services of audiology and speech-language pathology.

The IDEA ensures that educators and parents are provided with the tools—whether technical advancements, media support, or research and personnel preparation—necessary to support the provisions of the law. The law defines an assistive technology device as "any item, piece of equipment, or product system, whether acquired commercially off the shelf, modified, or customized, that is used to increase, maintain, or improve functional capabilities of a child with a disability," and assistive technology service as "any service that directly assists a child with a disability in the selection, acquisition, or use of an assistive technology device."

The provision of services for children with a hearing impairment are clearly identified in the IDEA. The inclusion and justification of amplification devices (FM systems, closed caption decoders for the classroom, and in certain situations hearing aids) in a child's individualized education plan (IEP) would mandate the implementation of such services. Audiologic rehabilitation services would be necessary to ensure the appropriateness of amplification selection; training and education of students, teachers, and family; auditory training; speechreading; and counseling.

Part H of the IDEA, the Early Intervention Program for Infants and Toddlers with Disabilities, identifies the importance of early identification and intervention of children with disabilities from birth onward. Children identified with any condition resulting in disability are provided services through a service coordinator as part of an individualized family service plan (IFSP). Hearing impairment is one of the conditions identified in Part H of the IDEA warranting the provision of services from an audiologist, the qualified provider. The provision supports the use of assistive technology and provides financial entitlement to families for a child with hearing impairment. Assistive technology would include hearing aids, assistive listening devices, and the services necessary for selecting and fitting the devices. Family counseling and individual rehabilitation services are also covered under Part H of the law.

The ADA of 1990 was designed to protect individuals with disabilities from discrimination in employment, transportation, public accommodations, state and local government, and telecommunications. Audiologic rehabilitation can become an important component in the implementation of the ADA. The audiologist serves as a patient advocate, counselor, and industry advisor. Employment counseling, assessment of the communication environment, family support, and employer education and training can be part of a rehabilitation strategy. Rehabilitation technology is an important component in the creation of a barrier-free environment for improved communication in the workplace, in telecommunication, or in areas of public access (Montano, 1994).

Legislative developments offer opportunities for audiologists to expand their role in the provision of rehabilitative service. It becomes our responsibility to define that role and demonstrate its importance. Unfortunately, a factor that has been frequently cited as a reason for limited availability of audiologic rehabilitation services is the lack of third-party reimbursement.

Financial Considerations

Third-party reimbursement for audiologic rehabilitation is limited. Considering the provision of audiology services in the diagnostic domain using the medical model of services delivery, financial remuneration is widely available. Audiologists are frequently reimbursed for hearing evaluations, electrophysiology examinations, and ENG (electronystagmography) with rehabilitation services scrutinized and rejected. It is an exception to the rule to find hearing aid delivery, hearing counseling, and auditory training as reimbursable services.

Under the federal Medicare program, audiologic rehabilitation may be a covered service when rendered under Part A to hospital inpatients or when an audiologist is employed by a physician and providing the service as part of cochlear implant management. The only audiologic rehabilitation service specifically identified through the Medicare program is speechreading, and it is only the speech-language pathologist who is identified as the provider of this service. Auditory training is not specified as a service permitted under Medicare.

The Social Security Act Amendments of 1994 (P.L. 103-432) directly addressed the role of the audiologist and audiology services permitted under the program. Although identifying the audiologist as an authorized provider was a desirable outcome of the law, it did not include the coverage of audiologic rehabilitation services. The passage of the amendment actually clarified existing practice and did not increase or propose any new benefits.

Considerable efforts have been and will continue to be made on behalf of audiologists to educate the public, service providers, third-party insurers, and our professional peers on the value and importance of rehabilitative audiology. We profess the importance of rehabilitation for the client with hearing loss but seem to acknowledge quickly the limited availability of the services. Providing the service as a component of a rehabilitation model of delivery clears any ambiguity one may have regarding our professional purpose. Erdman et al. (1994) suggest that if we are accountable for our services and can demonstrate their efficacy, reimbursement will not be a concern. Ross (1997) states that "the more doubts we have, the less we actually practice A/R, then the less likely it is that A/R will be a part of our professional future."

Marketing

Unlike what many audiologists appear to believe, marketing is not a dirty word. In fact, it is critical to survival. Especially in these difficult times, it is critical that all programs market their services. This begins by determining what the markets are and then determining what strategies will best meet the needs of those markets with the available resources.

It is very useful to begin by surveying the community. What services are available and what services are missing? What does your program offer that is unique? What services do you provide that are very satisfactory to your clients? What do your clients want that is not currently being provided either at your facility or in the community?

Each program has several markets. These include clients, referral sources, insurers, and state and federal payers. Each market needs to be addressed differently. Clients (both patient clients and referral sources) need to be made to believe that they need our services and that we are the providers of choice. Insurers and other payers need to be convinced that we, as providers, provide only those services that are critical to their clients and that we provide them in a cost-efficient manner. Many of our clients do not know who audiologists are and why we are the providers of choice for persons with hearing loss. Any marketing needs to address that critical issue.

Marketing comes in two formats—paid marketing and free marketing. Paid marketing includes advertisements in the yellow pages, newspaper advertisements, and other media including television and radio. Television and radio can be very expensive, especially in large cities. Public interest stories can draw the attention of the media and can result in what is essentially free advertising. This includes information about special clients or stories related to better hearing and speech month activities.

Talks and letters to professional groups, such as local pediatricians, otolaryngologists, or general medicine specialists, is another form of advertising to remind them of your presence in the community. Community groups are always seeking speakers, and your presence and willingness to be

available will likely be remembered when audiology services are needed. Talks to schools, parent groups, senior centers, and local business groups are an important way to reach clients. Many audiologists find newsletters a good use of time and money.

Marketing is not a one-time activity; it is on-going. It happens every time a patient comes into your office and every time someone in your office answers the telephone. It happens every time a report is mailed out and when a thank you note is sent to a referral source following a patient visit. If we do not handle these services well, we have failed in an opportunity to market.

Conclusion

Rehabilitation is an exciting part of the practice of audiology. It can be included in most if not all audiology programs, and doing so will make the practice more interesting for the staff and improve the quality of services for the clients. Regardless of our work environments, audiologic rehabilitation services can be incorporated into our programs. Identifying the environment of care as well as the needs of the individual with hearing impairment and the significant communication partners, can aid the audiologist in developing and implementing the numerous components of audiologic rehabilitation. Whether it is a program developed for patients in long-term care or the child with hearing impairment in the mainstream classroom, audiologic rehabilitation is crucial to the goal of improved communication.

There are many obstacles to the provision of audiologic rehabilitation services. Justifying our services with appropriate outcome measurements will help improve the audiologist's accountability and increase our visibility in the ever-changing health care arena. Health care reform will continue to have an effect on our profession. The outcome measures we develop for our profession must reach beyond the "ordinary clinical criteria, into the lifestyle and quality of life areas" (Hyde and Riko, 1994). We must prepare, through our rehabilitative services, to place people back into the workplace, the social structure, and the living environments they are part of and to advocate on their behalf. We have the knowledge base, we have the motivation, we have some of the legislative support, and most importantly we have the patients who need our assistance.

REFERENCES

ASHA. Spotlight on special interest division 7. Audiologic Rehabilitation, ASHA, 1992, vol 34:8, 18.

Binnie C. The future of audiologic rehabilitation: overview and forecast. In: Gagne JP, Tye-Murray N, eds. Research in audiological rehabilitation: current trends and future directions. J Acad Rehab Audiol 1994;27(Monogr Suppl): 13–25.

Crandell CC. An update on counseling instruction within audiology programs. J Acad Rehab Audiol 1997;30:77–86.

Demorest M, Erdman SA. Development of the communication profile for the hearing impaired. J Speech Hearing Res 1987;52:129–143.

Erdman SA, Wark DJ, Montano JJ. Implications of service delivery models in audiology. J Acad Rehab Audiol 1994; 27:45–60.

Flexer C. Neglected issues in educational audiology. J Acad Rehab Audiol 1989;20:61–66.

Gagne JP, Hetu R, Getty L, et al. Towards the development of paradigms to conduct functional evaluative research in audiological rehabilitation. J Acad Rehab Audiol 1995; 28:7–25.

Hyde ML, Riko K. A decision-analytic approach to audiological rehabilitation. In: Gagne JP, Tye-Murray N, eds. Research in audiological rehabilitation: current trends and future directions. J Acad Rehab Audiol 1994;27(Monogr Suppl):337–374.

Jennings MB, Head BG. Development of an ecological audiologic rehabilitation program in a home-for-the-aged. J Acad Rehab Audiol 1994;27:73–88.

Lubinski R. Speech, language and audiology programs in home health care agencies and nursing homes. In: Beasley D, Davis GA, eds. Aging communication processes and disorders. New York: Grune & Stratton, 1981:339–356.

Lubinski R, Morrison, E, Rigrodsky S. Perception of spoken communication by elderly chronically ill patients in an institutional setting. J Speech Hear Dis 1981;46:405–412.

Madell JR. Hearing aid orientation: a new experience. Hear J 1973; August:5.

Malinoff R, Kisiel D, Kisiel S, et al. The dispensing of hearing instruments: a study on industry structures and trends. Hear Instruments 1990;41:12–14.

Montano J. Knowledge and needs of nursing personnel regarding hearing impairment and hearing rehabilitation of long term care patients. Unpublished dissertation. Teachers College, Columbia University, 1993.

Montano J. Rehabilitation technology for the hearing impaired. In: Katz J, ed. Handbook of clinical audiology. 4th ed. Baltimore: Williams & Wilkins, 1994:638–656.

National Center for Health Statistics. Current estimates from the National Health Interview Survey, United States, 1986. Vital Health Stat 1987 Series 10 No. 164.

Noble W, Hetu R. An ecological approach to disability and handicap in relation to impaired hearing. Audiology 1994; 33:117–126.

Ross M. A retrospective look at the future of aural rehabilitation. J Acad Rehab Audiol 1997;30:11–28.

Schow RL, Balsara NR, Smedley TC, et al. Aural rehabilitation by ASHA audiologists: 1980–1990. Am J Audiol 1993;2:28–37.

Tye-Murray N, Witt S, Schum L, et al. Feasible aural rehabilitation services for busy clinical settings. Am J Audiol 1994;3:33–37.

Ventry I, Weinstein B. (1982). The hearing handicap inventory for the elderly: a new tool. Ear Hear 1983;3:128–134.

Wayner D. The hearing aid handbook: clinician's guide to client orientation. Washington, DC: Gallaudet University Press, 1990.

Weinstein B, Clark L. An aging society. ASHA 1989;31: 67–69.

SUGGESTED READINGS

Alpiner J. Educational audiology. J Acad Rehab Audiol 1974;7:50–54.

Carson AJ, Pichora-Fuller K. Health promotion and audiology: the community-clinic link. J Acad Rehab Audiol 1997;30:29–51.

Erickson JG, Garstecki DC. Practicum in aural rehabilitation in a university training program. J Acad Rehab Audiol 1973;6:9–12.

Goldberg-Citron L. Inservice education: one role of the audiologist in Public Law 94–142. J Acad Rehab Audiol 1979;12:21–26.

Israelite NK, Jennings MB. Participant perspective on group aural rehabilitation: a qualitative inquiry. J Acad Rehab Audiol 1995;28:26–36.

Madell JR, Montano J, Malinoff RL. Developing an aural rehabilitation program in a non-rehabilitation facility. Academy of Rehabilitative Audiology Summer Institute, June 12, 1992, Austin, TX.

O'Neill J. The school-educational audiologist. J Acad Rehab Audiol 1974;7:31–39.

Roberts SD, Bryant JD. Establishing counseling goals in rehabilitative audiology. J Acad Rehab Audiol 1992; 25:81–97.

Ross M. Aural rehabilitation revisited. J Acad Rehab Audiol 1987;20:13–24.

Sykes S, Tucker D, Herr D. Aural rehabilitation and graduate audiology programs. J Am Acad Audiol 1997;8: 314–321.

Teter DL. Personal reflections on aural rehabilitation: past, present and future. J Acad Rehab Audiol 1989;20:11–14.

AUDIOLOGIC REHABILITATION: CHILDREN

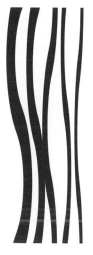

Early Identification: Principles and Practices

Dianne H. Meyer, Ph.D.

Unidentified hearing loss may have devastating effects on a child and the affected family. A child's speech and language development, psychosocial skills, academic progress, and vocational opportunities may all be negatively impacted. Fortunately, these unfavorable effects can be avoided or reduced if the hearing loss is identified early and followed promptly by appropriate intervention. The expertise and technology exist today to achieve the critical challenge of early identification.

This chapter presents issues and practices related to identification of hearing loss among newborns. First, the dual influences of U.S. health policy and developing technology are considered. Next, performance characteristics of screening tests and current screening methods are discussed. The chapter also describes programmatic issues, including goals, screening protocols, performance criteria, data management, and follow-up. Finally, the status of newborn hearing screening as a national initiative is considered.

Health Policy and Technologic Influences

NATIONAL HEALTH PRIORITIES

Over the past 20 years, health practices in the United States have undergone dramatic changes, including an important shift to health promotion and disease prevention.

Because many infectious diseases have been controlled (e.g., rubella, polio), the nation's health focus today is on ways to promote good health and to prevent chronic disease and disability. In its 1991 tutorial on prevention, the American Speech-Language-Hearing Association (ASHA) described types of prevention activities and discussed prevention strategies for audiologists and speech-language pathologists (American Speech-Language-Hearing Association, 1991). *Primary* prevention refers to the reduction or elimination of the onset of a disease or disorder. An example is the use of ear protection to prevent noise-induced hearing loss. *Secondary* prevention is early detection and treatment to reduce the negative effects of the disorder. Screening for hearing or speech problems is an example. *Tertiary* prevention, which is the type most commonly provided by audiologists and speech-language pathologists, refers to rehabilitation of the disabled individual who has realized some residual problem as a result of the disorder. Within this context, newborn hearing screening is viewed as a valuable strategy for secondary prevention of the consequences of infant hearing loss. Infants who are identified early benefit from prompt treatment and the reduction or elimination of speech and language delays.

Another factor that has led to increased interest in newborn hearing screening is national emphasis on early intervention to address the needs of handicapped infants. The Individuals with Disabilities Education Act (IDEA), formerly known as the Education of the Handicapped Act of 1986 (PL 99–457), requires that evaluation and early intervention services be provided to newborns and young infants with known or suspected disabilities, including hearing loss. Federal funding has provided support and incentives for states to identify these infants early and to provide appropriate, comprehensive intervention for infants and their families. The concept of newborn hearing screening fits in with states' goals to develop screening, diagnostic, and management programs.

HEALTHY PEOPLE DOCUMENTS

The national agenda for prevention can be found in the Healthy People documents published by the Surgeon General's office. The first report, released in 1979, called for establishing national health goals and monitoring the progress made in reaching those goals (U.S. Department of Health, Education and Welfare, 1979). *Healthy People 2000* was released in 1990 as a comprehensive agenda with 319 objectives organized into 22 priority areas (U.S. Department of Health and Human Services, 1990). Included in the document was the objective to "reduce the average age at which children with significant hearing impairment are identified to no more than 12 months." At that time it was estimated that the average age of identification in the United States was 24 to 30 months. This important objective became a catalyst for public health efforts and related technologic developments in the area of newborn hearing screening.

Healthy People 2010 aims to build on the improvements realized in the previous 10 years. The draft document points out that the average age of identification of infant hearing loss in the United States is well above other countries such as Israel and Great Britain, where the average age of identification is 7 months. Noting that the knowledge and technology are available, the draft document calls for all newborn infants to be screened for hearing loss by 1 month of age, to have diagnostic follow-up by 3 months, and to be enrolled in appropriate intervention services by 6 months (U.S. Department of Health and Human Services, 1998).

THE JOINT COMMITTEE ON INFANT HEARING (JCIH)

Undoubtedly, the activities of the JCIH have been the most important influence on the development of national policy regarding infant hearing. Established in 1969, this committee was charged with making recommendations concerning newborn hearing screening programs and the early identification of children with hearing loss or with risk factors related to hearing loss (Diefendorf and Finitzo, 1997). Its multidisciplinary membership has been composed of representatives from audiology, otolaryngology, pediatrics, nursing, deaf education, and state health and welfare agencies. Over the years, the JCIH has published a series of position statements that have included recommended preferred practices for the early identification and appropriate intervention with newborns and infants who either have or are at risk for a hearing loss. In its early years, the JCIH recommended identification of infants at risk for hearing loss in terms of specific risk factors and suggested a follow-up audiologic evaluation until an accurate assessment of hearing could be made. The JCIH 1990 position statement expanded the list of risk factors and recommended that newborns with one or more risk criteria should be screened before discharge from the newborn nursery but no later than 3 months of age. Auditory brainstem response (ABR) was recommended for the initial screening (Joint Committee on Infant Hearing, 1991). In 1994, the JCIH expanded its position further by stating that high-risk factors (i.e., indicators) play an important role in early detection but that the goal should be *universal* detection of infants with hearing loss. (American Academy of Pediatrics, 1995). Table 4.1 lists the JCIH indicators associated with sensorineural and/or conductive hearing loss.

Table 4.1
JCIH indicators associated with sensorineural and/or conductive hearing loss

Family history of hereditary childhood sensorineural hearing loss
In utero infection, such as cytomegalovirus, rubella, syphilis, herpes, and toxoplasmosis
Craniofacial anomalies, including those with morphologic abnormalities of the pinna and ear canal
Birth weight less than 1500 g (3.3 lb)
Hyperbilirubinemia at a serum level requiring exchange transfusion
Ototoxic medications, including but not limited to the aminoglycosides, used in multiple courses
 or in combination with loop diuretics
Bacterial meningitis
Apgar scores of 0 to 4 at 1 minute or 0 to 6 at 5 minutes
Mechanical ventilation lasting 5 days or longer
Stigmata or other findings associated with a syndrome known to include a sensorineural and/or
 conductive hearing loss

JCIH, Joint Committee on Infant Hearing.
From Joint Committee on Infant Hearing 1994 Position Statement. *Pediatrics* 1995;95:152–156.

The JCIH had developed a draft statement for year 2000 at the time that this chapter was prepared (American Speech-Language Hearing Association, 1999). The draft statement called for screening of all newborns, followed by confirmation of hearing loss by 3 months of age and referral to interdisciplinary intervention by 6 months of age. It endorsed the development of family-centered, community-based early hearing detection and intervention (EHDI) systems. Interested readers are urged to contact ASHA for information about the most current JCIH statement.

NATIONAL INSTITUTES OF HEALTH (NIH) CONSENSUS STATEMENT

In early 1993, the NIH convened a Consensus Development Conference on the Early Identification of Hearing Impairment in Infants and Young Children. Cosponsors of the conference were the National Institute on Deafness and Other Communication Disorders, the Office of Medical Applications of Research, the National Institute of Child Health and Human Development, and the National Institute of Neurological Disorders and Stroke. The NIH uses such conferences to evaluate available scientific information and to develop statements that are to be useful to health professionals and the public. The conference brought together specialists from a variety of health care and scientific disciplines as well as representatives from the public. Following two days of expert presentations and discussion, the independent consensus panel noted that screening based on high-risk criteria fails to identify more than 50% of children born with significant hearing impairment and that recent technologic developments had produced efficient screening methods for newborns. The consensus panel concluded that universal screening should be implemented for all infants within the first 3 months of life and preferably before discharge from the newborn nursery. The panel further recommended that the preferred model for screening should begin with an evoked otoacoustic emissions (EOAE) test, followed by an ABR test for infants who fail the EOAE. Infant caregivers and primary health care providers should be educated on the early signs of hearing impairment, and there should be ongoing surveillance for hearing loss throughout infancy and early childhood (National Institutes of Health, 1993). By emphatically recommending universal screening and a specific screening protocol, the NIH Consensus Statement sparked considerable debate among audiologists and pediatricians (Bess and Paradise, 1994; Northern and Hayes, 1994). It also significantly increased public and professional awareness of the importance of early identification of hearing loss and helped to increase the number of universal screening programs in the United States.

THE AMERICAN ACADEMY OF PEDIATRICS (AAP)

In 1999 the Task Force on Newborn and Infant Hearing of the AAP released the statement, *Newborn and Infant Hearing Loss: Detection and Intervention* (American Academy of Pediatrics, 1999). The AAP statement supported the implementation of universal newborn hearing screening and reviewed critical issues related to screening, tracking and follow-up, identification and intervention, and program evaluation. In addition, the statement included recommendations that state chapters of the AAP lead state-based efforts to develop universal screening and that educational materials about effective screening programs be developed and disseminated. Appendix 4.1 contains the complete text of the AAP statement.

ADDITIONAL POSITION STATEMENTS

ASHA, AAA, and the Directors of Speech and Hearing Programs in State Health and Welfare Agencies (DSHPSHWA) each participated as a member organization during the development of the JCIH 1994 position statement. While fully supporting the 1994 statement, each organization has developed supplemental recommendations and positions related to identification of infant hearing loss. For example, ASHA's 1988 position statement on prevention urged audiologists and speech-language pathologists to be involved in activities of early detection and treatment (American Speech-Language-Hearing Association, 1988). ASHA's 1996 document, *Guidelines for Audiologic Screening,* included a chapter on screening neonates and young infants that built on the JCIH 1994 statement. The guidelines gave recommended parameters for ABR and EOAE testing as well as specifications for maximum allowable ambient noise levels during screening (American Speech-Language-Hearing Association, 1996).

In the AAA position statement, *Early Identification of Hearing Loss in Infants and Children* (1998), audiologists were encouraged to develop alternative and innovative approaches to early identification programs, especially if the goal of universal screening was not feasible for a particular facility. Among other recommendations, AAA urged that mechanisms be established to promote compliance with recommended follow-up and that the success of hearing screening programs be periodically evaluated. Recently, AAA developed a draft document that considers the use of support personnel for newborn hearing screening. The draft guidelines included qualifications of support personnel, training, duties and responsibilities, and supervision (American Academy of Audiology, 1998).

In 1996, DSHPSHWA developed its position statement, *Universal Hearing Detection* (Directors of Speech and Hearing Programs in State Health and Welfare Agencies, 1998). While reaffirming its endorsement of universal newborn and infant hearing detection, this group also pointed out that most states do not have an organized statewide newborn hearing screening program. The DSHPSHWA recommended that either ABR or EOAE be used to screen infants and stressed that universal hearing screening programs should be community-based and family-centered. This group recommended that the financial support for universal hearing screening be included in individual and group health insurance coverage and in national health care reform.

DEVELOPING TECHNOLOGY

Early methods of infant hearing screening relied on behavioral changes to indicate if the infant responded appropriately to sound. Methods such as behavioral observation, the Crib-o-gram, and the auditory response cradle presented infants with high-intensity signals and compared the infant's prestimulus state to the poststimulus state (Downs and Hemenway, 1969; Simmons and Russ,

1974; Bennett, 1979). A measurable change in the infant's behavior, such as generalized body movement or changes in respiration rate, resulted in a pass for the hearing screening. These procedures could be effective in identifying infants with profound hearing loss, but were less sensitive to mild and moderate degrees of hearing loss and to unilateral hearing loss. In addition, behavioral techniques resulted in a large number of false-positive results, which necessitated follow-up efforts for many infants who were later found to have normal hearing.

The emergence of the electrophysiologic methods, ABR and EOAE, to assess infant auditory function has provided tools for identifying even mild to moderate hearing impairments and the ability to obtain separate-ear results. Technologic advancements incorporating ABR and EOAE procedures have resulted in portable, automated screeners that can be used easily by a variety of health care workers. These new screening methods are more sensitive, rapid, and easily administered than behavioral methods, making the implementation of universal newborn hearing screening feasible.

Performance Characteristics of Screenings

Approximately 4 million infants are born in the United States each year. With such a large population to be screened, procedures must be both effective and efficient. The results of newborn hearing screening should show that few, if any, hearing-impaired infants are missed and that the number of normal hearing infants who mistakenly fail the screening is minimal. How well the screening procedure achieves this goal is represented by its performance characteristics. The audiology literature includes several excellent discussions about performance characteristics, including their relation to infant hearing screening (Jerger, 1983; Turner and Nielsen, 1984; Northern and Downs, 1991; Turner, 1991). The following concepts are based on those discussions.

A decision matrix is a straightforward and convenient way to evaluate the performance of a hearing screening procedure. As shown in Table 4.2, a decision matrix is a two-by-two table that summarizes how effectively the screening test differentiates

Table 4.2
A decision matrix and performance characteristics for a presumed screening of 5000 newborns

Test Result	Hearing-Impaired	Normal Hearing	Total
Refer	True Positive 19	False Positive 300	319
Pass	False Negative 1	True Negative 4680	4681
Total	20	4980	5000

Sensitivity	19/20	= 95%
Specificity	4680/4980	= 94%
Predictive value		
Positive result	19/319	= 6%
Negative result	4680/4681	= 99.9%
Efficiency	4699/5000	= 94%

hearing-impaired infants from normal-hearing infants. Table 4.2 also includes results for a presumed screening of 5000 newborns. These numbers will be used to demonstrate hypothetically the performance characteristics of a test. Ideally, a screening test would correctly identify all infants as either normal or hearing-impaired, but, in practice, screening tests will have some degree of error. The decision matrix in Table 4.2 shows that four outcomes are possible. The screening test will have either a *pass* or *refer* result, and the infants screened will have either *hearing impairment* or *normal hearing*. The refer results on the screening test are reported as true-positives when they are found with hearing-impaired infants and as false-positives when they are found with normal-hearing infants. Pass results on the screening are referred to as true-negatives when they occur with normal infants and as false-negatives when they occur with hearing-impaired infants. By considering data in this way, the performance characteristics of *sensitivity, specificity, predictive value,* and *efficiency* can be specified for any procedure.

The hypothetical data in Table 4.2 will help the reader to understand these four characteristics. Sensitivity refers to how well the procedure identifies those infants who truly are hearing-impaired. In this example, 20 of the 5000 infants had hearing impairments. The procedure was 95% sensitive because it correctly identified 19 of 20 hearing-impaired infants. There was one false-negative result, meaning that one hearing-impaired infant erroneously passed the screening. Newborn hearing screening programs must strive for high sensitivity and minimal false-negative rates. The error of passing a hearing-impaired infant may have serious consequences on the child's development, especially if the eventual identification of the hearing loss is delayed beyond critical speech/language periods.

Screening tests must also be able to identify correctly, or pass, infants with normal hearing. In the example, a pass result was obtained for 4680 of 4980 infants with normal hearing. Specificity, or the ability to correctly identify true-negatives, was 94%.

Specificity is important because of its effect on follow-up. With high specificity, relatively few normal-hearing infants are referred for additional services. On the other hand, low specificity indicates that relatively more normal-hearing infants are referred. Having to provide additional screening or diagnostic services to normal-hearing infants who erroneously fail a screening involves additional time and expense, not to mention possible parental stress and anxiety.

The combination of high sensitivity and high specificity is the ideal. Often, these two characteristics have a reciprocal relationship in that increasing one may result in decreasing the other. For example, it may be possible to increase sensitivity by lowering the decibel level of the screening stimulus. Such a change, however, may decrease specificity by making it more difficult for a normal-hearing infant to respond.

The concept of predictive value relates to how the pass and refer results are interpreted. Most infants who fail a screening will later be found to have normal hearing, so the question arises as to what is the probability that hearing loss is present if a refer result is obtained. Similarly, if a pass result is obtained, what is the likelihood that hearing is actually normal? In the hypothetical example, 319 infants had a refer result, and 19 of those infants had hearing loss. Therefore, the predictive value of a positive result (i.e., refer) was 6%. In the example it is evident that a refer result did not necessarily mean that the infant had hearing loss. In fact, the probability was far greater that the infant had normal hearing (94%). On the other hand, the predictive value of a negative result (i.e., pass) was nearly 100%. Of the 4681 infants who passed the screening, only 1 was later found to have hearing loss. When a pass result occurred, the probability was very high that hearing was normal.

Predictive value is significantly influenced by prevalence, which refers to the number of individuals per 100,000 who have the disease (i.e., hearing loss) at the time of the study. If a disease is common within a given population, then it follows that the predictive value of a positive result will also be higher. For example, consider the results of a screening test that is applied to two different populations, one with 50% prevalence of the disease and one with 1% prevalence. The chances of a positive result being a true-positive is far greater for the first population than for the second because so many more individuals in the first group have the disease. The reported prevalence of newborn hearing loss is low, in the range of 3 to 6 per 1000 births (Brackett et al., 1993). With such a prevalence rate, it is expected that most infants who fail the screening will actually be showing false-positive results. Newborn hearing screening programs that use procedures with good sensitivity and specificity typically have estimated high predictive values for pass results and low predictive values for refer results.

Efficiency refers to the overall accuracy of the screening test results. It gives the percent of all results that are correct, whether pass or refer. Efficiency was very high (94%) in the example.

To determine accurately a given test's performance characteristics, it would be necessary to verify at a later time if the screening results were correct. One would need to evaluate diagnostically all individuals screened to determine the correct number of true-positive, false-positive, false-negative, and true-negative results. In the case of newborn hearing screening, programs attempt to provide follow-up testing for referred infants but rarely conduct follow-up on the large number of infants who pass the screening. It is usually assumed that pass infants are showing true-negative results unless otherwise shown to have hearing loss. In the case of referred infants, programs typically are not able to achieve 100% follow-up. For these reasons, the performance characteristics for newborn hearing screening are often based on a combination of the screening's results and generally accepted prevalence data.

Current Screening Methods

A significant factor in the widespread acceptance of newborn hearing screening has been the development of valid, rapid screening methods. At the present time, three approaches are widely used in newborn hearing screening, often in combination. These include the high-risk register, ABR, and EOAE.

HIGH-RISK REGISTER

The appeal of a high-risk register (HRR) is that it reduces the number of infants who need screening and/or follow-up by theoretically targeting those infants who are most likely to have hearing loss. Moderate to profound hearing loss is estimated to occur in 2.5 to 5% of a high-risk group, yet only approximately 10 to 12% of the newborn population have one or more risk factors (Hosford-Dunn et al., 1987; Epstein and Reilly, 1989). As already noted, the JCIH has described a list of 10 indicators associated with sensorineural and/or conductive hearing loss (Table 4.1). The ASHA guidelines for screening newborns added three indicators to that list: parent/caregiver concern regarding hearing and/or developmental delay, head trauma associated with loss of consciousness or skull fracture, and recurrent or persistent otitis media with effusion for at least 3 months (American Speech-Language-Hearing Association, 1996).

For many programs in the United States, the HRR has been a reasonable and cost-effective approach to identifying hearing loss. The disadvantage of using an HRR is that restricting the number of infants screened also reduces the number of hearing-impaired infants who are identified. Experience has shown that only approximately 50% of children identified with sensorineural hearing loss exhibit any JCIH risk factors at birth (Mauk et al., 1991). This fact alone is a strong argument for implementing universal screening whenever possible.

ABR

For more than 25 years, the ABR has played a dominant role in the evaluation of infant hearing, including newborn screening. As an electrophysiologic procedure, ABR does not directly measure hearing but does measure a process that is highly related to hearing sensitivity (i.e., function of the eighth nerve and/or auditory brainstem pathway). ABR offers the advantage of less subjective interpretation than traditional behavioral methods and the ability to detect even mild and unilateral hearing losses. Multiple studies have demonstrated its validity, reliability, and predictive efficiency in identifying infant hearing loss (Schulman-Galambos and Galambos, 1979; Galambos et al., 1982).

Despite its good performance, ABR also presents some limitations for newborn screening. Conventional ABR involves relatively long test times and is costly to implement due to equipment expenses and the need for trained clinicians. The recent development of screening equipment for ABR, especially automated equipment, has addressed these concerns. The most widely used automated ABR screener, the ALGO (Natus Medical, San Carlos, CA), can be used by a variety of personnel and features built-in artifact rejection that halts data collection if testing conditions are unfavorable. The electrodes and earphones are designed for easy application, and a pass or refer result is automatically provided at the end of each test. Table 4.3 summarizes the major advantages and other considerations related to the use of automated ABR (AABR).

Herrmann et al. (1995) summarized performance data on an early version of the ALGO. Combined data from several studies that compared ALGO to conventional ABR showed the specificity of the ALGO to be 96% and the sensitivity 98%. The AABR method has continued to perform well when used in large universal screening programs. Mason and Herrmann (1998) reported results for more than 10,000 infants screened over a 5-year period. Fifteen infants were identified with bilateral hearing loss, ranging from mild to profound. Specificity was estimated at 96%. Mehl and Thomson (1998) described a state-wide program in Colorado that relied primarily on AABR to screen more than 40,000 newborns. Sensitivity was at or near 100%, and specificity was approximately 94%. Positive predictive value, which ranged between 5 and 19% depending on the hospital, ex-

ceeded the values for most other newborn genetic screenings in the state.

With the current momentum toward universal newborn hearing screening, it is expected that AABR technology will continue to improve. Manufacturers are working toward low-cost, user-friendly devices that combine AABR and EOAE capabilities. More detailed information about AABR devices is available at the Web site for the National Center for Hearing Assessment and Management, which is listed in Table 4.4.

EOAE

Otoacoustic emissions are sounds recorded in the ear canal that are associated with normal cochlear function. They do not measure hearing sensitivity directly, but their presence is highly related to normal cochlear function. Although they may occur spontaneously, the most common clinical application is to measure the emissions in response to an evoking stimulus. Transient evoked otoacoustic emissions (TEOAE), which occur after the presentation of a brief stimulus like a click, typically are measured if auditory thresholds do not exceed 30 dB HL. Distortion product otoacoustic emissions (DPOAE) are produced by the ear in response to two simultaneous pure tones. They are present in ears if auditory thresholds do not exceed 50 dB HL (Lonsbury-Martin and Martin, 1990).

Once clinical instrumentation was developed, it did not take long for EOAE to become as valued as ABR in the evaluation of infants, including in newborn hearing screening. The Rhode Island Hearing Assessment Project (RIHAP) was the first large-scale clinical study designed to evaluate the feasibility, validity, and cost-efficiency of using TEOAE in universal newborn hearing screening (White et al., 1993). The study's initial report on 1850 screened infants indicated excellent sensitivity, in that 11 infants were identified with sensorineural hearing loss and 37 infants with persistent fluctuating conductive hearing losses. Of concern, however, was the procedure's unacceptably high fail rate of 27%. Nonetheless, the researchers concluded that TEOAE screening was simple, fast, econom-

Table 4.3
Some advantages and other considerations for two newborn hearing screening methods

Screening Method	Advantages	Other Considerations
Automated ABR	Very good sensitivity and specificity for mild to profound losses	
	Does not require personnel highly skilled in audiologic assessment	Costs associated with disposables
	Short training period	
	Procedure is quick	Procedure requires patient preparation time
	Objective analysis of results	Auditory information is partially frequency specific
	Noninvasive	
	Usually has safeguards for acoustic and electrical interference	Requires the infant to be in a quiet test state
	Not affected by minimal middle ear influences	May be influenced by neuromaturational factors or neurologic abnormalities
Otoacoustic emissions	Automated technology is becoming available	
	Very good sensitivity for mild to profound losses	Some studies have initially high failure rates
	May not require personnel highly trained in audiologic assessment	Proper placement of insert in the ear canal is essential
	Procedure is quick	
	Provides frequency information	
	Low supply costs	
	Not affected by electrical interference	Affected by acoustic interference (ambient noise)
	Not affected by neuro-maturational influences or neurologic abnormalities	May be affected by minimal middle ear influences

Adapted from (1) Mauk GW, Behrens TR. Historical, political, and technological context associated with early identification of hearing loss. *Semin Hear* 1993;14:1–17. (2) Stach BA, Santilli CL. Technology in newborn hearing screening. *Semin Hear* 1998;19:247–262. (3) Illinois Newborn and Infant Hearing Screening Work Group, personal communication, 1998.

ical, noninvasive, and accurate. The RIHAP data influenced the development of the 1993 NIH Consensus Statement that recommended the combined use of TEOAE (high sensitivity) with ABR (high specificity) in a two-tiered screening process. Since that time, better performance characteristics for TEOAE have been reported due to improvements in test technique and modifications in equipment and software (Maxon et al., 1995). In 1998, Vohr et al. reported TEOAE results for more than 50,000 infants screened in Rhode Island over a 4-year period. Sensitivity continued to be high (95%), while the fail rate on initial screening improved to 10%.

Several manufacturers have equipment available for measurement of TEOAE and DPOAE. Screening devices have become more user-friendly with the development of better-fitting ear probes and even hand-held units. Just as with ABR, the incorporation of automated procedures into EOAE equipment is enabling more widespread use. Additional information about EOAE equip-

Table 4.4
Selected Web sites that provide information and links about newborn hearing screening

Site	Address	Content
American Academy of Audiology	www.audiology.com	Professional resources, position statements
American Speech-Language-Hearing Association	www.asha.org	Professional resources, position statements
Centers for Disease Control and Prevention	www.CDC.GOV/nceh/programs/CDDH/ehdi.htm	Monthly teleconferences of the Ad Hoc Group for Early Hearing Detection and Intervention; links to other newborn hearing screening and impairment resources
Marion Downs National Center for Infant Hearing	www.Colorado.EDU/slhs/mdnc/	Includes program goals, technologies, state programs, upcoming events
National Center for Hearing Assessment and Management (NCHAM)	www.usu.edu/~ncham/	Information about NCHAM, equipment, HI-TRACK software, *Sound Ideas,* and other topics
O.Z. Systems	www.oz-systems.com/	Patient management services for universal newborn hearing screening; includes SIMS software

ment can be found at the National Center for Hearing Assessment and Management Web site listed in Table 4.4.

The EOAE method offers several advantages and some limitations for neonatal screening (Table 4.3). The responses can be measured objectively, enabling the development of automated procedures. Compared with AABR, there is little or no time spent in preparing the infant, and the test itself can be completed quickly. In addition, there are no expenses associated with electrodes and other disposables. On the other hand, it can be difficult to obtain EOAE in the nursery setting because of high ambient noise levels. Two conditions that often occur in newborns, debris in the ear canal or the presence of a nonpatent ear canal, can obscure measurement of the EOAE. These limitations can result in high fail rates.

Elements of Effective Screening Programs

Successful newborn hearing screening programs, whether local or statewide, re-quire careful planning and continuous monitoring. Goals and desired outcomes should be specified clearly so that appropriate screening and follow-up protocols can be designed. Fortunately, as newborn hearing screening has become more widespread, there is a growing base of experience from which to learn. The following sections consider issues related to screening goals, protocols, performance criteria, and data management and follow-up.

GOALS OF NEWBORN HEARING SCREENING

All newborn hearing screening programs strive to identify hearing loss early, but specific goals for programs may vary. For example, one program may work to identify all congenital sensorineural hearing loss, whereas another may aim to identify sensorineural and conductive loss. The JCIH draft statement for the year 2000 targeted permanent unilateral or bilateral hearing loss, averaging 30 dB HL or more in the frequency region important for speech recognition (approximately 500 through 4000

Hz). Both conductive and sensorineural hearing losses were included (American Speech-Language-Hearing Association, 1999). The ASHA guidelines urged the identification of hearing loss greater than 20 dB HL and included unilateral or bilateral sensorineural and/or conductive loss (American Speech-Language-Hearing Association, 1996). The recent statement of the AAP (1999) recommended identification of bilateral hearing impairment greater than 35 dB HL.

A program's goals are influenced by the availability of resources. If personnel, time, equipment, and follow-up services are sufficient, then a program can more easily choose to screen universally for various types and degrees of hearing loss. On the other hand, if resources are limited the program must carefully weigh issues such as degree of hearing loss or high-risk versus universal screening. In some cases, identification of mild and unilateral hearing loss may be of less concern to ensure that resources are available for more serious hearing losses (Mason and Herrmann, 1998). Because attempts to identify all auditory problems, no matter how minimal, would be costly and unrealistic, most programs focus on identifying losses that have serious effects and for which treatment is available (Stach and Santilli, 1998).

SCREENING PROTOCOLS

Successful screening programs use a variety of different protocols and equipment. Screening tests are used singly or in combination, by persons with different types of training and experience, at different times of the day or night, and in different locations in the hospital (White, 1998). There is no one "best" protocol. Rather, the program must design a protocol that is most suitable in relation to its goals, resources, and the characteristics of the newborn population to be screened. Most importantly, the program should consistently monitor outcomes in terms of pass/fail rates, follow-up success, number of infants identified with hearing loss, and costs. If outcomes are not satisfactory, protocols should be reviewed and modified. As more states begin universal screening and larger databases are available, it is becoming easier for programs to obtain benchmarks for their performances.

The process we used at our hospital to determine the screening method in the neonatal intensive care unit (NICU) is an example of developing a protocol that is appropriate for a given population and environment. As a Level III Perinatal Center, our hospital cares for some of the sickest and most fragile newborns in the state. Hearing screening was initiated in our NICU more than 25 years ago. Beginning with behavioral screening methods, the program has progressively used the Crib-o-gram, conventional ABR, and most recently AABR. We wanted to consider use of TEOAE, because that method could potentially provide time and cost savings if the pass/refer results were similar to what we obtained by AABR. At the time, many published reports on TEOAE methods were based on well-baby populations or on infants who had been screened under controlled acoustic environments. In contrast, our infants are medically involved and moving them from the NICU to a quieter screening environment was not an option.

To evaluate the potential effects of changing our screening method, 64 infants (128 ears) who had passed the screening by AABR (ALGO-2, Natus Medical) were also screened by TEOAE (Meyer et al., 1998). This group of newborns had a mean birth weight of 1398 g, average gestational age of 30 weeks, and average postconceptional age (at time of screening) of 35 weeks. The ILO-92 (ILO Otodynamic Analyzer, Institute for Laryngology and Otology, London, England) was used to obtain TEOAE at four frequency regions: 1600 Hz, 2400 Hz, 3200 Hz, and 4000 Hz. Using the Quick Screen Option, a TEOAE response was defined as $\geq$50% reproducibility and $\geq$3 dB S/N. Just as with AABR, the infants were screened in open cribs while resting quietly or in natural sleep. Ambient noise was reduced as much as possible by turning off audio alarms, removing nearby equipment, and asking caretakers to speak and work quietly.

The most striking result was that 30 ears

(23%) had no measured TEOAE at any frequency region even though they had passed the AABR screening. For those ears that did have TEOAE, the pattern of response was examined in an effort to identify an efficient pass/refer criterion. Figure 4.1 shows the number of ears with a TEOAE response at each frequency region. Responses were present most often in the higher frequency regions (i.e., 2400, 3200, and 4000 Hz). The lower number of measured responses at 1600 Hz probably reflected the effects of low-frequency and mid-frequency ambient noise because the infants were screened in open cribs in the NICU setting. Figure 4.2 illustrates how the number of ears that passed the screening changed as the pass/refer criterion was altered. The criterion was varied according to the number of frequency regions at which a response was present. A response was present at one or more frequency regions, two or more, three or more, or at all four frequency regions. Even with the most lax criterion (i.e., ≥1 frequency), only 64% of these infants (82 of 128) would have passed the TEOAE screening.

The last parameter examined was the noise level in the infants' ear canals, as measured by the ILO at the time of screening. Compared with an ideal level of <40 dB SPL (Culpepper, 1997), the mean level measured in our infants was 42 dB SPL.

Based on this experience, we concluded that the TEOAE procedure would result in an unacceptably high fail rate in our NICU

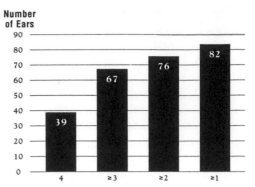

Figure 4.2. Number of infant ears in which a transient evoked otoacoustic emission (TOAE) response was present as a function of the number of frequency regions. A response was present at one or more frequency regions, two or more, three or more, or at all four frequency regions (n = 128 ears)

setting. The infants have multiple risk factors and are difficult to test, and noise levels from both the infants and the environment are relatively high. At the present time, we continue to use AABR as the preferred method in the NICU. Our experience underscores the point that the performance of screening tests will likely vary under different clinical conditions and that protocols require careful consideration of multiple factors. Well-baby nurseries and NICUs certainly present different conditions for screening. Even among NICUs, infant characteristics and test conditions may differ quite a bit from one hospital to another.

The National Institute on Deafness and Other Communication Disorders has addressed the complex question of protocols by funding a large, multicenter, collaborative project to evaluate EOAE and ABR in neonatal screening and to validate each procedure's accuracy by behavioral audiometry (Norton, 1997). The core site is Children's Hospital Medical Center and the University of Washington in Seattle. These data should help in understanding the variety of factors that influence test performance and in developing protocols with known performance characteristics for a given population and for a given degree of hearing loss.

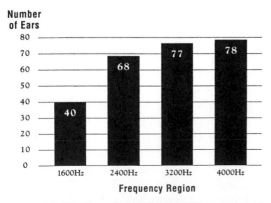

Figure 4.1. Number of infant ears with a transient evoked otoacoustic emission (TOAE) as a function of frequency region (n = 128 ears).

PERFORMANCE CRITERIA

A newborn hearing screening program is evaluated by its outcomes. As pointed out earlier, an effective program uses screening methods with high sensitivity and specificity. It achieves good follow-up of infants who are referred for further testing, and the number of infants identified is in keeping with prevalence data. The AAP (1999) has proposed goals that effective programs should screen ≥95% of newborns, maintain a false-positive rate of ≤3%, achieve 100% follow-up of referred infants, and ideally have a false-negative rate of 0.

Recent published studies, based on large-scale screenings, are valuable in understanding the results that programs should expect. Table 4.5 summarizes some reported data on percentage of newborns screened, refer rate, follow-up percentage, and number of infants identified. The data show some variability, but it appears reasonable to expect experienced programs to screen at least 90% of births, to maintain low follow-up rates, and to achieve follow-up testing on at least half of the infants referred.

Evaluating the performance of screening programs is approached as a quality issue in Texas (Albright and Finitzo, 1997). In the Sounds of Texas Project, four quality indicators are monitored: (1) the percentage of newborns screened before discharge, (2) the percentage of newborns who fail the birth admission screen, (3) the percentage who return for rescreening as outpatients and the follow-up rate, and (4) the identification or incidence of newborns with hearing loss. Established programs in that state are expected to screen 95% of the newborns, and failure rate targets have been set at <9% for TEOAE and ≤5% for AABR.

Tharpe and Clayton (1997) advised that screening programs can improve performance and reduce errors by establishing and following clear guidelines for quality assurance. Policies and procedures should be developed to minimize the possibility of missed cases, inadequate follow-up, and other potential problems. Programs that perform well are extremely beneficial. Poorly performing programs discredit themselves and may be vulnerable to litigation.

DATA MANAGEMENT AND FOLLOW-UP

With more hospitals and states becoming involved in newborn hearing screening, the need for effective information management has become increasingly apparent. Identifying information, screening results, and often

Table 4.5
Results from some large scale newborn hearing screening programs

Study	No. Screened (% of births)	Method	Initial Refer (%)	Follow-Up (%)	No. Identified
Finitzo et al. (1998)	52,508 (96.8%)	Screening ABR or EOAE or both	3.4	68.5	113
Mason and Herrmann (1998)	10,372 (96.3%)	AABR	4	90	15
Prieve (1997)	25,200 (94.7%)	TEOAE followed by AABR	2–7	61	46
		TEOAE	5–7		
Thomson (1997)	50,066 (81%)	AABR	≤3	48	133
		OAE	7–15		
		OAE followed by AABR	1		
Vohr et al. (1998)	52,659 (99%)	TEOAE or TEOAE followed by screening ABR	10	85	111

risk factors must be maintained for all infants screened, and follow-up data must be recorded for referred infants. As the number of screened infants increases, the challenge of organizing and accessing this informa-tion grows. Some conditions even confound good data collection, such as when the infant's name and/or address change after discharge from the hospital or when the infant lives too far to return to the original site for follow-up.

With the help of carefully collected and organized data, it is possible to improve and evaluate the effectiveness of programs on a local, state, and national level. Even simple measures such as pass/refer rates and follow-up rates rely on careful records and ease of data retrieval. The JCIH (American Academy of Pediatrics, 1995) and DSH-PSHWA (1998) have stressed the need for a uniform state and national database and for development of an infant tracking system. An organized tracking system will help ensure that newborns identified with or as at risk for hearing loss have access to evaluation, follow-up, and intervention services. Such a system could help locate and identify local services for an infant who is seemingly "lost" because the family has relocated to another area. Fortunately, several commercial and customized information management systems exist for newborn hearing screening, and others will undoubtedly be developed as universal screening becomes more widespread (Finitzo and Diefendorf, 1997).

If the goal of early identification and intervention is to be met, referred infants must receive prompt follow-up testing and management. In many cases, however, the link between screening programs and coordinated follow-up services is weak. Strickland and McPherson (1998) point out that often the very network of services to which infants and families are referred presents barriers such as insufficient insurance coverage, lack of transportation, inadequate child care, limited office hours, and difficult-to-find services. They urge that fragmentation and duplication of services be reduced and that newborn hearing screening programs nationwide be integrated with the community system of services.

Because such statewide follow-up systems are not yet available, individual screening programs must design their own follow-up protocols. Initially, the process appears to be straightforward. One must inform families about the screening results, explain the need for further testing, arrange follow-up appointment(s), and refer patients to appropriate intervention programs. In reality, several factors can and do complicate the process, including changes in the infant's name and address, lack of family understanding about the importance of follow-up, and costs for additional tests. Considerable effort, requiring both time and personnel, is needed to schedule and coordinate return appointments, to locate infants who become "lost," and to work with noncompliant families.

One of the most important strategies a program can use to help with follow-up is monitoring and improving its refer rate. It is obvious that the higher the refer rate, the greater the number of infants who will need to be followed. The challenge is to minimize the number of infants who are referred, most of whom will have normal hearing, while maintaining the screening's sensitivity. Rescreening before hospital discharge and changes in screening protocols and methodology often help to reduce the refer rate. By using such methods, hospitals in Colorado reduced the overall state average of 6% refer rate to 3% or less (Thomson et al., 1998).

Follow-up percentage refers to the percentage of infants who are successfully followed until diagnostic testing (Turner, 1991). With a higher follow-up percentage, more infants receive diagnostic testing and more hearing-impaired infants are identified. Follow-up percentage varies substantially across programs, presumably due to local demographics and the availability of resources. For example, the initial screening program in Rhode Island benefited from the fact that 70% of the births were at a single hospital and that more than 90% of patients lived within 40 miles of the hospital (Johnson et al., 1993). With the help of a computer-based tracking system, the program successfully followed 94% of screening failures. On the other hand, Colorado experienced a 48% return percentage and implemented such measures as transportation assistance and physician/hospital staff education to improve the follow-up rate (Thomson, 1997). Programs may also face unique circumstances that can affect follow-up. Some hospital programs in New York state have needed separate contracts for each county with which they interface because early intervention programs were run by individual counties (Prieve, 1997). Hospital programs in Illinois, which is just beginning to fund newborn hearing screening, must work with two agencies to coordinate follow-up services, the Illinois Department of Public Health and the University of Illinois at Chicago Division for Specialized Care for Children.

Each screening program faces situations unique to its location and population, making it imperative that the availability of follow-up and intervention services be evaluated before screening is initiated (Tharpe and Clayton, 1997). Good follow-up requires as much, if not more, planning than the actual screening itself.

Status of Newborn Hearing Screening in the United States

Some of the most current information about the status of newborn hearing screening and related issues can be found at various Web sites. The sites included in Table 4.4 are not exhaustive but do provide information and data from each organization's own perspective as well as important links to other organizations. They are a valuable source of updated information for those involved in newborn hearing screening.

The number of newborn hearing screening programs is increasing so rapidly that it is difficult to know the exact number. Since 1990, many states have mandated universal newborn hearing screening and several others have pending legislation. Other states have mandates to provide a system of newborn screening, often based on high-risk registries. Typically, these mandates vary in their requirements and are often implemented on a voluntary basis. Still other

states have initiated activities without legislation, such as training and consultation, financial sponsorship of pilot projects, development of written materials about hearing loss, and data management (Penn and Abbott, 1997).

As of 1998, approximately 20% of infants nationwide were screened for hearing loss before hospital discharge (White, 1998). As more hospitals initiate screening programs, especially smaller hospitals, there will be a need for financial, personnel, and technical assistance. One valuable resource for hospitals is the National Center for Hearing Assessment and Management (NCHAM), established at Utah State University (Table 4.4). This funded center conducts research, develops training materials, provides training and technical assistance, and disseminates information about early identification and management of hearing impairment. Since 1995, NCHAM has helped numerous hospitals initiate universal newborn hearing screening programs.

The challenge of providing appropriate follow-up and intervention has become increasingly evident as the amount of screening activity has increased. The Marion Downs National Center for Infant Hearing has undertaken an impressive effort to implement universal newborn hearing screening and coordinate follow-up in 17 states (Table 4.4). Established by a grant from the U.S. Public Health Service to the University of Colorado at Boulder, this project seeks to establish universal hearing screening (85% of births) in the 17 states by the year 2000. Among the Center's goals are the identification of hearing loss by 3 months of age, provision of amplification as early as possible, and intervention services by 6 months of age. In addition, the Center plans to measure the effect of early identification of deafness and hearing loss on development.

The issue of reimbursement is one of the most critical issues challenging the continued growth of universal newborn hearing screening. With the emergence of managed care in the United States, major emphasis has been placed on cost-containment in health care. Strickland and McPherson (1998) stress that newborn hearing screening must be seen by managed care companies as a valuable benefit that will contribute to the child's health and well-being as well as avoid future costs. If newborn hearing screening and follow-up are not included as benefits, it may be difficult for screening programs to be sustained. Programs may need to be creative in seeking other methods of support.

Another challenge relates to the establishment of programs in small and rural hospitals in which audiologic services may not be available. These hospitals need support and information to begin hearing screening and to link with diagnostic and management centers.

Conclusion

In many ways, the issue of early identification of infant hearing loss is an example of the adage, "Good things come to those who wait." It has taken more than 30 years to reach the right combination of events and circumstances that enable the implementation of newborn hearing screening in the United States. To quote another saying, we must now "keep the ball rolling." Additional states must begin screening, improved tracking methods must be developed, and follow-up services must be easily accessed. The challenge of early identification will not be met effectively until all newborns are routinely screened for hearing loss.

REFERENCES

Albright K, Finitzo T. Texas hospitals' quality control approach to universal infant hearing detection. In: Finitzo T, Roizen N, Sininger Y, eds. Joint Committee on Infant Hearing forum. Am J Audiol 1997;6(Suppl):88–90.

American Academy of Audiology. Early identification of hearing loss in infants and children. URL: www.audiology.com/infant/aaaposstminfant.htm. 1998.

American Academy of Audiology. Use of support personnel for newborn hearing screening (proposed guidelines). Audiol Today 1998;(Special Issue):21–23.

American Academy of Pediatrics. Joint Committee on Infant Hearing 1994 position statement. Pediatrics 1995;95:152–156.

American Academy of Pediatrics. Newborn and infant hearing loss: detection and intervention. Pediatrics 1999;103:527–530.

American Speech-Language-Hearing Association. Draft Joint Committee on Infant Hearing year 2000 position statement. Rockville, MD, 1999.

American Speech-Language-Hearing Association. Position statement on prevention of communication disorders. ASHA 1988;30:61.

American Speech-Language-Hearing Association. The prevention of communication disorders tutorial. ASHA 1991;33(Suppl 6):15–41.

American Speech-Language-Hearing Association. Guidelines for audiologic screening. Rockville, MD: ASHA, 1996.

Bennett MJ. Trials with the auditory response cradle: I. neonatal responses to auditory stimuli. Br J Audiol 1979;13:125–134.

Bess FH, Paradise JL. Universal screening for infant hearing: not simple, not risk-free, not necessarily beneficial, and not presently justified. Pediatrics 1994;98:330–334.

Brackett D, Maxon AB, Blackwell PM. Intervention issues created by successful universal newborn hearing screening. Semin Hear 1993;14:88–104.

Culpepper NB. Neonatal screening via evoked otoacoustic emissions. In: Robinette MS, Glattke TJ, eds. Otoacoustic emissions. New York: Thieme, 1997.

Diefendorf AO, Finitzo T. Foreword to the 1996 invited forum. In: Finitzo T, Roizen N, Sininger Y, eds. Joint Committee on Infant Hearing forum. Am J Audiol 1997;6(Suppl):70.

Directors of Speech and Hearing Programs in State Health and Welfare Agencies. 1996 position statement universal hearing detection. URL: http://www.audiology.com/infant/200017.16dshpshwa.htm. 1998.

Downs MP, Hemenway WG. Report on the hearing screening of 17,000 neonates. Int Audiol 1969;8:72–76.

Epstein S, Reilly JS. Sensorineural hearing loss. Pediatr Clin North Am 1989;36:1501–1519.

Finitzo T, Diefendorf AO. The state of the information. In: Finitzo T, Roizen N, Sininger Y, eds. Joint Committee on Infant Hearing forum. Am J Audiol 1997;6(Suppl):91–94.

Finitzo T, Albright K, O'Neal J. The newborn with hearing loss: detection in the nursery. Pediatrics 1998;102:1452–1460.

Galambos R, Hicks G, Wilson M. Hearing loss in graduates of a tertiary intensive care nursery. Ear Hear 1982;3:87–90.

Herrmann BS, Thornton AR, Joseph JM. Automated infant hearing screening using the ABR: development and validation. Am J Audiol 1995;4:6–14.

Hosford-Dunn H, Johnson S, Simmons B, et al. Infant hearing screening: program implementation and validation. Ear Hear 1987;8:12–20.

Jerger S. Decision matrix and information theory analyses in the evaluation of neuroaudiologic tests. Semin Hear 1983;4:121–132.

Johnson MJ, Maxon AB, White KR, et al. Operating a hospital-based universal newborn hearing screening program using transient evoked otoacoustic emissions. Semin Hear 1993;14:46–56.

Joint Committee on Infant Hearing. 1990 position statement. ASHA 1991;33(Suppl 5):3–6.

Lonsbury-Martin BL, Martin GK. The clinical utility of distortion-product otoacoustic emissions. Ear Hear 1990;11:144–154.

Mason JA, Herrmann KR. Universal infant hearing screening by automated auditory brainstem response measurement. Pediatrics 1998;101:221–228.

Mauk G, White KR, Mortensen LB, et al. The effectiveness of screening programs based on high-risk characteristics in early identification of hearing impairment. Ear Hear 1991;12:312–319.

Maxon AB, White KR, Behrens TR, et al. Referral rates and cost efficiency in a universal newborn hearing screening program using transient evoked otoacoustic emissions. J Am Acad Audiol 1995;6:271–277.

Mehl AL, Thomson V. Newborn hearing screening: the great omission. Pediatrics 1998;101:1–6.

Meyer DH, Austin K, Turetgen D. Selected factors that may influence TOAE screening outcomes. Poster session presented to annual convention of the American Academy of Audiology, Los Angeles, 1998.

National Institutes of Health. Early identification of hearing impairment in infants and young children. NIH Consensus Statement 1993;11:1–24.

Northern JL, Downs MP. Hearing in children. 4th ed. Baltimore: Williams & Wilkins, 1991.

Northern JL, Hayes D. Universal screening for infant hearing impairment: necessary, beneficial, and justifiable. Audiol Today 1994;6:10–13.

Norton S. The researcher's perspective on newborn hearing screening. In: Finitzo T, Roizen N, Sininger Y, eds. Joint Committee on Infant Hearing forum. Am J Audiol 1997; 6(Suppl):103–104.

Penn TO, Abbott SE. Public health and newborn hearing screening. Am J Audiol 1997;6:11–16.

Prieve BA. Establishing infant hearing programs in hospitals. In: Finitzo T, Roizen N, Sininger Y, eds. Joint Committee on Infant Hearing forum. Am J Audiol 1997; 6(Suppl):84–87.

Schulman-Galambos C, Galambos R. Brainstem evoked response audiometry in newborn hearing screening. Arch Otolaryngol 1979;105:86–90.

Simmons FB, Russ FN. Automated newborn hearing screening, the Crib-o-gram. Arch Otolaryngol 1974;100:1–7.

Stach BA, Santilli CL. Technology in newborn hearing screening. Semin Hear 1998;19:247–262.

Strickland B, McPherson M. Universal newborn hearing screening: a national goal. Semin Hear 1998;19:301–314.

Tharpe AM, Clayton EW. Newborn hearing screening: issues in legal liability and quality assurance. Am J Audiol 1997;6:5–12.

Thomson V. The Colorado newborn hearing screening project. In: Finitzo T, Roizen N, Sininger Y, eds. Joint Committee on Infant Hearing forum. Am J Audiol 1997; 6(Suppl):74–77.

Thomson V, Rose LB, O'Neal J, et al. Statewide implementation of universal newborn hearing screening. Semin Hear 1998;19:287–300.

Turner RG. Modeling the cost and performance of early identification protocols. J Am Acad Audiol 1991;2:195–205.

Turner RG, Nielsen DW. Application of clinical decision analysis to audiological tests. Ear Hear 1984;5:125–133.

U.S. Department of Health and Human Services. Healthy people 2000. Washington, DC: U.S. Government Printing Office, 1990.

U.S. Department of Health and Human Services. Healthy people 2010 objectives: draft for public comment. Washington, DC: U.S. Government Printing Office, 1998.

U.S. Department of Health, Education and Welfare. Healthy people: the Surgeon General's report on health promotion and disease prevention. Washington, DC: U.S. Government Printing Office, 1979.

Vohr BR, Carty LM, Moore PE, et al. The Rhode Island Hearing Assessment program: experience with statewide hearing screening (1993–1996). J Pediatr 1998;133: 353–357.

White KR. Five years after the NIH consensus conference. Sound ideas, 2, 2. Logan, UT: National Center for Hearing Assessment and Management, 1998.

White KR, Vohr BR, Behrens TR. Universal newborn hearing screening using transient evoked otoacoustic emissions: results of the Rhode Island Hearing Assessment project. Semin Hear 1993;14:18–29.

APPENDIX 4.1 American Academy of Pediatrics Task Force on Newborn and Infant Hearing Newborn and Infant Hearing Loss: Detection and Intervention[1]

Abstract

This statement endorses the implementation of universal newborn hearing screening. In addition, the statement reviews the primary objectives, important components, and recommended screening parameters that characterize an effective universal newborn hearing screening program.

Abbreviations

UNHSP, universal newborn hearing screening program; EOAE evoked otoacoustic emissions; ABR, auditory brainstem response; CDC, Centers for Disease Control and Prevention.

Significant hearing loss is one of the most common major abnormalities present at birth and, if undetected, will impede speech, language, and cognitive development.[1–7] Significant bilateral hearing loss is present in ~1 to 3 per 1000 newborn infants in the well-baby nursery population, and in ~2 to 4 per 100 infants in the intensive care unit population. Currently, the average age of detection of significant hearing loss is ~14 months. The American Academy of Pediatrics supports the statement of the Joint Committee on Infant Hearing (1994), which endorses the goal of universal detection of hearing loss in infants before 3 months of age, with appropriate intervention no later than 6 months of age.[8] Universal detection of infant hearing loss requires universal screening of all infants. Screening by high-risk registry alone (eg, family history of deafness) can only identify ~50% of newborns with significant congenital hearing loss.[9,10] Reliance on physician observation and/or parental recognition has not been successful in the past in detecting significant hearing loss in the first year of life.

To justify universal screening at least five criteria must be met:

1. An easy-to-use test that possesses a high degree of sensitivity and specificity to minimize referral for additional assessment is available.
2. The condition being screened for is otherwise not detectable by clinical parameters.
3. Interventions are available to correct the conditions detected by screening.
4. Early screening, detection, and intervention result in improved outcome.
5. The screening program is documented to be in an acceptable cost-effective range.[11,12]

Although additional studies are necessary, review of both published and unpublished data indicates that all five of these criteria currently are achievable by effective universal newborn hearing screening programs (UNHSP).[5,13,15–28] Therefore, this statement endorses the implementation of universal newborn hearing screening. In addition, this statement reviews the primary objectives, important components, and recommended screening parameters that characterize an effective UNHSP.

The Academy recognizes that there are five essential elements to an effective UNHSP; initial screening, tracking and follow-up, identification, intervention, and evaluation.[13,14] The child's physician and parents, working in partnership, make up the child's medical home and play an important role in each of these elements of a UNHSP.[29]

---

[1]The recommendations in this statement do not indicate an exclusive course of treatment or serve as a standard of medical care. Variations, taking into account individual circumstances, may be appropriate. Reprinted from PEDIATRICS (ISSN 0031 4005). Copyright © 1999 by the American Academy of Pediatrics.

Screening[11,13,14]

The following are guidelines for the screening element of a UNHSP:

- Universal screening has as its goal that 100% of the target population, consisting of all newborns, will be tested using physiologic measures in both ears. A minimum of 95% of newborns must be screened successfully for it to be considered effective.[16,19,21]
- The methodology should detect, at a minimum, all infants with significant bilateral hearing impairment, ie, those with hearing loss ≥35-decibel in the better ear.[1,6,19]
- The methodology used in screening should have a false-positive rate, ie, the proportion of infants without hearing loss who are labeled incorrectly by the screening process as having significant hearing loss, of ≤3%. The referral rate for formal audiologic testing after screening should not exceed 4%.[16,17,19–21]
- The methodology used in screening ideally should have a false-negative rate, ie, the proportion of infants with significant hearing loss missed by the screening program, of zero.[21,23]
- Until a specific screening method(s) is proved to be superior, the Academy defers recommendation as to a preferred method. Currently, acceptable methodologies for physiologic screening include evoked otoacoustic emissions (EOAE) and auditory brainstem response (ABR), either alone or in combination. Both methodologies are noninvasive, quick (<5 minutes), and easy to perform, although each assesses hearing differently. EOAE measures sound waves generated in the inner ear (cochlea) in response to clicks or tone bursts emitted and recorded via miniature microphones placed in the external ear canals of the infant. Although EOAE screening is even quicker and easier to perform than ABR, EOAE may be affected by debris or fluid in the external and middle ear, resulting in referral rates of 5% to 20% when screening is performed during the first 24 hours after birth. ABR measures the electroencephalographic waves generated in response to clicks via three electrodes pasted to the infant's scalp. ABR screening requires the infant to be in a quiet state, but it is not affected by middle or external ear debris. Referral rates <3% may be achieved when screening is performed during the first 24 to 48 hours after birth. Referral rates <4% are generally achievable with EOAE combined with automated ABR in a two-step screening system or with automated ABR alone.[16,17,19–21] In a two-step system using EOAE as the first step, referral rates of 5% to 20% for repeat screening with ABR or EOAE may be expected. The second screening may be performed before discharge or on an outpatient basis within 1 month of age. Screening should be conducted before discharge from the hospital whenever possible.
- Each birthing hospital should establish a UNHSP with a designated medical (physician) director and sufficient staff to perform the following:

1. Develop the screening protocol and select the screening method(s).
2. Provide appropriate training and monitoring of the performance of staff responsible for performing hearing screening.
3. Provide the parents or guardians information concerning the screening procedure, costs, potential risks of hearing loss, and the benefits of early detection and intervention.
4. Establish a system that ensures confidentiality and allows the parents or guardians the opportunity to decline hearing screening. In most institutions, general hospital consent obtained at time of admission is considered to be inclusive of routine care, such as newborn hearing screening.
5. Ensure that all individuals performing hearing screening are trained properly in the performance of the tests, the risks including psychological stress for the parents, infection control practices, and the general care and handling of infants in hospital settings according to established hospital policies and procedures.[30]

6. Establish clear guidelines for responsibility of documenting the results of the screening procedure.
7. Develop mechanisms for communicating results of screening in a sensitive and timely manner to the parents and the child's physician(s). If repeat screening is necessary after discharge from the hospital, ensure that appropriate follow-up is provided.
8. Work with local, state, and national monitoring systems to identify all cases of significant hearing loss occurring in infants designated initially as free of hearing impairment by the UNHSP (false-negatives).
9. Secure funding for the program. Funding through third-party reimbursement is essential to cover the costs of the UNHSP, including the initial screen(s), as well as of diagnostic and intervention services. The cost of complete screening in statewide programs ranges from ~$7 to $26 per infant screened.[13] Additional studies (some of which are ongoing) are necessary to quantify costs of tracking, diagnostic, and intervention services.[26–28]
10. Collect critical performance data to ensure that each UNHSP meets the criteria specified in this statement. These data should be reported in a regular and timely manner to a statewide central monitoring program.

Tracking and Follow-up[13–16, 26–28]

The following are guidelines for the tracking and follow-up elements of a UNHSP:

• Universal screening has as its goal that there will be 100% follow-up of all infants referred for formal audiologic assessment and for all infants not screened initially in the birthing hospital whose parents did not refuse screening. A minimum of 95% successful follow-up is required for a UNHSP to be considered an effective screening program.
• State departments of health, in coordination with programs mandated by Part C of the Individuals with Disabilities Education Act, should:

1. Establish and maintain a central monitoring system for all hearing screening programs within the state. Critical performance data, including number of infants born; the proportion of all infants screened; the referral rate; the follow-up rate; the false-positive rate; and the false-negative rate should be collected in a timely manner.
2. Establish and maintain a tracking program that monitors all referrals and misses. Monitoring should ensure that children with significant hearing loss are not missed, ie, all children designated as free of hearing loss by the UNHSP, but who are later detected to have significant hearing loss, are identified by the statewide tracking program.
3. Develop mechanisms for communicating results of follow-up activities with the parents/guardians and the child's physician(s), audiologist, and speech language therapist.[29]
4. Ensure that hearing screening is performed on all out-of-hospital births.
5. Report the screening performance parameters of individual hospital-based UNHSPs within the state in a timely manner.
6. Report critical performance data of each UNHSP (without personal identifiers) to a national Early Hearing Detection and Intervention monitoring program established by the Centers for Disease Control and Prevention (CDC).

Identification and Intervention[13–15, 26–28]

The following are guidelines for the identification and intervention element of a UNHSP:

• Universal screening has as its goal that 100% of infants with significant congenital hearing loss shall be identified by 3 months of age and shall have appropriate and necessary intervention initiated by 6 months of age.[5–7]

- Appropriate and necessary care for the infant with significant hearing loss should be directed and coordinated by the child's physician within the medical home, with support from appropriate ancillary services.[29]
- A regionalized approach to identification and intervention for infants with significant hearing loss is essential, ensuring access for all children with significant hearing loss to appropriate expert services. It is recognized that professionals with demonstrated competency to provide expert services in the identification and intervention of significant hearing loss in young infants are not available in every hospital or community. The child's physician, within the medical home, working with the state department of health must ensure that every infant with significant hearing loss is referred to the appropriate professional(s) within the regionalized system.
- It is anticipated that there will be increased demand for qualified personnel to provide age-appropriate identification and intervention services for young infants with significant hearing loss. As a result, there will be a need for the training and education of additional expert care providers.

Evaluation[13–15, 26–28]

The following are guidelines for the evaluation element of a UNHSP:

- The UNHSPs should be evaluated on an ongoing and regular basis by the state monitoring system for performance with regard to parameters enumerated in "Screening" above.
- Tracking and follow-up should be evaluated on an ongoing and regular basis by the state monitoring system, as well as through a national monitoring system to be established by the CDC.
- Intervention services should be evaluated on an ongoing and regular basis by the state department of health to ensure that sufficient expert services are available for children identified with significant hearing loss, that the services are accessible to the children in need, and that outcomes from interventions provided are effective.

Other Recommendations and Issues

The following are additional recommendations of the Academy for developing a UNHSP:

- The Academy recommends that each American Academy of Pediatrics chapter assume a leadership role in state-based efforts to promote optimal implementation of UNHSPs. Effective state-wide programs require broad-based support and collaboration. Collaboration should include (but not be limited to) appropriate professional organizations, parent advocacy groups, deaf and hard-of-hearing adults, physicians, audiologists, speech and language therapists, nurses, administrators, payers, legislators, and state departments of health and special education.
- The Academy shall identify, develop, and disseminate educational materials regarding effective hearing screening programs.[13]
- To promote additional research and the development of the needed infrastructure to provide universal newborn hearing screening, the Academy recommends the following:

1. The National Institutes of Health support ongoing research to improve the efficacy of screening, identification, and intervention.
2. The Health Resources and Services Administration promote the development of a state-based early hearing loss identification and intervention network.
3. The CDC establish and maintain a national monitoring and evaluation program for early hearing loss identification and intervention.

- Physicians should provide recommended hearing screening, not only during early infancy but also through early childhood for those children at risk for hearing loss (eg, history of trauma, meningitis) and for those demonstrating clinical signs of possible hearing loss.[9,14] Although most hearing loss in children is congenital (ie, present at birth), a significant portion of hearing loss is acquired after birth.[2-4] Regardless of the age of onset, all children with hearing loss require prompt identification and intervention by appropriate professionals with pediatric training and expertise.

TASK FORCE ON NEWBORN AND INFANT HEARING, 1998–1999

Allen Erenberg, MD
AAP Delegate to Joint Committee on Infant Hearing
James Lemons, MD
Chairperson, AAP Committee on Fetus and Newborn
Calvin Sia, MD
Chairperson, Project Advisory Committee for the Medical Home Program for Children With Special Needs
David Tunkel, MD
Chairperson, AAP Section on Otolaryngology-Bronchoesophagology
Philip Ziring, MD
Chairperson, AAP Committee on Children With Disabilities

CONSULTANTS

Mike Adams, MD
Associate Director for Program Development, Centers for Disease Control and Prevention
June Holstrum, PhD
Behavioral Scientist, Centers for Disease Control and Prevention
Merle McPherson, MD
Director, Division of Services for Children With Special Health Care Needs, Maternal and Child Health Bureau
Nigel Paneth, MD
Professor of Pediatrics and Epidemiology and Chairperson of the Department of Epidemiology at Michigan State University
Bonnie Strickland, PhD
Chief, Habilitative Services, Division of Services for Children With Special Health Care Needs, Maternal and Child Health Bureau

REFERENCES

1. Northern JL, Downs MP. *Hearing in Children.* 3rd ed. Baltimore, MD: Williams & Wilkins; 1984:89.
2. Centers for Disease Control and Prevention. Serious hearing impairment among children aged 3–10 years—Atlanta, Georgia, 1991–1993. *MMWR,* 1997, 46:1073–1076.
3. Parring A. Detection of the infant with congenital/early acquired hearing disability. *Acta Otolaryngol Suppl (Scand).* 1991;482;111–116. Discussion, p. 117.
4. Sorri M, Rantakallio P. Prevalence of hearing loss at the age of 15 in a birth cohort of 12000 children from northern Finland. *Scand Audiol.* 1985:14:203–207.
5. Yoshinaga-Itano C, Sedey AL, Coulter DK, Mehl AI. Language of early- and later-identified children with hearing loss. *Pediatrics.* 1998:102:1161–1171.
6. Robinshaw HM. Early intervention for hearing impairment. *Br J Audiol.* 1995;29:315–334.
7. Robinshaw HM. The pattern of development from non-communicative behavior to language by hearing-impaired infants. *Br J Audiol.* 1996;30:177–198.
8. AAP, Joint Committee on Infant Hearing 1994 position statement. *Pediatrics.* 1995;95:152–156.
9. Davis A, Wood S. The epidemiology of childhood hearing impairment: factors relevant to planning of services. *Br J Audiol.* 1992:26:77–90.

10. Watkin PM, Baldwin M, McEnery G. Neonatal at risk screening and the identification of deafness. *Arch Dis Child.* 1991;66:1130–1135.
11. Fletcher RH, Fletcher SW, Wagner EW. *Clinical Epidemiology: The Essentials.* 2nd ed. Baltimore, MD: Williams & Wilkins; 1988.
12. Sackett DL, Haynes RB, Tugwell J. *Clinical Epidemiology: A Basic Science for Clinical Medicine.* 2nd ed. Boston, MA: Little, Brown and Company; 1991.
13. Spivak LG, ed. *Universal Newborn Hearing Screening.* New York, NY: Thieme, 1998.
14. Davis A, Bamford J, Wilson I, Ramkalawan T, Forshaw M, Wright S. A critical review of the role of neonatal hearing screening in the detection of congenital hearing impairment. *Health Technol Assess Winch Engl.* 1997;1ii–iv, 1–176.
15. White KR. Realities, myths, and challenges of newborn hearing screening in the United States. *Am J Audiol.* 1996;6:95–99.
16. Barsky-Firsker L, Sun S. Universal newborn hearing screenings: a three-year experience. *Pediatrics.* 1997;99(6). www.pediatrics.org/egl/content/full/99/G/e4. Accessed October 8, 1998.
17. Downs MP. Universal newborn hearing screening—the Colorado story. *Int J Pediatr Otorhinolaryngol.* 1995;32:257–259.
18. Lubrum MI, Davis AC, Fortnum HM, Wood S. Field sensitivity of targeted neonatal hearing screening by transient evoked otoacoustic emissions. *Ear Hear.* 1997;18:265–276.
19. Mason JA, Herrmann KR. Universal infant hearing screening by automated auditory brainstem response measurement. *Pediatrics.* 1998;101:221–228.
20. Mehl AL, Thomson V. Newborn hearing screening: the great omission. *Pediatrics.* 1998;101(1). www.pediatrics.org/cgi/content/full/101/1/e4. Accessed October 8, 1998.
21. Vohr BR, Carty LM, Moore PE, Letourneau K. The Rhode Island Hearing Assessment Program: experience with statewide hearing screening (1993–1996). *J Pediatr.* 1998;133:353–357.
22. Watkin PM, Outcomes of neonatal screening for hearing loss by otoacoustic emission. *Arch Dis Child Fetal Neonat Educ.* 1996;75:F158–F168.
23. Watkin PM. Neonatal otoacoustic emission screening and the identification of deafness. *Arch Dis Child Fetal Neonat Educ.* 1996;74:F16–F25. Comments.
24. Windmill IM. Universal screening of infants for hearing loss: further justification. *J Pediatr.* 1998;133:318–319.
25. Johnson JL, Mauk GW, Takekawa KM, Simon PR, Sia CJ, Blackwell PM. Implementing a statewide system of services for infants and toddlers with hearing disabilities. *Semin Hearing.* 1993;14:105–119.
26. Downs MP. The case for detection and intervention at birth. *Semin Hearing.* 1994;15:76–83.
27. Stevens JC, Hall DM, Davis A, Davies CM, Dixon S. The costs of early hearing screening in England and Wales. *Arch Dis Child.* 1998;78:14–19.
28. Maxon AB, White KR, Vohr BR, Behrens TR. Using transient evoked otoacoustic emissions for neonatal hearing screening. *Br J Audiol.* 1993;27:149–153.
29. AAP. The medical home. *Pediatrics.* 1992;90:5. Statement addendum. *AAP News.* November 1993.
30. American Academy of Pediatrics/American College of Obstetricians and Gynecologists. *Guidelines for Perinatal Care.* 4th ed. Washington, DC: American Academy of Pediatrics/American College of Obstetricians and Gynecologists; 1997.

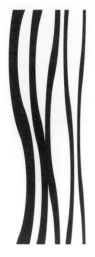

Amplification for the Hearing-Impaired Child

Ruth A. Bentler, Ph.D.

According to the Office of Demographic Studies, approximately 1 in 1000 children is born with severe or profound bilateral sensorineural hearing impairment; relative to mild or moderate hearing loss, ". . . estimates range from 6 children per 1000 to 16 per 1000, depending upon who you include" (Matkin, cited in Mahon, 1987). With improved objective measures of auditory function, the process of identification and remediation can begin with greater certainty. In fact, Ross most aptly states it: "By starting earlier, we have the opportunity to employ a developmental rather than a remedial approach to training" (1996, p. 13). Any audiologist involved with the pediatric population needs to become cognizant of the issues surrounding amplification decisions for the hearing-impaired child, whatever the age or degree of impairment. This chapter examines some of those issues.

Limited Data to Define Hearing Loss

It is often the attentive parent who gets the first clue that a newborn or young child is not responding appropriately to environmental stimuli. Nevertheless, Elssman et al. (1987) have reported that across all socioeconomic levels and degrees of hearing loss, the average age of formal identification is 19 months with a 6-month average delay before amplification. Other investigators have re-

ported similar findings (Bergstrom, 1976; Shah et al., 1978; Simmons, 1980; Benoit, 1994). Diagnostic evaluation of the very young child must be viewed as an ongoing process whereby the audiologist uses a battery of test procedures appropriate to the age and abilities of the client, including conditioned play audiometry, tangible reinforcement audiometry, and visual reinforcement audiometry (see Chapter 4 for an overview of diagnostic procedures). If, in fact, the child is too young or manifests any of a number of mental or physical limitations, a more objective approach may be needed to ascertain hearing levels.

Urgency

Northern and Downs (1991) and Ross and Seewald (1988) provide reviews of studies of sensory deprivation in animals. Findings of incomplete maturation of brainstem auditory neurons (Webster and Webster, 1977), pathologic changes in the brainstem (Evans et al., 1983), inability to resolve differences in sound patterns (Tees, 1967), and an increase in the latency of the auditory neural response and abnormal binaural interaction (Clopton and Silverman, 1977; Silverman and Clopton, 1977) provide convincing evidence of the urgency of early intervention. Although there are few human studies corroborating these findings (e.g., Dobie and Berlin, 1979), recent investigations of the effect of temporary auditory deprivation, such as can occur with prolonged otitis media in infants and young children, require consideration (Gravel and Wallace, 1992; Downs, 1995).

In addition to sensory deprivation and its physiologic consequences, the effect on language acquisition during this critical period is of great concern. Northern and Downs (1991) define the critical period as "certain period(s) in development when the organism is programmed to receive and utilize particular types of stimuli and that subsequently the stimuli will have diminishing potency in effecting the organism's development in the function represented" (p. 117). Although some controversy exists as to the exact timing of the period (Greenstein et al., 1976), most investigators pinpoint the time before age 2 as being essential to development of auditory functioning and speech/language development.

Matkin (1986) poses another potential deprivation possibility: "Does the lack of auditory input during early developmental periods have detrimental effects with respect to the hearing impaired child's psychosocial development?" (p. 172). The evidence is overwhelming that the earlier the intervention is initiated (regardless of the degree of impairment), the greater the likelihood of success. To deny an infant some amplification system due to limited audiologic information rather than approaching the entire diagnostic/rehabilitative process as an ongoing process is without merit. The advice of Ross and Lerman (1967) many years ago still holds true: ". . . denying a child a hearing aid during the critical language years may only be saving his or her hearing for no good purpose" (p. 60).

Candidacy

Any child with a significant hearing loss is a candidate for amplification. Although a number of authors have attempted to describe candidacy in terms of the degree or configuration of the hearing loss, the rules are not easily defined (e.g., Pediatric Working Group, 1996). Hearing-impaired children are a heterogeneous group, and the effects of hearing impairment on intellectual status, academic achievement, and social skills vary from child to child (Davis et al., 1986). Davis et al. (1986) have indicated that "even minimal hearing loss places children at risk for language and learning problems" (p. 53). Further, they found a concern among hearing-impaired children of all degrees and ages about being accepted by their peers (50% of the hearing-impaired group compared with 15.5% of normal-hearing children). Any hearing loss that places a child at a disadvantage in an academic, social, or (in the case of the older child) occupational setting warrants amplification consideration. Candidacy cannot be dictated a priori on the basis of thresholds.

Candidacy for the profoundly hearing-impaired child may become an issue as well. With the advent of cochlear implantation of children and vibrotactile units of multichannel design, the candidacy for a variety of amplification systems must be considered (see Chapter 15 for further discussion of cochlear implantation and vibrotactile stimulation).

One cannot discuss candidacy issues without considering the plight of the unilaterally hearing-impaired child. Incidence of monaural hearing impairment ranges from 2 per 1000 to 13 per 1000 (Bess, 1985; Oyler et al., 1988). Whether the unilateral loss is conductive or sensorineural, evidence is growing as to the potential for academic failure, lower language performance, and behavioral disorders (see entire monograph, *Ear and Hearing*, 1986;7). Auditorily, the following problems are obvious (Mueller and Hawkins, 1990):

1. Binaural summation. With two equally sensitive ears, threshold is 3 dB better than with either ear alone; relative to loudness judgments, a stimulus presented simultaneously to both ears at 40 dB sensation level (SL) will require a 46 dB SL presentation level for equal loudness when presented to either ear alone. As pointed out by Bess and Tharpe (1986), this "advantage becomes rather

substantial when one considers the effect on speech recognition." Eighteen to 30% improvement in speech recognition can be expected from binaural listening over monaural listening, depending on the stimulus used (Konkle and Schwartz, 1981).

2. Head shadow effects. Head shadow refers to the reduction in signal intensity that occurs as the signal moves from one side of the head to the other; this effect is more substantial in the high frequencies. For the unilaterally hearing-impaired child, any signal presented on the side of the impaired ear may be attenuated 10 to 16 dB above 1000 Hz by the time it reaches the functional ear (Festen and Plomp, 1986). Obviously, this magnitude of attenuation can have significant effects on speech intelligibility (Mueller and Hawkins, 1990), because that area of the speech spectrum may account for 60% of speech intelligibility (Bess and Tharpe, 1986).

3. Localization. The importance of localization, or directionality, is generally considered to be a binaural phenomenon, the result of interaural time and intensity differences. For low-frequency stimuli, the primary cue for localization is the interaural time difference, whereas for high frequencies (above 1500 Hz), the primary cue is the interaural intensity difference.

The typical clinical management approach until the past decade had been relatively nonaggressive; that is, children with unilateral hearing loss were provided preferential seating with an occasional referral for a contralateral routing of signals (CROS) type hearing aid (Bess and Tharpe, 1986). It was generally assumed that because one ear was normal, normal cognitive, academic, and social development would prevail. Recently, a more aggressive approach has been taken toward management of the unilaterally hearing-impaired child. Preferential seating and/or use of amplification will not restore these auditory deficits, but closer monitoring of potential areas of weakness may preclude more serious ramifications.

Gain/Frequency Response Considerations

Children younger than 10 or 12 years of age cannot be expected to provide extensive input into the hearing aid fitting process (see Chapter 11 for adult hearing aid selection procedures). As a result, a formula approach toward determining and setting frequency response characteristics may be necessary.

With the advent of probe microphone technology, a clearer understanding of the results of our hearing aid fitting efforts is possible. Measurements of individually derived acoustic transformations allow for more precise setting of gain and output. Of particular interest is the external ear resonance measure or real ear unaided response (REUR). Shaw (1974) compiled data from 12 contemporary investigations to show the average sound pressure transformation from a free field. His data for frontal incidence (0° azimuth) indicate that the primary resonance of the adult ear is approximately 2600 Hz, with an average pressure gain of 17 dB. Probe microphone measures of hearing aid performance (in particular, gain) require some initial measure of this transformation.

Kruger (1987) noted that the external ear resonant frequency is higher at birth (note in Figure 5.1 the resonant peak at approximately 6000 Hz) and deceases with age to adult values by the second year. Other investigators (Bentler, 1989; Dempster and MacKenzie, 1990) have studied the change in resonant frequency and peak amplitude and reported that beyond age 3 there is only a slight relationship between age and changes in resonant frequencies. Both investigations showed wide variability in results and cautioned for the need for individual ear resonance measures. The use of average transformation values rather than individually derived values continues to be challenged (Mueller, 1989; Byrne and Upfold, 1991). As Byrne and Upfold (1991) point out, if one child exhibits a higher external ear resonant peak than is typical, then sounds will have to be amplified to a higher level in that frequency range to achieve the same insertion gain values. Instead, the au-

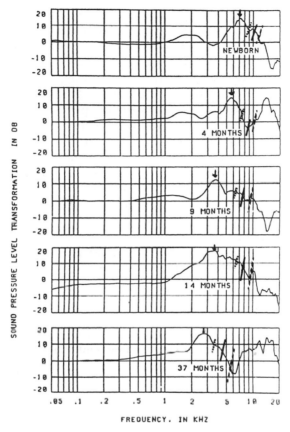

Figure 5.1. Diffuse field to ear canal transformation for a newborn and 4-, 9-, 14-, and 37-month-old children. (Reprinted with permission from Kruger B. An update on the external ear resonance in infants and young children. Ear Hear 1987;85:74–81.)

thors continue, we should be thinking of transmission gain, or the increase in the aided signal level relative to the unaided level, using an in situ gain rather than an insertion gain target. Byrne and Upfold conclude that "insertion gain versus transmission gain is a complex issue that requires further thought and, if prescriptions were made in transmission gain, then there should be no correction for individual differences in ear canal resonance" (p. 40).

The real-ear-to-coupler transformation or difference, as a function of age, has also been investigated. It has long been documented (Sachs and Burkhard, 1972; Bruel et al., 1976; Bergman and Bentler, 1990; Hawkins et al., 1990) that more sound pressure may be generated in an occluded ear canal than in the standard 2-cc coupler. For example, if the hearing aid manufacturer reports that a par-

ticular model has a high-frequency average output of 120 dB SPL in a 2-cc coupler, one might assume the output in an average ear may be 10 dB higher. For small children that difference may be even higher! Feigin et al. (1989) obtained ear canal sound pressure levels for 31 children from the ages of 4 weeks to 5 years. Twenty-one adult subjects, ages 17 through 48, served as controls. Using a constant 10-mm depth insertion of the probe tube from the ear canal entrance, the output was measured in each ear canal for 11 pure tones presented with insert earphones. The output of the insert earphone at each of the 11 frequencies was measured, and the coupler-to-real-ear differences were computed. As shown in Figure 5.2, at all frequencies, the real-ear-to-coupler difference (RECD) for the children exceeded that measured for adults. It was further noted by these investi-

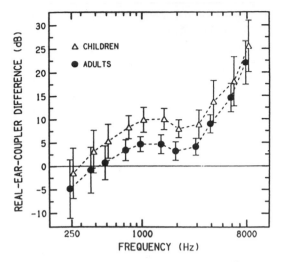

Figure 5.2. Real ear-to-coupler difference (in dB) measured as a function of frequency (in Hz) for children and adult subjects. Error bars represent ± one standard deviation from the mean. (Reprinted with permission from Feigin J, Kopun J, Stelmachowicz P, et al. Probe-tube microphone measures of ear-canal sound pressure levels in infants and children. Ear Hear 1989;10:254–258.)

gators that the transformation values decrease as a function of age, as shown in Figure 5.3, and could be predicted to fall within 1 standard deviation (SD) of the adult mean values by age 7.7. The clinician must always be cognizant of the probability that output from a prescribed hearing aid on a young child will be higher than that shown on manufacturer's specification sheets, and use caution in determining appropriate SSPL90 values. Obviously, excessive output can cause further deterioration of hearing, yet unduly limiting the output will reduce the child's dynamic range of listening and may result in excessive distortion if the hearing aid is continually operated in saturation.

A number of gain-targeting approaches have been forwarded over the years, including the Berger (Berger et al., 1977), prescription of gain and output (POG) (McCandless and Lyregaard, 1983), and National Acoustics Laboratory (NAL) (Byrne and Dillon, 1986) procedures, to name a few. Each formula purports to provide the elec-

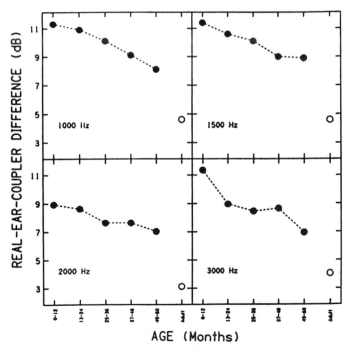

Figure 5.3. Real ear-to-coupler difference (in dB) measured as a function of age (in months). Open circles represent adult means at each frequency. (Reprinted with permission from Feigin J, Kopun J, Stelmachowicz P, et al. Probe-tube microphone measures of ear-canal sound pressure levels in infants and children. Ear Hear 1989;10:254–258.)

Table 5.1
Formula for calculating required real-ear gain (insertion gain or functional gain) for volume control setting 15 dB below maximum

1. Calculate $X = 0.05 (H_{500} + H_{1k} + H_{2k})^a$
2. $G_{250}^{b} = X + 0.31 H_{250} - 17b$
   $G_{500} = X + 0.31 H_{500} - 8$
   $G_{750} = X + 0.31 H_{750} - 3$
   $G_{1k} = X + 0.31 H_{1k} + 1$
   $G_{1.5k} = X + 0.31 H_{1.5k} + 1$
   $G_{2k} = X + 0.31 H_{2k} - 1$
   $G_{3k} = X + 0.31 H_{3k} - 2$
   $G_{4k} = X + 0.31 H_{4k} - 2$
   $G_{6k} = X + 0.31 H_{6k} - 2$

[a]H, HTL (ISO standard).
[b]G, insertion gain.

troacoustic characteristics necessary for maximizing speech intelligibility, yet different response characteristics are typically derived from each formula for the same audiogram. The clinician is often in the situation of determining which formula most favorably suits which client. For the pediatric population, the theoretical considerations of the NAL approach deserve consideration.

The NAL formula derived by Byrne and Tonisson (1976) was originally developed for use with young children (Byrne and Fifield, 1974). A later revision of that prescriptive approach was provided by Byrne and Dillon (1986). The premise of the approach is to amplify the long-term speech spectrum so that it is most comfortably loud and equally loud across frequency. That is, the speech spectrum is shaped so that each frequency band contributes equally to its loudness; this, presumably, will lead to maximum intelligibility. As shown in Tables 5.1 and 5.2, insertion gain targets (or functional gain targets, if a probe microphone system is not accessible) are derived based on the degree of hearing loss at each frequency. Table 5.2 also provides a formula for converting these gain values to 2-cc coupler values, if necessary, to select hearing aids from manufacturer's specifications. Although the required insertion gain will be the same regardless of aid style—body, behind-the-ear (BTE), or in-the-ear (ITE)—the coupler gain required to give that insertion gain will vary,

as a result of different microphone locations on the different styles.

Other investigations (Byrne and Cotton, 1988; Pascoe, 1998; Schwartz et al., 1988; Byrne et al., 1990, 1991) have suggested that for severely impaired listeners (adults and children), more gain may be required than is prescribed by this formula. In Table 5.3, a modification of the NAL prescriptive formula is shown for losses in excess of 60 dB HL. Preferred gain was typically found to be approximately 10 dB greater than the NAL prescribed gain for hearing losses greater than 60 dB HL (Byrne et al., 1991). In addition, approximately half of their subjects who exhibited steeply sloping hearing losses, as shown in Figure 5.4, preferred more low-frequency gain than prescribed by the formula, based on judgments of intelligibility, home trials, and speech recognition testing.

A recent modification of this prescriptive scheme has been developed for use with nonlinear or dynamic range compression[a] hearing aids that maintain the original intent of providing comfortable and equally loud speech across frequencies (NAL-NL1) (Dillon, 1998). This software-driven formula provides for inputs of air conduction and bone conduction data, choice of type of hearing aid (BTE, ITE, in-the-canal [ITC] or completely in-the-canal [CIC]), number of desired compression channels (1 to 4), and modifications due to tubing acoustics. RECD and REUR values can be entered or will be predicted to result in closer proximity to target gain and output values. Any or all input values from 40 to 90 dB (in 10-dB steps) can be viewed simultaneously. In addition, any of the following screens can be viewed during the fitting and verification stages:

- 2-cc Coupler response (dB SPL).
- 2-cc Input/output curve (dB SPL).
- Audiogram.
- Ear simulator response (dB).
- Ear simulator I/O curve (dB SPL).
- Real ear insertion response (dB).
- Real ear aided response (dB SPL).

[a]The use of compression in hearing aids is not covered in this chapter. The reader is referred to Chapter 11 for that overview.

Table 5.2
Formulas for calculating required 2-cc coupler and ear simulator gain

			2-cc Coupler[a]			Ear Simulator		
			BTE	ITE	Body	BTE	ITE	Body
1. Calculate $X = 0.05\ (H_{500} + H_{1k} + H_{2k})^b$								
2. G_{250}	=	$X + 0.31\ H_{250} + 1$	−1	0	5		2	0
G_{500}	=	$X + 0.31\ H_{500} + 9$	9	2	13		12	6
G_{750}	=	$X + 0.31\ H_{750} + 12$	13	8	17		16	12
G_{1k}	=	$X + 0.31\ H_{1k} + 16$	16	13	22		21	19
$G_{1.5k}$	=	$X + 0.31\ H_{1.5k} + 13$	14	22	19		21	28
G_{2k}	=	$X + 0.31\ H_{2k} + 15$	14	25	24		23	35
G_{3k}	=	$X + 0.31\ H_{3k} + 22$	15	26	29		25	33
G_{4k}	=	$X + 0.31\ H_{4k} + 18$	13	17	24		25	23
G_{6k}	=	$X + 0.31\ H_{6k} + 12$	4		21		19	

Reprinted with permission from Byrne D, Dillon H. The National Acoustics Laboratories (NAL) new procedure for selecting the gain and frequency response of a hearing aid. *Ear Hear* 1986;7:257–265.

[a] *H*, HTL (ISO standard).

[b] *G*, insertion gain.

Table 5.3
Modifications to NAL hearing aid selection procedure (Byrne and Dillon, 1986)
for application to severe/profound hearing losses

1. $X = 0.05 \times HTL\ (0.5 + 1 + 2k)$ up to 170 dB (i.e., 3FA = 60 dB) + 0.116 × combined HTL in excess of 180 dB.
2. Where the 2000 Hz HTL is 95 dB or greater, add the following

2 kHz HTL	250	500	750	1k	1.5k	2k	3k	4k	6k
95	4	3	1	0	−1	−2	−2	−2	−2
100	6	4	2	0	−2	−3	−3	−3	−3
105	8	5	2	0	−3	−5	−5	−5	−5
110	11	7	3	0	−3	−6	−6	−6	−6
115	13	8	4	0	−4	−8	−8	−8	−8
120	15	9	4	0	−5	−9	−9	−9	−9

Reprinted with permission from Byrne D, Parkinson A, Newall P. Modified hearing aid selection procedure for severe/profound hearing loss. In: Studebaker G, Bess F, Beck L, eds. The Vanderbilt hearing aid report II. Parkton, MD: York Press, 1991.

- Speech-o-gram (dB SPL).
- Aided thresholds (dB SPL).

A number of other fitting schemes are based on the philosophy of making as much of the speech spectrum audible as possible without exceeding discomfort (Version 3.1 MSU Prescription Formula, Cox, 1983, 1985; CID Phase IV, Popelka, 1983, 1988, Popelka and Engebretson, 1983; DSL V 4.1, Seewald et al., 1997). The difference in these approaches is subtle. Whereas the original NAL prescription places the speech spectrum at approximately one-half the hearing loss for mild to moderate hearing losses (0.46 HTL) and at equal loudness across the frequency range, these approaches attempt to make as much of the speech spectrum audible as possible—presumably at a preferred listening level—without exceeding discomfort. The underlying difference here is that the audiologist is working with measured sensation levels of amplified speech spectra, rather than the targeting of some gain values derived from threshold estimates. Thresholds of hearing do not change with the use of amplification; therefore, it may be more practical to begin to look at how the amplified speech range fits into the child's usable hearing range.

A prescriptive formula of this nature used extensively in pediatric fittings is the desired sensation level (DSL) approach, originally proposed by Seewald et al. (1985) and recently modified to include dynamic range compression hearing aids (Cornelisse et al., 1994, 1995; Seewald et al., 1997). Based on the premise that "suprathreshold dimensions of auditory perception" in young children lack reliability and validity, these authors attempt to place the long-term speech spectrum between the child's threshold and loudness discomfort level (LDL) across the frequency range. In generating a long-term average speech spectrum (LTASS) specifically related to children, Seewald et al. (1991) considered two issues. First, the relationship between the hearing aid microphone and the source of the speech; second, the self-monitoring that children do of their own vocalizations. Typically, the spectral characteristics of speech used in the calcula-

tion of amplification characteristics are obtained from recordings taken directly in front of a talker rather than at the ear level of the hearing-impaired listener (Byrne and Dillon, 1986; Cox and Moore, 1988). As Cornelisse et al. (1991) point out, the hearing-impaired child must monitor his or her own voice as well, and any algorithm based on the former LTASS may result in inappropriate gain characteristics for self-monitoring of speech. In fact, these investigators found that ear-level measures of LTASS taken for three groups of subjects (adult males, adult females, and children) consisted of more low-frequency energy (below 1000 Hz) and less high-frequency energy (above 2500 Hz) than previous estimates obtained directly in front of the talker. As a result of the findings, the DSL approach incorporates a speech spectrum that comprises the average of male/female/child recordings of speech obtained directly in front of the talker and recordings taken at the ear level of the child. This speech spectrum has an overall level of 70.9 dB SPL and is shown in Figure 5.5. The relative weightings of the prescribed sensation levels for this spectrum

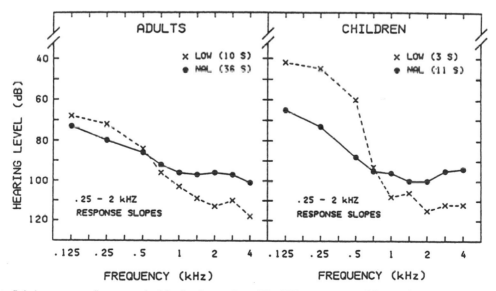

Figure 5.4. Average audiograms of subjects who preferred the NAL response and those who required more low-frequency amplification. (Reprinted with permission from Byrne D, Parkinson A, Newall P. Modified hearing aid selection procedures for severe/profound hearing loss. In: Studebaker G, Bess F, Beck L, eds. The Vanderbilt hearing aid report II. Parkton, MD: York Press, 1991.)

are similar to Pascoe's (1978) "perceived speech spectrum" with two exceptions: reduced low-frequency emphasis and slightly increased mid-frequency emphasis (1500 to 3000 Hz). The latter is intended to restore natural amplification associated with external ear resonance in that range, but which is eliminated with an occluding mold.

The DSL v 4.1 computerized procedure involves several stages. In the first stage, thresholds obtained using insert earphones, circum-aural earphones, or sound field presentation are entered. The program will make calculations on entered thresholds only; no interpolation at other frequencies is done. If the child's REUR and RECD values are known, those values are entered as well. If no measures are available, the program will use default age-appropriate values for children (Kruger, 1987) or adult values (Shaw, 1974; Shaw and Vaillancourt, 1985). Loudness discomfort values, if available, are also entered. Default values for adults (Skinner, 1988) are used for the calculation of a prescribed saturation sound pressure level with a 90-dB input (SSPL90) and real ear saturation response (RESR). During this stage, the program determines the amount of gain required to place the idealized speech spectrum at the DSLs for each of nine frequency regions. The prescribed RESR at each frequency is selected on the basis of the prescribed level of amplified speech. As with the MSU method, these maximum output values are related to threshold levels and fall below the median LDL values for differing degrees of loss as reported by Kamm et al. (1978). Because the program provides for recommended electroacoustic specifications of gain and output as well as preferred sensation and real ear output levels, all prescribed values are corrected for their 2-cc equivalent (Feigin et al., 1989; Hawkins et al., 1990). As shown in Figure 5.6, the amplified long-term speech spectrum target and prescribed output at 1000 Hz are derived from threshold values.

If a probe microphone system is used, the derived in situ gain necessary for preferred sensation levels across frequency can be plotted as real ear targets, and adjustments can be made to the hearing aid to match the desired target with minimal cooperation from the child. Output measures can also be verified quickly using the probe system. The DSL program is optimally useful when interfaced with a probe microphone system. In that way, thresholds and individual transformation values entered into the hearing aid software program will result in target values for probe microphone measures without having to enter these target values manually.

One issue that may never be resolved involves the choice of speech spectrum used for setting gain and output. Obviously, the primary goal of any amplification system should be to make the speech signal audi-

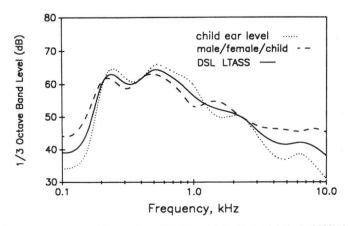

Figure 5.5. The long-term average speech spectrum (LTASS) used by Seewald et al. (1991a,b) in the desired sensation level (DSL) hearing aid fitting strategy composed of the average of male/female/child recordings obtained directly in front of the talker (1 m) and recordings taken at ear level of a child.

DSL 3.0: 1000 Hz

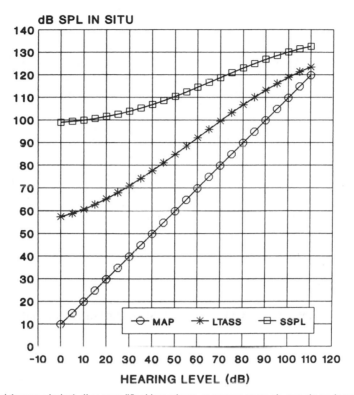

Figure 5.6. Threshold (open circles), the amplified long-term average speech spectrum target levels (asterisks), and the desired maximum real-ear sound pressure levels (open squares) in dB SPL at the eardrum as a function of dB HL for the 1000 Hz frequency region, as prescribed by desired sensation level (DSL). (Reprinted with permission from Seewald RC, Zelisko DLC, Ramji K, et al. Computer assisted implementation of the DSL approach: version 3.0. Poster presentation at the International Hearing Aids Conference, Iowa City, Iowa, 1991.

ble; logically, one should be able to assume that the chosen target speech spectrum is representative of what the child actually hears. What are the characteristics of that speech signal? As Olsen et al. (1987) have pointed out, the particular speech spectrum used depends on the sex, age, and vocal effort of the talker; the choice of speech material; the length of the sampled interval (and whether silent intervals between words were included in the measurement); distance; and azimuth of the microphone relative to the talker.

Stelmachowicz (1991) has attempted to describe speech spectra in more typical parent-child positions. For example, the intensity difference from the typical 1-m distance from the talker to the ear position for a child placed at the mother's shoulder has been shown to be as much as 15 to 20 dB. Stelmachowicz points out that for adults we can expect level effects, due to proximity of talker and listener, but that distance is typically greater, not lesser, than it may be with a child placed on the shoulder or cradled in the arms of the talker/parent. As a result of her efforts, a software-driven verification scheme has been developed for use in estimating the audibility of the primary speech signal (Stelmachowicz et al., 1994). This Situational Hearing Aid Response Profile (SHARP) provides a graphic display of any of 13 LTASS depicting the amplified signal in relation to the audiometric thresholds. Of particular concern to these investigators is the concern that linguistic cues and "world knowledge" are not likely to facilitate speech perception in children to the same degree as for adults (Nittrouer and Boothroyd, 1990). For this reason, the optimal frequency/gain characteristics of the pediatric hearing aid fitting may necessitate more high-frequency emphasis. This assumption is based on previous research efforts indicating that low frequencies contribute more to intelligibility than do high frequencies for highly contextual material (Studebaker et al.,

1987), while high frequencies contribute more to intelligibility for reduced context material (ANSI, S3.5; American National Standards Institute, 1997). Because the pediatric hearing aid user is presumably attempting to learn speech and language through the amplified signal, the frequency/gain characteristics should differ for that population. As shown in Figure 5.7, the audibility across frequency for a variety of speech spectra can be visualized with this verification scheme.

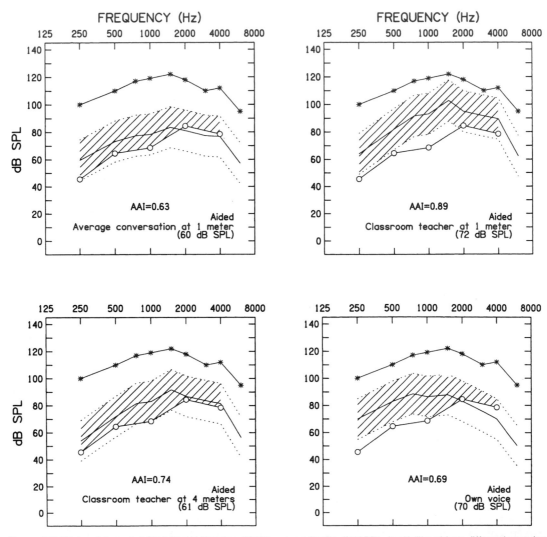

Figure 5.7. Print-out from the Situational Hearing Aid Response Profile (SHARP). Audibility of four different spectra (average conversation at 1 m, classroom teacher at 1 and 4 m, and a child talking) are shown relative to a child's threshold values. Aided articulation index (AAI) values are calculated for each condition.

Output Considerations

The saturation sound pressure level (SSPL) of a hearing aid refers to its maximum output regardless of input level. Related to the SSPL of any amplification system are the concerns of (1) creating additional hearing loss as a result of overexposure or overamplification, and (2) exceeding the threshold of discomfort for the hearing aid user. It is often not clear to the clinician that exceeding threshold of discomfort might not cause additional hearing loss (although the hearing aid may get yanked) and levels of overamplification might not cause discomfort! Yet, both issues need careful consideration.

With children, setting appropriate output levels is especially critical. Young children often cannot express that a hearing aid is allowing some incoming sounds to "hurt"; parents may react to any rejection as being

caused by other factors, such as stubbornness, anxiety, etc. Obtaining thresholds of discomfort in young children is often impossible due to the cognitive level required to complete the task (Kawell et al., 1988; Macpherson et al., 1991), and "observing the level which elicits the eye blink reflex" (Liden and Harford, 1985) is generally not acceptable! In an attempt to address this need, Kawell et al. (1988) designed a procedure to be used with children 7 years and older, using a methodology adapted from Hawkins et al. (1987). The following instructions, along with the labeled drawing (Fig. 5.8), were presented:

We're going to see how loud this hearing aid makes sound. You will hear some whistles and I want you to tell me how loud the whistle is. When the sounds are "Too Loud," this is where you want the hearing aid to stop and you do not want the sounds to get any louder. Now, for every whistle, tell me how loud it sounds (p. 136).

Data were obtained in a sound field with warble tone stimuli for 20 hearing-impaired subjects (7 to 14 years of age) wearing a high-output BTE style hearing aid. Their results indicated that thresholds of discomfort could be obtained reliably from children as young as 7 years of age. Comparing the results obtained using a similar procedure for 20 hearing-impaired adults showed no systematic differences in mean thresholds of discomfort (or SDs) for the two groups. Stuart et al. (1991) reported similar success with the Kawell et al. procedure; however, their method used an insert earphone coupled to the child's own earmold delivery system. Using this form of coupling, according to the authors, eliminates the potential error of sound field measures and provides for output values that can be compared directly to hearing aid SSPL90 specifications. A limitation in the maximum linear output of the insert earphones was noted, however.

Macpherson et al. (1991) attempted to develop a procedure with cognitive and language requirements appropriate for younger children. Their procedure used four initial training tasks to teach the concept of "too

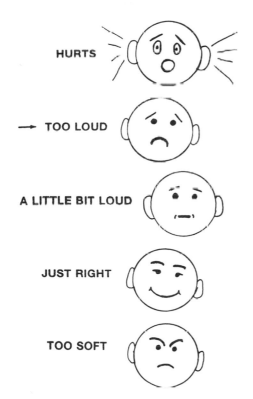

Figure 5.8. Verbal and pictorial representation of the loudness categories used with children 7 to 14 years of age. (Reprinted with permission from Kawell ME, Kopun JG, Stelmachowicz PG. Loudness discomfort levels in children. Ear Hear 1988;9:133–136.)

much"; a fifth task was then used to obtain thresholds of discomfort under supra-aural earphones for pure tones at octave frequencies, although any stimulus type would be appropriate. These investigators were attempting to match the task demands to the conceptual abilities of the child. Piagetian literature suggests that beginning around the age of 5 or 6, children can begin to recognize equivalencies between two distinct orderings of magnitude (Ginsburg and Opper, 1969). They point out that "children younger than age six (may) have not yet developed the cognitive ability to order different magnitudes of loudness stimuli as required in the Kawell et al. procedure" (Macpherson et al., 1991, p. 184). In fact, whereas 5-year-old normal-hearing subjects were able to perform the task with fair reliability, younger children with mental age levels younger than 5 years were not.

For younger or less cooperative children, more objective alternatives have been suggested for obtaining discomfort levels, including attempting to make predictions of discomfort based on recordings of auditory brainstem responses (ABRs) (Gorga, 1988), acoustic reflex measures (Greenfield et al., 1985), and degree of hearing loss (Cox, 1985; Kawell et al., 1988; Ross and Seewald, 1988). Results have been inconclusive.

Issues of stimulus type, psychophysical method, and manner of presentation for determining discomfort levels have been discussed in great detail (Hawkins, 1980; Beattie and Sheffler, 1981; Cox, 1983; Cox and Sherbecoe, 1983; Mueller and Bentler, 1994). Of particular concern to the clinician should be the validation of the resultant SSPL90 settings. If the hearing aid is adjusted appropriately to match some threshold of discomfort contour based on frequency-specific stimuli, it would be expected that the child would not experience discomfort with any level of input. Some typical clinical procedures, such as jiggling keys or banging on the examination table, may give a rough estimate of the validity of the settings, but probe microphone validation procedures may provide the most accurate assessment. Regardless of the procedure implemented, frequency-specific discomfort measures should be obtained and the hearing aid output set just below those levels. Validation should be accomplished using frequency-specific input signals as well. Stelmachowicz (1991) points out that to check the SSPL settings using a wide-band or speech-weighted noise may give an inaccurate picture of the maximum output of the hearing aid. As shown in Figure 5.9, the SSPL90 curves obtained for a swept pure-tone input suggest possible output levels that are 15 to 20 dB higher than those obtained from the same hearing aid using a speech-weighted complex noise. Although the overall rms output would agree with the high-frequency SSPL90 ob-

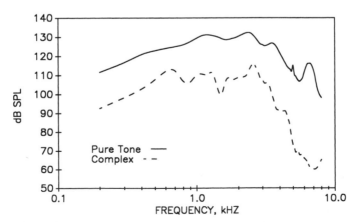

Figure 5.9. Comparison of 2-cc coupler output from a hearing aid (Oticon E38P) obtained in response to 90 dB inputs of complex and pure-tone stimuli.

tained with a pure-tone input, the output at any one frequency for the complex stimulus will appear to be lower. It may not be obvious to the clinician that the broad-band input may underestimate the output level that would be realized with other environmental inputs. Stelmachowicz (1991) further measured the output from a hearing aid with a variety of environmental inputs. Although measures of gain (difference in unaided and aided condition) may be accurately obtained with a wide-band complex, validation of maximum output necessitates use of a pure-tone input so that the maximum possible output in any frequency region can be compared with the discomfort threshold at the same frequency. In this way, complex environmental stimuli will not exceed discomfort even in those peak frequency regions.

Until a protocol is developed that results in reliable, valid measures of discomfort in very young children, a conservative (yet realistic) approach must be taken in setting hearing aid maximum output. If hearing aids are too conservatively limited, the child may be listening to all incoming information with the aid in saturation. The DSL and MSU fitting strategies prescribe relatively conservative maximum output levels based on degree of loss, whereas many of the other procedures require additional measures be taken. Matkin (1986) has suggested the following 2-cc values for output: 110 dB SPL for mild loss, 120 dB SPL for moderate loss, and no more than 125 dB for profound loss. More recently, he has revised those values to account for the age of the child, due to the size of the ear canal: 100 dB plus one-fourth the hearing loss at 1000, 2000, and 4000 minus 5 dB for a preschooler, or 10 dB for an infant or toddler (Matkin, cited in Bebout, 1989). Based on the Sachs and Burkhard (1972) transformation data, those values at the eardrum may be 10 dB higher in the upper frequency range. In recent years, the increased implementation of probe microphone systems has provided a means to determine output levels at the eardrum of the child with hearing amplification.

Effect on Residual Hearing

For more than 50 years, there has been concern about the possibility of hearing aid use causing additional hearing impairment (for example, Berry, 1939; Holmgren, 1940). Since the first studies of overamplification appeared in the literature, there has been little consensus as to what constitutes safe output levels. Although reports of changes in hearing that can be attributed directly to hearing aid use are relatively rare (Mills, 1975; Hawkins, 1982; Macrae, 1985), the literature is replete with evidence of potential harm (Naunton, 1957; Belletleur and Van Dyke, 1968; Hine and Furness, 1975; Darbyshire, 1976; Markides and Ayree, 1978; Markides, 1980; Rintlemann and Bess, 1988). Of more current debate is the issue of sensory deprivation of the unaided ear. This "late-onset auditory deprivation" (see Neuman, 1996 for review) may be manifested in reduced speech recognition scores in the unaided ear of unilaterally or bilaterally hearing-impaired listeners (Gelfand et al., 1987; Gatehouse, 1989a,b; Silverman, 1989; Stubblefield and Nye, 1989; Hood, 1990). In fact, some investigators have reported improved speech recognition scores in the aided ear and decreased scores in the unaided ear (Markides and Aryee, 1978, 1980). Hattori (1993) reported that children who were monaurally aided had poorer speech recognition performance in the unaided ear than those who alternated their single aid from ear to ear. Gelfand and Silman (1993) showed actual decrement in the unaided ears of 10 monaurally aided children compared with a matched group of children who were binaurally aided for the same period. The implications of these investigations for early identification and binaural aiding are portentous.

Verification Issues

Quantifying benefit from amplification implies a determination that the amplification characteristics have resulted in the availability of more of the speech spectrum and thus the potential for improved communication skills. Benefit from an amplification system is typically measured using probe microphone systems, functional gain measures, speech recognition measures, or some form of questionnaire or inventory. Often done in a clinical setting, the audiologist attempts to explain the overall benefit of a hearing aid in terms of how much it improves the audibility of speech sounds. Seewald et al. (1992) compared two commonly used methods of estimating the sensation level of amplified speech: the sound field aided audiogram approach, and an approach using a probe microphone system.

Sound field aided thresholds are used clinically to provide an aided audiogram, or measured thresholds in a sound field obtained while wearing the desired amplification system. A frequent misconception of those using this method of determining hearing aid benefit is that a hearing aid improves thresholds, but this is not the case. Incoming signals are amplified; the child's thresholds are not changed. In fact, due to the nonlinear characteristics of some hearing aids, providing functional gain measures may indicate more gain than the child is actually receiving for moderate input signals. This is due to the fact that in the aided condition, sound field aided thresholds are often obtained using low SPL levels, whereby in a typical communicative setting, higher input may activate an input compression circuit, resulting in less usable gain than was indicated by the functional gain measure.

Seewald et al. (1992) compared the sensation level (SL) of speech obtained by sound field functional gain measures with that obtained with a probe microphone measure of insertion gain. They found that the two methods were in agreement for SL estimates only 58% of the time. "For the remaining 42% of comparisons, the majority were in the direction of higher SL estimates produced by the aided audiogram approach relative to SL estimates observed with the electroacoustic method" (p. 142). The authors suggest caution in providing aided information to parents and/or educators that may, in fact, overpredict hearing levels and abilities. Hearing aids using some input compression circuitry will provide differing

gain dependent on the level of the input stimulus.

More objective attempts to measure hearing aid benefit have been suggested, including use of acoustic reflex thresholds (ARTs) and auditory evoked responses (AERs) including ABR, middle latency response (MLR), and 40 Hz event-related potentials (ERPs). Mueller and Grimes (1987) review these approaches, noting that their usefulness lies in the fact that they are objective rather than subjective measures of hearing aid benefit. In view of the increasing use of probe microphone systems, however, such objective tests are currently used more for threshold determination than in pediatric hearing aid evaluation.

Successful use of amplification suggests that the child for whom a particular amplification strategy has been chosen is indeed using the available information successfully in communicative attempts. For the profoundly hearing-impaired child, the options for sensory input may include vibrotactile stimulation, cochlear implantation, or more traditional acoustic stimulation via an analog hearing aid. The audiologist must balance the need to find the best sensory aid for the child—as soon as possible—with the need to give the child enough time to show proof of successful use of that benefit (covered in more detail in Chapters 15 and 19). For many children an unresolvable question remains: what constitutes an adequate trial period? Degree, configuration, etiology, onset, cognitive abilities, and other factors may affect the length of time it takes to adjust to, and derive benefit from, an amplification system. In view of the differing degrees of intervention used, establishing any guidelines becomes impossible. In addition, "the time course of auditory perceptual learning can vary from one hour to one year, depending on the task, the complexity of the sounds, and the level of stimulus uncertainty under which the tasks are learned" (Watson, 1980, p. 96). With this issue comes the question of the need for auditory training or the choice of audiologic rehabilitation strategies to enhance the newly provided information. Although it is beyond the scope of this chapter to outline such remediation strategies, it can only be assumed that the advantageously deafened child has more potential for the new perceptual learning tasks confronting him or her.

Some Style Issues

The standard rules relative to size, style, direct input capabilities, etc., still apply despite our rapidly advancing technology. That is, regardless of how limited our audiometric information, the recommended hearing aid should have the flexibility to allow for changes in frequency response and output as further audiometric data become available. The "ideal" hearing aid for a child does not differ substantially from the "ideal" choice for an adult (see Chapter 11 for more information on basic styles and components). A hearing aid with output and tone adjustment capabilities; strong telecoil, directional, or multimicrophone design; high fidelity/low distortion; and direct input capabilities should be sought for any child. Although the size of the device is frequently scrutinized for cosmetic reasons, it should be considered only in how well it fits over the smaller pinna of the child. This is especially true when the hearing aid must compete for space with eyeglasses. BTE style hearing aids continue to be the style of choice for children from infancy through adolescence. On a rare occasion, good-intentioned parents will press the issue of a (more discrete) ITE or canal style hearing aid. Northern and Downs (1991) point out that the child's pinna and concha may continue to grow and change in shape until the age of 9, resulting in the necessity of recasing every 3 to 5 months. As the professional to whom parents turn for delineation of options, such information regarding frequency and cost of recasing, need for loaner devices, and so on must be conveyed.

The decision relative to the choice of a directional microphone needs to be more often considered. In his review of research comparing directional microphone hearing aids to omnidirectional hearing aids, Mueller (1981) noted that regardless of the measuring tool (electroacoustic, speech recognition measures, or listener ratings), the directional microphone hearing aid "either rated superior or equal to the omnidirectional hearing aid but never worse" (p. 19). Nevertheless, he goes on to acknowledge that directional microphones are used in only 20% of BTE hearing aids, the unfortunate result of "indifference" on the part of the clinician (Mueller and Grimes, 1987). Recently, there has been renewed emphasis on use of this feature (Valente et al., 1995; Agnew and Block, 1997; Voss, 1997; Killion et al., 1998; Ricketts and Dahr, 1999). An improvement of 5 to 8 dB in signal-to-noise ratio for 50% performance has been reported with the newer designs, depending on variables such as vertical and horizontal azimuth placement of talker and background interference, noise type, microphone port spacing, and alignment. These factors are currently under investigation. Presumably, the attention to and efficacy of directional hearing aid designs applies to the pediatric population as well.

Occasionally, the need for a bone conduction (BC) hearing aid still arises. The child with chronic otitis media or atretic ear canals may derive great benefit from an amplification system but is not able to use the traditional earmold for reasons of hygiene or structural abnormalities. BC transducers worn with a headband and powered by a BTE style hearing aid can be recommended successfully.

Frequency Modulated (FM) Systems

Auditory trainers can be construed as another style option. The term "auditory trainer" has traditionally been used to refer to any personal amplification system—hard-wired, FM, infrared—other than a personal hearing aid. FM systems are the most accepted systems used today. They were first developed in the 1940s in an effort to provide the hearing-impaired child direct access to the teacher's voice, thus reducing the deleterious effects of background noise and reverberant classrooms (Table 5.4). The

Table 5.4
Mean monosyllabic word discriminations scores of the normal-hearing children (loudspeaker-aided) and the hearing-impaired children

Reverberation Time (sec)	Message-to-Competition Ratio (dB)	Groups		
		Normal (Loudspeaker-Aided)	Hearing-Impaired (Loudspeaker-Aided)	Hearing-Impaired (Hearing Aid-Aided)
0.0	+∞	94.5	87.5	83.0
	+12+	89.2	77.8	70.0
	+6	79.7	65.7	59.5
	0	60.2	42.2	39.0
0.4	+∞	92.5	79.2	74.0
	+12	82.8	69.0	60.2
	+6	71.3	54.5	52.2
	0	47.7	28.8	27.8
1.2	+∞	76.5	61.8	45.0
	+12	68.8	50.2	41.2
	+6	54.2	39.5	27.0
	0	29.7	15.3	11.2

Reprinted with permission from Finitzo-Hieber T, Tillman T. Room acoustics effect on monosyllabic word discrimination ability for normal and hearing impaired children. *J Speech Hear Res* 1978;21:440–458.

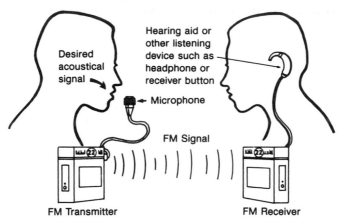

Figure 5.10. Schematic of FM transmission system. (Reprinted with permission from Compton CL. Assistive devices: doorways to independence. Washington, DC: Gallaudet University, 1989.)

early devices were intended for severely and profoundly hearing-impaired children. They were characterized by broad and flat frequency responses and were seldomly fit "to match the amplification needs of the child" (Bess and Gravel, 1981, p. 24). Current systems are composed of a teacher's (or some other talker's) microphone, often a small lapel style wireless microphone, an FM transmitter, and an FM receiver (Fig. 5.10). These portable and wireless systems are now frequently adjustable (gain and output characteristics) and typically provide signal transmission within a 300- to 600-foot radius outdoors and a 100-foot radius indoors. They operate in the 72 to 76 MHz band-width region originally designated by the Federal Communication Commission (FCC) for "educational assistance devices for the hearing impaired" (Hammond, 1991). Thirty-two frequencies are available within that band, allowing for multiple systems to be operating at one time within a single school building.

An FM system may be one of two types: self-contained or personal. A self-contained system is worn in place of a hearing aid. Like the personal hearing aid, it has adjustable controls for different degrees and configurations of hearing loss. As shown in Figure 5.11, this system can be coupled to personal hearing aids, headphones, earbuds, or even a BC transducer. The personal FM system is more often used in conjunction with the child's own hearing aids. This system typically does not have its own internal controls (although it may have a separate volume control wheel) but allows for the response and output shaping of the personal hearing aids. Alternately, the personal FM system can be used with earphones or earbuds, as long as the output characteristics are known and monitored (Lewis, 1994b).

A number of investigators have questioned the effect of the various coupling systems on the electroacoustic characteristics of the personal hearing aid. Matkin and Olsen (1970, 1973) looked at the effect of the induction loop on hearing aid performance. They reported "undesirable" changes in performance and noted that "interference of other radio signals was periodically quite audible" (p. 77). Sung and

Hodgson (1971) also reported differences in electroacoustic characteristics between microphone and telecoil modes, both in frequency response and total harmonic distortion levels. Other investigators (Freeman et al., 1980; Van Tasell and Landin, 1980; Hawkins and Van Tasell, 1982; Gladstone, 1985; Hawkins and Schum, 1985; Thibodeau and Saucedo, 1991) have demonstrated significant variability in electroacoustic measures across all coupling methods.

Rather than coupling an FM receiver to the child's hearing aid, another option is now available from a number of manufacturers. An integrated BTE FM receiver/hearing aid, which can be used as the primary amplification system, is available for mild, moderate, severe, and profound degrees of hearing loss. This style of FM system (shown in Fig. 5.12) looks like a typical, although slightly larger, BTE hearing aid and has an antenna that can be adjusted for further reception. Many have three operational modes: FM only, hearing aid only, and combined FM/hearing aid. One investigation of the effect of the BTE antenna

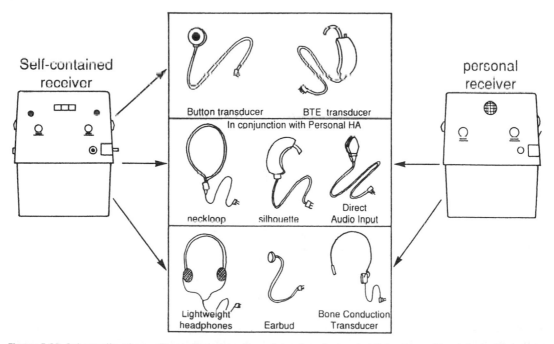

Figure 5.11. Schematic of coupling options for self-contained and personal FM systems. (Reprinted with permission from Lewis D. Assistive devices for classroom listening. Am J Audiol 1994a;3:58–69.)

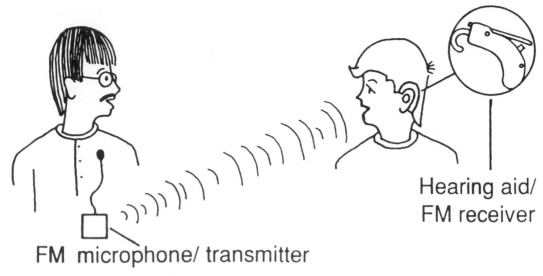

Figure 5.12. Schematic of ear-level hearing aid/FM system combination. (Reprinted with permission from Lewis D. Assistive devices for classroom listening. Am J Audiol 1994a;3:58–69.)

placement on transmission range (Chase and Bess, 1996) found that the maximum transmission range (81 feet) occurred with the antenna fully extended and with a lavaliere rather than a lapel-clipped microphone. Although these investigators did not assess the potential benefit of the boom microphone (shown in Fig. 5.13), they did recommend lavaliere microphones over the lapel microphones because of the reduced opportunity for "inadvertent poor placement."

Although FM systems have been standard equipment for children with hearing loss in educational environments for many years, no validated measurement procedures currently exist for fitting or monitoring these systems. In 1994, the American Speech-Language-Hearing Association (ASHA) first published guidelines for the fitting and monitoring of personal and self-contained FM systems (ASHA, 1994). The guidelines offer preselection considerations, fitting, and monitoring guidelines as well as electroacoustic and real ear measurements of performance. Considerable debate has ensued relative to the "optimal" relationship of the transmission (or teacher's) microphone sensitivity relative to the environmental microphone sensitivity. As a result, a revised set of guidelines has been proposed (ASHA,

1999) that offers additional recommendations of conserving the signal-to-noise benefits of the FM microphone by adjusting for equal gain from both microphones rather than equal output. Outlines for adjusting FM systems and assessing speech perception with an FM system are available in Appendices 5.1, 5.2, and 5.3.

One potential source of concern for FM system use in schools has not been well investigated. It has long been recognized that electromagnetic interference may affect FM use when personal or classroom loop coupling is used. Electrical outlets, fluorescent lights, and computer systems have all been shown to generate potentially disruptive electromagnetic interference (Harder, 1971; Beaulac et al., 1989; Beck and Nance, 1989; Bevacqua et al., 1989; Carlson, 1990). With the increasing use of personal and classroom amplification systems, which often include loop coupling, the interference in the classroom setting from any of these sources may be detrimental. Although the FCC has developed regulations for radiated emissions from computing devices (Violette et al., 1987), it is still unclear whether permissible levels may still interfere with hearing aid telecoil/loop function. More research is necessary in this area.

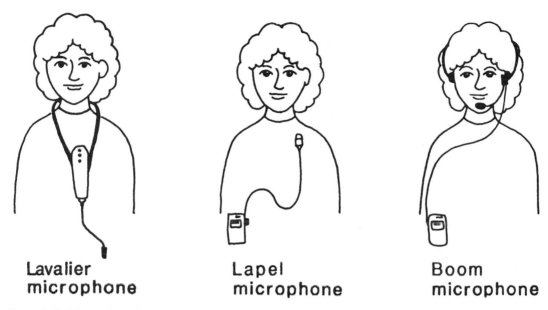

Lavalier
microphone

Lapel
microphone

Boom
microphone

Figure 5.13. Schematic of FM microphone/transmitter options. (Reprinted with permission from Lewis D. Assistive devices for classroom listening. Am J Audiol 1994a;3:58–69.)

Binaural Versus Monaural

The advantages of binaural hearing have long been established (Langford and Faires, 1973; Ross, 1977, 1980; Maxon, 1981; Liden and Harford, 1985; Mueller, 1986; Northern et al., 1990). Other investigators have noted only situational benefits (Grimes et al., 1981; Brooks, 1984; Hawkins, 1984) In addition to the benefits of binaural summation, elimination of head shadow, and localization (discussed earlier as unilaterally hearing-impaired children's deficits), other subjective reports of "ease of listening," improved speech intelligibility in noise, spatial balance, and enhanced sound quality reports from adult hearing aid users suggest that additional subjective benefits are possible. In fact, in a nationwide survey of current pediatric fitting practices used by audiologists, 90% reported always recommending binaural fittings across all age groups (Hedley-Williams et al., 1996).

Obviously, the child with bilaterally symmetrical thresholds may appear to be the most likely candidate, although any child with usable hearing in each ear should be considered a potential binaural candidate. Although probe microphone measures of insertion gain may indicate that the input to

each cochlea is equivalent, the assumption that the child is getting true binaural advantage cannot be made. The audiologist may refer to the cost, limited audiologic information, risks, parental resistance, and so on as contraindicators; of particular interest is the current evidence of auditory deprivation in monaurally aided adults (see previous discussion).

Appropriateness of "Higher-Tech" Hearing Aids

The current hearing aid market is besieged with claims of new and improved circuitry resulting in significant improvements to the hearing aid user. The "new" signal processing schemes for noise reduction have not conclusively shown enhanced speech recognition in noisy backgrounds, although anecdotally "ease of listening" may be improved (Preves and Sigelman, 1989; Bentler, 1991, 1993; Bentler et al., 1993a,b). When considering programmable hearing aids for the pediatric population, the options must be assessed relative to the needs and abilities of the child. Those options include use of the remote control, multiple versus single memory, multiple versus single channel, compression parameters, and cost, to name a few. Because nearly all the current digitally programmable hearing aids use some form of input and/or output compression, the clinician needs to assess carefully the effect of adjustment of the various compression parameters on the intended signal's audibility. Although compression in hearing aids has been scrutinized for many years (see monograph by Braida et al., 1979), it is still unclear what the optimal compression thresholds and time constants should be. Because the effect of altering release time as a function of frequency may be subtle, the clinician may have to depend on adult-derived data to direct clinical decision-making. The effect of varying these compression parameters on speech perception is currently under debate. Except for extreme amounts of compression, it appears that neither speech intelligibility nor sound quality is enhanced or compromised in adult listeners by these nonlinear processors (Souza and Turner, 1996, 1998; Bentler and Duve, submitted). As the signal processing schemes become more complex, the audiologist will have to rely on adult-derived efficacy data to determine the course of amplification management.

Digital hearing aids have been available for several years from a number of manufacturers. Unlike the digitally programmable hearing aids, or digitally controlled analog (DCA) circuits (Agnew, 1997), "true" digital hearing aids actually convert the analog acoustic signal to discrete time and discrete amplitude signals represented by binary numbers (see Schweitzer, 1997 for tutorial). As with the earlier DCA hearings aid, digital signal processing (DSP) hearing aids offer a number of advantages in the pediatric population. Perhaps the most advantageous feature of the programmable hearing aid is its flexibility. Because the diagnostic process for the pediatric client is typically ongoing and amplification cannot be postponed until a complete audiogram is obtained, the flexibility of these computer-adjusted hearing aids allows for early fitting with subsequent changes in gain and/or output without manufacturer replacement. The parents are not faced with repeated purchases during the

first 5 years, although the initial cost may be substantially more. As with other higher-tech features, the audiologist must again rely on the efficacy data obtained from adult subjects to determine appropriateness for this population (Bentler, 1998).

Special Applications

Diefendorf has suggested that 30 to 45% of hearing-impaired children have one or more additional disabilities (Mahon, 1987). Whether that additional disability refers to chronic middle ear effusion or some degree of mental or physical impairment, the effects must be assessed for successful hearing aid use. The child with chronic or fluctuating conductive hearing loss has previously been discussed as a good candidate for amplification. Consideration must also be given to the child with hearing impairment confounded by physical and/or mental impairments. The neurologically impaired child should not be overlooked, but rather the cognitive level carefully considered in the fitting stages. The terminally ill child, likewise, should be considered a potential candidate unless immediate crises deter the process. Parents may choose to deal with one impairment at a time due to emotional and financial drains. Ultimately, that is their decision to make. For the physically impaired child, other considerations must be made. If the child exhibits motor impairments that may preclude control of the hearing aid's operation, in-services to teachers and caretakers must be provided in addition to orienting parents. A minimally physically impaired child may derive more benefit from a body style hearing aid for which the controls are more easily manipulated.

Elfenbein and Logemann (1992) were concerned with the effect head and neck support systems might have on the acoustic signal arriving from different azimuths. Headrests and head wings, as used for motor-impaired, wheelchair-bound individuals, were shown to affect signal level at the ear by as much as 20 dB for frequencies of 2000 and 4000 Hz. Consideration of these azimuth effects on signal transmission must be made for children in academic settings. Critical speech cues may be lost for signals from the rear (e.g., during classroom discussions) as a result of such unintentional sound barriers. Use of an FM system may reduce or eliminate the detrimental effects of these barriers.

In addition to the uses discussed previously, auditory trainers (FM systems) have been advocated for three other unique groups: (1) moderately to profoundly hearing-impaired preschoolers for home use, (2) learning disabled/auditory processing dysfunctional children for personal and sound field use, and (3) school-age children with mild and/or fluctuating hearing loss.

Proponents of FM use for the first group contend that during this critical period of language development, the improved signal-to-noise ratio will enhance language learning significantly. An additional benefit of the arrangement is encouraging parent/child acceptance of the system in a familiar background (Benoit, 1989). Opponents of FM use at home for this moderately to profoundly hearing-impaired group point out the unnaturalness of the stimulation and/or absence of typical environmental input when a child is using an FM system (in FM condition only) at home. Part-time use of the environmental or hearing aid microphone should alleviate some of that concern. More research is needed to determine the efficacy of such an amplification strategy.

Relative to the second group, the use of auditory trainers has also been advocated for essentially normal-hearing children who have learning disabilities, attention problems, or auditory processing problems (Willeford and Billger, 1978; Loose, 1984; Blake et al., 1986, 1991). In a report prepared by the Committee on Amplification for the Hearing Impaired of the American Speech-Language-Hearing Association (1991), concerns related to safety and efficacy in the use of amplification for "individuals with normal peripheral hearing" were raised. Because published articles to date on this topic have not typically provided specific information on the gain or output provided by the amplification systems, the cumulative wearing time, or the method of selection or fitting, the committee cautioned against overinterpreting the reported benefits.

Relative to the third group, the child with the fluctuating or mild hearing loss has been found to be at risk for academic achievement (Davis et al., 1986). Auditory trainers and other forms of classroom amplification have been proposed as management strategies. Careful medical and audiologic monitoring is necessary with this group as well to ensure appropriate output limitation.

Parent Counseling

As Davis has pointed out (in Mahon, 1987), no one is more influential in the habilitative process of a hearing-impaired child than are the parents. Because "parents come in all shapes and sizes when it comes to their attitudes about and their degrees of involvement" (p. 10), it is the responsibility of the clinician to provide ongoing counseling to whatever degree required. It is paramount that the clinician understands the process parents pass through while learning to accept, cope, and manage the hearing impairment, regardless of its severity. Counseling is a major component of the rehabilitation amplification process (see Chapter 9 for an in-depth discussion of the counseling process).

Follow-Up

Although appropriate hearing aid recommendation and use constitute a major component in the pediatric rehabilitative process, it must be acknowledged that it is only one component. In addition to further decision making regarding speech and language remediation, auditory training, and academic placement (discussed elsewhere in this chapter), the audiologist must plan for ongoing audiologic follow-up as well. It is not clear how much follow-up constitutes sufficient follow-up, but it is clear that close monitoring for threshold shifts and hearing aid function (including any classroom amplification system) are minimally required. Liden and Harford (1985) suggest audiologic follow-up be scheduled at least every 6 to 8 weeks for the first 3 months; every 3

Table 5.5
Suggested components for a training program designed to teach children effective monitoring practices

Training Program
Instruction by audiologist
Instruction by THI, SLP, or others
Establishment of age-appropriate criterion referenced IEP goals
Familiarity with resources: equipment and personnel
Development of strategies for coping when hearing aids are nonfunctional

Reprinted with permission from Elfenbein JL, Bentler RA, Davis J, et al. Status of school children's hearing aids relative to monitoring practices. *Ear Hear* 1988;9:212–215.

THI, teachers of the hearing impaired; *SLP,* speech-language pathologists; *IEP,* individualized education plan.

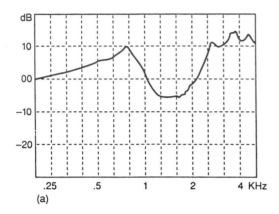

(a)

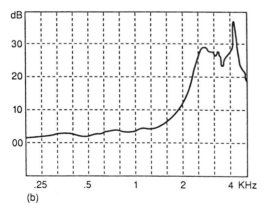

(b)

Figure 5.14. Real ear unaided responses (REURs) obtained before (a) and after (b) closure of a tympanic membrane perforation. (Reprinted with permission from Moryl CL, Danhauer JL, DiBartolomeo JL. Real ear unaided responses in ears with tympanic membrane perforations. J Am Acad Audiol 1992;3:60–65.)

Elfenbein et al. (1988) surveyed available data over the past 20 years related to incidence of malfunction in hearing aids used by children in various settings. They found 27 to 92% malfunction rates at any given time, depending on the particular criteria used. Of even more interest was the fact that the teachers of the hearing impaired—the individuals most likely to have responsibility for monitoring—believed that such malfunctions rarely occur! In their own investigation of three groups of mainstreamed children, a similar incidence of malfunction occurred even with "conscientious parental and professional monitoring." Active participation of both the parent and the child may be the best available solution. As shown in Table 5.5, a training program designed to teach children effective monitoring practices should begin with the audiologist. The audiologist should provide information relative to simple monitoring tasks (such as cleaning the earmold, checking battery voltage, performing visual inspections) to the child as well as the parent and teachers; this training should continue into the classroom and/or therapy room. Children should be familiarized with available resources, both equipment for monitoring their hearing aids and contact persons for reporting malfunctions. Parents should also become active participants in the monitoring process. Many parents, however, lack the equipment and/or skills necessary to accomplish this task (Elfenbein, 1994). Parents and their children should be considered partners in the management plan.

Even when the hearing aid is functioning

months until the age of 3; every 6 months until school age; and then annually. Although this may be a good rule of thumb for most situations, any extenuating circumstances may require more or less frequent monitoring.

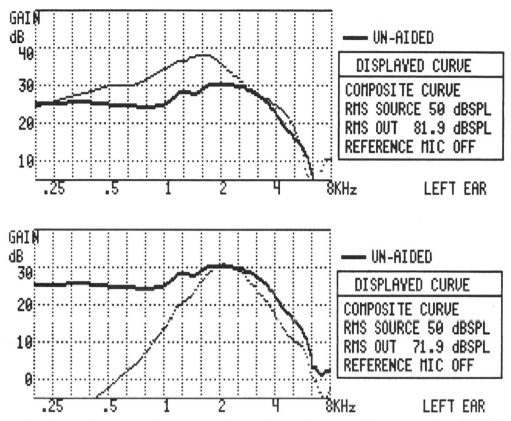

Figure 5.15. Real-ear-to-coupler differences (RECDs) obtained using Moodie, Seewald and Sinclair (1994) procedure on a FONIX 6500 probe microphone system (Frye Electronics), shown with a well-fitting earmold (top panel) and after physical changes in the child and ear canal resulted in a poorly fitting system (bottom panel).

adequately, changes in middle ear status, earmold fit, or even minor electroacoustic modifications can affect the benefit derived from the chosen amplification scheme (Bentler and Niebuhr, 1999). Figure 5.14 shows REURs obtained before (upper panel) and after (lower panel) closure of a tympanic membrane perforation. Because current fitting schemes for children provide input of the REUR values for better approximation of gain/output targets, the audiologist must be cognizant of the effects that middle ear effusion, tympanic membrane abnormalities, or even foreign bodies in the external canal can have on the REUR. Gerling et al. (1997) reported decreases in primary and secondary peaks and concomitant shifts in both peaks to higher frequencies as a result of varying amounts of cerumen accumulation.

Figure 5.15 shows the effect of an ill-fitting earmold on the RECD measurement taken at the fitting session (top panel). Although the initial RECD values were consistent with those expected for a young child, the subsequent growth resulted in the earmold becoming loose. The RECD values used to set the gain of the hearing aid are no longer valid, and the child is actually receiving less than optimal speech input across the frequency range.

Figure 5.16 shows the effects of small changes in the SSPL setting on distortion levels. The top panel shows the total harmonic distortion measured across frequency before a 2-dB adjustment in the maximum output of the hearing aid. An adjustment in the opposite direction would have resulted in high levels of unwarranted distortion. In each example, consistent monitoring of the

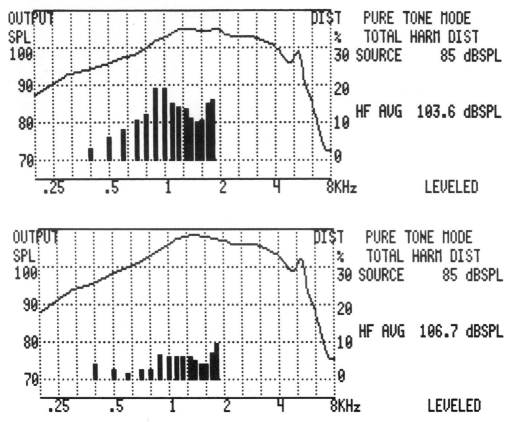

Figure 5.16. Bar graph illustration of total harmonic distortion before (lower panel) and after (lower panel) a small adjustment of the SSPL upward.

status of the ear, as well as the electroacoustic function of the hearing aid, could alleviate the detrimental consequences.

Summary

The issues surrounding amplification for the hearing-impaired child are relatively straightforward; the answers are not. As we search for a better understanding of what constitutes optimal gain/output and optimal speech spectrum characteristics (as well as an understanding of the extent that one can generalize adult data to infants and children), we should continue to question our process. Just as the diagnostic and rehabilitative processes need to be ongoing, our critical evaluation of the proposed solutions needs to be ongoing also. Newer signal processing schemes offer additional challenges in determining efficacy for the pediatric population. We cannot be complacent in our management of the pediatric population; rather, we must strive to understand better how these patients differ from adults in both size and auditory needs.

REFERENCES

Agnew J. Binaural hearing for understanding speech in noise with hearing aids. Semin Hear 1997;18:355–373.

Agnew J, Block M. HINT thresholds for dual microphone BTE. Hear Rev 1997;4:29.

American National Standards Institute. American National Standard methods for the calculation of the speech intelligibility index, ANSI, S3.5. New York: American National Standards Institute, 1997.

American Speech-Language-Hearing Association. Amplification as a remediation technique for children with normal peripheral hearing. ASHA 1991;33(Suppl 3):22–24.

American Speech-Language-Hearing Association. Guidelines for fitting and monitoring FM systems. ASHA 1994;36:1–9.

American Speech-Language-Hearing Association. Guidelines for fitting and monitoring FM systems (Draft). ASHA, 1999.

Beattie RC, Sheffler MV. Test-retest stability and effects of psychophysical methods on the speech loudness discomfort level. Audiology 1981;20:143–156.

Beaulac D, Pehringer J, Shough L. Assistive listening devices: available options. Semin Hear 1989;10:11–30.

Bebout JM. Pediatric hearing aid fitting: a practical overview. Hear J 1989;42:13–20.

Beck L, Nance G. Hearing aids, assistive listening devices, and telephones: issues to consider. Semin Hear 1989;10:78–89.

Bellefleur PA, Van Dyke RC. The effect of high gain amplification on children in a residential school for the deaf. J Speech Hear Res 1968;11:343–347.

Benoit R. Home use of FM amplification systems during the early childhood years. Hear Instr 1989;40:8–12.

Benoit R. Infant hearing screening task force work paper. Newington, CT: Newington Children's Hospital, 1994.

Bentler RA. External ear resonance characteristics in children. J Speech Hear Disord 1989;54:264–268.

Bentler RA. Clinical implications and limitations of current noise reduction circuitry. In: Studebaker G, Bess F, Beck L, eds. The Vanderbilt hearing aid report II. Parkton, MD: York Press, 1991.

Bentler RA. Satisfaction with current noise reduction circuits. Am J Audiol 1993;2:51–53.

Bentler RA. Outcome measures: where should the emphasis be? Hear J 1998;51:46–51.

Bentler RA, Duve M. Hearing aids through the ages. (submitted).

Bentler RA, Niebuhr D. Verification: issues and implementation. Trends Amp 1999;4:90–102.

Bentler RA, Anderson CV, Niebuhr D, et al. A longitudinal study of hearing aid effectiveness. Part I: objective measures. J Speech Hear Res 1993a;36:808–819.

Bentler RA, Anderson CV, Niebuhr D, et al. A longitudinal study of hearing aid effectiveness. Part II: subjective measures. J Speech Hear Res 1993b;36:820–831.

Berger K, Hagberg N, Rane R. Prescription of hearing aids. Kent, OH: Herald Publishing, 1977.

Bergman BM, Bentler RA. Relating hearing aid output to measures of volume and immittance. Paper presented at the American Speech-Hearing-Language Association annual meeting, Seattle, Washington, 1990.

Bergstrom L. Congenital deafness. In: Northern J, ed. Hearing disorders. Boston: Little, Brown, 1976.

Berry G. The use and effectiveness of hearing aids. Laryngoscope 1939;49:912.

Bess F. The minimally hearing impaired child. Ear Hear 1985;6:43–47.

Bess F, Gravel J. Recent trends in educational amplification. Hear Instr 1981;32:24–29.

Bess F, Tharpe AM. An introduction to unilateral sensorineural hearing impaired children. Ear Hear 1986;7:14–19.

Bevacqua F, Cipollone F, Morviducci A, et al. Advances in understanding of E.M. emissions from computing devices. Paper presented at the IEEE National Symposium on Electromagnetic Compatibility, Denver, Colorado, 1989.

Blake R, Torpey C, Wertz P. Preliminary findings: effect of FM auditory trainers on attending behaviors of learning disabled children. Minneapolis, MN: Telex Communications, 1986.

Blake R, Field B, Foster C, et al. Effect of FM auditory trainers on attending behaviors of learning-disabled children. Lang Speech Hear Serv Schools 1991;22:111–114.

Braida LD, Durlach NI, Lippman RP, et al. Hearing aids—review of past research on linear amplification, compression amplification, and frequency lowering. ASHA monograph 19. Rockville, MD: ASHLA, 1979.

Brooks DN. Binaural benefit—when and how much? Scand Audiol 1984;13:237–141.

Bruel P, Frederiksen E, Rasmussen G. Investigations of a new insert earphone coupler. Hear Instr 1976;34:22–25.

Byrne D, Cotton S. Preferred listening levels of sensorineurally hearing-impaired listeners. Aust J Audiol 1988;9:7–14.

Byrne D, Dillon H. The National Acoustics Laboratories (NAL) new procedure for selecting the gain and frequency response of a hearing aid. Ear Hear 1986;7:257–265.

Byrne D, Fifield D. Evaluation of hearing aid fittings for infants. Br J Audiol 1974;8:47–54.

Byrne D, Tonisson W. Selecting the gain of hearing aids for persons with sensorineural hearing impairments. Scand Audiol 1976;5:51–62.

Byrne D, Upfold G. Implications of ear canal resonance for hearing aid fitting. Semin Hear 1991;12:34–41.

Byrne D, Parkinson A, Newall P. Hearing aid gain and frequency response requirements for the severely/profoundly hearing impaired. Ear Hear 1990;11:40–49.

Byrne D, Parkinson A, Newall P. Modified hearing aid selection procedures for severe/profound hearing loss. In: Studebaker G, Bess F, Beck L, eds. The Vanderbilt hearing aid report II. Parkton, MD: York Press, 1991.

Carlson E. Corrosion concerns in EMI shielding of electronics. Materials Perform 1990;29:76–80.

Chase PA, Bess FH. Behind-the-ear FM systems: new technology for children. In: Bess FH, Gravel JS, Tharpe AM, eds. Amplification for children with auditory deficits. Nashville: Bill Wilkerson Center Press, 1996.

Clopton BM, Silverman MS. Plasticity of binaural interactions. II. Critical periods and changes in midline response. J Neurophysiol 1977;40:1275–1280.

Compton CL. Assistive devices: doorways to independence. Washington, DC: Gallaudet University, 1989.

Cornelisse LE, Gagne J-P, Seewald RC. Ear level recordings of the long-term average spectrum of speech. Ear Hear 1991;12:47–54.

Cornelisse LE, Seewald RC, Jamieson DG. Fitting wide dynamic range compression hearing aids: the DSL[1/o] approach. Hear J 1994;47:23–29.

Cornelisse LE, Seewald RC, Jamieson DG. The input/output (I/o) formula: a theoretical approach to the fitting of personal amplification devices. J Acoust Soc Am 1995;97:1854–1864.

Cox RM. Using ULCL measures to find/gain and SSPL90. Hear Instr 1983;34:17–21.

Cox R. Hearing aids and rehabilitation: a structural approach to hearing aid selection. Ear Hear 1985;6:226–239.

Cox RM, Moore JN. Composite speech spectrum for hearing aid gain prescriptions. J Speech Hear Res 1988;31:102–107.

Cox R, Sherbecoe R. Effect of psychophysical method on the repeatability of loudness discomfort levels. Paper presented at the American Speech and Hearing Association Convention, Cincinnati, Ohio, 1983.

Darbyshire JD. A study of the use of high power hearing aids by children with marked degrees of deafness and the possibility of deterioration in auditory acuity. Br J Audiol 1976;10:74–82.

Davis JM, Elfenbein JL, Schum R, et al. Effects of mild and moderate hearing impairments on language, educational, and psychosocial behavior of children. J Speech Hear Disord 1986;51:53–62.

Dempster JH, MacKenzie K. The resonance frequency of the external auditory canal in children. Ear Hear 1990;11:296–298.

Dillon H. The NAL-NL1 hearing aid fitting strategy. Presentation at Jackson Hole Rendezvous, Jackson Hole, Wyoming, 1998.

Dobie RA, Berlin CI. Influence of otitis media on hearing and development. Ann Otol Rhinol Laryngol 1979;88 (Suppl 60):48–53.

Downs M. Contribution of mild hearing loss to auditory language learning problems. In: Roeser R, Downs M, eds. Auditory disorders in school children. New York: Thieme Medical Publishers, 1995.

Elfenbein JL. Monitoring preschoolers' hearing aids: issues in program design and implementation. Am J Audiol 1994;3:65–70.

Elfenbein JL, Logemann JM. Measuring the effects of head and neck support systems on signals transmitted to the ear. Ear Hear 1992;15:368–371.

Elfenbein JL, Bentler RA, Davis J, et al. Status of school children's hearing aids relative to monitoring practices. Ear Hear 1988;9:212–215.

Elssman SF, Matkin ND, Sabo MP. Early identification of congenital sensorineural hearing impairment. Hear J 1987;40:13–17.

Evans W, Webster D, Cullen J. Auditory brainstem responses in neonatally sound deprived CBA/J mice. Hear Res 1983;10:269–277.

Feigin J, Kopun J, Stelmachowicz P, et al. Probe-tube microphone measures of ear-canal sound pressure levels in infants and children. Ear Hear 1989;10:254–258.

Festen J, Plomp R. Speech reception threshold in noise with one and two hearing aids. J Acoust Soc Am 1986;79: 465–471.

Finitzo-Hieber T, Tillman T. Room acoustics effect on monosyllabic word discrimination ability for normal and hearing impaired children. J Speech Hear Res 1978;21:-440–458.

Freeman B, Sinclair J, Riggs D. Electroacoustic characteristics of FM auditory trainers. J Speech Hear Disord 1980; 45:16–26.

Gatehouse S. Apparent auditory deprivation of late-onset: the effects of presentation level. Br J Audiol 1989a;23:167.

Gatehouse S. Apparent auditory deprivation effects of late onset: the role of presentation level. J Acoust Soc Am 1989b;86:2103–2106.

Gelfand SA, Silman S. Apparent auditory deprivation in children: implications of monaural versus binaural amplification. J Am Acad Audiol 1993;4:313–318.

Gelfand SA, Silman S, Ross L. Long-term effects of monaural, binaural and no amplification in subjects with bilateral hearing loss. Scand Audiol 1987;16:201–207.

Gerling IJ, Boester K, Yu JH. The transient effect of cerumen on the external ear resonance. Poster presented at the annual conference of the American Academy of Audiology, Ft. Lauderdale, Florida, 1997.

Ginsburg H, Opper S. Piaget's theory of intellectual development. Englewood Cliffs, NJ: Prentice Hall, 1969.

Gladstone V. Variables affecting hearing aid telephone induction coil performance. Hear Instr 1985;36:18–21.

Gorga M. Clinical applications of auditory evoked potentials. Lecture presented at the University of Iowa, Iowa City, Iowa, October 1988.

Gravel JS, Wallace IF. Listening and language at 4 years of age. Effects of early otitis media. J Speech Hear Res 1992;35:588–595.

Greenfield DG, Wiley TL, Block MG. Acoustic-reflex dynamics and the loudness-discomfort level. J Speech Hear Disord 1985;50:14–20.

Greenstein JM, Greenstein BB, McConville K, et al. Mother infant communication and language acquisition in infants. New York: Lexington School for the Deaf, 1976.

Grimes AM, Mueller HG, Malley JD. Examination of binaural amplification in children. Ear Hear 1981;2:208–210.

Hammond L. FM auditory trainers: a winning choice for students, teachers, and parents. Minneapolis, MN: Gopher State Litho, 1991.

Harder J. Digital computer systems. In: Ficchi R, ed. Practical design for electromagnetic compatibility. New York: Hayden Book, 1971;165–182.

Hattori H. Ear dominance for nonsense-syllable recognition ability in sensorineural hearing-impaired children: monaural versus binaural amplification. J Am Acad Audiol 1993;4:319–330.

Hawkins DB. The effect of signal type on the loudness discomfort level. Ear Hear 1980;1:38–41.

Hawkins DB. Overamplification: a well-documented case report. J Speech Hear Disord 1982;47:382–384.

Hawkins DB. Comparisons of speech recognition in noise by mildly-to-moderately hearing impaired children using hearing aids and FM systems. J Speech Hear Disord 1984;49:409–418.

Hawkins D, Schum D. Some effects of FM-system coupling on hearing aid characteristics. J Speech Hear Disord 1985;50:132–141.

Hawkins D, Van Tasell D. Electroacoustic characteristics of personal FM systems. J Speech Hear Disord 1982;47: 355–362.

Hawkins D, Walden B, Montgomery A, et al. Description and validation of an LDL procedure designed to select SSPL90. Ear Hear 1987;8:162–169.

Hawkins DB, Cooper WA, Thompson DJ. Comparison among SPLs in real ears, 2 cm^3 and 6 cm^3 couplers. J Am Acad Audiol 1990;1:154–161.

Hedley-Williams A, Tharpe AM, Bess FH. Fitting hearing aids in the pediatric population: A survey of practice procedures. In: Bess FH, Gravel JS, Tharpe AM, eds. Amplification for children with auditory deficits. Nashville: Bill Wilkerson Center Press, 1996.

Hine WD, Furness HJS. Does wearing a hearing aid damage residual hearing? Teacher Deaf 1975;73:261–271.

Holmgren L. Can the hearing be damaged by a hearing aid? Acta Otolaryngol 1940;28:440.

Hood JD. Problems in central binaural integration in hearing loss cases. Hear Instr 1990;41:6–11.

Kamm C, Dirks DD, Mickey MR. Effect of sensorineural hearing loss on loudness discomfort level and most comfortable loudness judgments. J Speech Hear Res 1978; 21:668–681.

Kawell ME, Kopun JG, Stelmachowicz PG. Loudness discomfort levels in children. Ear Hear 1988;9:133–136.

Killion M, Shulein R, Christenesen L, et al. Real-world performance of an ITE directional microphone. Hear J 1998;51:24–38.

Konkle D, Schwartz D. Binaural amplification: A Paradox. In: FH Bess, BA Freeman, Sinclair S, eds. Amplification in Education. Washington, D. C.: Alexander Graham Bell Association, 1981.

Kruger B. An update on the external ear resonance in infants and young children. Ear Hear 1987;8:333–336.

Langford SE, Faires WL. Objective evaluation of monaural vs. binaural amplification for congenitally hard-of-hearing children. J Audiol Res 1973;13:263–267.

Lewis D. Assistive devices for classroom listening. Am J Audiol 1994a;3:58–69.

Lewis D. Assistive devices for classroom listening: FM systems. Am J Audiol 1994b;3:70–83.

Liden G, Harford ER. The pediatric audiologist: from magician to clinician. Ear Hear 1985;6:6–9.

Loose F. Learning disabled students use FM wireless systems. Minneapolis MN: Telex Communications, 1984.

Lurquin P, Rafhay S. Intelligibility in noise using multi-microphone hearing aids. Acta Otorhinolaryngol Belg 1996;50:103–109.

Macpherson BJ, Elfenbein JL, Schum RL, et al. Thresholds of discomfort in young children. Ear Hear 1991;12: 184–190.

Macrae JH. Temporary and permanent threshold shift associated with hearing aid use. Aust J Audiol 1985;7:45–54.

Mahon W. Hearing care for infants and children. Hear J 1987;40:7–10.

Markides A. The effect of hearing aid amplification on the user's residual hearing. In: Libby ER, ed. Binaural hearing and amplification. Chicago: Zenetron, 1980;2:341–355.

Markides A, Aryee DT-K. The effect of hearing aid use on the user's residual hearing: a follow-up study. Scand Audiol 1978;7:19–23.

Markides A, Aryee DT-K. The effect of hearing aid use on the user's residual hearing II: a follow-up study. Scand Audiol 1980;9:55–58.

Matkin N. Hearing aids for children. In: Hodgson W, ed. Hearing aid assessment and use in audiologic habilitation. 3rd ed. Baltimore: Williams & Wilkins, 1986.

Matkin N, Olsen W. Response of hearing aids with induction loop amplification systems. Am Ann Deaf 1970;115: 73–78.

Matkin N, Olsen W. An investigation of radio frequency auditory training units. Am Ann Deaf 1973;118:25–30.

Maxon AB. Binaural amplification of young children: a clinical application of Ross' Theory. Ear Hear 1981;2: 215–219.

McCandless G, Lyregaard PE. Prescription of gain/output (POGO) for hearing aids. Hear Instr 1983;34:16–21.

Mills JH. Noise and children: a review of literature. J Acoust Soc Am 1975;58:768–779.

Moodie KS, Seewald RC, Sinclair ST. Procedure for predicting real-ear performance in young children. Amer J Audiol 1994;3:23–31.

Moryl CL, Danhauer JL, DiBartolomeo JR. Real ear unaided responses in ears with tympanic membrane perforations. J Am Acad Audiol 1992;3.60–65.

Mueller HG. Directional microphone hearing aids: a ten year report. Hear Instr 1981;32:18–20.

Mueller HG. Binaural amplification: attitudinal factors. Hear J 1986;39:7–10.

Mueller HG. Individualizing the ordering of custom hearing instruments. Hear Instr 1989;40:18–22.

Mueller HG, Bentler RA. How loud is allowed. Hear J 1994;47:42–44.

Mueller HG, Grimes A. Amplification systems for the hearing impaired. In: Alpiner J, McCarthy P, eds. Rehabilitation audiology: children and adults. Baltimore: Williams & Wilkins, 1987:115–160.

Mueller HB, Hawkins DB. Three important considerations in hearing aid selection. In: Sandlin R, ed. Handbook of hearing aid amplification. Boston: College Hill Press, 1990;2.

Naunton RF. The effect of hearing aid use upon the user's residual hearing. Laryngoscope 1957;67:569–576.

Neuman AC. Late-onset auditory deprivation: a review of past research and an assessment of future research needs. Ear Hear 1996;17(Suppl).3–13.

Nittrouer S, Boothroyd A. Context effects in phoneme and word recognition by young children and older adults. J Acoust Soc Am 1990;87:2705–2715.

Northern JL, Downs MP. Hearing in children. 4th ed. Baltimore: Williams & Wilkins, 1991.

Northern JL, Gabbard SA, Kinder DL. Pediatric considerations in selecting and fitting hearing aids. In: Sandlin RE, ed. Handbook of hearing aid amplification. Boston: College Hill Press, 1990;2.

Olsen WO, Hawkins DB, Van Tasell DJ. Representations of the long-term spectra of speech. Ear Hear 1987;8(Suppl 5):100–107.

Oyler RF, Oyler AL, Matkin ND. Unilateral hearing loss: demographics and educational impact. Lang Speech Hear Serv Schools 1988;19:201–210.

Pascoe DP. An approach to hearing aid selection. Hear Instr 1998;29:12–16.

Pediatric Working Group of the Conference on Amplification for Children with Auditory Deficits. Amplification for infants and children with hearing loss. Am J Audiol 1996;5:53–68.

Popelka GR. Program for hearing aid selection and evaluation: PHASE IV. St. Louis: Central Institute for the Deaf Publication, 1983.

Popelka GR. The CID method: phase IV. Hear Instr 1988; 39:15–16, 18.

Popelka GR, Engebretson AM. A computer-based system for hearing aid assessment. Hear Instr 1983;34:6–9.

Preves DA, Sigelman JA. A questionnaire to evaluate signal processing hearing aids. Hear Instr 1989;40:20–21, 24.

Ricketts T, Dhar S. Comparison of performance across three directional hearing aids. Am Acad Audiol 1999;10:180–189.

Rintelmann WF, Bess FH, High-level amplification and potential hearing loss in children. In: Bess FH, ed. Hearing impairment in children. Parkton, MD: York Press, 1988: 278–309.

Ross M. Binaural versus monaural hearing aid amplification for hearing impaired individuals. In: Bess FH, ed. Childhood deafness: causation, assessment and management. New York: Grune and Stratton, 1977:235–249.

Ross M. Binaural versus monaural hearing aid amplification for hearing impaired individuals. In: Libby ER, ed. Binaural hearing and amplification. Chicago: Zenetron, 1980;2.

Ross M. Amplification for children: the process begins. In: Bess FH, Gravel JS, Tharpe AM, eds. Amplification for children with auditory deficits. Nashville: Bill Wilkerson Center Press, 1996;1–28.

Ross M, Lerman J. Hearing aid usage and its effects upon residual hearing: a review of the literature and an investigation. Arch Otolaryngol 1967;86:57–62.

Ross M, Seewald RC. Hearing aid selection and evaluation with young children. In: Bess F, ed. Hearing impairment in children. Parkton, MD: York Press, 1988:190–213.

Sachs RM, Burkhard MD. Making pressure measurements in insert earphone couplers and real ears. J Acoust Soc Am 1972;51:140(A)

Schwartz D, Lyregaard PE, Lundh P. Hearing aid selection for severe/profound hearing loss. Hear J 1988;41:13–17.

Schweitzer C. Development of digital hearing aids. Trends Amp 1997;2:41–77.

Seewald RC, Ross M, Spiro MK. Selecting amplification characteristics for young hearing-impaired children. Ear Hear 1985;6:48–53.

Seewald RC, Zelisko DLC, Ramji K, et al. Computer assisted implementation of the DSL approach: version 3.0. Poster presentation at the International Hearing Aids Conference, Iowa City, Iowa, 1991.

Seewald RC, Hudson SP, Gagne J-P, et al. Comparison of two methods for estimating the sensation level of amplified speech. Ear Hear 1992;13:142–149.

Seewald RC, Cornelisse LE, Ramji K, et al. DSL 4.1 for windows: a software implementation for fitting linear gain and wide-dynamic-range compression hearing instruments. London, Ontario, CA: The University of Western Ontario,1997.

Shah CP, Chandler D, Dale R. Delay in referral of children with impaired hearing. Volta Rev 1978;80:206–215.

Shaw E. Transformation of sound pressure level from the free field to the eardrum in the horizontal plane. J Acoust Soc Am 1974;56:1848–1861.

Shaw EAG, Vaillancourt MM. Transformation of sound pressure level from the free field to eardrum presented in numerical form. J Acoust Soc Am 1985;78:1120–1123.

Silverman CA. Auditory deprivation. Hear Instr 1989; 40:26–32.

Silverman MS, Clopton BM. Plasticity of binaural interaction: I. Effect of early auditory deprivation. J Neurophysiol 1977;40:1266–1274.

Simmons FB. Diagnosis and rehabilitation of deaf newborns. Part II. ASHA 1980;22:475.

Skinner M. Hearing aid evaluation. Englewood Cliffs, NJ: Prentice Hall, 1988.

Souza PA, Turner CW. Effect of single-channel compression on temporal speech information. J Speech Hear Res 1996;39:315–326.

Souza PA, Turner CW. Multichannel compression, temporal cues, and audibility. J Speech Hear Res 1998;41:315–326.

Stelmachowicz PG. Clinical issues related to hearing-aid maximum output. In: Studebaker G, Bess F, Beck L, eds. The Vanderbilt hearing aid report II. Parkton, MD: York Press, 1991.

Stelmachowicz P, Lewis D, Kalberer A, et al. User's manual situational hearing-aid response profile. Omaha: Boys Town National Research Hospital, 1994.

Stuart A, Durieux-Smith A, Stenstrom R. Probe tube microphone measures of loudness discomfort levels in children. Ear Hear 1991;12:140–143.

Stubblefield J, Nye C. Aided and unaided time-related differences in word discrimination. Hear Instr 1989;40:38–43, 78.

Studebaker GA, Pavlovic CV, Sherbecoe RL. A frequency importance function for continuous discourse. J Acoust Soc Am 1987;81:1130–1138.

Sung R, Hodgson W. Performance of individual hearing aids utilizing microphone and induction coil input. J Speech Hear Res 1971;14:365–371.

Tees RC. The effects of early auditory restriction in the rat on adult duration discrimination. J Audiol Res 1967;7: 195–207.

Thibodeau L, Saucedo K. Consistency of electroacoustic characteristics across components of FM systems. J Speech Hear Res 1991;34:628–635.

Valente M, Fabry D, Potts LG. Recognition of speech in noise with hearing aids using dual microphones. J Am Acad Audiol 1995;6:440–449.

Van Tasell D, Landin D. Frequency response characteristics of FM mini-loop auditory trainers. J Speech Hear Disord 1980;45:247–258.

Violette J, White D, Violette M. Electromagnetic compatibility handbook. New York: Van Nostrand Reinhold, 1987.

Voss T. Clinical evaluation of multi-microphone hearing instruments. Hear Rev 1997;4:45–46, 74.

Watson CS. Time course of auditory perceptual learning. Ann Otol Rhinol Laryngol 1980;89(Suppl 74):96–102.

Webster DB, Webster M. Effects of neonatal conductive hearing loss on brain stem auditory nuclei. Ann Otol Rhinol Laryngol 1979;88:684–688.

Willeford J, Billger J. Auditory perception in children with learning disabilities. In: Katz J, ed. Handbook of clinical audiology. 2nd ed. Baltimore: Williams & Wilkins, 1978:410–425.

APPENDIX 5.1 *Outline for Adjusting Gain in the FM Channel for a Personal FM System Used as an Accessory to an Existing Hearing Aid[a]*

1. Ensure that the Volume control, Tone control, Saturation Sound Pressure Level, and any compression characteristics of the hearing aid are adjusted as normally used and that the aid is functioning properly.
2. Measure output into a 2-cm³ coupler for an input to the hearing aid microphone of 65 dB SPL at a frequency of 1000 Hz, as illustrated in Figure 5.1.A.

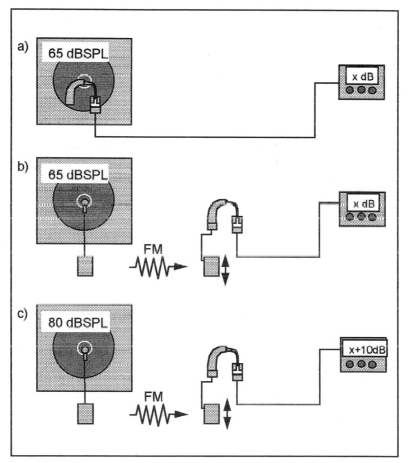

Figure 5.1.A. Suggested procedure for adjusting FM gain so as to preserve a 10 dB FM advantage. **a.** Using a 1 kHz tone, measure output for 65 dB SPL input to the local microphone. **b.** Provide 65 dB SPL input to the remote microphone and adjust FM gain to give the same output (the two channels now have equal gain). **c.** Increase input to 80 dB SPL. If the output increases by 10 dB, the process is complete. If it does not, increase FM gain to give an FM advantage of between 5 and 7 dB (see text).

[a]Reprinted with permission from the American Speech-Language-Hearing Association. Guidelines for fitting and monitoring FM systems (Draft). ASHA working group, 1999.

3. Couple the FM receiver to the hearing aid in the manner that is to be used. If using a standard neck loop, make sure the shape and orientation of the loop, and the distance and orientation of the aid in relation to the loop, are the same as in actual use.
4. Adjust the FM volume control of the FM receiver so that a 65 dB SPL, 1000 Hz input to the remote microphone generates the same output from the hearing aid as measured with the local microphone, as illustrated in Figure 5.1.A.
5. Increase the input to 80 dB SPL. You should find that the output from the hearing aid increases by at least 10 dB. If so, then the adjustment can stand.
6. If the increase was 15 dB, you may reduce the FM volume control of the FM receiver so that the output into the 2-cm^3 coupler falls by 5 dB.
7. If the increase was only 5 dB, increase the FM volume control of the FM receiver to provide an additional 2 or 3 dB of output (giving a 7 or 8 dB FM advantage rather than a 10 dB advantage).
8. If there was no increase of output when the input changed from 65 to 80 dB SPL, you may assume that the FM transmitter has a very low compression threshold. In this case, increase the FM volume control of the FM receiver to provide a 5 dB increase of output (giving a 5 dB FM advantage).

When dealing with a self-contained FM system, in which the FM receiver and amplifier are in a single unit, first adjust the characteristics of amplification via the local (environmental) microphone to match those of the users' personal hearing aid (which we assume to have been fitted properly). Then follow the procedure just outlined.

Depending on the nature of the audiologist's test equipment, it may be easier to carry out the above procedure with a swept tone or speech-weighted noise input so as to produce a complete curve showing output as a function of frequency. In this case, the focus should be on output in the 500 to 2000 Hz range rather than just at 1000 Hz.

APPENDIX 5.2 *Outline for FM System Electroacoustic Confirmation*[a]

A. Recommendations for 2-cc coupler assessment
1. Attach the hearing aid, or the receiver/amplifier of a self-contained FM system, to the 2-cc coupler and place in the test box with the microphone in the calibrated position.
2. Using swept tones or a complex noise, measure output as a function of frequency following standard procedures. The results should include:
   a. An estimate of maximum output as a function of frequency.
   b. An estimate of full-on gain as a function of frequency.
   c. An estimate of actual gain as a function of frequency at user settings for conversational input (65 dB SPL).
   d. If the aid incorporates full dynamic range compression—estimates of user gain as functions of frequency for low (50 dB SPL), typical (65 dB SPL), and high (80 dB SPL) input levels.
   e. Estimates of distortion as a function of frequency under normal conditions of use.
3. Remove the hearing aid, still attached to the coupler, from the test box.
   a. If this is a personal FM system, couple the FM receiver to the personal hearing aid.

---

[a]Reprinted with permission from American Speech-Language-Hearing Association. Guidelines for fitting and monitoring FM systems (Draft). ASHA working group, 1999.

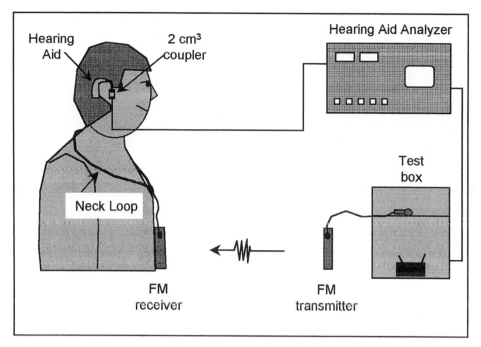

Figure 5.2.A. Suggested arrangement for electroacoustic assessment of a personal FM system that uses neck loop coupling.

Note that if Direct Audio Input is being used, the sensitivity of the hearing aid microphone may change. The system should, therefore, be retested with input to the hearing aid microphone before assessing FM input.

   b. If neck loop coupling is being used, make sure that the configuration of the loop, and the position and orientation of the aid in relation to the loop, represent real conditions of use. The ideal way to meet this requirement is to place them on the actual user (Fig. 5.2.A). An alternative is to use another person, or a manikin. With all three options, it may be necessary to support the weight of the coupler as it hangs in front of the ear.

4. Place the FM microphone in the test box in the calibrated position.

   a. If possible, turn off the local ("environmental" or hearing aid) microphone. If it is not possible, the measurements must be done in a quiet environment such as the audiometric test booth. Note that, when testing a self-contained FM system in which the environmental microphone can be turned off, the receiver/amplifier can remain in the test box.

5. Set all volume controls to their normal use positions.

6. Repeat the output measurements to obtain:

   a. An estimate of gain, as a function of frequency, for a high input level (80 dB SPL).

   b. An input-versus-output curve to obtain an estimate of compression threshold in the FM transmitter.

B. Real-ear assessment

If electroacoustic confirmation is to be carried out using output measurements in the ear canal of the user, rather than in a 2-cm³ coupler, the audiologist should follow standard procedures for testing via the local or hearing aid microphone. When testing via the FM microphone, this should be placed as close as possible to the location of the reference microphone (see Sullivan, 1987; Seewald et al., 1991; Hawkins, 1992, 1993).

C. Limitations of aided sound field threshold as a means to estimate gain

While behavioral measurements of real-ear performance such as functional gain have been recommended by some investigators (Turner and Holte, 1985; Van Tasell et al., 1986; Madell, 1992b), several distinct limitations of this approach have been described recently (Lewis et al., 1991; Seewald and Moodie, 1992). The major problem with the functional gain approach is that the input levels to the FM microphone at the aided threshold will typically be quite low during the measurement procedure. These lower input levels would not be representative of the talker's voice entering the FM microphone during actual use of the FM system. These input level differences, combined with the fact that most FM microphone-transmitters incorporate input compression, make the aided sound field threshold values difficult to interpret. The sound-field threshold values do represent the lowest intensity signal that the user can detect with the FM system. Unfortunately, they lead to an overestimate of both the amount of gain for the FM signal under normal use conditions and the sensation level at which speech is presented to the user (Lewis et al., 1991; Seewald and Moodie, 1992; Seewald et al., 1992).

APPENDIX 5.3 *Outline for Monitored Live-Voice Assessment of Speech Perception With an FM System*[a]

---

1. Select an appropriate speech recognition test with consideration given to the user' developmental age, language skills, and primary language.
2. Make sure that all controls on the FM system are set for customary use and that the system is working.
3. Place the FM microphone on yourself in the position normally worn but turned off.
4. Place the hearing aid(s) and personal FM receiver (or self-contained FM receiver/amplifier) on the client.
5. Place the user in the calibrated sound field and yourself at the audiometer controls, as shown in Figure 5.3.A. Note that the loudspeakers are located at ±45° azimuths[5].
6. Measure speech perception in quiet and noise via the local microphone(s):
   a. Set the speech level to 55 dB HL (68 dB SPL) and obtain a speech perception score through the loudspeaker (FM microphone off).
   b. Turn on speech-shaped noise at 50 dB HL (63 dB SPL), producing a S/N ratio of +5 dB. Obtain a second speech perception score.
7. Measure speech perception in quiet and noise via the FM microphone(s):
   a. Without making any other changes, turn ON the FM microphone and obtain a third speech perception score via Aid plus FM in noise.
   b. Turn OFF the noise and obtain a final speech perception score via Aid plus FM in quiet.
8. Evaluate the results:
   a. The score obtained in quiet by Aid alone should be commensurate with other speech perception scores for this client obtained either aided or under headphones.
   b. The score obtained in noise by Aid alone should be poorer than that obtained in quiet.
   c. When the FM microphone is turned on, the score in noise should return to a value that is not significantly lower (and may be higher) than that obtained in quiet by aid alone. If the score remains below that obtained by Aid alone in quiet, the gain in the FM channel is probably too low.

---

[a]Reprinted with permission from American Speech-Language-Hearing Association. Guidelines for fitting and monitoring FM systems (Draft). ASHA working-group, 1999.

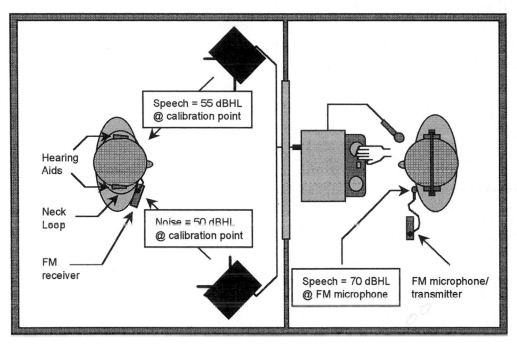

Figure 5.3.A. Suggested test arrangement for speech perception assessment with an FM system using monitored live voice.

  d. Turning off the noise in the Aid plus FM condition should not produce a significant change of score. If there is a significant increase of score, the gain in the FM channel is probably too low.
9. At all points in the test process, confirm with the client that the speech levels are within an acceptable range of loudness and perceived quality—making due allowance for the negative effects of the noise.

REFERENCES

Hawkins D. Selecting SSPL90 using probe microphone measurements. In: Mueller H, Hawkins D, and Northern J (Eds). Probe Microphone Measurements: Hearing Aid Selection and Assessment. San Diego, CA: Singular Press, 1992:145–158.

Hawkins, DB. Assessment of hearing aid maximum output. Am J Audiol 1993;2:36 37.

Lewis D, Feigin J, Karasek A, Stelmachowicz P. Evaluation and assessment of FM systems. Ear Hear 1991;12:268–280.

Madell JR. FM systems for children birth to age 5. In: Ross M (Ed.). FM auditory training systems: Characteristics, selection, and use. Timonium, MD: York Press, 1992b:157–174.

Seewald R, Hudson S, Gagne J, Zelisko D. Comparison of two methods for estimating the sensation level of amplified speech. Ear Hear 1992;13;142–149.

Seewald R, Moodie K. Electroacoustic considerations. In: Ross M (Ed.). FM auditory training systems: Characteristics, selection and use. Timonium, MD: York Press, 1992:75–102.

Seewald R, Zelisko D, Ramji K, Jamieson D. DSL 3.0 User's Manual. London, Ontario, Canada: University of Western Ontario, 1991.

Sullivan R. Aided SSPL90 response in the real ear: A safe estimate. Hear Instruments 1987:36,38.

Turner C, Holte L. Evaluation of FM amplification systems. Hear Instruments 1985:36;6–12,56.

Van Tasell D, Mallinger C, Crump E. Functional gain and speech recognition with two types of FM amplification. Lang Speech Hear Services in Schools 1986:17;28–37.

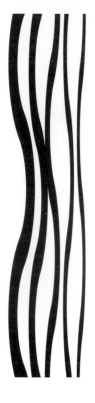

Assessment and Intervention With Preschool Children Who Are Deaf and Hard-of-Hearing

Christine Yoshinaga-Itano, Ph.D.

The future of education of deaf and hard-of-hearing (D/HH) children in the United States is being altered dramatically as universal newborn hearing screening programs are developed throughout the nation. As of writing this chapter, there are 20 states with legislation mandating newborn hearing screening and 5 states with the governor's signature pending. More than a dozen more have legislation in process. By the beginning of the next century, more than half the newborns born in the United States may be screened for hearing loss before discharge from the hospital.

The Effects of Early Identification of Hearing Loss on the Assessment and Intervention of D/HH Children

LANGUAGE CHARACTERISTICS

Receptive and expressive language skills—birth to 3 years

Studies by Yoshinaga-Itano et al. (1998) indicate that children with normal cognitive ability identified as D/HH before 6 months of age who receive immediate and appropriate intervention services have developed language

skills within normal limits in early childhood. Their cognitive abilities are commensurate with their language skills. They maintain age-appropriate language skills from 12 months through 3 years of age, regardless of degree of hearing loss, gender, ethnicity, socioeconomic status, age at testing, or mode of communication. Preliminary data on children aged 3 to 6 years indicate that these findings from the infant-toddler period are consistent through the preschool years (Figs. 6.1 and 6.2).

Expressive and receptive language skills of later-identified children are one standard deviation (SD) lower than those of early-identified children. Children with normal cognitive ability who are later identified maintain about a 60 developmental language quotient throughout their early childhood years. There is some tendency for this level to drop to developmental quotients below 50 as the children age.

Children with hearing loss identified after 6 months of age but before 30 months of age had similar language quotients when identification of hearing loss was followed by immediate and appropriate intervention. They were significantly lower than in children

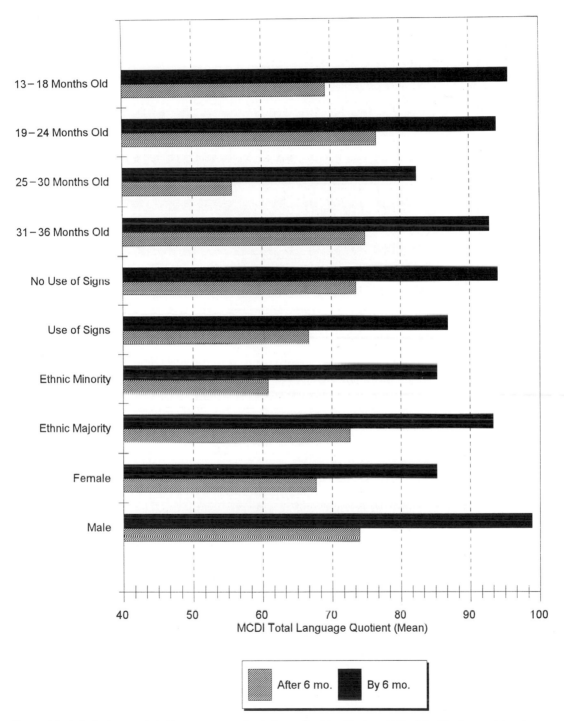

Figure 6.1. Adjusted mean total language quotients for earlier-identified and later-identified groups by demographic category for children with normal cognition. (Reprinted with permission from Pediatrics 1998;102: 1161–1171.)

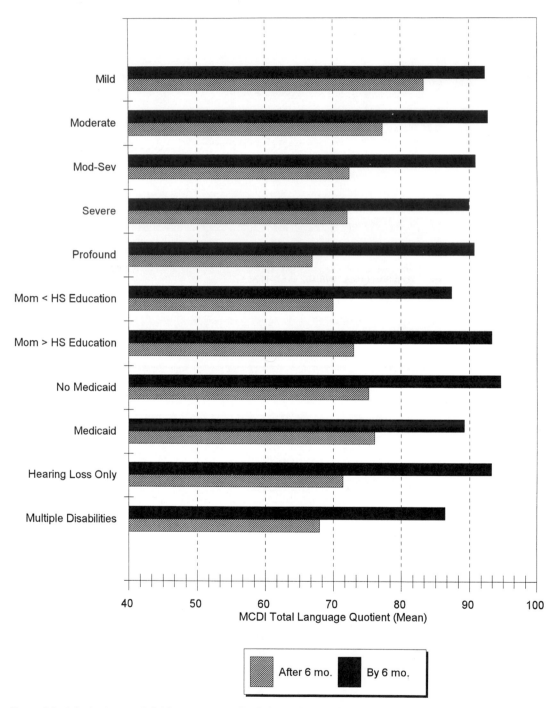

Figure 6.2. Adjusted mean total language quotients for earlier-identified and later-identified groups by demographic category, Medicaid status, and Mom's education for children with normal cognition. (Reprinted with permission from Pediatrics 1998;102:1161–1171.)

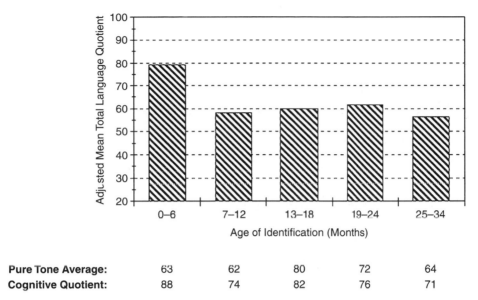

Pure Tone Average:	63	62	80	72	64
Cognitive Quotient:	88	74	82	76	71

Figure 6.3. Adjusted mean total language quotients for groups based on age at identification of hearing loss. (Reprinted with permission from Pediatrics 1998;102:1161–1171.)

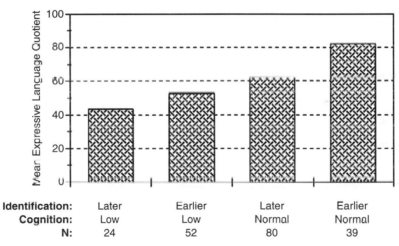

Identification:	Later	Earlier	Later	Earlier
Cognition:	Low	Low	Normal	Normal
N:	24	52	80	39

Figure 6.4. Mean expressive language quotient by age at identification of hearing loss and cognition for children 3 to 6 years of age.

with hearing loss identified before 6 months of age (Fig. 6.3).

Receptive/expressive language skills—preschool

In a preliminary study of 83 preschool-aged D/HH children with normal cognitive abilities (Yoshinago-Itano, 1999a), 47 were identified before 6 months of age, and 46 were identified after 6 months of age. The children were tested between 34 and 50 months of age. Developmental quotients for the early-identified children were within the low normal range, indicating that the developmental scores obtained in the infant/toddler period remained stable during the preschool period (Fig. 6.4). Moeller (1996) reported similar findings for early-identified preschool-aged children with signficant hearing loss.

Vocabulary skills—birth through 3 years

Early-identified D/HH children with normal cognitive ability had expressive vocabulary lexicons similar to their normal-hearing peers. In a study of 90 D/HH children, Carey reported that vocabulary inventories of the 50th percentile of the distribution fell at the 25th percentile of the hearing distribution. (Carey A. The language development of young hearing-impaired children using the MacArthur Communicative Developmental Inventories. Unpublished master's thesis. Boulder, CO: University of Colorado, 1995) Mayne et al. (in press) updated these statistics in 1998 to include 200 children with similar results. The children ranged in age from 12 to 36 months (Fig. 6.5).

No differences by degree of hearing loss, mode of communication, gender, ethnicity, or

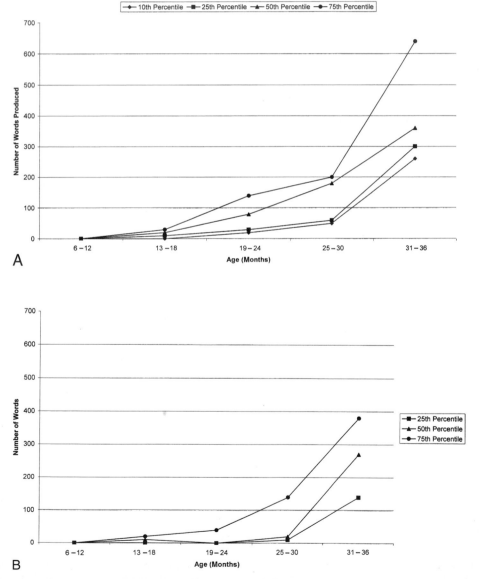

Figure 6.5. Expressive vocabulary: children with normal cognition who were identified with hearing loss (**a**) at or younger than 6 months of age and (**b**) older than 6 months of age.

socioeconomic status were found. A remarkable similarity between the vocabulary sizes of children with normal cognition who were later identified and children with low cognition who were early identified was noted.

Vocabulary skills—preschool

A preliminary study of 159 children between the ages of 34 and 51 months was conducted. (Yoshinaga-Itano, 1999b). Sixty-three children were identified as deaf or hard-of-hearing by 6 months of age, and 96 were identified after 6 months of age. Results indicate that significant development in vocabulary occurs between 3 and 4 years of age. A significant number of children have lexical inventories approaching 1000 words (Table 6.1).

Pragmatic language skills—preschool

Very little information is available about the pragmatic language abilities of children with hearing loss. At the preschool level, the categories suggested by Halliday (1975) can be used to assess pragmatic language abilities. These specific pragmatic language skills are reported to be developed during the preschool period for typically developing children. Halliday (1975) discussed pragmatic language skills in seven categories: (1) instrumental or "I want"—requests for objects or actions; (2) regulatory, "Do as I tell you"—the command; (3) interactional, "Me and you"—conversational strategies; (4) personal, "Here I come"—expressions of feelings; (5) heuristic, "Tell me why"—requests for information; (6) imaginative,

"Let's pretend"—the creative strategy; and (7) informative, "I've got something to tell you"—the commenting strategy. Preschool-aged D/HH children may have age-appropriate vocabularies and even syntactic skills. However, many of them experience difficulties in applying their language knowledge in socially appropriate situations.

A study of 54 preschool-aged D/HH children, 24 3-year-olds, and 30 4-year-olds was conducted (Yoshinaga-Itano, 1999c). Because these data were collected at a time when universal newborn hearing screening programs were just beginning in Colorado, there are fewer early-identified (before 6 months) children at the 4-year-old level (10%) than the 3-year-old level (50%). Teachers indicated the presence of the following pragmatic categories in the observed language of the preschool children. It may be possible that the pragmatic language skills of the preschool-aged child will change if hearing loss is identified earlier as a result of universal newborn hearing screening. Teachers rated the following pragmatic skills in the following categories: no ability, occasionally present, and regularly present in seven pragmatic categories: (1) instrumental, (2) regulatory, (3) international, (4) personal, (5) heuristic, (6) imaginative, and (7) informative (Tables 6.2 to 6.9).

Validity and reliability of the pragmatic checklist

The ability to develop age-appropriate pragmatic language skills is highly related to the

Table 6.1
Total group: number of words produced[a]

Group	Age in Months	No.	Number of Words Produced				
			Percentile Rank				
			10	25	50	75	90
Total group	34–39	114	5.0	50.2	164.5	380.8	551.0
	46–51	61	58.8	238.5	412.0	579.0	662.6
Identified by 6 months	34–39	48	5.0	56.5	324.5	474.2	655.2
	46–51	15	13.8	181.0	489.0	605.0	679.4
Identified after 6 months	34–39	62	3.3	22.0	125.5	287.2	409.1
	46–51	34	50.0	255.0	396.5	565.5	619.5

[a]MacArthur Communicative Development Inventories age norms for children who are deaf or hard-of-hearing.

Table 6.2
Percentage of children at ages 3 and 4 whose language indicates that the iInstrumental ("I want") categories are not present or regularly present

	Age 3, Not Present	Age 4, Not Present	Age 3, Regularly Present	Age 4, Regularly Present
Polite requests	0%	11%	32%	67%
Gives directions	38%	17%	12%	21%

Table 6.3
Percentage of children at ages 3 and 4 whose language indicates that the regulatory ("do as I tell you") categories are not present or regularly present

	Age 3, Not Present	Age 4, Not Present	Age 3, Regularly Present	Age 4, Regularly Present
Polite commands	35%	19%	24%	48%
Gives directions for arranging objects	75%	36%	5%	32%
Gives directions for sequential tasks, making something	67%	37%	5%	32%
Gives directions when participating in a simple game	57%	43%	4%	29%

Table 6.4
Percentage of children at ages 3 and 4 whose language indicates that the interactional ("me and you") categories are not present or regularly present

	Age 3, Not Present	Age 4, Not Present	Age 3, Regularly Present	Age 4, Regularly Present
Interacts socially and graciously	17%	9%	26%	43%
General poise in use of social rules (greeting, farewell, thank you)	8%	12%	25%	54%
Apologies and explanations of behavior	46%	30%	15%	22%

Table 6.5
Percentage of children at ages 3 and 4 whose language indicates that the conversational skills categories are not present or regularly present

	Age 3, Not Present	Age 4, Not Present	Age 3, Regularly Present	Age 4, Regularly Present
Initiation of a topic	28%	12%	24%	44%
Maintenance of a topic	38%	12%	14%	40%
Taking conversational turns	20%	23%	24%	41%
Relevant answers to questions	28%	12%	20%	38%
Revision of unclear message	75%	50%	0%	15%
Respect for alternative points of view	64%	48%	9%	24%

Table 6.6
**Percentage of children at ages 3 and 4 whose language indicates that the personal ("here I come")
categories are not present or regularly present**

	Age 3, Not Present	Age 4, Not Present	Age 3, Regularly Present	Age 4, Regularly Present
Expression of a state of mind/health/attitude ("I'm angry/my side hurts")	45%	32%	9%	27%
Expression of feelings (one-word statements: happy, sad)	32%	12%	32%	62%
Explanation of feelings ("I'm really mad because . . ." "I'm really hurt because . . .")	76%	42%	8%	17%
Tells an adult what is not understood in an accusation (e.g., "It wasn't Tommy, Johnny hit from first") (kindergarten competency)	81%	48%	5%	10%
Offers an opinion on an issue and supplies a supportive statement for the opinion ("I like that because . . ." "That movie was great because . . .") (kindergarten competency)	86%	42%	4%	12%
Supplies basic identification and biographic data (such as birthday, address, full name, parents' occupation) (kindergarten competency)	74%	34%	11%	21%

Table 6.7
**Percentage of children at ages 3 and 4 whose language indicates that the heuristic ("tell me why") categories
are not present or regularly present**

	Age 3, Not Present	Age 4, Not Present	Age 3, Regularly Present	Age 4, Regularly Present
Asks questions for clarification: is it the big one?	81%	41%	8%	22%
Asks questions to gather information systematically: 20 questions (kindergarten competency)	46%	32%	19%	36%

ability to understand and produce language and the number of words in the expressive lexicon. Additionally, pragmatic language skills are highly related to the development of personal-social skills.

The pragmatic checklist had significant and strong relationships to the Minnesota Comprehension-Conceptual subtest (a mea-sure of receptive language), the Minnesota Expressive Language subtest, and the MacArthur Communicative Development Inventory: Level III (Dale, 1997) subtest at both the 3-year-old and 4-year-old levels. At the 3-year age level, the pragmatic checklist sub-tests were not significantly related to the MacArthur Communicative Development In-

Table 6.8
Percentage of children at ages 3 and 4 whose language indicates that the imaginative ("let's pretend") categories are not present or regularly present

	Age 3, Not Present	Age 4, Not Present	Age 3, Regularly Present	Age 4, Regularly Present
Engages in role-playing	26%	12%	30%	52%
Creates a story that has a beginning, logical events, and a conclusion	76%	46%	8%	23%

Table 6.9
Percentage of children at ages 3 and 4 whose language indicates that the informative ("I've got something to tell you") categories are not present or regularly present

	Age 3, Not Present	Age 4, Not Present	Age 3, Regularly Present	Age 4, Regularly Present
Organized description of a situation or object	57%	41%	4%	23%
Interprets and relates 4- to 6-frame picture story sequence (relates story to wordless picture book)	64%	43%	14%	35%
Observation of cause/effect details	53%	43%	14%	17%
Use of precise noun/pronoun referents (that boy, he, she)	67%	46%	7%	12%
Improves story quality after exposure to model story	58%	32%	17%	32%
Explanation of the relationship between two objects (toothbrush/toothpaste)—they go together because . . .	52%	36%	11%	24%
Compares and contrasts attributes of 2 objects, vehicles, or events—they are alike or different because . . . (kindergarten competency)	56%	44%	13%	19%
Engages in evaluation of one object in contrast to another ("I like this better because . . .") (emerges in preschool/kindergarten competency)	64%	43%	16%	19%
Evaluates the quality of an event ("That party/game was great, boring, bad . . .")	82%	63%	9%	11%

ventory: Level III (Dale, 1997). The pragmatic language skills were significantly related to the Minnesota Child Development Inventory subtests and ranged from r = 0.45 to 0.84. They ranged from r = 0.69 to 0.85 for the Minnesota subtests and r = 0.55 to 0.84 for the MacArthur subtest at the 4-year age level. The seven pragmatic categories were highly related to the Personal-Social subtest of the Minnesota at the 4-year level r = 0.49 to 0.81; at the 3-year level, only three of the seven categories had significant relationship to the Personal-Social subtest (instrumental [r = 0.45], heuristic [r = 0.59], imaginative [r =

0.58]). This finding may indicate that the interaction between social interaction and pragmatic language skills becomes stronger as the child ages, as does the relationship between vocabulary and pragmatic language skills.

Syntax and morphology—preschool

A study of 50 3-year-old D/HH children was conducted (Yoshinaga-Itano, 1999d). The mean length of utterance from a 30-minute videotape of parent-child interaction was coded. Early identification (EID) of hearing loss resulted in significantly higher mean length of utterance than did later identification (LID) for these 3-year-old children for morphemes (EID = 1.7, LID = 1.3; $p < 0.01$), words (EID = 1.8, LID = 1.3; $p < 0.05$), total number of words used (EID = 274, LID = 144; $p < 0.05$), and total number of different words used (EID = 74, LID = 42; $p < 0.05$). There were no significant differences between the two groups in their developmental ages on the Situation Comprehension (EID = 29.5, LID = 28.9) or Self-Help (EID = 32.3, LID = 30.6) subtests of the Minnesota Child Development Inventory.

Children who are later-identified with hearing loss have previously been described in the literature. Most preschool-aged children had one-word and two-word utterances, and their sentence structure was described using semantic cases and categories. Traditional means of language sample analysis could not be done on the later-identified preschool population because they did not yet formulate sentences beyond the two-word stage. Because mean length of utterance has been so restricted in children with later-identified hearing loss, Curtiss et al. (1979) reported that mean length of utterance (MLU) was insensitive to communicative development in the preschool age group.

Syntax and pragmatic language interaction

In a study by Lartz and McCullom (1990), it was found that a mother of twins used 42% more questions with the hearing twin than with the deaf twin. These findings are similar to Goss (1970) and Matey and Kretschmer (1985). The deaf twin had significantly lower language level and primarily used one-word utterances. There were both quantitative and qualitative language differences when comparing the 3.6-year-old twins.

Lartz (1993) found that the MLU of a child appears to influence the amount and types of maternal questions. Mothers of children with hearing loss use significantly fewer questions than mothers of hearing children. There were 5 subjects between 3.1 and 4.3 years of age with MLU ranging from 1.54 to 1.93, and the total number of utterances ranged from 17 to 196.

Phonologic development— birth through preschool

Findings related to phonologic development for birth through preschool are as follows:

- D/HH children who were early-identified (before 6 months) have significantly greater numbers of consonants, consonant blends, and vowels compared with children from the same hearing loss category who are later-identified.
- Degree of hearing loss and age at identification predict speech intelligibility from 12 months through the preschool years. The relationship between babble in the first year of life and later speech intelligibility. (Wallace V, Menn L, Yoshinaga-Itano C [1998] unpublished manuscript. Boulder, CO. University of Colorado, 1998).
- Children between birth and 36 months with mild through severe hearing losses have similar phonologic development when identified early. They have significantly higher phonetic repertoires than children with profound hearing losses.

Personal-social development— birth through preschool

Findings related to social development from birth through preschool are as follows (Yoshinaga-Itano, 1998):

- Personal-social skills of children with early-identified hearing loss are significantly higher than those of children with later-identified hearing loss.
- A significant proportion of the variance in

personal-social skills can be predicted by symbolic play ability, expressive language, and degree of hearing loss. Later-identified children with milder hearing loss had poorer personal-social skills than children with moderate through profound hearing loss (Fig. 6.6).

- Language development of early-identified children is significantly more advanced than in later-identified children. Language development is highly related to emotional availability.
- Emotional availability of mother to child and child to mother predicts later language ability.
- Children with better language skills have parents who report less parental stress.
- Children who are early-identified with better language development than later-identified children have a better sense of self.
- The raw score of the personal-social subtest is significantly and strongly related to the subtests of the Meadow-Kendall Social

Adjustment Inventory: The Social-Communicative Behavior Scaled Score ($r = 0.574, p < 0.01$) (Meadow, 1983) the Impulsivity Domain Behavior Scaled Score ($r = 0.511, p < 0.01$), and the Developmental Lags Scaled Score ($r = 0.654. p < 0.01$), but not to the Anxiety, Compulsivity Behavior Scaled Score ($r = 0.241, p > 0.05$) or the Specific Items Deafness Scaled Score ($r = 0.306, p > 0.05$).

Cognitive symbolic play skills

Children with early-identified losses have cognitive skills that are comparable to their language skills whether they have normal cognitive skills (Fig. 6.7) or low cognitive skills (Fig. 6.8). Cognitive ability was measured by the Play Assessment Questionnaire. Children with normal cognitive abilities who are later identified have similar language at 31 to 36 months compared with children with low cognitive abilities who are early-identified (Fig. 6.9).

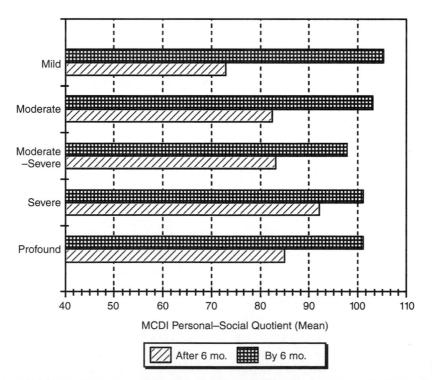

Figure 6.6. Adjusted mean personal-social quotients for the earlier-identified and later-identified groups.

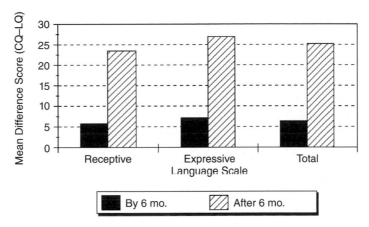

Figure 6.7. Discrepancy between cognitive quotient and language quotient by age at identification of hearing loss for children with normal cognition.

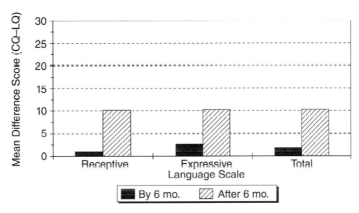

Figure 6.8. Discrepancy between cognitive quotient and language quotient by age at identification of hearing loss for children with low cognition.

An evaluation of symbolic play can provide a nonverbal assessment of thinking abilities that are parallel to language development in children with normal hearing as well as those who are deaf or hard-of-hearing.

PLAY CHARACTERISTICS

The relationship between play and language

Studies of the relationship between play and language have resulted in several findings.

- McCune (1995) found that the onset and independence levels of specific aspects of symbolic play were related to language development of typically developing children.

- Casby and Ruder (1983) found no difference in symbolic play when children who were developmentally delayed (ages 2 to 11 years) were matched by MLU to children with normally developing language (ages 19 to 32 months).

- Eisert and Lamorey (1996) found a relationship between play and language skills at 20 months of age with typically developing children. This study also found that expressive language was the best predictor of play development between the ages of 14 and 36 months.

- Terrell et al. (1984) compared symbolic play behavior of 15 children with normally developing language and 15 children with delayed expressive language skills. The play skills of the children with

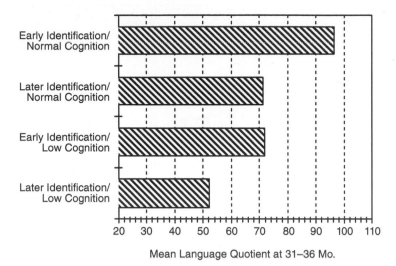

Figure 6.9. Mean total language quotient scores at 31 to 36 months by age at identification of hearing loss and cognition.

delayed expressive language were significantly less advanced than those of the children with normally developing language.

- Lombardino et al. (1986) reported differences in mean length of play sequences when comparing children with normally developing language and children with significant language impairment who were matched for MLU, indicating that measures of play may be more sensitive measures than MLU.

Play behavior and communication development of D/HH children

Findings that relate play behavior to communication development in hearing-impaired children include the following:

- Schirmer (1989) reported a significant relationship between imaginative play and language development as measured by Brown's stages, although imaginative play was not significantly related to chronologic age in a sample of 20 severely to profoundly deaf children between 3 and 6 years of age. Stage I children did engage in some imaginary play (MLU of 1.00 to 1.99). The presence of rule-based utterances in the subject's language corresponded to use of planned pretend play.
- Higginbotham and Baker (1981) and Darbyshire (1977) both reported less mature

play and significantly less time in dramatic play. Mann (1984) reported similar play behaviors in 3- to 6-year-old D/HH children but a lower frequency of their play behaviors.

- Casby and McCormack (1985) reported that higher symbolic play scores for D/HH children ages 3 to 5–9 were highly related to more developed communication skills.

The relationship between play and social behaviors

Children's social behaviors and play partners do not differ according to hearing status (Arnold and Tremblay, 1979; Vandell and George, 1981; Lederberg et al., 1986). However, D/HH preschool-aged children segregate themselves even in integrated settings (Arnold and Tremblay, 1979; Levy-Shiff and Hoffman, 1985; Minnett et al., 1994). Likewise, hearing children actively choose hearing playmates, avoiding D/HH peers (Arnold and Tremblay, 1979; Vandell and George, 1981; Vandell et al., 1982; Minnett et al., 1994). The degree of hearing loss in preschool children was not found to be related to social development (Musselman et al., 1988), nor was it related to social interactions with other children who are deaf or hard-of-hearing (Antia and Kreimeyer, 1988).

Minnett et al. (1994) summarized the number of reasons provided in the literature for the lack of integrated play of D/HH preschool children:

1. Low communication skills of D/HH children (Brackett and Hennings, 1976; Lederberg, 1991).
2. Hearing children's poor motivation to interact with D/HH peers (Lederberg et al., 1996).
3. Hearing children's persistence in inappropriate communication to D/HH peers (Vandell and George, 1981)
4. Social skills delays of D/HH children in auditory environments (Higginbotham and Baker, 1981).
5. Social skills delays of D/HH children in total communication (TC) environments (Lederberg et al., 1987; Vandell and George, 1981).
6. Degree of hearing loss—the greater the hearing loss, the less likely the child will interact with hearing children (Levy-Skiff and Hoffman, 1985).

Other findings on the relationship between play and social behaviors include the following:

• D/HH children play more together outdoors (Minnett et al., 1994) than in the preschool classrooms.
• Spencer et al. (1994) reported that deaf and hearing preschool children communicated with both same hearing status and different hearing status peers, but more frequently with same status peers.
• Deaf and hearing children with higher language levels engaged in more communicative interactions with hearing peers compared with children with lower language levels.
• Two- and three-year-old hearing children appear to be capable of adjusting their communicative modalities to fit the need of interactive partners, both peers and adults.
• Cornelius and Hornett (1990) reported higher levels of social play (functional, constructive, dramatic, and social were measured) and lower levels of aggres-

sion in sign-based class than oral-based class in a study of 20 D/HH children between the ages of 5.4 and 6.3 years. Sign-based children engaged in more dramatic play.

Play behavior and narrative development

Schirmer (1989) found that as children used multiword expressions, they combined units of play into sequences (i.e., story line). There was wide subject variation on this variable.

Play Assessment Procedures

Play in the preschool period can be measured through a variety of criterion-reference assessments. Westby (1988), McCune-Nicolich (1981), and Linder (1990) offer different methods to accomplish this goal. The assessment of play in the preschool period provides a nonverbal reflection of skills required for language development and can be extremely helpful in designing interventions.

WESTBY PLAY SCALES

Westby (1988) developed an assessment that yielded developmental ages scores for play and language development. Westby's model uses parallel stage levels for play and language to evaluate a child's progress.

• Stage I: 17 to 19 months—tool use; requires life-like props; familiar, everyday activities; single pretend action; self as agent. Beginning of functional and semantic relations such as recurrence, existence, rejection, denial, location, etc.
• Stage II: 19 to 22 months—combination of two actions or toys in pretend; child acts on doll; beginning of word combinations.
• Stage III: 2 years—elaborate single play schemas representing daily life experiences. Beginning of phrases and use of morphologic markers.
• Stage IV: 2.5 years—schemas that are

pleasurable or traumatic but less frequently occurring personal events; responds to questions.

- Stage V: 3 years—reenactment of experienced events; unplanned but multiple schema sequences. Language includes reporting, predicting, narrating or storytelling, and using future and past tense.
- Stage VI: 3 to 3.5 years—carries out pretend play activities; play sequences in which child observed but was not personally involved; toy used as character, participant; expresses desires; changes speech according to listener; reasoning.
- Stage VII: 3.5 to 4 years—uses props to invent scene; builds three-dimensional block structures; schemas and scripts are planned; child or doll has many roles; uses language to take roles; appearance of modals; responds to why and how questions.
- Stage VIII: 5 years—uses language to set the scene; action and roles in play; highly imaginative schemes (outer space, castles, fantasy); several sequences of pretend play; relational terms such as then, first, last, before, after.

MCCUNE-NICOLICH SYMBOLIC PLAY LEVELS

McCune-Nicolich (1981) uses a hierarchical progression of symbolic play behavior that is consistent with the developmental theories of Piaget and Inhelder (1969). Level 1 is presymbolic play, which may include pretending to drink from a cup or eat with a fork. Level 2 is autosymbolic play, the level at which children begin to use toys with respect to their own bodies. Level 3 is directed symbolic play. The child begins to use dolls in play instead of just the self. The child engages in one scheme at a time. Level 4 is combinatorial symbolic play. At this stage, the child combines schemes. Level 5 is internally directed symbolic play. Children begin to demonstrate some planning in their play behavior rather than play emerging as a characteristic of an object. At 30 months, most children are able to engage in internally directed symbolic play. This development is completed in most children by 30 months of age.

TRANSDISCIPLINARY PLAY-BASED ASSESSMENT

The transdisciplinary play-based assessment (TPBA) is an evaluation conducted in an arena style in which the child's parents and professionals representing a variety of disciplines observe a child in both structured and unstructured play. Information from the TPBA identifies concerns in the areas of communication and language, social-emotional, and sensorimotor domains. This assessment is designed for children developmentally functioning between infancy and 6 years of age and can be used with children who have disabilities and those who do not (such as children at risk). The outcome of a TPBA is an individualized report and program plan for the child, the family, and the professionals who will be working with the child (speech-language pathologists, psychologists, and physical and occupational therapists).

I. Cognitive component
  A. Attention span
    1. Length of attention span
    2. Sensory preference
    3. Internal stimuli and attention span
    4. Distractibility
  B. Schema use
    1. Number and level of schema
    2. Range of schema
    3. Schema use and generalization
    4. Symbolic object use
    5. Symbolic play schema
    6. Problem-solving schema
  C. Imitation
    1. Gestural imitation
    2. Timing of imitation
    3. Context of imitation
    4. Type of imitation
  D. Discrimination/differentiation
    1. Classification
    2. One-to-one correspondence
II. Communication component
  A. Forms of communication

1. Primary and supplementary forms
2. Quantity and quality
3. Cognitive/correlative skills
B. Functions
   1. Stage
   2. Communicative intent
   3. Discourse skills
C. Level of understanding of word/symbols
   1. Average length of utterance
   2. Type of words used
   3. Level of knowledge
   4. Level of cognition
D. Structure usage
   1. Grammatical structure
   2. Overgeneralization and word error
E. Sound system
   1. Preverbal skills
   2. Developmentally normal pronunciation
   3. Intelligibility
   4. Intonation and prosody
F. Echolalia
   1. Type
   2. Function
G. Receptive language skills
   1. Responses
   2. Understanding of parts of speech and word categories
   3. Comprehension of questions
III. Social-emotional component
   A. Temperament
      1. Activity level
      2. Approach or withdrawal
      3. Adaptability
      4. Threshold of responsiveness
      5. Intensity of reaction
      6. Quality of mood
   B. Attachment-separation-individuation
      1. Attachment to parent
      2. Separation from parent
      3. Individuation, self-identity
   C. Social-relatedness to others
      1. Relation to adults
      2. Relation to peers in dyad
      3. Relation to peers in group
      4. Sense of humor
      5. Awareness of social conventions

IV. Sensorimotor component
   A. Neurologic responses
      1. Primitive (neonatal reflexes)
      2. Mature responses (righting reactions, protective extension)
      3. Equilibrium response
      4. Tone
   B. Gross motor skills
      1. Overall quality of movement
      2. General performance
      3. Static postures
   C. Fine motor skills
      1. Qualitative assessment during fine motor tasks
      2. General performance of fine motor skills (bilateral development, grasping patterns, release, reach patterns, specific object manipulation abilities)
   D. Sensory integration
      1. General characteristics
      2. Tactile responses
      3. Auditory responses
      4. Vestibular and proprioceptive response
      5. Motor planning

The transdisciplinary assessment is very useful in the assessment of difficult-to-assess children who are multiply disabled. Intervention goals can be set using a cooperative transdisciplinary interaction, and progress toward those goals can be measured.

Language Assessment Strategies: Effect of Early Identification

Because it can result in significantly higher language levels, the early identification of D/HH children will have significant effects on the assessment and intervention strategies from infancy through the preschool years. Most children with early-identified hearing loss have language skills that can be assessed through traditional language development tools. Children who are later-identified typically must be assessed through either language tests designed for younger children (infants and toddlers) or criterion reference checklists.

ASSESSMENT FOR LATER-IDENTIFIED CHILDREN WITH NORMAL COGNITIVE ABILITY OR EARLY-IDENTIFIED CHILDREN WITH LOW COGNITIVE ABILITY

Assessment approaches include the following:

1. Assessing Linguistic Behaviors (ALB) (Olswang et al., 1987). These infant observational scales include five subsections: (a) cognitive antecedents to word meanings, (b) communicative intentions, (c) play behaviors, (d) language comprehension, and (e) language expression and phonologic development scales. The nondirective, observational tasks are illustrated on a videotape, which can be used for examiner training. Samples of normally developing infants are used to train coders.

2. Communication and Symbolic Behavior Scales (CSBS) (Wetherby and Prizant, 1990). This scale includes a caregiver questionnaire that surveys parents' observations of the child's presymbolic and early symbolic communicative behaviors. The second portion of the assessment involves videotaping the infant during playful interactions with the parents and examiner. The videotape is later scored, using scales of communication (functions, means, reciprocity, and social/affective signaling) and symbolic behavior (verbal and nonverbal).

3. MacArthur Communicative Development Inventory (Dale and Thal, 1989). This inventory of early lexical attainments relies on parent report, in a manner similar to parent diary studies. Checklists prompt parents to recall whether the child understands and/or produces a range of early appearing words from varied semantic classes. Because young children often have difficulty demonstrating optimal or usual performance in a structured clinical setting, this tool recruits useful observations from the home setting. The infant scale is designed for use with 8- to 16-month-old infants. The scale also appraises use of actions and gestures. A form for toddlers is designed for use between 16 and 30 months of age. A D/HH child's vocabulary size can be compared with normative data collected on 659 infants and 1130 toddlers with normal hearing (Fenson et al., 1993) and with normative data on D/HH infants and toddlers by age at identification and cognitive status from 12 through 36 months of age.

4. Minnesota Child Development Inventory (Ireton and Thwing, 1972). This inventory is a parent-report questionnaire that includes the areas of general development, gross motor skills, fine motor skills, self-help abilities, personal-social abilities, expressive language capabilities, conceptual comprehension, and situational comprehension. This standardized measure can be used from birth through 7 years of age.

5. Play Assessment Questionnaire (Calhoun's 1987 adaptation of the Play Assessment Scale; Calhoun D. A comparison of two methods of evaluating play in toddlers. Unpublished master's thesis. Ft. Collins, CO: Colorado State University, 1987) (Yoshinaga-Itano et al., 1998; Snyder and Yoshinaga-Itano [in press], Yoshinaga-Itano and Snyder [in press]). This measure of symbolic play can be used with children whose developmental levels are between birth and 30 months of age.

EVALUATION STRATEGIES FOR CHILDREN WITH AGE-APPROPRIATE LANGUAGE DEVELOPMENT

The following assessment materials and strategies are particularly suited to identifying children's cognitive/linguistic development. The information obtained is useful in setting goals and monitoring progress.

1. Child Assessment Record (CAR) (High/Scope Press, Ypsilanti, Michigan). The High/Scope curriculum contains forms that allow clinicians/teachers to record daily objective observations of children's responses across key experience areas

(e.g., representation, seriation, classification, number, space, time, social). This objective record helps the interventionist track progress and is also critical for planning future sessions.

2. Preschool Language Assessment Instrument (PLAI) (Blank et al., 1978). This instrument evaluates children's understanding of questions posed on four distinct levels of semantic abstraction, from simple to abstract. Simple level questions (Level I) require that children apply language to what they see in the immediate context (e.g., what is that?). Level II questions require children to focus selectively on features of what they see (e.g., what is happening here?). At Level III, children must restructure their perceptions to respond (e.g., find the things that are not . . . ; what will happen next?). Level IV requires the child to reason—to predict, explain, or find a logical solution. This requires the child to go beyond immediate context and perceptions.

This assessment tool has been adapted easily to use with D/HH children. A picture is provided with most of the prompts, which is helpful in establishing the topic for the young D/HH child, amid several topical shifts. Clinicians use the assessment results to determine what levels of questions are straightforward for the child, which are emerging, and which are too complex. The clinician then provides numerous opportunities for the child to respond to tasks and questions at levels appropriately challenging for the individual child. The assessment strategy can also be used to monitor change in response to long-term intervention. Figure 6.10 shows the results from a class of eight profoundly D/HH preschoolers who participated in the intervention program. Four of eight children (represented by group 1) approximated the response levels of hearing age-mates at the posttest interval. All the children demonstrated developmental patterns of responses.

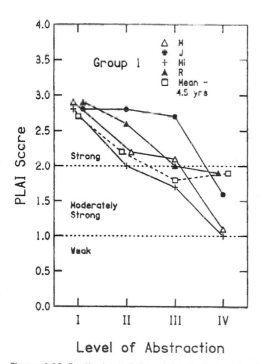 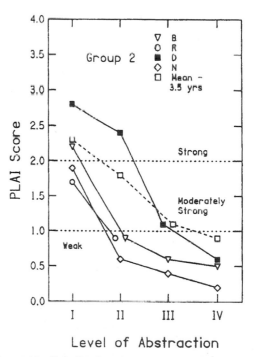

Figure 6.10. Posttest results for eight deaf preschoolers (ages 4 to 6) on the Preschool Language Assessment Instrument compared with mean scores for children ages 3.5 and 4.5.

3. Spontaneous language sampling. Spontaneous language sampling is a vital component of the evaluation battery. Emergence of personal narrative skills is tracked by taking dictation during recall and sharing time routines. These samples are analyzed using Systematic Analysis of Language Transcripts (SALT) (Miller and Chapman, 1983).

4. Observational checklist during play. Social behaviors are often reflected in children's play. Westby's (1988) play scale offers a structured observational checklist for evaluation of social, cognitive, and language skills during symbolic play.

5. Task analysis. One of the most valuable assessment tools is the astute clinician, who continually analyzes tasks and responses during intervention. Skilled clinicians constantly ask, "Is there something about this task that is preventing the child from attending to the concept? How can I restructure the learning situation to enhance his or her performance?" Skilled clinicians are also able to determine the basis of children's responses. For example, the clinician may ask, "Did John respond to that question on the basis of linguistic cues, or did he predict the correct response because of situational context? Perhaps I can manipulate the number of context cues available and see how this influences his responses." Systematically applied task analysis is fundamental to the process of individualization.

Intervention Strategies

PRESCHOOL PROGRAMMING: A COGNITIVELY ORIENTED FRAMEWORK FOR LANGUAGE ENHANCEMENT

Components of a cognitively oriented approach

Cognitively oriented approaches share several common features. Moeller's conceptualizations of key features of this approach are described in Table 6.10. Although the approach is eclectic, its foundations were heavily influenced by a cognitively oriented curriculum designed for early childhood education by the High/Scope Educa-tional Research Foundation (Weikart et al., 1971; Hohmann et al., 1979). Moeller has adapted this developmental curriculum for use with D/HH preschoolers. Adaptations were particularly necessary in the following areas.

Schema-based content units (vocabulary)

Because of the language-learning needs of D/HH children, attention has been given to developing content units that support children's expansion of schemata. Yoshinaga-Itano and Downey (1986) point out that D/HH children often have gaps or incomplete world/word knowledge. They stress the need to help children expand their knowledge of scripts and schemata as a basis for comprehension of conversation and written texts. Strategies for developing schema-based units will be discussed later in this chapter.

Targeted language structures (syntax and grammar)

Some creative manipulation of discourse has been required to obligate the use of targeted language structures and give children sufficient, appropriate practice with targeted forms/functions. Interactive modeling using two clinicians who participate in a team-teaching situation in a group intervention setting is recommended. This allows the adults to use the powerful strategy of interactive modeling, providing children with multiple opportunities to see language used interactively understand social language rules. Interactive models have been particularly necessary with signing children who see only one primary signer at home. Clinicians create functional contexts for eliciting target behaviors and then use strategies such as semantically contingent expansions and visual and verbal scaffolds. Scaffolding (Bruner, 1978) refers to techniques adults use to reduce task complexity or support the child's effort. This might include increasing nonlinguistic support to allow the child to concentrate on the linguistic demands of the task. The clinicians also hold children accountable for representative language behaviors and routinely "up the ante." These

Table 6.10
Components of a cognitively oriented approach to language intervention

Theoretical Premise	Strategy Component	References
Contemporary views of learners emphasize the active learning process. Children construct meaning as they form and test our hypotheses	Experiences are designed to provoke mentally active participation; to encourage children to explore, question, and make discoveries	Piaget and Inhelder, 1969; Weikart et al., 1971; Bruner, 1975; Stone, 1980; Wells and Nicholls, 1985
Acquisition of knowledge structure (schemata and scripts) guide comprehension of discourse and print. Vocabulary learning is enhanced when children "anchor" a new word to existing knowledge.	Content units and teaching strategies are designed to expand children's word and world knowledge. Associative learning strategies help children link new and established concepts.	Pearson, 1984; Kail and Leonard, 1986; Yoshinaga-Itano and Downey, 1986
Language acquisition is facilitated when adults use a collaborative rather than a directive style. Semantic contingency to literacy-related behaviors is related to literacy attainment.	Clinicians use open-ended strategies of (1) presenting or capitalizing on problems, (2) asking divergent questions, (3) commenting to expand children's discoveries, and (4) commenting on children's preliteracy observations.	Weikart et al., 1971; Grammatico and Miller, 1974; Masur, 1982; Barnes et al., 1983; Snow, 1983; Wells and Nicholls, 1985; Tomasello and Farrar, 1986
As a child's language matures, discourse demands become increasingly decontextualized and less tied to immediate contexts or perceptions. This process of decontextualizations is important to literacy attainment.	Implementation of a classroom discourse model supports gradual and systemic "upping of the ante" in semantic abstraction. Social routines such as Plans-Do-Recall help children develop personal narrative kills (beginning decontextualized language use).	Blank et al., 1978; Weikart, 1979; Hohmann et al., 1979; Westby, 1985
Interactive models in rich social contexts may aid children's ability to formulate and respond to questions. Question-asking is a critical tool for active learners/hypothesis testers.	Adults verbalize their own curiosities, inferences, and discoveries; they make implicit knowledge explicit and scaffold children's attempts to express questions. These strategies are incorporated during storytelling and other functional routines.	Snow, 1983; Constable and van Kleeck, 1985; Yoshinaga-Itano and Downey, 1986
Systematic daily routines support children's ability to predict and plan up-coming events and to recall past activities. Classroom time starts to be understood as a series of predictable events.	Daily routines capitalize on opportunities to plan and predict upcoming events, to learn and express time relations, and to reflect on past experiences. These activities are also relevant to the process of distancing language from immediate context.	Hohmann et al., 1979; Westby, 1985

continued

Table 6.10–Continued
Components of a cognitively oriented approach to language intervention

Theoretical Premise	Strategy Component	References
Key experiences, based on characteristics of pre-operational thinkers, can serve as a framework from which clinicians can extend and broaden opportunities. Key experiences may build a foundation for later logical thinking.	Curricular design (based in High/Scope principles) provides systematic exposure to key experiences in the areas of classification, seriation, number concepts, spatial relations, and time concepts.	Hohmann et al., 1979; Moeller and McConkey, 1984; Moeller et al., 1985
Effective parents recognize their role in supporting and encouraging children's self-activated learning. Parents and children often engage in rich social interactions, in which there is shared negotiation of meaning.	Family members are given opportunities to learn to use open-ended and thought-provoking strategies with their children during natural, daily routines.	Wells and Nicholls, 1985

strategies are known to enhance both language and preliteracy skills (Snow, 1983).

Emphasis on question-asking behaviors (pragmatics)

Yoshinaga-Itano and Stredler-Brown (1992) reported that D/HH infants and toddlers are significantly delayed in the acquisition of verbal and nonverbal question-asking behaviors. Nonverbal questioning was found to be significantly related to total verbal communicative intentions. Question-asking is an essential skill children use in making sense out of their world. Thus, Moeller and Carney (1993) enhanced the curriculum by integrating a model of classroom discourse that would strengthen children's question-responding and question-asking skills (Blank et al., 1978). Clinicians also explicitly verbalize their own thinking process to model for children how they can express their own natural curiosity.

Family members are a critical component

Family members are critical to the success of intervention methods. When rich discourse occurs at home, children are accustomed to exploring the meaning of events around them and are in an ideal position to take advantage of rich experiences presented to them at school. Within a total communication program, weekly family classes support the parental role by focusing on signing skills, language facilitation strategies, and positive parenting techniques.

D/HH children represent a heterogeneous group, requiring individualized management. Ongoing evaluation of the child's emerging cognitive, linguistic, and social skills is critical to the process of individualization of the curriculum. The next section briefly addresses evaluation strategies that uniquely support curriculum objectives.

CHARACTERISTICS OF SUCCESSFUL PROGRAMS

Early-intervention programs that have identified successful outcomes for early-identified children have several characteristics in common.

Parent partnership

Parent involvement in early intervention for D/HH children was promoted by several model demonstration programs in the early 1970s. These programs included the SKI-HI project in Utah, the Project Parent Child in

Colorado, and the Northcutt Preschool Program in Minnesota, to name a few. Since that time, the role of parents has evolved from the client who is to be educated and counseled, to an equal partner with professionals in the decision-making process, with a trend toward parent-directed teacher/clinician supported decision-making.

In the infant/toddler period, most intervention involves direct service to the family unit rather than therapeutic intervention directly with the child. Parents and other family members learn techniques to incorporate auditory, language, and speech goals into their everyday life. Many families add direct service in the preschool period through preschool programs and individual therapy.

Parent programs in the preschool period are, unfortunately, de-emphasized once the child enters the traditional school system. Because the role of the parent in the infant-toddler period is so significant, it is hoped that future changes in educational programming for D/HH children will include greater involvement and inclusion of parent-partnerships from infancy through the school-age period.

Data-driven approaches

Early-identified children have demonstrated the ability to maintain age-appropriate language skills in early childhood. Before this time, language skills were so significantly delayed when late-identified children began receiving intervention services that the use of standardized tests that compared D/HH children with their peers with normal hearing was not possible. As a result, criterion reference checklists became the most common mode of assessing a child's progress.

Both the Boys Town and Colorado programs used comprehensive 6-month evaluations to assist parents and educators in their decision-making. Parent involvement in the evaluation process was facilitated through the use of parent questionnaires of various aspects of development. These comprehensive evaluations helped the parents identify the next steps in the child's developmental progression.

The 6-month evaluations helped parents

determine whether the choices they made had produced the outcomes they desired. They could alter their approaches and decisions depending on their child's needs. Objective evaluation of intervention outcome is accomplished in part through language sample analysis and use of formal evaluation instruments. Particularly useful to this process are recently developed communicative scales that incorporate parental observations and noninvasive, naturalistic techniques.

Developmentally appropriate approaches

All the approaches used with families and their D/HH children were developmentally appropriate techniques. Children with typical development and normal hearing benefited from the use of these educational techniques. During the preschool period, identifying developmentally appropriate goals and ensuring that the children have focused experiences that enable them to learn incidentally are priorities. This often involves games and activities that have repetitive language patterns. Participation in these activities ensures mass practice of some language skills that have frequently been identified as problems for D/HH children. The key to successful programming is to incorporate these goals in natural and age-appropriate activities.

Parent facilitators with specialized training and significant years of experience

The educators in both the Boys Town and Colorado programs had Master's degrees in deaf education, speech/language pathology, or audiology. Most had 10 to 15 years of experience in parent-infant intervention. In addition, these providers received intensive in-service education in specialized areas such as auditory skill and speech development for very young children, sign language development in the early years, diagnostic evaluation, and intensive counseling training.

Facilitators with counseling skills

Incorporating families into the educational process requires that the educator/facilitator have skills in counseling. The facilitator needs to develop the ability to assist families in grief resolution. They need to have experience with a wide variety of families from diverse cultural and socioeconomic backgrounds. The Colorado Home Intervention Program has provided training in theories of family systems and therapies associated with these theories (Minuchin, 1974, 1984; Minuchin and Fishman, 1981) as well as the Circumplex model of families, which discusses 16 types of marital and family systems based on two dimensions: adaptability (rigid, structured, flexible, chaotic) and cohesion (disengaged, separated, connected, enmeshed) (Olson and McCubbin, 1989). A situational leadership model adapted from Hershey and Blanchard (1988) has been helpful in providing parent-intervention facilitators with some guidelines on adjusting their interactional style according to the ability of the family to utilize resources. This model recommends four interaction styles: (1) providing direction for families with low levels of resources and motivation, (2) assisting or coaching families with low levels of resources but high levels of motivation, (3) encouraging/supporting families with a high level of resources and a low level of motivation, and (4) delegating for families with a high level of both resources and motivation.

A pragmatic/socially oriented approach

It is critically important that the social use of language be addressed during the preschool period, in addition to a focus on conceptual understanding, the development of play both symbolically and socially, the development of semantics and growth of vocabulary understanding and expression, and the development of understanding and use of grammatic constructions. Children with significant hearing loss, even those with strong lexical knowledge and sizable vocabularies, seem to require more direct instruction of pragmatic language than children with normal hearing. Many of the social nuances of conversation that are frequently learned through incidental learning seem to require explicit instruction if children who are D/HH are to master these skills at developmentally appropriate stages.

The Language Arts Curriculum (Lower and Middle School [see Gjerdingen, 1996]) from the Clarke School for the Deaf provides excellent examples of how pragmatic, semantic, and syntactic skills can be integrated and infused into the language curriculum for a school-aged population. The challenge will now be to lower-extend these principles to the preschool age group. Stone (1986) provides lessons for school-aged children to facilitate the development of pragmatic language skills.

Assessment of Speech Production

Early identification, coupled with higher language development, has also affected the way in which speech is assessed and developed in young children who are D/HH. This section deals first with evaluation/assessment procedures for speech production and auditory skills and then with intervention strategies and curricula that can be used for the development of speech and audition.

LING PHONETIC EVALUATION

Although originally developed for school-aged children (5 years and older), this criterion reference assessment can be done with preschool children who can imitate speech production on command. The Ling Phonetic Evaluation requires oral imitation of each phonetic item. The evaluation assesses phonemes in the initial, medial, and final positions; pitch differentiation; and alternating syllable combinations. Consonants are assessed according to manner, place, and voicing. Consonant blends are assessed in the initial, medial, and final positions.

LING PHONOLOGIC EVALUATION

The Ling Phonologic Evaluation was developed for the school-aged population but has been used successfully with spontaneous speech as an assessment from infancy (Yoshinaga-Itano et al., 1992). The Ling

Phonologic Evaluation relies on a speech sample of spontaneous speech typically in a 20- to 30-minute period. The evaluator simply indicates the number and type of different phonemes in the spontaneous speech sample. Consonants are recorded by manner, place, and voicing. Consonant blends in initial, medial, and final positions are recorded.

In a study of 128 preschool-aged children with mild to profound sensorineural hearing loss, significant differences by degree of hearing loss were found for the number of vowels, consonants, initial blends, and final blends in a spontaneous speech sample. Three hearing loss categories were identified: (1) mild and moderate, (2) moderate-severe and severe, and (3) profound (Table 6.11).

Sixty-nine percent of the variance in the number of consonants plus blends in spontaneous speech production can be accounted for by three variables: expressive language development, degree of hearing loss, and age at identification at this age.

REDUCED ASPECT FEATURE TRANSCRIPTION (RAFT) (CARNEY, 1991)

This test assesses (1) percentages of consonant productions at the front, mid, and back portions of the vocal tract, (2) percentages of use of manner categories (stop, continuant, nasal, and unknown), and (3) voicing categories (voiced, voiceless, and unknown).

The test uses the following procedure.

- Each syllable is transcribed according to its syllabic makeup (i.e., ba/ba/ba = CVCVCV).
- Vowel-like and vocalic segments (V) are coded globally according to vowel height (high, mid, low), vowel place (front, back, mid), and vowel resonance (full, nasal, quasiresonant).
- Closant or consonant-like segments (C) are coded according to place of articulation (front, mid, back), manner of articulation (stop, continuant, nasal, unknown), and voicing (voiced, voiceless, and unknown).

SPEECH INTELLIGIBILITY RATING SCALE

In a study of 126 preschool children with mild to profound sensorineural hearing loss, approximately 35% were rated by a trained phonologist as having very intelligible speech, and 35% did not have enough speech to rate intelligibility or were unintelligible. In contrast, parents rating their own children responded that 44% of the children were highly intelligible, whereas only 25% did not have enough speech to rate intelligibility or were unintelligible.

When children with profound hearing loss were analyzed separately, the speech intelligibility of those with mild through severe hearing loss was rated very highly, with 50% having very intelligible speech and only 15% (parent rating) to 25% (phonologist rating) having unintelligible speech. The coding system was a numeric rating from 1 to 6: 1 = always or almost always understand; 2 = almost always understand; however, I need to listen carefully; 3 = I typically understand 50% of the child's speech; 4 = I typically understand 25% of the child's speech; 5 = the child's speech is very hard to understand; I typically understand only occasional, isolated

Table 6.11
Number of vowels, consonants, and initial and final blends (means and standard deviations) of 128 deaf and hard-of-hearing preschool-aged children (mean age, 48 months)

Degree of Hearing Loss	Vowels	Consonants	Initial Blends	Final Blends
Mild	14 (3)	19.5 (7.4)	7.1 (4.3)	4.3 (4.1)
Moderate	13 (3)	19.3 (6.7)	4.8 (4.7)	3.1 (3.3)
Moderate-severe	12 (4.8)	15.9 (8.8)	4.0 (4.7)	2.5 (3.4)
Severe	11.8 (4.4)	13.7 (7.4)	2.0 (2.8)	0.85 (1.7)
Profound	8.9 (4.4)	8.8 (6.2)	0.52 (1.5)	0.45 (1.2)

Table 6.12
Mean speech intelligibility ratings (standard deviations) of a phonologist, parents, and therapists at a mean age of 48 months

Hearing Loss	Intelligibility		
	Phonologist	Parents	Therapists
Mild	2.5 (1.9)	2 (1.4)	1.7 (1.4)
Moderate	3 (1.8)	1.7 (1.6)	3.4 (1.4)
Moderate-severe	3.6 (1.8)	3 (1.9)	3.5 (1.9)
Severe	4.8 (1.7)	4.1 (1.6)	5.0 (1.1)
Profound	5.3 (1.2)	4.8 (1.6)	5.3 (1.3)

words and/or phrases; and 6 = I never or almost never understand the child's speech (Table 6.12).

DIAGNOSTIC SPEECH INVENTORY (DSI) (CAROTTA ET AL., 1990)

The diagnostic speech inventory uses real words that have either a CV, VC, or CVC makeup. Test items are elicited through repetition, both immediate and delayed. Test plates have manipulable pictures and objects to encourage children to produce the number of repetitions desired and to provide them with a concrete referent for their speech.

MEANINGFUL USE OF SPEECH SCALE (MUSS) (ROBBINS AND OSBERGER, 1994)

This scale consists of a 10-item questionnaire with a possibility of 40 points. Each item is scored on a 0- to 4-point scale: 0 = never spontaneously uses voice; 1 = rarely vocalizes (less than 50% of the time); 2 = occasionally uses vocalization alone (at least 50% of the time); 3 = frequently uses vocalizations alone (at least 75% of the time); and 4 = always uses vocalization alone (100% of the time). The items range from "The child uses vocalizations to attract others' attention" to the child spontaneously uses appropriate oral repair and clarification strategies when speech is not understood by people unfamiliar with him or her. Three items evaluate the child's use of voice to gain attention, and to control the use of suprasegmentals to communicate effectively. Four items evaluate the use of

speech with familiar people about familiar and unfamiliar topics, in social situations, and persistence in being understood. Three items evaluate the child's use of speech with unfamiliar people in spontaneous use, intelligibility, and persistence in making speech understood.

SPEECH DEVELOPMENT OF YOUNG D/HH CHILDREN

Toddlers

Obenchain et al. (in press) reported that most early-identified children with mild through severe hearing loss became effective vocal communicators, indicating that hearing status in the second year of life is significantly related to whether children develop vocal competence. He studied 20 children with their first speech recording between 16 and 22 months of age. Of these early-identified children, 7 were judged to be experts, 7 novices, 3 prosodic specialists, and 3 articulatory specialists. The following participant variables were analyzed: mode of communication, degree of hearing loss, age at identification, and motor difficulties or delayed development.

The vocal competence criteria were (1) prosodic—intonation patterns match intentions of child's utterance, (2) articulation—having no systematic or regular inaccuracies beyond those in the typical speech development of children in the fourth year, and 3) syntactic—ability to speak in complete sentences. Experts met all of the criteria. Novices met none of the criteria. Prosodic specialists failed to meet the articulation criterion, and articulatory specialists failed to meet the prosodic criterion.

Obenchain et al. (in press) used the following variables to measure the speech ability in the second year of life:

I. Phonologic-segmental variables
   A. Total segmental inventory—number of different speech sounds
   B. Vowel inventory—number of vowel sounds
   C. Consonant inventory—number of consonant sounds
   D. Diphthong inventory
   E. Syllable structure
II. Phonologic-prosodic variables
   A. Total nuclear tones, nuclear tones in speech
   B. Nuclear tones in jargon, percentage of jargon
   C. Stress
   D. Duration
   E. Phonation
   F. Intonational utterances
III. Semantic variables
   A. Lexical inventory
   B. Mean length of utterance
   C. Intentional utterances
   D. Percentage of speech
   E. Syntactic variables
   F. Use of phrases
   G. Use of affixes
IV. Other variables
   A. Utterances per minute
   B. Syllable per utterance

Obenchain et al, (in press) reported that intelligible speech was a factor of the following variables:

1. Degree of hearing loss: mild through severe.
2. Early identification of hearing loss (by age 2), although much later identification is possible.
3. No motor or other developmental delay.
4. High frequency of utterances (more than 4.5 in 25 minutes).
5. High mean length of utterance (more than 0.1).
6. Relatively large lexical inventory (more than 9).
7. Large phonetic inventory, especially consonants (9 or more).
8. High percentage of rising tones (20% or more).
9. Relatively high percentage (approximately 30%) of intonational utterances of speech and/or jargon.
10. Tendency to show intention even in utterances with no semantic content, and this intention would be demonstrated by associating gestures (pointing, showing, reaching, and offering with utterances).
11. Complex syllable types would be present with a relatively large percentage (more than 50%) of syllables containing consonants.

Yoshinaga-Itano and Sedey (in press) found that the majority of early-identified children with mild to severe hearing loss were reported to communicate through intelligible oral speech and language by the end of their preschool years.

Preschool years

Significant differences in the speech production of the number of vowels, consonants, consonants and simple blends, initial blends, final blends, and overall speech intelligibility differ by three categories of hearing: (1) mild to moderate, (2) moderate-severe to severe, and (3) profound. Three variables account for 70% of the variance in the production of consonants and blends. Fifty-nine percent of this variance is accounted for by the variable expressive language development. Age at identification accounts for an additional 6% of the variance, and degree of hearing loss accounts for an additional 5% of the variance (Yoshinaga-Itano, 1999).

ASSESSING AUDITORY SKILLS OF PRESCHOOL-AGED CHILDREN WITH AGE-APPROPRIATE LANGUAGE

Variables to consider when choosing auditory diagnostic tests include the following.

1. Age of the child/developmental age. Does the child have the developmental ability necessary to perform the task? Is the child capable of raising his or her hand when he or she hears a tone? This skill typically develops toward the end of the preschool years. Is the child capable of pointing to pictures when named? This skill typically develops in the 2- to 3-year period of life, although it can be seen in some children between 12 and 24 months of age. Before picture pointing, the young child is capable of pointing at real objects or at miniature replicas of objects. Is the child capable of understanding same/different and verbally labeling these differences? This skill typically is demonstrated at the kindergarten level in hearing children.

2. Oral language level of the child is required for auditory/speech tasks. Does the child have the auditory and oral skills for the language stimulus? If the child does not have the vocabulary in the receptive and expressive lexicon, then the task becomes a nonsense task rather than a symbolic task. Later-identified children typically demonstrate much greater delays in language than earlier-identified children.

3. What is the degree of hearing loss, configuration, and type of hearing loss? At what level should the stimuli be presented?

4. Auditory skill developmental level. What is the level of auditory skill development? Is the child able to be conditioned? Is the child able to demonstrate a conditioned response to the presence of sound? Can the child say the word? Can the child discriminate suprasegmental elements of speech such as stress patterns, inflection, intonational contours? Can the child discriminate fine speech sounds such as vowels, consonants, or consonant blends? Can the child discriminate gross environmental sounds such as a telephone ringing, a doorbell ringing, a car honking, or a toilet flushing?

Northwestern University-Children's Perception of Speech Test (NU-CHIPS) (Elliott and Katz, 1981)

This test uses 50 monosyllabic words. These words are within the recognition vocabulary of the typical child older than 2.5 years of age. There are 65 word pictures and interchanges, 50 words as test items, and foil items within a 4-alternative picture set.

Children must have auditory language and language comprehension commensurate to age-matched peers as well as vocabulary ages older than 2.5 years. Chermak et al. (1984) reports reliability issues when NU-CHIPS is administered in a noisy background.

Word intelligibility picture identification (WIPI) test (Ross and Lerman, 1970)

This picture identification task is appropriate for children aged 3.5 years to approximately 5.5 years. The test is composed of 25 picture plates with 6 pictures per plate. The lists have high reliability.

This test can be used successfully with children who have auditory language and vocabulary levels commensurate with their age-matched hearing peers. If D/HH children do not have auditory language sufficient to understand the words, poor performance may be an indication of language delay, not necessarily auditory development.

Pediatric Speech Intelligibility (PSI) Test (Jerger et al., 1980, 1981)

This test is composed of 20 monosyllabic words and a 10-sentence procedure. The word list consists of simple nouns and two types of sentence construction identified as Format I and Format II. This test is applicable to children 2.5 to 6 years of age and has been used successfully with children who have had chronic otitis media and children with suspected central auditory dysfunction.

Assessment of Auditory Skills: Minimal Auditory Language Skills

SOUND AWARENESS

Ling Five-Sound Test

The Ling Five-Sound Test (a/i/u/s/sh) is a criterion reference assessment for detection of five speech sounds. Ability to detect these five speech sounds indicates auditory capability to detect all sounds of the English language. The response consists of a simple motor act such as placing checkers on a board, placing rings on a stick, dropping bears in a can, raising a finger, or raising a hand (in older children).

Glendonald Auditory Screening Procedure (GASP) (Erber, 1982)

This criterion reference test is designed to evaluate speech perception in three areas: (1) phoneme detection, (2) word identification, and (3) sentence completion. Performance is described by the number correct as well as the number and type of adaptations necessary to help the child succeed.

- Phoneme detection: children respond with a yes or point to a "yes" picture if they hear something and nod "no" or point to a "no" picture if they do not hear anything. Ten consonants intermingled with a silent oral articulation are presented auditorially.
- Word identification: this test is designed to determine whether children identify words on the basis of intensity patterns or spectral qualities. A set of 12 pictured nouns are used. These words represent four different stress patterns: three monosyllabic words, three trochaic words, and three trisyllabic words. Children are asked to point to the word they hear.
- Sentence comprehension (questions): children are asked 10 simple questions without objects or prompts. Most hearing-impaired 6-year-olds can answer the question stimuli.

EVALUATION OF PERCEPTION REPRESENTATION

SCIPS: Screening Inventory of Perception Skills (SCIPS) (Osberger et al., 1991)

This test consists of four subtests in which the task is to pick out a target word from a string of words. The child does not have to identify or recognize the word.

1. The target is a monosyllabic word (i.e., "ball") and the two foils are three-sylla-

ble words such as "birthday cake" or "lemonade."
2. The target is a monosyllabic word contrasted with bisyllabic words ("ball" versus "popcorn" and "ice cream").
3. The target is a monosyllabic word contrasted with other monosyllabic words ("ball" versus "shoe" and "cup").
4. The target is a bisyllabic word contrasted against other bisyllabic words ("baseball" versus "hot dog" and "ice cream").

The goals of this test are to determine whether the child can attend to the changing suprasegmental structure in words for the first two subtests and to changing segmental structure when syllables are kept constant for the second two subtests.

This test is based on the "Go-No-Go" paradigm and includes three different forms (A, B, and C) at different test intervals. Each of the three forms contains Level I and Level II. Level I tests whether the child can identify the same one-syllable word each time it is presented among three-syllable foils. The test requires the child to identify another one-syllable word each time it is presented among two-syllable foils. The test is designed to determine whether the child can listen for and focus on identification of the target item. Level II is designed to determine whether the child can identify the same two syllable word presented with other two-syllable foils. At this level, the words have the same number of syllables but have different acoustic patterns.

Three-Interval Forced-Choice Test of Speech Pattern Contrast Perception (THRIFT) (Boothroyd et al., 1988)

The task in this test consists of "same versus different" in a complex discrimination task. The child must indicate which interval (one, two, or three) contains the odd stimulus. The stimuli are nonsense syllables in a three-alternative forced-choice task. Two syllables are the same, and one is different.

- A single suprasegmental or segmental feature is assessed in each subtest (such as consonant voicing, manner, place).

• Each feature is assessed in a variety of phonetic contexts (i.e., voicing differences are contrasted for several different stops and fricatives with a variety of vowels).

This test was designed for children ages 6 or older, particularly if there is severe to profound hearing loss.

Change-No Change (Sussman and Carney, 1989)

This task consists of a string of nonsense syllables. The stimuli are fixed acoustic differences for a speech contrast pair that is maintained throughout a subtest. In a no-change condition, all syllables in the string are the same (ba/ba/ba/ba). In a change condition, the first half of the syllables in the string are identical to each other (ba/ba/ba), followed by a second set of contrasting syllables (da/da/da).

The child indicates detection of change by a simple motor task (such as the type of response used in play audiometry). No response is made for no-change trials. Use of a linguistic response—same or different—can be used with some children. Any type of speech contrast can be used, such as suprasegmental contrasts (short versus long, high versus low) or segmental contrasts (such as ba versus da).

For the child to perform this task, he or she must be able to make a same-different response. This skill usually develops in typical children at the end of the preschool years/beginning of kindergarten. The chance score for this test is 50%.

Early Speech Perception Battery: Low-Verbal Version (Geers and Moog, 1989)

The task for this test consists of two play alternatives, a train on a track and a rabbit. The training component trains the child to recognize the train as a continuous stimulus "aahh" and the rabbit as an interrupted stimulus "hop hop hop." The child is required to determine whether the stimulus is a continuous or interrupted stimulus, using the "aahh" or "hop hop hop" distinction.

The low-verbal version consists of the following: (1) pattern perception training for ("aahh" versus hop hop, trochees, and

three-syllable words), (2) pattern perception subtest, and (3) word identification subtest (spondees and monosyllable identification). The low-verbal version is designed for children from 3 to 6 years of age.

Early Speech Perception Battery: Standard Version

The standard version is designed to be used with profoundly deaf children with limited oral vocabulary and language skills, typically 6- to 7-year-olds. The test is designed to place children into four speech perception categories: (1) no pattern perception, (2) pattern perception, (3) some word identification, and (4) consistent word identification. The standard version is usually administered in 20 minutes or less and consists of colored picture cards and interesting toys for the words on both the standard and low-verbal version. The standard version consists of three subtests: (1) pattern perception subtest, (2) word-spondee identification subtest, and (3) word-monosyllabic identification subtest.

Functional Auditory Skills Test (FAST) (Moeller, 1984)

Moeller (1984) has developed elicitation tasks for use with very young children to assess auditory skill development. The tasks can be administered in a home or clinical setting.

DISCRIMINATION OF SPEECH SOUNDS IN WORDS

Minimal Pairs Test (Robbins et al., 1988)

This task consists of the presentation of two pictures that vary by one segmental feature for both consonant and vowel contrast pairs. Words are scored as either "word correct" or "feature correct." The purpose of this test is to determine vowel and consonant discrimination. The test is appropriate for children with severe and profound hearing loss.

Discrimination by Identification of Pairs Test (DIP/TIP) (Siegenthaler and Haspiel, 1966)

This test consists of 48 cards with 2 pictures on each card. Chance performance can result in high scores, because there are only two choices per presentation. Selection of the test items were on the basis of contrasting acoustic dimensions rather than phonemic balancing. The test was standardized on 295 normally hearing children between 3 and 8 years of age. The DIP-TIP is administered at sensation levels of 0, 5, and 10 dB.

Monosyllable-Trochee-Spondee (MTS) Test (Erber, 1982)

The task is a test of word recognition using a closed-set format with 12 words including monosyllables, trochees, and spondees. The test is scored for "words correct" and "stress pattern correct." There is an expansion of this test in the GASP.

The Auditory Numbers Task is an expansion of this task for younger, less verbal children. The Early Speech Perception battery uses the same approach.

Hoosier-Auditory-Visual Enhancement (HAVE) Test (Renshaw et al., 1988)

This task consists of individual test items presented once in a combined auditory-visual mode. The stimuli are a three-alternative picture format, two words that are homophenous with a third rhyming but nonhomophenous foil. Responses are scores as both "word correct" and "visual correct."

Common Phrases Test (Indiana University School of Medicine) (Osberger et al., 1991)

This test consists of 6 lists with 10 items each. The test is designed to assess understanding of familiar phrases spoken in everyday situations. The test was developed based on the clinical impression that children could recognize familiar phrases better than monosyllabic words in an open-set format. The common phrases are either declarative statements or questions containing simple syntactic structures and vocabulary familiar to children who are profoundly deaf. This test can be administered in three conditions: (1) with audition only, (2) with vision only, and (3) with audition plus vision.

CHILDREN WITH RECEPTIVE LANGUAGE AGES YOUNGER THAN 4 YEARS OR ORAL LANGUAGE PERCEPTION AND PRODUCTION LIMITATIONS

Auditory Perception of Alphabet Letters (APAL) Test (Ross and Randolph, 1988)

This test is for use with children with oral language limitations who know the oral alphabet. This test was developed for children with hearing loss who do not have the vocabulary levels sufficient for the WIPI, NU-CHIPS, or phonetically balanced kindergarten (PBK) tests. The stimuli for this test are the names of the letters of the alphabet. The test consists of a closed set response of the 26 letters of the alphabet. Live presentation of the test is used for training, but the actual testing should be conducted with the recorded version of the APAL test. There are five test forms, and the first four stimuli in each list are used as practice items. Scoring is dependent on how closely the response matches the acoustics of the correct answer. The APAL test incorporates a weighted error score.

Ross and Randolph (1990) administered the test to 73 severely and profoundly hearing-impaired children between the ages of 4.1 and 18 years of age. The test-retest reliability was very high at $r = 0.95$. The construct validity was high compared with the WIPI and PBK. Speech discrimination scores from the WIPI were very similar to the APAL ($r = 0.80$ [weighted version], $r = 0.82$ [unweighted version]), as were the PBK scores ($r = 0.76$ [weighted version], $r = 0.78$ [unweighted version]). The APAL has no floor effect attributed to chance performance, whereas the WIPI chance correct score is 16.75%. The APAL was designed to be more difficult than the WIPI (a closed-set test) but easier than the PBK (an open-set test).

Auditory Numbers Test (Erber, 1980)

This test is for use with children with oral language limitations who know oral numbers one through five. This test was designed for children with severe and profound hearing loss and to distinguish perception of spectral aspects of speech and gross temporal acoustic patterns. It is administered via live voice. The child must identify counted sequences and individual numbers. The child must be able to count to five and be able to apply these numbers to sets of one through five. Picture cards depict one to five ants with corresponding numerals and are color-coded.

Sound Effects Recognition Test (SERT) (Finitzo-Hieber et al., 1980)

This is for use with children with oral language limitations who know environmental sounds. The test is composed of three equivalent sets. Each test is composed of 10 familiar environmental sounds such as a baby crying, a toilet flushing, hammering, etc. The test results provide a standardized measure of auditory discrimination for environmental sounds.

The child listens to gross environmental stimuli presented through an audiocassette recording and points to one of four pictures per page. Presentation is usually set between 25 and 40 dB in relationship to the speech awareness threshold.

The SERT includes 30 test items and is composed of 3 equivalent 10-item subtests. This test of discrimination has been most commonly used with children between the ages of 3 and 6 years.

SKI-HI Auditory Skills Checklist (Tonelson and Watkins, 1979)

This criterion reference checklist can be used with infants and toddlers as a gross measure of auditory skill developmental level.

Developmental Approach to Successful Listening (DASLII) Test (Stout and Windle, 1994)

This test of auditory skill development can be used with children and consists of 13 subskills in sound awareness, 54 subskills in phonetic listening, and 58 subskills in auditory comprehension. Sound awareness is designed to assess the child's care of the hearing aid and awareness of sound through amplification. Phonetic listening assesses the ability of the child to listen to speech and voice characteristics. Auditory comprehension assesses the ability of the child to understand the auditory message. The test provides some norms for children with varying degrees of hearing loss. It can successfully be administered to children from 3 years of age.

The information from 10 children of preschool age was provided in the DASL (Stout and Windle, 1994). No demographic information, such as age at identification of hearing loss, was provided (Table 6.13).

Table 6.13
DASL (adapted from manual) results of 10 children aged 3 through 5 years

Degree of Hearing Loss	Sound Awareness (13 subskills)	Phonetic Listening (54 Subskills)	Auditory Comprehension (58 Subskills)
Age 3			
Profound, 90–100 dB	5	1	0
Profound, <500 Hz	3	0	0
Age 4			
Moderate, 44–69 dB	9	22	3
Profound, 90–100 dB	8	18	14
Profound, >100 dB	6	1	0
Profound, <500 Hz	1	0	0
Age 5			
Severe, 70–90 dB	11	34	36
Profound, 90–100 dB	8	15	11
Profound, >100 dB	7	10	8
Profound, <500 Hz	5	9	1

Test of auditory comprehension (TAC) (Trammel, 1981)

This test of auditory discrimination was designed to be used in conjunction with the Auditory Skills Curriculum and is for children ages 4 to 17 years. The TAC is composed of 10 subtests. Subtests one through three assess a suprasegmental discrimination, speech versus nonspeech, and speech differing in rhythm, stress, and intonational patterns. Subtests four through six assess discrimination and memory-sequencing abilities for messages containing one, two, and four critical elements. Subtests seven and eight assess comprehension abilities and auditory-cognitive integration, including comprehension of simple to complex stories. Subtests nine and ten assess auditory figure-ground abilities at a signal-to-noise ratio of 0 dB. The standardization data include information on 169 preschool children, 21 4-year-olds, 71 5-year-olds, and 77 6-year-olds. In the preschool age group, 21 had moderate losses (41 to 55 dB), 29 had moderately severe losses (56 to 70 dB), 53 had severe losses (71 to 90 dB), and 67 had profound losses (91 dB+). The TAC has a total of 139 items (Table 16.14).

Preschool SIFTER: screening instrument for targeting educational risk (Anderson and Matkin, 1993)

The preschool form of the SIFTER is a teacher questionnaire that can be used with children who are D/HH and are educated in regular classrooms. The SIFTER is particularly useful in determining whether children in regular classrooms require in-depth assessment. Behaviors that are assessed are class standing, achieving potential, distractibility, attention span, ability to follow oral directions, comprehension, vocabulary, storytelling, ability to volunteer information, completion of work on time, difficulty starting, exhibiting unusual behaviors, whether the child frustrates easily, and ability to get along with others. This instrument provides information about (1) preacademics, (2) attention, (3) communication, (4) class participation, and (5) behavior. Referral for further diagnostic assessment is recommended for scores below 9 for preacademics and attention, scores below 6 for communication, scores below 7 for class participation, and scores below 9 for behavior.

PARENT QUESTIONNAIRE FOR AUDITORY SKILL DEVELOPMENT OF CHILDREN WITH SEVERE/PROFOUND HEARING LOSS

Meaningful auditory integration scale (MAIS) (Robbins et al., 1991)

The MAIS is a 10-item parent questionnaire with ratings assigned on a 5-point scale: 0 = no skill, 1 = skill shown less than 50% of the time, 2 = skill shown more than 50% of the time, 3 = skill shown more than 75% of the time, 4 = child consistently exhibits the skill. Two questions evaluate the child's use of amplification, wearing of the aid, and reporting about functioning. Five questions evaluate the ability to detect sound, to respond to their name in quiet and noisy situations, and to be alert to environmental sounds at home, outside the home, and in the classroom. Three questions evaluate the child's ability to discriminate suprasegmental aspects of speech, different voice, speech versus nonspeech, and the association of intonation and meaning.

Table 6.14
Average TAC score adapted from manual by degree of hearing loss for 4- to 6-year-olds

Degree of Hearing Loss	Subtests Passed	Total Raw Score
Moderate (n = 21)	6.6 (SD = 2.2)	100.8 (73%)
Moderate-severe (n = 29)	5.3 (SD = 2.0)	84.7 (61%)
Severe (n = 53)	3.4 (SD = 2.3)	56.5 (41%)
Profound (n = 67)	1.1 (SD = 1.2)	25.6 (18%)

Infant-toddler meaningful auditory integration scale (IT-MAIS) (Zimmerman-Phillips et al., 1997)

This parent questionnaire of children's auditory skills was designed to assess the auditory functioning of children with cochlear implants. The questionnaire is composed of 10 questions rated on a 0 to 4 scale (0 = never, 1 = rarely, 2 = occasionally, 3 = frequently, 4 = always). The questions survey the child's vocal behavior and speech; the response to his/her name in quiet and in background noise; the ability to respond to environmental sounds; the ability to discriminate two speakers; the ability to distinguish speech vs. non-speech; and vocal tone associations for emotions such as anger or excitement.

Auditory Training Curricula

AUDITORY SKILLS CURRICULUM, PRESCHOOL SUPPLEMENT (Head, Fendorak, Gibbons et al.,1978)

This curriculum can be used with children as young as 2 years of age. This curriculum was developed for the Parent Infant Resource Systems of the Lexington School for the Deaf by Head et al. (1986). The tasks are divided into three categories: discrimination, memory-sequencing, and auditory feedback. There are 16 discrimination subskills, 14 memory-sequencing subskills, and 31 subskills in auditory feedback. The discrimination objectives include discrimination of (1) nonverbal sounds, (2) speech on the basis of suprasegmental features, (3) linguistic messages with contextual cues, and (4) words on the basis of segmental features. The memory-sequence objectives include the ability to (1) recall and sequence critical elements in a message, (2) demonstrate auditory/cognitive skills within a structured listening set (follows multielement directions), and (3) demonstrate auditory/cognitive skills in conversation. Auditory feedback objectives include the ability to (1) engage in preverbal behavior such as vocalizing for attention or on demand, (2) imitate vocal production, (3) modify vocal production independently, (4) demonstrate audi-

tory skills at varying distances in a quiet classroom, (5) demonstrate auditory skills at varying distances in a classroom with a normal noise level, (6) demonstrate auditory skills at varying distances in a noisy classroom, and (7) demonstrate auditory skills in the presence of a verbal distraction.

The curriculum offers lists of contrasting word pairs to discriminate between words in which (1) the consonants are identical and the vowels differ, (2) the vowels are identical and the consonants differ in manner and place of articulation and in voicing, (3) the vowels are identical and the consonants differ only in manner of articulation, and (4) the vowels are identical and the consonants differ only in voicing.

DEVELOPMENTAL APPROACH TO SUCCESSFUL LISTENING (DASL) (Stout and Windle, 1994)

This curriculum has been used with children as young as 2 years of age with severe to profound hearing losses. The DASL curriculum divides activities and objectives into sound awareness, phonetic listening, and auditory comprehension. The DASL consists of a Placement Test, an Auditory Checklist, and an Observation Checklist for Listening Skills. Resources for the curriculum include the Ling (1976) *Speech for the Deaf Child,* Erber's (1982) *Auditory Training,* and the Test of Auditory Comprehension (Trammel, 1981). The curriculum provides auditory activities that closely parallel the sequence recommended by Ling for speech development. Because the Ling approach for teaching speech was developed for school-aged children 5 years and older, the sequence of objectives may have to be adapted to be appropriate developmentally for the preschool-aged child.

SPEECH PERCEPTION INSTRUCTIONAL CURRICULUM AND EVALUATION (SPICE) (Moog, Biedenstein, and Davidson, 1995)

The SPICE was developed for children aged 3 years and older and is a guide for auditory lessons with sequential listing of skills in the expected order of development. The lessons are designed for 15 minute daily sessions and the goals are listed in 4 categories: Detection, Suprasegmental Perception, Vowels and Consonants, and Connected Speech. SPICE can be used to document the child's present auditory skill level, to identify instructional objectives and measure progress towards these objectives.

PARENT EDUCATION CURRICULA

SKI-HI resource manual: family-centered home-based programming for infants, toddlers, preschool-aged children with hearing impairment (Clark and Watkins, 1993)

The SKI-HI resource manual provides parent instructional materials for auditory skill, language, and speech development.

Parent infant habilitation

This is a comprehensive approach to working with hearing-impaired infants and toddlers and their families (Schuyler and Rushmer, 1998). The Infant Hearing Resources curriculum offers auditory skill activities for parents as well as language and speech stimulation techniques that can be incorporated into home activities.

John Tracy clinic correspondence course (1983)

This correspondence course is available to parents to learn to stimulate auditory development, language, and speech. For more information, write to The John Tracy Clinic Correspondence Course, 806 West Adams Boulevard, Los Angeles, CA 90007.

Components of Successful Speech and Auditory Skills Development Programs

The main components of successful speech and auditory skills development programs include the following:

- Skilled providers. Auditory skills development should be provided through the intervention of individuals who have had extensive experience with young children with a variety of different levels and types of hearing losses.

- Hierarchical curriculum. Successful auditory skills development has been the result of curricula that follow a hierarchy of skills. Mastery of lower level skills is required as a basis for the more advanced and difficult auditory skills.

- Mass practice. Speech production and speech perception development require mass practice within typical development. It is a reasonable assumption that without mass practice of the targets, speech will not become automatic. Speech production should become automatic and unconscious rather than being consistently and consciously cognitively mediated. Fluent speakers do not think about where their articulators should be or whether they are producing the sound with the correct aspects of production.

- Unisensory stimulation. The child must have some experience with sound that has no interference from the visual modality. Visual information can, in some instances, confuse the auditory perception, as has been demonstrated by the McGurk effect (McGurk and MacDonald, 1976). In this classic experiment, there was a mismatch between the lip movements and the auditory signal (ga/ba confusions), and the perception that resulted was ta/da. However, once the perception/production has been mastered, the child needs an opportunity to demonstrate mastery of the skill in a multimodality natural environment. Unisensory experiences should be provided in the most natural settings. Parents sitting beside the child or behind the child can often provide auditory stimulation in very natural situations.

- Parent partnership. Whether in individualized or group instruction, speech therapy and auditory skill development typically focus on cognitively mediated production and perception, thinking about how to do it and what is being heard. Generalization of these skills and automaticity can be accomplished only if the preschool-aged child incorporates the skills into everyday life. Because the preschool-aged child spends the vast majority of time in the family setting, it is imperative that a strong parent partnership is developed. When parents can identify natural situations in which auditory and speech stimulation are appropriate, the progress of the child's development will be optimal.

• Integrated activities into daily living. The primary focus of speech production and auditory skills development is on communication. Unless speech production and auditory skills are used in daily living, the skills will not become automatic and unconscious and will not generalize. For example, sound awareness becomes more meaningful when the sounds signal something of importance to the child, such as the refrigerator door opening and closing, the car engine starting, or the telephone ringing. Identifying the voice of the speaker in a conversation has importance to the child when the conversation deals with information that the child wants.

• Integrated auditory activities with language. Auditory perception and speech production drills that deal with nonsense syllables provide direct instruction to the child for sounds and combinations that are essential for intelligible speech production but are not common in everyday speech. The primary goal of auditory perception is to develop auditory skills for the production of speech and language. Therefore, speech and auditory skills should be integrated as quickly as possible into language production. Degree of hearing loss, language level, and age at identification are the primary predictors of speech production of D/HH children from infancy through preschool. An emphasis on speech and audition to the detriment or exclusion of language development could have deleterious effects in early childhood for D/HH children. A coordinated program that does not sacrifice one aspect of development for another will result in optimal outcomes for D/HH children. The ability to close language delays becomes increasingly difficult as the child ages. In contrast, children with no

speech production, even to 5 years of age, have been shown to have the capability of developing intelligible speech through cochlear implant research. The critical period for development of language skills appears shorter than the critical period for the development of speech skills for D/HH children.

When the skills of the provider are comparable, the use of any method of communication can promote the development of intelligible speech production. If an auditory skills curriculum and speech development curriculum are appropriate and children have similar demographic characteristics (i.e., degree of hearing loss, socioeconomic status, ethnicity, gender), the use of sign language has no negative effect on speech outcome (Yoshinaga-Itano and Sedey, in press).

Acknowledgments

The author acknowledges Mary Pat Moeller for permission to include portions of her chapter published in the previous edition of this book.

REFERENCES

Anderson K, Matkin N. Preschool SIFTER: screening instrument for targeting educational risk. Danville, IL: Interstate Printers and Publishers, 1993.

Antia Kreimeyer KH. Maintenance of positive peer interaction in preschool hearing-impaired children. Volta Rev 1988;90:325–337.

Arnold D, Tremblay A. Interaction of deaf and hearing preschool children. J Commun Dis 1979;12:245–251.

Blank M, Marquis MA. Directing discourse. Tucson, AZ: Communication Skill Builders, 1987.

Blank M, Rose S, Berlin L. The language of learning: the preschool years. New York: Grune & Stratton, 1978: 8–21.

Boothroyd A, Springer N, Smith I, et al. Amplitude compression and profound hearing loss. J Speech Hear Res 1988;31:362–376.

Brackett D, Henninges M. Communicative interactions of preschool hearing impaired children in an integrated setting. Volta Rev 1976;97:197–208.

Bruner J. The ontogenesis of speech acts. J Child Lang 1975;2:1–20.

Bruner JA. Learing how to do things with words. In JS Bruner, RA Garton (Eds.) Human Growth and Development. Oxford, UK: Oxford University Press, 1978.

Carney AE. (1991). Reduced Aspect Feature Transcription (RAFT) as an index of speech intelligibility. Journal of the Acoustical Society of America 1990;87(Supple.), S89(A).

Carotta C, Carney A, Dettman D. Assessment and analysis of speech production in hearing-impaired children. ASHA 1990;32:59(A).

Casby M, McCormack S. Symbolic play and early communication development in hearing-impaired children. J Commun Disord 1985;18:67–78.

Casby M, Ruder K. Symbolic play and early language development in normal and mentally retarded children. J Speech Hear Res 1983;26:404–411.

Chermak GD, Pederson CM, Bendel RB. Equivalent forms and split-half reliability of the NU-CHIPS administered in noise. J Speech Hear Disord 1984;49:196–201.

Clark T, Watkins S. SKI-HI resource manual family-centered home-based programming for infants, toddlers, and preschool-aged children with hearing impairment. Logan, UT: Hope, 1993.

Constable CM, van Kleeck A. From social to instructional uses of language: Bridging the gap. Submitted for presentation at the Amerian Speech-Language-Hearing Association. Annual Convention, Washington, DC (1985).

Cornelius G, Hornett D. The play behavior of hearing-impaired kindergarten children. Am Ann Deaf 1990;135:316–321.

Curtiss S, Prutting CA, Lowell EL. Pragmatic and semantic development in young children with impaired hearing. J Speech Hear Res 1979;22:534–552.

Dale P. MacArthur communicative development inventory: Level III. Unpublished assessment. University of Washington, Seattle, Washington, 1997.

Dale P, Thal D. MacArthur communicative development inventory. San Diego: Center for Research in Language, UCSD, 1989.

Darbyshire J. Play patterns in young children with hearing impairment. Volta Rev 1977;79:19–26.

Eisert D, Lamorey S. Play as a window on child development: the relationship between play and other developmental domains. Early Educ Dev 1996;7:221–234.

Elliott LL, Katz DR. Northwestern University children's perception of speech test (NUCHIPS). St. Louis: Auditec of St. Louis, 1981.

Erber NP. Use of the auditory numbers test to evaluation speech perception abilities of hearing-impaired children. J Speech Hear Disord 1980;45:527–532.

Erber NP. Auditory training. Washington, DC: A.G. Bell Association for the Deaf, 1982.

Fenson L, Dale P, Reznick J, et al. MacArthur communicative development inventories: user's guide and technical manual. San Diego: Singular Publications, 1993.

Finitzo-Hieber T, Malkin N, Cherow-Skalka E, et al. Sound effects recognition test. St. Louis: Auditec of St. Louis, 1980.

Geers A, Moog J. Factors predictive of the development of literacy in profoundly hearing-impaired adolescents. Volta Rev 1989,91.69–86.

Gjerdingen DB. Language arts curriculum. Northampton, MA: Clarke School for the Deaf/Center for Oral Education, 1996.

Goss RN. Language used by mothers of deaf children and mothers of hearing children. Am Ann Deaf 1970;115:93–96.

Grammatico L, Miller S. Curriculum for the preschool deaf child. Volta Rev 1974;79:1926.

Halliday MAK. Learning how to mean. London: Edward Arnold, 1975.

Head J, Fendorak L, Gibbons D, et al. Auditory skills curriculum preschool supplement. North Hollywood: Foreworks, 1986.

Hershey P, Blanchard KH. Management of organizational behavior: utilizing human resources. 5th ed. Englewood Cliffs, NJ: Prentice Hall, 1988.

Higginbotham D, Baker B. Social participation and cognitive play differences in hearing-impaired and normally hearing pre-schoolers. Volta Rev 1981;83:135–149.

Hohmann M, Banet B, Weikart D. Young children in action. Ypsilanti, MI: High Scope Press, 1979.

Ireton H, Thwing E. The Minnesota child development inventory. Minneapolis: University of Minnesota, 1972.

Jerger S, Lewis S, Hawkins J, et al. Pediatric speech intelligibility test. I. Generation of test materials. Int J Pediatr Otorhinolaryngol 1980;3:217–230.

Jerger S, Jerger J, Lewis S. Pediatric speech intelligibility test. II. Effect of receptive language age and chronological age. Int J Pediatr Otorhinolaryngol 1981;3:101 118.

John Tracy Correspondence Course. Los Angeles: John Tracy Clinic, 1983.

Kail R, Leonard L. Word-finding abilities in language-impaired children. ASHA Monograph, 25, Rockville, MD: ASHA, 1986.

Lartz MN. A description of mothers' questions to their young deaf children during story book reading. Am Ann Deaf 1993;138:322–330.

Lartz MN, McCullom J. Maternal questions while reading to deaf and hearing twins: a case study. Am Ann Deaf 1990;135:235–240.

Lederberg AR. Social interaction among deaf preschoolers: the effects of language ability and age. Am Ann Deaf 1991;136:35–59.

Lederberg AR, Chapin S, Rosenblatt V, et al. Ethnic, gender, and age preferences among deaf and hearing preschool peers. Child Dev 1986;57:375–386.

Lederberg AR, Rosenblatt VR, Vandell DL, et al. Temporary and longterm friendships in hearing and deaf preschoolers. Merrill-Palmer Quart 1987;33:513–533.

Lederberg AR, Ryan HB, Robbins BL. Peer interaction in young deaf children: the effect of partner hearing status and familiarity. Dev Psychol 1996;22:691–700.

Levy-Skiff R, Hoffman M. Social behavior of hearing impaired and normally hearing preschoolers. Br J Educ Psychol 1985;55:111–118.

Linder T. Transdisciplinary play-based assessment: a functional approach to working with young children. Baltimore: Paul H. Brookes, 1990.

Ling D. Speech for the deaf child. Washington, DC: A.G. Bell Association for the Deaf, 1976.

Lombardino LJ, Stein JE, Kricos PB, et al. Play diversity and structural relationships in the play and language of language-impaired and language-normal preschoolers: preliminary data. J Commun Disord 1986;19:475–489.

Mann L. Play behaviors of deaf and hearing children. In: Martin D, ed. International symposium on cognition: education and deafness. Washington, DC: Gallaudet University Press, 1984.

Masur EF. Mothers' responses to infants' object-related gestures: influences on lexical development. Journal of Child Language 1982;9:23–30.

Matey C, Kretschmer R. A comparison of mother speech to Down's syndrome, hearing-impaired, and normal hearing children. Volta Rev 1985;87:205–213.

Mayne A, Yoshinaga-Itano C, Sedey A, Carey A, et al. Expressive vocabulary development of infants and toddlers who are deaf or hard-of-hearing, The Volta Rev (in press).

McCune-Nicolich L. A normative study of representational play at the transition to language. Dev Psychol 1995;31:198–206.

McCune-Nicolich L. Toward symbolic functioning: structure of early pretend games and potential parallel with language. Child Dev 1981;52:785–797.

McGurk H, MacDonald J. Hearing lips and seeing voices. Nature 1976;264:746–748.

Meadow K. The revised social emotional adjustment inventory manual (forms for school age and preschool students). Washington, DC: Gallaudet Press, 1983.

Miller J, Chapman R. Systematic analysis of language transcripts. Madison: University of Wisconsin, 1983.

Minnett A, Clark K, Wilson G. Play behavior and communication between deaf and hard of hearing children and their hearing peers in an integrated preschool. Am Ann Deaf 1994;139:420–429.

Minuchin S. Families and family therapy. Cambridge: Harvard Press, 1974.

Minuchin S. Family kaleidoscope. Cambridge: Harvard Press, 1984.

Minuchin S, Fishman HC. Family therapy techniques. Cambridge: Harvard Press, 1981.

Moeller MP. Assessing hearing and speechreading in hearing-impaired children. In: Sims D, ed. Deafness and communication: assessment and training. Baltimore: Williams & Wilkins, 1984:127–140.

Moeller MP. Early intervention of hearing loss in children. Presentation at the fourth international symposium on Childhood Deafness. Kiawah Island, South Carolina, October 11, 1996.

Moeller MP, Carney AE. Assessment and intervention with preschool hearing-impaired children. In: JG Alpiner and PA McCarthy (Eds.). Rehabilitative audiology: Children and adults (2nd ed.). Baltimore, MD: Williams and Wilkins, 1993:106–135.

Moeller MP, McCondey AJ. Language intervention with preschool deaf children: A cognitive/linguistic approach. In: WH Perkins (Ed.). Current therapy of communication disorders. New York, NY: Thieme-Stratton, 1984: 11–25.

Moeller MP, Osberger MJ, Morford J. Enhancing the communicative skills of hearing-impaired children. In: J. Alpiner and P McCarthy (Eds.). Rehabilitative audiology: Children and adults. Baltimore, MD: Williams & Wilkins, 1985.

Moog JS, Biedenstein JJ, Davidson LS. SPICE: Speech perception instructional curriculum and evaluation. St. Louis, MO: Central Institute for the Deaf, 1995.

Musselman CR, Wilson AK, Lindsay PH. Effects of early intervention on hearing impaired children. Except Child 1988;55:222–228

Obenchain P, Menn L, Yoshinaga-Itano C. Can speech development at thirty-six months in children with hearing loss be predicted from information available in the second year of life? *The Volta Rev* (in press).

Obenchain P, Menn L, Yoshinaga-Itano C. Factors and linguistic predictors of competence in speech development by children with hearing loss. Volta Rev (submitted).

Olson DK, McCubbin HI. Families: what makes them work. Beverly Hills: Sage Publications, 1989.

Olswang L, Stoel-Gammon C, Coggins T, et al. Assessing linguistic behavior (ALM). Seattle, WA: University of Washington Press, 1987.

Osberger MJ, Miyamoto RT, Zimmerman-Phillips S, et al. Independent evaluation of the speech perception abilities of children with the nucleus 22-channel cochlear implant system. Ear Hear 1991;12(Suppl):665–805.

Pearson P. A primer for schema theory. In: RE Kretschmer (Ed.). Reading and the hearing-impaired individual. Volta Rev 1982;84(5);25–35.

Piaget J, Inhelder B. The Psychology of the Child. London: Routledge & Kegan Paul, 1969.

Renshaw J, Robbins AM, Miyamoto RT, et al. Hoosier auditory visual enhancement test. Indiana University School of Medicine, Department of Otolaryngology-Head and Neck Surgery, 1988.

Robbins A, Osberger MJ. Meaningful use of speech scale. Indiana University School of Medicine, Department of Otolaryngology-Head and Neck Surgery, 1994.

Robbins AM, Renshaw J, Miyamoto RT, et al. Minimal pairs test. Indiana University School of Medicine, Department of Otolaryngology-Head and Neck Surgery, 1988.

Robbins AM, Renshaw J, Berry S. Evaluating meaningful auditory integration in profoundly hearing-impaired children. Am J Otol 1991;12:(Suppl):144–150.

Ross M, Lerman JA. A picture identification test for hearing-impaired children. J Speech Hear Res 1970;13:44–53.

Ross M, Randolph K. Auditory perception of alphabet letters test (APAL). St. Louis: Auditec, 1988.

Ross M, Randolph K. A test of the auditory perception of alphabet letters for hearing-impaired children: the APAL test. Volta Rev 1990;92:237–244.

Schirmer BR. Relationship between imaginative play and language development in hearing-impaired children. Am Ann Deaf 1989;134:219–222.

Schuyler V, Rushmer N. Parent infant habilitation: a comprehensive approach to working with hearing-impaired infants and toddlers and their families. Portland, OR: IHR Publications, 1998.

Siegenthaler B, Haspiel G. Development of two standardized measures of hearing of speech by children. Cooperative Research Program, project no. 2372, contract OE-5-10-003. Washington, DC: U.S. Department of Health, Education, and Welfare, U.S. Office of Education, 1966.

Snow CE. Literacy and language: relationships during the preschool years. Harvard Educ Rev 1983;53: 165–189.

Snyder L, Yoshinaga-Itano C. Specific play behaviors and the development of communication in children with hearing loss. Volta Rev (in press).

Spencer P, Koester LS, Meadow-Orlans K. Communicative interaction of deaf and hearing children in a day care center. Am Ann Deaf 1994;139:512–518.

Stone P. Developing communicative competency. Washington, DC: A.G. Bell Association for the Deaf, 1986.

Stone P. Developing thinking skills in young hearing-impaired children. Volta Rev 1980;82(6);345–353.

Stout G, Windle J. Developmental approach to successful listening II. Englewood, CO: Resource Point, 1994.

Sussman JE, Carney AE. Effects of transition length on the perception of stop consonants by children and adults. J Speech Hear Res 1989;32:151–160.

Terrell BY, Schwartz RG, Prelock PA, et al. Symbolic play in normal and language impaired children. J Speech Hear Res 1984;27:424–429.

Tomasello M, Farrar MJ. Joint attention and early language. Child Development 1986;57;1454–1463.

Tonelson S, Watkins S. Auditory skills checklist. Logan, UT: SKI-HI Institute, 1979.

Trammel J. Test of auditory comprehension. North Hollywood: Foreworks, 1981.

Vandell DL, George LB. Social interaction in hearing and deaf preschoolers: successes and failures in initiations. Child Dev 1981;52:627–635.

Vandell DL, Anderson LD, Erhardt G, et al. Integrating hearing and deaf preschoolers: an attempt to enhance hearing children's interaction with deaf peers. Child Dev 1982; 53:1354–1363.

Wallace V. Is babble the gateway to speech for all children? A longitudinal study of deaf and hard-of-hearing infants. Volta Rev (in press).

Wells G, Nicholls J. Language and Learning: An Interactional Perspective. London: Falmer Press, 1985.

Weikart DP, Rogers L, Adcock C, et al. The cognitively oriented curriculum. Urbana, IL: University of Illinois Press, 1971.

Westby C. Assessment of cognitive and language abilities through play. Lang Speech Hear Serv School 1980;3: 154–163.

Westby C. Children's play: Reflections of social competence. Seminars in Speech and Language 1988;9:1–14.

Westby C. Learning to talk-talking to learn: oral-literate language difference. In: CS Simon (Ed.). Communication skills and classroom success. San Diego, CA: College-Hill Press, 1985:181–219.

Wetherby A, Prizant B. Communication and symbolic behavior scales. San Antonio: Special Press, 1990.

Yoshinaga-Itano C. Predictors of successful outcomes of deaf and hard-of-hearing children of hearing parents. 7th Annual International Pediatric Amplification Conference. Denver, CO, July 22–25, 1998.

Yoshinaga-Itano C. (1999a) Language of early- and later-identified preschool-aged children with hearing loss. Preliminary analysis.

Yoshinaga-Itano C. (1999b) Expressive vocabulary levels of early- and later-identified preschool-aged children with hearing loss. Preliminary analysis.

Yoshinaga-Itano C. (1999c) Pragmatic language skills of three and four year old children with hearing loss. Descriptive analysis for this chapter.

Yoshinaga-Itano C. (1999d) Mean length of utterance of early- and later-identified oral preschool-aged children with hearing loss. Preliminary analysis.

Yoshinaga-Itano C. Predictors of successful speech and language development of children with severe and profound hearing loss. Controversial issues in pediatric amplification. New York: Long Island College Hospital, 1999.

Yoshinaga-Itano C, Downey D. A hearing impaired child's acquisition of schema: something's missing. Topics Lang Dis 1986;7:45–57.

Yoshinaga-Itano C, Sedey A. Interrelationships with language and hearing: Speech development of deaf and hard-of-hearing children in early childhood. Volta Rev (in press).

Yoshinaga-Itano C, Snyder L. The relationship between language and symbolic play in children with hearing loss. Volta Rev (in press).

Yoshinaga-Itano C, Stredler-Brown A. Learning to communicate: babies with hearing impairments make their needs known. Volta Rev 1992;94:107–129.

Yoshinaga-Itano C, Jancosek E, Stredler-Brown A. From phone to phoneme: can we find meaning in babble? Volta Rev 1992;94:283–314.

Yoshinaga-Itano C, Sedey A, Coulter D, et al. Language of early- and later-identified children with hearing loss. Pediatrics 1998;102:1161–1171.

Zimmerman-Phillips S, Osberger MJ, Robbins AH. Infant-toddler: meaningful auditory integration scale (IT-MAIS) 1997, Indiana University School of Medicine, Dept of Otolaryngology Head and Neck Surgery.

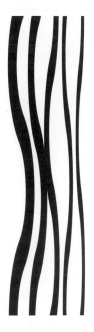

Auditory Learning, Assessment, and Intervention With School-Age Students Who Are Deaf or Hard-of-Hearing

Joan Laughton, Ph.D.,
and Suzanne M. Hasenstab, Ph.D.

Communication models for children who are deaf or hard-of-hearing (D/HH) proliferated during the 1990s and will come of age in the 21st century. The pragmatics revolution of the 1980s provided a framework for the metalinguistic and multicultural focus of the 1990s, which in turn brought light to the challenges of educating more children with hearing loss in mainstream or inclusive settings along with their hearing counterparts. To participate actively in learning, students must be competent in receiving and expressing the language of the classroom. In U.S. classrooms, that language most frequently is English. As more students have moved from schools for the deaf to public school inclusive settings, this challenge has heightened and presents now as a bilingual/bicultural issue with American Sign Language (ASL) and English spoken language in competition.

Providing rehabilitative services for children with hearing loss is subject to the same tumultuous changes that seem to be characteristic of our world in general. Where once there was solid ground, now there is shifting sand; what once was dogma may now be irrelevant; and the craft once mastered as a student continues to change, requiring updated information for competence and maintenance. This chapter first provides an overview of issues that promise to become focal points for more sweeping changes. Then a current model of each phase of auditory learning, in all its intricacies, is presented as a backdrop for a discussion of each facet of assessment and intervention requisite to comprehensive rehabilitation of school-age students with hearing loss. The chapter is designed to provide direction and answers where they exist; to direct readers away from complacency by provoking reflection on issues of controversy and benign neglect; to channel as much information as possible about new tools and conceptual schemes that may aid readers in their work; and finally to provide a sense of philosophical underpinning for those who seek it.

Areas of Focus

This chapter focuses on the school-age student with significant hearing impairment in any school setting, with particular emphasis on the integration of services required for effective intervention in mainstream or inclusive educational settings. The definition of "school-age" has experienced a downward extension, with the recent provisions for schooling for "preschool" children. However, the school-age referred to here begins at the kindergarten level and continues through the secondary school years. With recognition that rehabilitation needs continue at postsecondary levels—including vocational, technical, college, and university schooling—each bringing its own set of challenging conditions, these issues will be deleted from this discussion. The range of hearing loss under consideration includes the student with enough residual hearing to develop spoken language skills and the child who has met candidacy criteria and received a cochlear implant, as well as the functionally deaf child who uses sign language. Focus on the child with less severe, fluctuating, or unilateral hearing loss is detailed in another chapter of this text, as is the younger child (infancy through preschool). The areas of discussion here are based in prior evaluation of auditory functioning of the child (e.g., the auditory peripheral mechanism and auditory processing). Attention is directed toward (1) specific language and speech abilities, including receptive and expressive skills within the communication perspectives of pragmatics, semantics, syntax, morphology, and phonology as well as their integration, and their effect on the (2) overall development of the child, including cognitive abilities and academic performance.

Scope

The scope of this chapter centers around a model for auditory learning on which the assessment and intervention of communication, language, speech, and psychoeducational performance of school-age children with hearing disorders can be based. Rehabilitation or intervention should then focus on integration of all the assessed areas into a context-based program tailored to the school-age student's needs and environment. If assessment and intervention are not ongoing and holistic, and if the child receives a fragment of speech training here and a little language training there without follow-up across the environment, the service process becomes a disservice to the child.

Issues and Changes

A GUIDE FOR VIEWING THE CHANGING LANDSCAPE

The newly graduated communication disorders specialist, whether audiologist, speech pathologist, or educator of D/HH students, emerges from academia into the real world armed with the most up-to-date information that universities can offer. Veterans have already pledged their allegiance to documented systems of theory and practice. Now both groups may be assisted by a map of the terrain or a guide book, describing points of interest and caution. A multiplicity of forces—including technological, theoretical, political, and cultural—have changed the once familiar, if often conflict-ridden, landscape of rehabilitation of school-age D/HH children.

TECHNOLOGIES

Technology has added new dimensions to the resolution of long-standing issues, and new issues have emerged. Advancements in multichannel cochlear implants have brought new challenges and potential to intervention efforts for deaf children. The potential is for mastery of spoken language and the phonologic awareness requisite for learning to read. The challenges include breaking free from old categories (e.g., Parent: "Should I move my child from a total communication education setting to an oral communication setting?") and fine-tuning expectations so that each child is led to his or her growing edge. Expectations may be too low (e.g., Parent: "If my child can only hear car horns, I will be happy") and short-circuit success, or expectations may be too high (e.g., Parent: "He has had his cochlear implant for 3 months. He should have really clear speech now!") and foster frustration and a sense of failure. With the increased frequency of cochlear implant use for deaf children at an earlier age, the rehabilitation specialist is faced with a whole new population to serve.

Speech, often a source of frustration for teachers and D/HH students, has a new powerful friend in cochlear implants. This technology, especially if introduced at an early age, provides the opportunity for all speech strategies and programs of the past to be implemented successfully in the present. Enhancement of auditory experience, in turn, opens a new realm of possibilities for children who are D/HH to develop intelligible spoken language.

At no other time in history has audiologic audiology in theory and practice been more relevant or critical for children who are D/HH. Current technology in amplification systems (hearing aids, FM systems, assistive devices), tactile devices, and cochlear implants bring a powerful asset to habilitation of school-age children. Auditory training strategies have been used for many years, but the quality and quantity of input for auditory perception now available make the task of rehabilitation more hopeful.

CULTURAL AND REHABILITATION ISSUES

The issue here is not intended to be one of combat with the cultural view of deafness. The intent is not to cure or fix deafness, nor is it to cast negative implications on the community of deaf individuals. Rather, it is to view the multicultural aspects of deafness as an area in which access, choice, and acceptance of differing views and philosophies are embraced.

With new technologies, deaf empowerment, child language theory, and research, the long-standing manual versus oral debate has both changed and accelerated. In addition to a dichotomy between signed and spoken language, there is now a bridge composed of ASL and English sign systems instruction leading to learning English. Using second-language learning techniques, ASL and English are currently referred to in the bilingual-bicultural focus in education of deaf students. The new technologies, and especially cochlear implants, now provide substantial "hearing" for effective auditory strategies to develop auditory-based spoken language (such as English).

The modality and language issues reflect both the differences and the commonalties between interpersonal (face-to-face) and school (written and instructional) language. Further discussion is available in the native language (L1) and English as a Second Language (L2) literature (Wilbur, 1987; Kannapell, 1990; Paul and Quigley, 1990). Only recently has the relationship between ASL and English literacy been empirically documented (Strong and Prinz, 1997). An excellent review of sign language and sign systems used to facilitate language acquisition has been provided by Coryell and Holcomb (1997).

Deaf versus deaf

Cultural and political awareness have given the Deaf community a prominent place to express the Deaf perspective. The philosophical view is that Deaf is a point of cultural identity rather than a disability. Deafness unites deaf individuals in culture and language. As a unique culture, Deaf individuals should be accorded the rights and respect that are consistent within our multicultural world. They should not be victim to the subtle subjugation implicit in client-professional relationships in the past. They look to the Deaf world for their role models and measure themselves against Deaf, not hearing, standards. Audiology and speech-language pathology students are likely to have been exposed only to the deaf perspective in their training, where hearing loss is regarded as a handicap or a disability, and the primary issue is what to do to rehabilitate. Most deaf students have hearing parents who want their children rehabilitated into a hearing world. However, as hearing professionals assume roles in the real world and encounter the Deaf perspective, it becomes apparent that their education has only just begun. This confrontation is the prototypical, ethical dilemma. The choice is whether, on the one hand, to open to the sometimes unsettling process of self-searching, releasing old attitudes and expanding professionally, or, on the other hand, to shrink from the challenge and maintain the status quo in service delivery at the expense of the real needs of clients. Respect for the client's values and needs should remain paramount.

Cognitive/language research and the D/HH experience in the mainstream

In child language and cognitive research, normal language acquisition is viewed as a creative process. The child actively constructs meaning rather than merely assimilates externals into the linguistic system. Meaning is shared by individuals with similar experiences and the same fundamental knowledge of a given language. This construction of personal meaning by a child makes language a creative or generative process that applies across phonologic, morphologic, semantic, syntactic, and pragmatic rule systems or across content, form, and use categories. Deaf children also construct meaning, but the absence or restrictions of auditory input caused by hearing loss inhibit the coding of meaning by virtue of fragmented rule systems for the linguistic components of spoken English language.

The status of education of deaf students has been characterized as one of "creative confusion" (Quigley and Paul, 1984, p. xi). The creative component has led to significant change, but has this been translated to educational practice? We have come a long way since investigators were intrigued by the deaf as a pure research sample because they had no language, or have we? The relationship between language and thought is yet unresolved. Cognition has been described as the acquisition, organization, and application of knowledge (Sternberg, 1984). So cognition includes an acquisition or encoding phase to establish cognitive structures, and cognitive processes play active roles in the initial representation of knowledge (structure). Metacognition or an individual's awareness of thinking and reasoning is a more advanced and very powerful aspect of cognitive processing. Cognition then is composed of a structural, representational level, as well as a dynamic executive level for application of knowledge (Anderson, 1985; Paul and Quigley, 1990).

METALINGUISTICS AND THE SCHOOL-AGE STUDENT WITH HEARING LOSS

A child with or without hearing impairment must have multiple levels of linguistic and nonlinguistic knowledge to communicate effectively via face-to-face or written means. Knowledge of the rules for pragmatic, semantic, syntactic, morphologic, and phonologic use is necessary as a base. This knowledge is integrated and reflected in comprehension and performance in communication. At another level, a child who has knowledge and integration of these rules may discuss or reflect on language as a topic (i.e., have metalinguistic function).

School language requires metalinguistic competence for both spoken and written language. This level of awareness is critical for success in the academic setting whether the task involves listening, speaking, writing, understanding humor, or understanding figurative language. Children are expected to function independently in the use of receptive language (listening, reading) and expressive language (speaking, writing) by the fourth grade to support learning in the content subjects (i.e., comprehend the language of math, history, and other subjects) (Laughton and Hasenstab, 1986; Hasenstab and Laughton, 1995).

School systems attempt to facilitate school language development through language arts programs. Much of the categoric content addressed in such programs may be appropriate for students who are D/HH, but too often the programs neglect linguistic differences among children. They presuppose that all children have equal facility for mastering objectives and similar entry-level expertise. One child may appear to have a competent semantic-syntactic system and yet be unable to use that system in daily communication. Such a pragmatic problem will be reflected in the child's inability to accomplish expected communication goals. Another student may have phonologic problems that mask difficulties in semantic, syntactic, and pragmatic performance. In this case, it will be necessary to probe beyond sound production. As children move through school, metalinguistic expectations increase. Students are no longer coached through the language learning process but are instead expected to use language to synthesize information, solve problems, and generalize new learning.

The key to understanding these individual patterns of cognition lies in auditory learning, which is grounded in information processing. These processes have their beginnings long before birth and are shaped and qualified during the formative years.

INFORMATION PROCESSING

Information processing refers to a series of operations that allow external events to become meaningful. The purpose of information processing is to convert sensory input into some usable format (Kendler, 1995). The development of the ability to detect, process, organize, and use sensory stimuli in an efficient and effective manner has been an area of interest and investigation for many years. There are abundant theories of information processing, and new technology has opened the possibility of tracing and observing neural pathway activation and brain region stimulation during sensory experiences (Koch and Davis, 1994).

The study of how children process and use auditory information is particularly interesting because auditory information is the substance of spoken language (i.e., spoken language is an auditory code). This fascinating exploration of how sound is processed and treated by children with auditory systems that perform optimally is paralleled by interest in how this process operates in less than intact systems. The advent of cochlear implants for children now presents another area of investigation. The capacity of multichannel devices to provide enhanced auditory experiences, including spectral information reflecting patterns of the auditory linguistic code, offers a unique opportunity to observe the effects of introducing or reinstating auditory information during formative learning years.

Scientific models and taxonomies are impressive and necessary in understanding the operative nature of the sensory system and related areas of the brain, but there must also be a translation of information processing into a manageable explanation of function that can be used for understanding behavior, assessing performance capabilities, and developing strategies that will optimize auditory experiences made available through multichannel cochlear implants. The focus in this perspective is what a child "does" with in-coming information rather than the neurophysiology of the system.

ASSUMPTIONS

Every perspective has underlying assumptions. Although the following tenets relate to all avenues of sensory learning and utilization, here they are applied to the auditory modality.

1. Children have a limited capacity for recovery and processing information (i.e., they can address only so many events at one time). Adults are aware of this feeling of "overloading" from too many stimuli at once. The result is that we are unable to process and use the information effectively.
2. During an auditory experience, listeners select and make choices among available stimuli. Choices may be based on the value of the information either at that time or due to some existing principle, the uniqueness or novelty of the stimulus, or some extrinsic requirement such as the directive, "Pay attention!" Relevancy also plays a part in a child's selective operations, and what is relevant to anyone depends on many personal factors (age, experience, developmental levels).
3. Information processing is driven by properties of the auditory sensory event (intensity, frequency of occurrence, pat-

tern changes) and aspects of the child (mood, need, drive). If a child is involved in a certain behavior or activity, auditory events pertaining to that activity are more likely to be selected for processing.

4. Information that is consistent, something we "value," or somehow related to previously experienced events is more likely to be processed and used than information that is unfamiliar, irrelevant, or fragmented in some way. Information that is in phase with a child's ability to analyze an auditory event has the highest likelihood of being processed and used (i.e., "learned").

5. When information is processed successfully, there is an increased probability that additional information of similar or related content presented at a later time will also be processed successfully and used.

6. Accurate information processing permits optimal behavior related to internal needs and a child's depiction of external reality.

Auditory Processing and Auditory Learning

Communication is behavior. Although communication encompasses many operations, the reception and expression of the spoken linguistic code is primarily dependent on the intactness of the auditory modality. The ultimate purpose of communicative interaction is to exchange meaning. The reason we use any language system (spoken, written, signed, gestural) is to exchange knowledge, information, or feelings. Because very few of us are telepathic, we must rely on linguistic coding as our medium to exchange meaning. How sound patterns of speech are received and processed will affect how they are cognitively treated and linguistically understood and reproduced.

Lieberman (1984) emphasizes that as humans, speech perception and speech production are our evolutionary inheritance. Spoken language is a biologically determined human characteristic (Nelson, 1996). Thus, newborns are prepared to analyze their

world, including the language within the scope of their world. Children with intact auditory systems possess the ability to learn to analyze complex auditory stimuli, but the manner by which children process information depends on their age and developmental level. Auditory processing gradually emerges through and is dependent on experience and learning. A developmental model proposed by Aslin and Pisoni (1980) suggests that infants possess certain processing abilities at birth, others operate partially and must expand and mature as the child develops, and still others will emerge through later auditory learning experiences. Research indicates that very young children process information nonselectively, but throughout childhood there is a gradual, systematic move toward the ability to abstract relevant information rapidly and efficiently (Kendler, 1995). As young children experience auditory events, the analyses made by their auditory systems will provide the substance for initial cognitive representations of sounds and form the criteria against which new information is compared so that new or revised knowledge can occur. Thus, learning is a crucial factor in effective processing.

DEFINITION

There is a vast discrepancy in the definition of, reference to, and understanding of auditory processing. The critical nature of the auditory system in all learning and interactive situations has prompted clinicians and researchers in many specialties and disciplines to conceptualize the role of the auditory modality as it pertains to their orientation. Auditory processing has been viewed as a unitary function related to a larger operation or process such as language (Rees, 1972). However, it is most often described as consisting of several subcomponents, the nature and number of which are subject to variation. Auditory processing has been assigned components that include discrimination, memory, adaptation to novel speech sound tasks, interpretation of sound without orthography, resistance to distortion, masking and distraction, sound blending, closure, recognition, stimulus matching, sequencing, attention, figure-ground orientation, and other auditory "skills" (Hanley, 1956; Solomon et al., 1960; Hirsh, 1967; Bever, 1970; Piavio, 1971; Witkin, 1971; Witkin et al., 1977; Erber, 1982). These skills or mechanisms are usually considered hierarchical and/or part of a continuum.

For our perspective, auditory processing is the ability to analyze and make decisions concerning an auditory event. Thus, it is the foundation of auditory learning. Unless in-coming information is processed adequately, cognition operations cannot occur; thus, learning will not result. These analyses and resulting decisions are critical for the utilization of auditory information, including key aspects of knowledge acquisition and spoken communication. Feature representation in concepts and schemata as well as encoding and production in any spoken linguistic code is a reflection of a child's auditory processing analyses and decisions. Without these processing strategies, it is not possible to "make sense" of auditory coded information.

ANALYSIS AND DECISIONS FOR FOSTERING AUDITORY LEARNING

Although auditory processing is necessary for treatment and utilization of all sound events, emphasis in this discussion is on processing the auditory-linguistic code of spoken communication. The phases of auditory processing are examined individually but are in reality a series of interactive and interdependent operations. Auditory processing includes the following analyses and resulting decisions.

Detection analyses and decisions

Detection or awareness of sound is the entry level for all auditory events. This initial analysis is for the existence of sound. The decision involves sound versus no sound. Unless a child is aware that a sound has occurred, ceased, or changed in some way, auditory processing does not occur. Detection is the trigger for the entire auditory-cognitive-linguistic chain. When profound

hearing loss is present, awareness (if possible at all) usually occurs only at low intensity levels. If detection is partial, fragmented, or distorted in some way, further analyses and decisions will be based only on that information. Thus, if no high-frequency data are received, no high-frequency data will be processed. As a general rule, children with early onset of hearing loss clearly illustrate this reality. Essentially, the spoken output we hear from them is what they receive from hearing (with or without amplification), that is, the result of what they detect and subsequently process.

In our goals for the habilitation of children with hearing loss we may:

1. Provide a way to enhance or increase the auditory information they are receiving (amplification, cochlear implants);
2. Provide strategies to help them become aware of sound (auditory training, auditory-verbal therapy); or
3. Use other sensory avenues to offset the limits of auditory capabilities (sign language, tactile devices).

The first two strategies are based on providing and stimulating detection and awareness of sound. The third option circumvents the auditory system. Creating the availability of sound and the possibility of detection, as in cochlear implantation, does not alone ensure successful utilization of auditory information. However, further analyses are made possible, thus opening the option.

Attention analyses and decisions

Once a sound enters a child's awareness, a decision must be made to attend to or abandon the event. Attentional analyses are necessary for all sound and are especially essential to pragmatic aspects of spoken language. For example, rules for discourse and topic contracting rely on attentional decisions. The continuum of analyses and decisions related to attention include the following.

Localization. Localization is an orienting analysis and serves as a bridge from awareness to focus. It is a search to determine the source or reference of a sound. The ability to localize a sound is greatly influenced by the listening context. Aspects such as distance from the stimulus and the presence of intervening factors can influence a child's ability to locate the source of a sound. In communication, for example, localization of the speaker is best accomplished in face-to-face interaction or at close proximity. If the source of the linguistic message is moving around, turned away, at some distance, or separated from a listener by a field of interference, localization will be difficult. Localization is also enhanced by aspects of the sound itself, such as increased intensity over other sounds or novelty within the acoustic surroundings. Localization (i.e., finding a sound source) may seem basic and even a simple step in the listening process. However, considering the complexity of the auditory environment, this is not true. The analyses and resulting decisions concerning the source or reference for a sound stimulus at this phase are basic to other attentional and discrimination decisions.

Selective Attention. In any given context, there are many sources of auditory stimuli. However, because children (and adults) are limited-capacity information processors, a mechanism for choosing a priority sound source is necessary. A child may localize several sound sources at once, but no listener can attend to or focus on all of them; thus, selective attention is enacted. The ability to select and separate one sound from all other co-occurring sounds allows the child to prioritize an auditory event. This phase of processing is critical if the act of listening is to take place. If a child is unable to select a priority sound (such as a speaker's voice) from the vast choices available, further processing cannot occur. Selective attention is a figure ground determination or sound targeting behavior. This phase initiates focus on an auditory event (Assumption 2).

The importance of the figure ground determinations of selective attention is obvious in the frequent reports of listening diffi-

culty in the context of background noise for elderly persons, hearing aid and cochlear implant users, and children with auditory-based learning disabilities. Sound prioritization has been the motivation behind the technology that produces assistive listening devices and hearing aid and cochlear implant options designed to suppress competing sound.

Sustained Attention. This phase of attentional analyses is usually referred to as "attention span." Maintaining attention to a particular auditory event or activity for a sufficient period requires extended focus and following a sound or sound pattern over time. However, attention span implies some ideal static time frame. Processing requires time, but the required length of attention is dependent on the listener and the stimulus event or activity. Sustained attention is dictated by the nature and requirements of the task, its saliency or relevancy to the listener, and each individual's unique ability to process it. Young children, children with auditory-based problems, and elderly persons, for example, may need to sustain attention for longer periods to process information. Sustained attention is a requisite for linguistic interpretation of pragmatic discourse rules (turn-taking and turn-maintenance) and topic contracts (joint attention, topic constancy) (Assumption 3).

Attention Shift. In any listening activity, attention can be shifted from one stimulus to another. A same modality or different modality input may captivate and distract a listener's attention. The distraction may be an activity, environmental sound, or some linguistic message. Attention shifts may be very rapid and not significantly interrupt the processing flow or they may create a complete disruption of sustained attention so that a child will cease one activity and begin another as, for example, in losing a topic or flow of thought during a conversation (Assumption 1). The ability to refocus once a listener has been distracted is influenced by several factors and is also affected by developmental level (i.e., adults can shift easier and faster than children). The focus-distraction-refocus pattern may be altered by the value or interest of the focus versus that of the distraction. For example, a distraction may simply captivate a child more than what has been the focus of his or her attention and refocus will not occur, or the opposite may take place and attention will be refocused to the initial task or topic.

Implications. Attentional analyses and decisions can be fostered by controlling the auditory environment in the learning context and by practicing instructional and interactive behaviors that are conducive to encouraging and achieving children's attention. Nonverbal performatives (such as eye contact), communicative enhancement techniques (such as proximity), and linguistic strategies (such as direct coding of intent) will assist hearing-impaired children in their processing and use of auditory information.

Discrimination analyses and decisions

Processing information requires determination of the regularities and patterns of input. Once attentional decisions have been made, differential analyses of the auditory event occur. Auditory discrimination has received much attention because it is necessary for differentiations within any auditory pattern. It is generally included in all discussions of auditory processing and auditory learning and usually refers to differences between phonemes and phoneme patterns in word or syllable forms. However, discrimination also includes distinctions between larger linguistic patterns. Discrimination analyses and decisions provide the foundations for children to "crack the code" by analyzing the surface structure auditory-linguistic components of pragmatics, syntax, and phonology based on previous knowledge and semanticity. Two of the analysis phases (general determination and suprasegmental discrimination) are holistic and address distinctions in overall patterns. Acoustic differentiation and segmental discrimination target the discreet nature of acoustic parameters and phonemic characteristics, respectively.

General Determinations. Sounds are treated in different ways depending on their nature. For example, the actual sound of a fire truck is cognitized differently than the language coded word "fire truck" or the sentence, "I hear a fire truck." An early decision must be made regarding the nature of the auditory signal. Is it a sound emitted by an object or a sound represented in a code? Is it a familiar or novel sound? Does it have established meaning? General determinations of sound events influence and are influenced by a child's auditory and contextual experience, knowledge base, and linguistic semanticity. Because auditory processing is a continuum of analyses and decisions, this initial phase of discrimination will influence and is influenced by the foregoing attentional analyses. For example, a sound determined to be meaningful by a child will have more likelihood of being selected and receiving sustained attention (Assumptions 3 and 4).

Acoustic Differentiation. This phase of discrimination analyzes the acoustic parameters of the auditory stimulus (relative intensity, frequency, rate composition, and timing changes). These differentiations underlie a child's ability to understand, apply, and code auditory aspects of his or her spoken language system as produced by different speakers in different settings. Acoustic differentiation is necessary for mastery of pragmatic role requirements for intent, discourse rules, and meaning variations. Unfortunately, acoustic features of words, phrases, and sentences are not constant but vary in an envelope of acceptance. For example, phonemes influence and are influenced by other speech sounds produced in an utterance. Acoustic parameters also vary among speakers. Although we as adults recognize words produced by speakers from Brooklyn, Boston, Dallas, and Mobile as American English, the acoustic parameters vary greatly among these speakers. The ability to determine acoustic differences underlies a listener's facility in recognizing modulations of acoustic cues in daily conversation. If children are unable to differentiate within these acoustic parameters, the subtle underlying purpose and meaning of a language system cannot be realized. Acoustic differentiation is also the basis for interpreting and comprehending meaning beyond the literal definition of words. For example, a slight increase of intensity (stress) to one word within a sentence can alter the purpose and meaning conveyed (Assumption 3).

Suprasegmental Discrimination. Suprasegmental analysis is also called prosodic determination. This analysis phase permits decisions concerning phrasal contours and emotive stresses carried by timing, pitch, and loudness changes. Prosody is that aspect of language and music that represents "quality." The various language systems of our world cultures have characteristic suprasegmental patterns (French, Italian, German, etc.). Prosodic discriminations in spoken English are based on patterns of stress, pitch and loudness variation, rhythmic stress (intonation contours), and timing factors, including pauses. Suprasegmental analyses affect phonology and syntax and cue linguistic aspects such as question forms and phrase boundaries. It is an analysis of pattern rather than specific elements within the overall pattern. Therefore, a listener may recognize the flows and changes of a melody or language system but not the specific words.

Segmental Discrimination. Segmental discrimination is the analysis of phonemes and phoneme patterns and constitutes a very discrete analysis (e.g., the difference between the words "bid," "bed," and "bad"). This analysis phase may be viewed as the extension of acoustic differentiation and relates specifically to the linguistic code. The linguistic components of phonology and morphology are dependent on this phase of discrimination. It is generally believed that children's ability to analyze accurately the exact phoneme patterns of their native language is not complete until the mid-preschool years (approximately age 3). Speech production is assumed to mirror processing mastery for sound patterns of words, phrases,

sentences, and discourse. It would therefore seem that the processing functions must mature before accurate production is mastered. For example, older preschoolers are aware of mispronunciations made by others although they cannot correctly produce a phoneme precisely themselves. Linguistic encoding within the components of phonology and morphology reflect decisions of the segmental discrimination phase.

Implications. Discrimination analyses and decisions are the very substance of what we have traditionally called auditory training. Knowledge and production of speech elements is certainly necessary for auditory learning and mastery of a child's spoken language code. However, drill without substance cannot produce useful language for communication.

Organization analyses and decisions

The final phase of auditory processing analyses is organization so that the auditory event can be processed further in the cognitive and linguistic domains. Organization provides the framework for the auditory event as it has been received and processed. These phases reflect how a child has organized similar auditory experiences previously and the rules and demands of his or her spoken language code. The three phases of organization (retention, sequencing, synthesis) are sometimes assigned to cognitive mechanisms. However, in this perspective they are considered prerequisite to cognitive treatment.

Retention. This initial organization phase analyzes pattern boundaries of an auditory event according to learned timing criteria. Retention decisions reflect a culture's established linguistic boundaries of meaning units and phrases and syntactic complexities in coding formats (embedding, inversions, etc.). This organization phase is not memory. Memory is a cognitive dimension. Because the nature of the auditory signal is temporal, in-coming information (especially linguistic code data) must be held and accumulated for accurate pattern constriction. This accumulation process is brief, and once a recognized pattern is established, processing continues.

Sequencing. Ordering or sequencing is an analysis of position within patterns and is critical to structuring elements as in phrase and sentence formation. Sequencing reflects a language culture's learned organization for positional criteria. It is basic to a child's ability to determine the semantic role or function of a word according to where it occurs in the pattern. For example, the word "answer" may be a subject, predicate verb, object of a verb or preposition, or even an adjective depending on its position within a sentence. This analysis is also a requirement for determining patterns within patterns, such as phrases and clauses embedded in a primary sentence format.

Auditory sequencing is an organizational process that has received much attention as a skill necessary for mastery of reading, spelling, and following directions. It is often equated with immediate recall for sequential patterns. However, like retention, sequencing is not a memory function; it is an organizational process that permits or underlies pattern recall and is likewise modified by previous learning (as stored in memory) concerning sequential order. Syntactic rules of language (phrase and sentence patterning), phonemic order in words, and aspects of pragmatics influence and are influenced by this organizational phase of auditory processing.

Synthesis. Synthesis is a gathering and blending of existing information into a coherent form. Synthesis allows a decision concerning the completeness of the overall auditory event boundaries from beginning to end. It is the result of all the foregoing analyses and decisions and constitutes the quantity and quality of the auditory stimulus as it is received and processed. This phase of auditory processing also prepares the analyzed data for integration with sensory information from other contributing modalities. Synthesis represents the bridge from auditory processing to the cognitive treatment of auditory experiences.

Implications. In many cases the organizational phases of auditory processing are treated as discrete auditory skills. However, these key steps in processing are integral in organizing sequential auditory stimuli into a whole and integrated entity that constitutes language and represents meaning. Because meaning conveyed via spoken language is not just an orderly series of auditory parameters, there must be some level of organization that interfaces with linguistic rules that will prepare, so to speak, in-coming data for cognitive operations and language comprehension.

THE NEXT STEP

Sensory information is the raw material for learning, but sound does not merely enter children's ears, get processed, and exit from their mouths or evoke some action. Processing does not simply equal production. The ability to use auditory information from a specific environment and that which characterizes one's spoken linguistic code is also intimately bound to cognitive treatment of auditory events beyond the auditory processing phases. Behavior (including communication behavior) is based on decisions that result from the auditory processing analyses, the treatment of that information at a cognitive level, and finally the coding of that information according to the linguistic rules of a listener's spoken language system.

Communication behavior requires both cognitive and linguistic operations. As a child interacts with the environment, sounds begin to relate to objects, actions, and events. Sounds begin to have meaning for the child and illustrate the reality of something that exists or occurs in some context. For example, there are characteristic sounds that come from a car. Children and adults often use the sound of an object or action to communicate that reality (i.e., "rrrrr" for a car). Use of characteristic sounds allows us to convey a message about an object even if it is not immediately present, provided of course that the listener also shares the sound reference. Although sound illustration is an avenue of conveyance, it is limited to concrete objects or actions that produce a characteristic sound. Much of what we communicate requires a more sophisticated medium of exchange to share meaning, a spoken language code. Use of the code allows us to think in words and percepts. For example, we can use words to explain other words, such as "honesty" or "bravery," which exceed the limitations of sound illustrations. In the foregoing discussion, we have explored a proposal addressing a series of analyses and decisions that comprise auditory processing. Auditory processing is the initial operation in a child's attempt to derive meaning, acquire knowledge, and exercise communicative behavior.

The next section addresses cognitive treatment of in-coming information and experiences.

COGNITION

After an auditory event has been analyzed and decisions have been made concerning the various sound parameters of the stimulus, cognitive treatment takes place. Cognitive strategies or operations are mental plans for learning. The many cognitive theories that have contributed to our current grasp of cognition, including the influential works of Piaget, emphasize the role of cognition in learning and our acquisition of knowledge (Vygotsky, 1934, 1962; Hunt, 1961; Bruner, 1962; Flavell, 1963; Guilford, 1967). According to Piagetian theory (1952, 1954), the developing cognition is a child's internal adjustment to the external world. This adjustment is accomplished through the process of experience and discovery of his or her world, the assimilation of these interactions, and his or her resulting adaptions. The "job" of cognition is learning.

Piaget's theory has been modified and elaborated in the context of new discovery, but the basic premise of cognitive requirements for learning still hold true. Schema theory, for example, is an elaboration of Piaget's early work. This perspective has provided new insights on learning, especially as it pertains to written language. However, the principles of schema theory can also be applied to spoken language. An important conclusion that emerges from studies of schema theory is the role of schemata in understanding and comprehending indirect, implied, or nonliteral meaning in complex actions, events, and language (Pearson, 1979; Adams and Bertram, 1980; Durkin, 1981).

Definition

Cognition is a product of children's learning as they move through stages of development. It is constantly evolving throughout the life span, but this development is remarkably rapid in childhood. Cognition, like auditory processing, has been awarded a variety of operations. In a broad sense it is the process of obtaining, organizing, and using information (Kaplan and Sadlock, 1991) and involves all the mental operations that result in knowing. Cognitive operations encompass a child's ability to organize, categorize, represent, symbolize, interpret, store, and retrieve information received from the input modalities. These mechanisms are hypothesis-testing operations that permit learning and act as the vital link between input and output which is necessary for all behavior, including communication. Cognitive treatment does not occur in a vacuum but in the context of a continuous flow of new sensory data with previously acquired knowledge.

Underlying mechanisms

Cognitive operations involve many aspects, but at least two mechanisms are basic to the successful operation of all others in children's acquisition of knowledge. These two facets are memory and meaning.

Memory. Memory is a key underlying cognitive operation and constitutes a study of its own. However, for our purpose, we shall treat memory as the collective repository for experiences, including auditory experiences, that are the substance of percepts, concepts, and schemata. Percepts, concepts, and schemata are the knowledge structures that constitute organization of what we know. They are constantly modified by new experiences and input. Children's ability to acquire knowledge, recall information, make applications to new and familiar experiences, and understand relationships is a result of these knowledge structures filed in their memories.

Percepts. Percepts are the most basic knowledge structures and are thought to be sensory-specific (auditory percepts, visual percepts). Percepts reflect the modality-related features or characteristics of an object, action, or event. These constructs are created from whatever sensory-specific information is processed and introduced for cognitive treatment. Therefore, it is possible for a child with an altered sensory system to have no percept or one that is partial or inaccurate compared with the target characteristic of the external object, action, or event. An inaccurate or missing percept will affect the subsequent formation of concepts and schemata. Our goal in providing children with amplification or cochlear implants is to foster the development of sound percepts.

Concepts. Concepts are the mental building blocks that are essential to learning. These knowledge structures are frequently explained as sets of attributes or features of objects, actions, or events in reality. Thus, percepts combine to create concepts. Concepts may reflect our experience for concrete objects (house, dog, book), concrete actions (run, wait, eat), conditions and attributes (big, pretty, yellow), or locations (outside, home, school). Children develop these conceptual forms early because they are easily defined and classified by their specific features. In spoken language, such concepts are the first knowledge structures coded in words of young hearing children and are expressed as the semantic cases and relationships at one- and two-word utterance levels (12 to 24 months). Concepts are dynamic and expand and change as new examples are encountered. Characteristics are added, modified, or deleted according to experiences that each individual child encounters.

Schemata. Experiences with objects, actions, and events in the external world do not occur as isolated encounters. A child's in-teractions with aspects of reality are always placed in some context. Although there is a target factor (e.g., a house), all other surrounding conditions and objects create a context for that target object, such as trees, grass, the color of the house, whose house, the weather, and so on. A concept structure is not sufficient for knowing within multiple contexts. Thus, the theory of schematic structures is helpful.

Schemata are clusters of concepts that share common relationships. They reflect children's experiences for contexts and for more complex actions and events and they are also necessary for abstractions and ideas. Schemata are the most sophisticated constructs of knowledge and create a web of interrelationships. The connections are more than linear combinations of concepts and act as integrated systems in which the whole is greater than the sum of the parts.

Schematic structures thus allow children to transfer knowledge or generalize and apply previously acquired knowledge to new situations. Schemata are the meaningful filing systems of a child's related knowledge and experience as it pertains to some aspect of reality (Pearson and Johnson, 1978). They emerge through the depth and quality that a child experiences in interactions with objects, actions, and events. Schemata are unique to each individual based on experience yet share common features that permit exchange of meaning. The more extensive and relevant a child's schemata are to an experience, the easier it is to derive meaning. If previous experience is absent or limited (i.e., there is no existing schema), the new experience will have no foundation for meaning or relevance.

Meaning/semanticity

Meaning may be seen as the value that an object or ideal holds for someone, but it is also a person's definition of that reality. Although there is a common meaning (i.e., we all agree a dog is a dog), we also have personal meaning (i.e., one author's definition of a dog is a 65-lb, chow-collie mix named Sadie; the other author's is a 170-lb Saint Bernard named Mozart). The interface of meaning and our knowledge structures in memory creates the foundation of cognition. It is all that someone knows, ever has known, and influences what new knowledge will be acquired. The more meaning a child brings to a task, the larger the scope of reference for interaction within the situation.

Coded Meaning of Knowledge. The meaning carried within a language code is also based in this meaning-knowledge pool. Meaning coded in symbols such as words, mathematical formulas, or musical notation is semanticity. Thus the code stands for some real object or idea. However, meaning is more than word meaning or even the additive meaning of words in phrases or sentences. Words cast subtle influences on all other words within the linguistic context. The actual unit of meaning may be a single word, a phrase, a protosentence, a sentence, embedded sentences, or several sentences produced in a sequence. For example, "house" evokes a different meaning than "brick house" or "my aunt Julie's big brick house on Main Street." A speaker's meaning is also coded by variations in timing (pauses, increased rate), intensity (stress, accent), and pitch (changing contours).

Linguistic interaction (both spoken and written) that results in the exchange of knowledge is not just the speaker's (or writer's) meaning being conveyed to a listener (or reader). Communication occurs only when there is shared meaning. Recognizing the words but missing the message results from an absence or breakdown in shared meaning. When children listen to someone speak, shared meaning comes not only from the speaker's words, phases, and sentences, but from the individual child's own pool of knowledge. Listeners (both adults and children) actually construct meaning from a spoken message based on what they know. Meaning is everything one knows about something as it exists in their own percepts, concepts, and schemata.

Reaching a Level of Knowing. If the external world is to be understood, including auditory aspects of that world, there must be mechanisms to mirror, match, and designate meaning to that reality. One of the operations of cognition in the treatment of sensory information is a process of depiction or illustration. Based on the accuracy of sensory processing, a mental image of an external object, action, or event is created. The result is representation, the foundation for the creation of knowledge categories. If external realities are represented, there must be another strategy to determine if the in-coming sensory information is familiar or novel. Sensory data may verify, add to, modify, or require the creation of new knowledge categories. Finally, because the ultimate goal is learning and accumulation of knowledge, a determination of meaning (i.e., understanding) must occur. These cognitive mechanisms include representation, recognition, and understanding.

Representation. Representation is a cognitive operation that allows children to create a mental reflection of external reality. An accurate representation of objects, actions, or events usually requires integration of sensory information from several or all modality inputs. Koch and Davis (1994) suggest that there must be many levels in the actual representation system. Representation in persons with intact sensory systems results from a balance of unique input from each modality because most external experiences are characterized by parameters of several sensory systems. When one avenue (i.e., hearing) is affected, the balance of representation is altered. Anyone's representation is only as accurate as the input received and processed. Thus, the auditory aspects of representation for a child with a hearing loss are quantitatively and qualitatively different from those of a child with intact hearing. There are no auditory percepts or they are partial, fragmented, or distorted in some way. The processed information is not a true reflection of the auditory reality. How external reality is represented governs the creation of a child's knowledge categories. The parameters of these knowledge structures can only reflect what is represented (i.e., only the sensory information received and processed from input modalities). If in turn, our knowledge constructs are limited in some manner, subtle nuances of meaning will also be affected in some way.

Representation may be the most neglected cognitive operation in intervention strategies for developing auditory learning for children with hearing loss, or it is assumed to occur without much effort. Experience with deaf children initially programmed with cochlear implants, however, clearly attests to the fact that sound without a represented reference has no form, function, or relevance. Thus, step one is to relate the sound to its source. Although children who have gained some benefit from hearing aids may adjust more rapidly to referents that have been afforded through amplification, reality will be different and there will be many auditory events that are beyond the reaches of their hearing aids.

Recognition. It is an enormous task to determine or associate a represented structure within the continuous stream of sensory messages listeners receive. Recognition, which is frequently defined as an auditory skill, is actually a cognitive operation dependent on representation as it exists in one's knowledge structures. Recognition is testing an hypothesis to create a match. It is the awareness of familiarity in an in-coming event and emerges through repeated encounters with a stimulus or experience. The better a child's definition (i.e., what exists in his or her knowledge structure), the easier recognition occurs. Recognition taps into a child's existing percepts, concepts, and schemata to ascertain a preexisting reference for the represented reality. If a child possesses a well-developed conceptual formation and schema structure, a single attribute such as a sound can instantiate that concept or schema. For example, a dog bark opens an enormous reference for most of us. If some facsimile can be determined, understanding is possible. If not, the external reality may be confused, dismissed, or forgotten or require the instatement of a new concept that will develop over time.

Understanding. Only if recognition takes place can understanding occur. Understanding is a determination of meaning. It is knowing the object, action, or event in the external reality. The knowing may be simplistic or complex depending on a child's previous experiences as defined by his or her percepts, concepts, and schemata and stored in his or her memory files. Understanding expands and refines with repeated direct and related encounters with external events. Therefore, each time a child hears a dog bark, recognition becomes more efficient and understanding more automated. When there is new information accompanying recognition, understanding is expanded or modified. Thus, other animal sounds become differentiated (i.e., represented, recognized, and understood as referents for cats, wolves, and so on). Nonlinguistic information can be understood by these operations, but linguistic information requires different strategies.

Coded Knowledge. When an auditory stimulus is the spoken language code, cognitive treatment must be synchronous with linguistic rule interpretation. Treatment requirements beyond representation, recognition, and understanding are necessary because the reality is not an object, action, or event but an abstraction of that reality. There must first be a parallel for representation that reflects the symbols of the message code. Second, the symbols must be identified as familiar. They must also be decoded or interpreted and finally comprehended based on what we know. The cognitive mechanisms necessary for deriving meaning from spoken language are symbolization, identification, interpretation, and comprehension. These operations represent the interface of cognition and language. Without knowledge of the linguistic rule structure of a language code, these operations cannot occur.

Symbolization. Symbolization is the initial operation for coded input that allows language users to create an internal model for reality from a code. Symbolization is a code representation rather than the image of the external experience. The mechanism is a universal phenomenon for language users, but the symbols that are represented vary according to the phonemic rule system of the language code. Without the ability to symbolize, we would be unable to use linguistic code rules, perform mathematic operations, or write music. Symbols are not reality, they are arbitrary abstractions of a reality. Symbolization is the foundation for both decoding and encoding language. Without this cognitive operation, what is called speech perception and speech production cannot occur.

The ability to attach a symbol to a real entity is the crux of linguistic competence, both auditory symbols in spoken language and visual symbols for reading, writing, and mathematics. Children who are hearing, deaf, or hard-of-hearing may present with a learning deficit that inhibits or interferes with their ability to attach symbols accurately to real entities in any efficient manner. Thus, even the relatively "easy" task of assigning a word to an object is difficult. As mentioned, step one in aural (re)habilitation is relating a sound to its source. Step two is attaching a label (symbol/word) to its referent.

Symbolization also has important implications for reading instruction. Approaches in which the auditory and visual code elements (phonemes and letters) are paired, despite the mismatches between phonology and orthography, will create problems for children with symbolism deficits. In addition, overemphasis on "phonologic awareness" (i.e., successful auditory processing), may slow the progress of a child with hearing loss if such methodology is the sole avenue of instruction.

Identification. Once a child is able to attach symbols to referents, repeated exposure to the symbol will produce and refine identification. Identification is similar to recognition but it is a code match. It is recognizing the code whether that code is visual, auditory, or some other form of sensory symbolization. Identification requires familiarity with a symbol. In the case of a developing child, if there is no basis for a symbol-referent match, repeated experiences with the code will be required to form a knowledge base sufficient for identification, just as it is necessary in the process of recognition. The difference between recognition and

identification is that identification of symbols is identifying the code and the rules that govern the system rather than matching the sound to the actual object, action, or event. Identification may be inhibited even for adults if the symbol system is unknown, as in hearing a foreign language spoken. In this scenario the unfamiliar symbols will also have to be learned to access the existing knowledge pool.

Interpretation. Because spoken language is a code made up of symbols and not characteristic sounds of real objects, activities, or events, there must be an operation that translates the elements within the code once a match has been made. This phase is interpretation. Interpretation is the cognitive-linguistic mechanism for decoding the symbol and providing access to our knowledge structures. Interpretation cannot occur if symbols are not represented and recognized (symbolization and identification) or if there is no existing knowledge structure in memory. Interpretation enables a code interface with the knowledge pool (meaning). It is based on the match between a word and a represented entity. Interpretation of a linguistic code requires knowledge of that code and of reality constructs and is necessary for comprehension. Rote learning or parroting is an example of symbolization and identification without interpretation, thus symbols without meaning. A failure of interpretation also occurs when a child pronounces a word imitatively from an oral model, sees and articulates a word presented in written form, or phonetically recodes a word through a phonics approach, but cannot attach meaning to that symbol. In other words, the child may match the auditory code, recode the visual code, or not necessarily decode the symbol. Decoding always ends in meaning (i.e., comprehension).

Comprehension. Comprehension has long interested linguistic and cognitive psychologists in the pursuit of analyzing what occurs when spoken or written language is comprehended. It is fundamental to a child's ability to assess and make judgments about experience and create new learning structures or alter existing constructs from experiences and encounters. Comprehension is knowing the meaning contained in the code. It is not the ability to recognize and pronounce words. It is the child's process of attaching meaning to those words. The mechanism of comprehension enables developing children to construct meaning by extracting relevant data from a code as it pertains to their knowledge or references. It allows them to determine the implicit and explicit meaning of a speaker's (or writer's) message. Learners relate what they already know to the coded message. Thus, they are able to share meaning, which is the ultimate goal of communicative interaction.

Comprehension is a complex mechanism. For example, extracted meaning from the auditory linguistic code may require a literal knowing, an inferential knowing, or a creative knowing. Comprehension is thus very dependent on our mastery of the rules that govern our language system. In spoken language these rules are coded both as words and word clusters (i.e., auditory signals with acoustic and prosodic variations).

METACOGNITION

Metacognition is the ability to monitor one's own thoughts and activity as information is processed (Valletutti and Dummett, 1992). Metacognition allows learners to be aware of what they know and do not know and to regulate their cognitive operations. This mechanism also enables children to initiate strategies and resources to complete a task and to recognize success or to select alternative courses of action to overcome inhibitions or interference. A child's ability to weigh and evaluate facts and opinions and create hypotheses and assumptions within an encounter or task is likewise a facet of metacognition.

Metacognition is the operation that also enables children to be flexible in problem-solving strategies so that they can determine meaning or solutions in an efficient and effective manner. Metacognition is an internal monitoring system and results in inherent questioning. "Does this make sense? Have I met this experience before?" Metacognition

is therefore reflected in children's learning and communication style. It is the individualization of the mechanisms for achieving knowledge. One example of metacognition is cognitive inhibition. This phenomenon may be seen as the metacognitive parallel to sensory selective attention. Cognitive inhibition is the ability to suppress and eliminate irrelevant activity or processing and thus control or resist interference of potentially distracting thoughts. This ability represents a complex operation, but at a basic level inhibition processes control focus for a task, activity, interaction, or thought and confines attention to related aspects of the context so that learners are able to use only what is crucial and necessary (Bjorklund and Harnishfeger, 1995). If a child's inhibitory ability is inefficient, he or she experiences "wandering." This can create difficulty for children (or adults) in timed tasks or speech contexts. However, creative thought requires some relaxation of strict inhibition so that other avenues of thought can be explored. Balance of cognitive inhibition is necessary for learning. The efficiency of cognitive inhibition is developmental and increases during childhood, affecting not only thought but behavior and social interaction (Dempster, 1993a; 1993b; Diamond, 1991). For example, younger children have more difficulty staying with a task than do older children.

COGNITION AND LANGUAGE

Cognition and language share a vital interface which is meaning or knowledge. Language is the symbolic medium for coding what we know. As Smith et al. (1976, p. 111) state, "Language frames the thought . . . " Language is the medium that enables children (and adults) to encode the outcomes of their cognitive processes and becomes the form and content for cognitive operations and complex thinking. Language and cognition in children who are developing according to normal expectations expand and extend interactively and simultaneously. Nelson (1996, p. 325) states that between the ages of 2 and 6, a child's language and culture "take over the human mind." Although cognitive processes may initially form the basis for language by the creation of a basic knowledge pool, spoken language is ever-present and "heard" in the encounters of children with intact hearing. Therefore, spoken language becomes the vehicle for thought as children master the linguistic systems (i.e., they develop the ability to think in spoken words).

Language actually enhances a child's ability to organize knowledge. According to Bruner (1962), language is not just a vehicle for communication but a process for thought. If, however, there is no spoken word, knowledge and, therefore, thought must be different. In hearing-impaired children, cognitive development is not paralleled by auditory-linguistic development. Hearing-impaired children may know an object but not possess the auditory-linguistic symbol (spoken word) for it. In addition, cognitive development is quantitatively different when auditory parameters are distorted, fragmented, or completely absent. Part of the picture is missing. The internal and external realities for hearing and hearing-impaired children are not identical.

Implications for children who are D/HH

Improvements in amplification technology, including the availability of digital and programmable hearing aids and sophisticated FM systems, have made access to auditory experiences and information more of a possibility for children with hearing loss than ever before. In addition, use of multichannel 1986 FDA investigative studies with the Nucleus 22 device has opened vistas of auditory learning that were never dreamed possible for profoundly deaf children.

Currently, there are approximately 3000 children in the United States who are using cochlear implants. The capacity of these devices to provide auditory information to children with substantial hearing losses has far exceeded the expectations of many professionals. Based on the foregoing discussions of auditory processing and cognitive mechanisms, we will now explore implications this perspective may hold for children who receive cochlear implants or use hearing aids and/or FM systems.

Implications for children using cochlear implants

A perspective that emphasizes both a series of auditory processing analyses and decisions and cognitive treatment of an auditory event once these analyses are complete, has important implications for children with hearing loss who are in pursuit of mastery of the spoken linguistic code. New research examining areas of the brain that are active during various forms of auditory stimulation coupled with such a functional perspective may provide insights concerning what learning strategies and personal characteristics enhance a child's successful use of amplification or a cochlear implant. Understanding behaviors associated with the use of auditory input also may assist professionals in determining and developing changes in coding strategies for these devices and suggest applications for optimal programming of these devices.

Although the operations and mechanisms of auditory processing, cognition, and the linguistic rule systems may have general application (at least in theory), the content of these operations does not. Meaning and knowledge have commonalties but they are also unique to each individual adult or child. This principle also applies to children using amplification and cochlear implants. Studies have shown that children who use cochlear implants demonstrate improvement in speech perception (Cowan et al., 1990, 1995; Osberger et al., 1991; Staller et al., 1991; Tyler, 1993; Dowell et al., 1995; Clark et al., 1997). Reports also indicate that tasks designed specifically to promote listening practice can enhance and accelerate auditory benefits of a cochlear implant (Tye-Murray and Fryauf-Bertschy, 1992), and that children using cochlear implants as well as children using amplification systems indeed need assistance in developing their listening ability (Clark et al., 1997).

Child-centered variables

Auditory training directed toward auditory learning improves listening performance (Geers and Moog, 1994); however, all children using cochlear implants are not alike.

The child with hearing loss is more than a set of ears that do not function at full capacity. Children differ in regard to factors of hearing loss (e.g., etiology, age of onset, duration of hearing loss), personal profile (age, sex, developmental level), support structure (parents, family, school), and learning style (intellect, problem-solving strategies) Other variables specific to each child include:

• Other sensory avenues—especially vision, which is important for speechreading, learning strategies that require spatial processing, reading.
• Additional disabilities—for example, a learning disability that combines with hearing loss to produce a more complicated processing problem.
• Personality factors—motivation, independence, self-esteem.
• Learning styles—some D/HH children are able to use auditory information despite limitations imposed by hearing loss, as do hearing auditory learners.
• Communication model—what types, when initiated, how consistently used.
• Use of amplification—what types, when initiated, how consistently used.
• Educational history—school-age children bring baggage or success from earlier educational experiences, affected by setting, methodologies, extent, teacher styles.
• Family factors—parental attitudes, support, ability of the family to participate fully in planning and carrying out the child's educational plan.
• Life factors—access to services, advocacy, environmental issues.

All these variables interact to produce varying degrees and patterns of readiness for the social and academic challenges of school. These differences influence how each child will process newly introduced auditory experiences and how these experiences, both linguistic and nonlinguistic, will be treated cognitively.

The differences among children must be considered when applying any functional model. There is no such thing as "one rule for all." For example, the manner in which children process information differs with each phase of development. Preschoolers are less sophisticated in their ability to process input than school-age children. The experiential base of young children is constrained; thus, their knowledge structures and meaning are limited. In addition, they have not mastered the linguistic rule systems of their spoken language code and they are not capable of decoding or encoding nuances of language. Integration of auditory information, including language, is not the same task for all children, even children with normal hearing. All children make sense of the world by relating new information to previously existing knowledge. Therefore, any new information, including auditory experiences, must be deemed meaningful.

Children who are D/HH are first of all children, and, therefore, subject to all principles of learning and development that pertain to children in general. The additional factor of hearing loss can compromise these growth principles, but the introduction of amplification or a cochlear implant may offset or narrow discrepancies in learning. Each D/HH child is a constellation of characteristics, behavior, and experience that will affect the benefits any device can provide.

There are many children who use hearing aids quite successfully, and there is a large population of children using cochlear implants who function with auditory independence (open set capabilities). There are also many children who have significantly poorer performance levels, and factors related to etiology can contribute to the inhibition of progress. Meningitis, for example, may result in various sequelae that can restrict a child's use of auditory experiences in addition to hearing loss. Among the pediatric cochlear implant patients at the Medical College of Virginia Hospital, 25% of children present an auditory-based learning disability in addition to hearing loss. Although 35% of these cases fall into the "unknown-congenital" etiology, the vast majority of these children have etiologies of meningitis. Various etiologies can create a constellation of conditions. For example, cytomegalovirus can be associated with visual problems, developmental delay, cerebral palsy, and attention deficits. The children in our studies with hearing loss attributed to cytomegalovirus all have auditory processing deficits, attention-deficit/hyperactivity disorder, and/or cognitive organization problems in addition to hearing loss.

Coexisting conditions that share a common etiology with hearing loss are sometimes overlooked, as in the case of learning disabilities. Recognition of the hearing-impaired child with a learning disability has only been recently documented (Laughton, 1989). However, professionals have long been aware that some hearing-impaired children have learning deficits that are beyond what is expected from their degree of hearing loss alone. In a study of matched pairs of children using cochlear implants who had a documented learning disability and those who did not, we found significant differences in performance in all areas examined, including speech perception tasks, measures of speech production, and performance in auditory skill areas such as recall for sequential patterns. Despite improvements in auditory acuity, the children with learning disabilities showed characteristics typically associated with hearing children with auditory processing deficits (Hasenstab and Laughton, 1995).

Even if we could restore absolute normal hearing to D/HH children, we could still not eliminate the other deficits presented by some children, because these problems exist in addition to hearing loss. Parents of children with etiologies known to place them at risk for additional problems should be counseled concerning reasonable and realistic expectations before fitting of amplification or undergoing implant surgery. School personnel and other service providers should also be informed about and assisted in developing (re)habilitation goals and objectives for these children. This will require careful, ongoing, in-depth assessment of children before fitting hearing aids or both preoperatively and at regular intervals

following programming of the cochlear implants device. We do not know how extensive a coexisting deficit or deficit constellation would have to be to override completely any benefit of a cochlear implant, but we should realize that some impact will be made (Clark et al., 1997). This is likewise true for hearing aids. Any inhibitory effect on the auditory processing analyses and decisions and/or cognitive treatment and mechanisms will in turn affect utilization of auditory information.

New learning and relearning

Studies of prenatal development have shown that the auditory system is functional by the 20th gestational week. Despite the limited repertoire of auditory experiences in utero, babies do hear before they are born. However, exactly what they hear is somewhat uncertain. Studies show that neonates prefer their mother's voices to voices of other women and prefer the language of their own culture to other languages (De-Casper and Fifer, 1980; Spense and De-Casper, 1987; Bahrick and Pickens, 1988). These results suggest that auditory analyses and cognitive representation, recognition, and understanding have taken place. What is heard prenatally established familiarity with some aspects of the child's language. Mother's voice has meaning, is known, and is understood as different from other female voices (not to be confused with linguistic comprehension). The experience of auditory learning is therefore most likely to be the earliest form of sensory learning in infant development. From these early beginnings, auditory learning is a key facet of nearly all encounters with objects, actions, and events. As infants adapt to the world around them, early percepts play key roles in synthesizing sensory features from each encounter into new, more coherent forms. Prior experiences combine with new experiences to create new learning.

Relearning, on the other hand, requires us to "unlearn" a previously established construct and replace it with an alternative. The more entrenched we are in a given learned construct, the more difficult relearning becomes. Language learning provides an excellent example. As we become established and proficient in a language system throughout childhood, it becomes ever more difficult to retain the linguistic systems and assume the requirements of a different paradigm. It is not impossible to introduce and develop proficiency in new linguistic rule requirements, it is just more challenging because of the extent of relearning that is necessary.

It is obvious that whether a child has ever heard any meaningful sound before the introduction of a hearing aid or cochlear implant, other sensory input and processing have enabled learning and knowledge acquisition and meaning foundations have been established. However, auditory information is absent or partial. A central question in the decision and selection of amplification and cochlear implants is how will the child integrate these new auditory features into what he or she already knows and how will the addition of sound affect future learning. The auditory features of objects, actions, and events must be processed, represented, recognized, and understood. The linguistic code parameters must pass the cognitive mechanisms of symbolization, identification, interpretation, and comprehension. A child's efficiency in meeting the new demands of using auditory input is based at least in part on the need for new learning and the requirements for relearning according to existing and established knowledge structures.

As explained in the discussion concerning the development of cognition, new information must be integrated into previously constructed schemata. In the case of many children using amplification or cochlear implants, this is not the simple addition of new data. Adding auditory parameters (excluding spoken language for a moment) is not merely another experience with a familiar encounter. This process requires modification through fine-tuning and, in some cases, restructuring existing concepts and schemata. External reality has changed and has taken on an entire new set of features that must be infused into the representation of objects, actions, and events in the outside world. Sound features are not just tagged onto knowledge structures, they must be integrated into the child's concepts and schemata and become meaningful. Thus, relearning must take place if recognition and understanding are to occur. This relearning and realignment of knowledge structures will then serve as a basis for new learning. This will also be true for children who have worn hearing aids and subsequently receive cochlear implants. The quality and quantity of auditory experiences and information will be different.

Linguistic coding is more complex. Spoken language rule systems are based on the auditory linguistic code. D/HH children who are candidates for cochlear implants and have congenital hearing losses or other etiologies resulting in early onset of deafness have few or no auditory symbols represented in the linguistic formation of their schemata and an incomplete spoken linguistic rule structure at best. Language learning will entail much new learning. Children with slowly progressing hearing losses or those who lose their hearing after basic mastery of the linguistic code need to modify and restructure schemata and linguistic rule structure. New learning will be necessary but to a lesser degree, depending on the time length of the hearing loss. Language learning will thus require both relearning and new learning.

The introduction of auditory experiences to a child with hearing aids or cochlear implants will require both relearning or altering previous knowledge, and new learning through the introduction of novel information and experiences for which there is no previous exposure. Processing the abundance of new sounds and making sense of it is an enormous task. Just considering the aspect of hearing loss alone, factors such as age of the child at onset, length of time the child's hearing has been compromised, auditory profile, and nature of the hearing loss (i.e., progressive or stable) are important in determining the extent and quality of auditory learning that a child has accumulated before receiving a cochlear implant. Factors pertaining to hearing loss combined with the objectives, strategies, and outcomes of habilitation before implantation govern the extent of auditory learning and the paradigm that has been established cognitively for the child. Sensory experiences produce percepts that shape and color concepts and schemata. Therefore, the prior presence and quality of auditory percepts define whether the introduction of auditory information produced by a cochlear implant is new learning or relearning and redefining established knowledge structures. This issue pertains to both auditory learning and all subsequent knowledge accumulation following cochlear implantation.

Our ability to learn reflects the malleability of our information processing systems. We are able to alter or change what we have learned based on the significance of new stimuli and novel experiences. Learning is knowing what is relevant and what is not. The learning style and strategies that we use will contribute to or inhibit effective information processing. As children develop from infancy and attempt to make some sense of all that they encounter, they construct strategies to assist in organizing information or reaching some goal. Learning factors such as problem-solving strategies, coping mechanisms used in challenging situations and tasks, or modality-specific proficiencies are aspects of learning style that contribute to effective and efficient accumulation of knowledge.

Problem-solving strategies are essential to learning. Some strategies are more effective than others, and many seem to be developmental or typical of children at particular stages. The critical importance of learning strategies is the variety at the child's disposal and his or her flexibility in strategy application. One problem-solving strategy is trial and error. It is not usually the most efficient approach, although it may be effective. Another strategy is talking through a task. As children develop and learn, language is often used to guide them to a solution. Thus, language becomes an instrument for organizing data to solve a problem. No one else can know the world for us,

and learning style is as unique to an individual as personality, feelings, values, temperament, and so on. Yet we persist in trying to create the ultimate strategy for all children. Learning style will have a profound effect on how the D/HH child approaches experiences and will also reflect the child's perspective on the world.

Many children are described as aggressive learners. They are described as curious and as children who manipulate, investigate, and actively interact with their surroundings. Their style appears to emerge from a premise of attack and consume. Other children are seen as more passive learners. They are reported by parents and teachers to observe, evaluate, absorb, and thus learn in a less obvious manner. It is not fair to say that one learning style is better than another; however, the environment in any given learning context may foster success for one learning style over the other. Learning is a two-way proposition. It is an interaction of what the context provides and what the child brings to the situation. Elements of learning style, such as a child's repertoire of problem-solving strategies and coping mechanisms in difficult situations, can enhance or hinder learning.

Many parents and professionals assume that because a child has an extensive hearing loss, he or she is by nature a visual learner. This may or may not be true. Of course, the child is forced to rely extensively on visual information; however, it could be that our "gold standard" hearing aid and cochlear implant users are indeed auditory learners and are able to use even fragmented bits of auditory events optimally. Experience with hearing aids and now cochlear implants clearly illustrates that children do not perform equally well even when they appear to have comparable profiles and characteristics (Boothroyd, 1991; Dawson et al., 1992; Dowell and Clark, 1994; Miyamoto et al., 1994).

Communication style, attitudes, and affect

Just as children learn differently, they are motivated to communicate for different purposes. Communication fulfills many needs for us, but our needs and therefore our communication styles vary. For some children, gratification is a primary motivator. If someone or something is deemed necessary at a given moment, then communication may also be necessary. If there is no desire or the need can be fulfilled without assistance, there is no purpose for communication. Other children are extremely social and interactive and use communication as a vehicle to accomplish this objective. They simply enjoy communicative interaction and sharing that experience.

A child's interests, feelings, attitudes, and beliefs have a profound effect on learning. Although we recognize that these factors influence us as adults, we sometimes forget that children are also motivated or inhibited by their internal affective state. Children may seemingly possess "all the right stuff" to succeed with a cochlear implant, but the way a child feels about himself or herself, school, teachers, or the subject will influence learning and the fruition of intervention objectives.

It is important for parents and professionals to recognize communication uniqueness among children. Linguistic proficiency should be measured by how well it serves the child's purpose. Interest and attitude may undermine effort, and if a child determines any intervention attempt as unnecessary or unimportant, self-imposed blocks will counteract new learning and relearning.

COMMENTS

New, sophisticated amplification devices and multichannel cochlear implants provide a reasonable depiction of auditory reality. Appropriately fitted and programmed, they permit the transmission of sound with seemingly acceptable accuracy. However, merely opening the door to sound does not produce an immediate ability to know what to do with the information, how to interpret it, or to match existing meaning. Information processing is not directly observable; thus, it is inferred from what we can note under specified conditions. In addition, we do not know what degree of hearing or what pe-

riod of time for normal hearing is necessary before the onset of deafness to influence auditory learning or cognitive operations. Is there perhaps a threshold of quality and experience necessary? We divide children into groups based on the emergence of expressive spoken language relative to assumed onset of hearing loss (prelinguistic, perilinguistic, and postlinguistic). Thus, we use the production of spoken language as an indicator of auditory sophistication. Essentially we use the product or outcome as the measure, not auditory development per se. What we see in performance of children on speech perception tests and measures of speech production are results, not process. What we measure or observe are partial reflections of what really occurs in the auditory learning-cognitive-linguistic chain. For example, when children answer questions or perform a task as directed, we do not observe comprehension directly; rather, what we see is the product of comprehension.

We must be careful not to jump from stimulus input to output performance without addressing processing and cognitive-linguistic operations that develop and change in children using cochlear implants. Granted, it is no easy task. We do not fully realize the sophistication of cognition, and if we do not know and understand the operations, it is difficult to assess function completely. Intervention and (re)habilitation are more than the myopic study of auditory skills or phoneme production. Cognitive and cortical development are surely related; thus, behavior is surely related to physiology. Perhaps in the coming century, a mutual pursuit of scientists and behaviorists will allow our scientific investigations examining neurotransmission of sound and brain region activity to mirror clinical studies and observations of function and behavior.

School context variables

As more school-age students with hearing loss are included within hearing classroom settings, rather than in schools for the deaf as in the past (Moores, 1991; Brackett, 1997), it has become critical to develop appropriate rehabilitation programs to implement within that setting. Although mainstreaming and inclusion provide a rich opportunity, without comprehensive services (including ongoing assessment and intervention as well as effective collaboration) the opportunity is depreciated. Countless deaf students document the splintered world view that may be constructed in the absence of auditory language. Speech therapy 2 times a week for 30 minutes and fitting hearing aids or cochlear implants without adequate training to develop listening, language, and speech skills are exercises in futility. Specific speech targets must be integrated into a total curriculum for school-age D/HH students. Without carefully choreographed follow-up across the environment, speech therapy not only fails to provide any real auditory or linguistic improvement, but it leaves the child with yet another fragment of reality to integrate into a meaningful whole.

Supportive services necessary for inclusion of students with hearing loss into regular education settings have been well described (Brackett, 1997). Educational intervention and habilitation for D/HH children may be a compromise between what is needed to optimize a child's cognitive and auditory abilities and what is reasonably available through the educational agency. Options vary from state to state and from school system to school system. All options may not be available to all school-age students in all settings. If they were, appropriate placement would be relatively easy. A child may attend a residential school or a day school for deaf children because there is nothing else available and not because those options are appropriate for that child. Another child may receive only speech services or itinerant programming even though more intensive educational support is required, simply because such programming is the only available option in that child's local school system. For many deaf children, there is only one option reasonably available. That option may or may not coincide with the student's actual educational needs or choices of parents. Students in rural areas or smaller communities or in areas without regionalized programs may be especially affected by this lack of alternatives. Generally, more populated areas present a wider continuum of services. The role of the rehabilitation specialist includes acting as an advocate for the student's receipt of all services to which he or she is entitled. Some school context variables to consider are:

- Placement options (residential school, day school, public school resource, itinerant services).
- Support services (speech therapy, language therapy, counseling, learning disabilities resource, or other resources if additional disabilities are present).
- Competencies of professionals (teacher preparation and experience, counseling, and other competencies).
- School philosophy (general attitudes toward education, special education, and D/HH children).
- Curricula (regular education, modification of regular education specifically for D/HH children, availability of instructional/learning materials).
- Access (technology, facilities, and materials available to hearing students).
- Acoustics of the learning environment (classroom amplification, sound treatment).

Assessment

The assessment process should be largely a reflection and definition of the interplay of child and school variables for each individual student. A comprehensive assessment is essential to implement effective rehabilitation and/or instruction. Such an assessment should include analysis of the various contexts that constitute the child's world as well as a complete description of the child's communication, language, and speech systems used for learning in and out of school.

As Simeonsson (1987, pp. 195–196) aptly observes about testing children with hearing loss, "Their characteristics and needs cannot be adequately approached through traditional assessment practices. Any attempt to evaluate hearing-impaired children, therefore, mandates a thorough understanding of the methodological and procedural elements necessary to maximize the validity of assessment with this group."

The primary purpose of assessment of school-age students is to determine the nature and extent of the child's strengths and weaknesses so that appropriate intervention and education can follow. Assessment includes formal testing, use of informal measures, dynamic assessment, and review of case history and current performance in school and other social settings. The repertoire of formal tests, with specific guidelines to administer, score, and interpret results, is sparse with respect to inclusion of students with hearing loss in the standardization sample. These tests are norm-referenced; that is, they have a normative group for comparing a student's performance and yield several types of scores providing information about a student's performance relative to other students. Unfortunately, this is comparison relative to hearing students. Informal testing may be less structured and is used to determine present performance levels, student progress, and changes subsequent to direct instruction (McLoughlin and Lewis, 1990). Group and individual testing is common for hearing students, whereas individual testing will more likely be necessary for students with hearing loss. The five major purposes for assessment or administration of tests are:

1. Screening.
2. Placement.
3. Program planning.
4. Program evaluation.
5. Monitoring individual progress (Salvia and Ysseldyke, 1988).

These purposes are valid for assessment of the performance of D/HH students across communicative, language, speech, and psychoeducational domains. Assessment is necessary to extract information regarding a child's educational and auditory habilitation. Ongoing assessment provides parents and professionals with a fund of new information to expand and alter the child's program to nurture development.

GUIDELINES FOR ASSESSMENT RIGHTS

Public Law 94-142 and the Individuals with Disabilities Education Act (IDEA) provide clear guidelines regarding assessment of individuals with disabilities; these guidelines include the assessment of individuals with hearing loss. Assessment must be nondiscriminatory. To that end, assessment tools (tests) must be free from cultural or racial bias, be administered in the student's language, and not discriminate on the basis of the student's disability. Assessment should be comprehensive and multidisciplinary and should focus on the student's specific educational needs. A single measure may not be the only basis for special educational placement, and no area of educational performance may be omitted. Whereas D/HH students may be eligible for educational services based solely on their hearing loss, they are entitled to a comprehensive evaluation that should include vision, cognitive function, academic performance, communicative status, social/emotional status, motor abilities, and health.

The team of professionals evaluating the D/HH student's performance should include at least one individual knowledgeable about hearing impairment. Assessment tools must be technically sound (valid and reliable) and administered by appropriately trained and experienced professionals. This may be a problematic area within public school systems. Often the school psychologist and diagnostic team responsible for administration of intelligence and achievement tests have limited experience in testing students with significant hearing loss (Gibbins, 1989). The final aspect of assessment with respect to legislation involves rights: informed consent of parents, right to annual evaluation of progress, and reevaluation every 3 years. Most importantly, no student will be placed in special education unless a comprehensive assessment including evaluation of educational needs has occurred (McLoughlin and Lewis, 1990).

COMMUNICATION ASSESSMENT

The assessment of a school-age student's communication performance should include language, speech, and sign language (if used) in a variety of school contexts. Ying (1990) describes the components of a communication evaluation as including:

1. Reception (replicate the real-life background noise expected in school settings in addition to usual audiometric testing in sound-treated environments).
2. Comprehension (include evaluation of the amount of contextual support required for understanding within various classroom settings).
3. Production (acquire from spontaneous and elicited language samples).
4. Intelligibility (evaluate across increasingly complex language contexts).
5. Conversational competence (acquire from a diversity of conversational contexts).
6. Written language (acquire for analysis along with interpersonal language samples).

These areas are all critical for effective functioning in the academic mainstream. A criterion-referenced checklist that identifies the child's communication function that can be used very easily and effectively in school settings is the Kendall Communicative Proficiency Scale (in Thompson et al., 1987). The primary modalities used in communication should be evaluated. These include sign language readiness and proficiency, speech, and/or simultaneous use of sign and speech.

ASSESSMENT OF SIGN LANGUAGE PROFICIENCY

Few specific measures are available to assess this component of a school-age D/HH student's functioning. However, a rating of readiness and/or proficiency should be a part of the comprehensive evaluation for those students who use or may potentially use some form of sign language. A typical assessment includes measures of:

1. Manual dexterity and ability to form the hand shapes required for signing.
2. Receptive recognition and expressive performance of signs (Johnson, 1988).

Some schools for deaf students. such as Kendall Elementary and the Atlanta Area School for the Deaf have developed informal assessment tools for this purpose. Such tests as the Carolina Picture Vocabulary Test are useful receptive measures of picture sign recognition. Many language tests developed specifically for D/HH students recommend in their directions the use of signed or spoken language in presenting the items to the student being evaluated.

CHARACTERISTICS OF SPEECH

The landmark study of speech characteristics of deaf and severely hearing-impaired students was conducted by Hudgins and Numbers (1942). Their findings indicated a pervasive impact of severe to profound hearing impairment on all aspects of speech production. Later investigations, including those conducted by Markides (Markides A. The speech of deaf and partially-hearing children with special reference to factors affecting intelligibility. Unpublished thesis, University of Manchester, 1967; 1980), were consistent with earlier studies and showed the following frequently reported errors:

Vowels
1. Vowel substitution.
2. Vowel neutralization (substitution of schwa for vowel).
3. Vowel prolongation.
4. Vowel diphthongization.
5. Diphthong errors (prolongation or neutralization).

Consonants
1. Consonant omission.
2. Consonant substitution.
3. Consonant distortion.

Suprasegmental
1. Intonation.
2. Phrasing.
3. Pausing.
4. Rate.
5. Breath control.
6. Stress.

7. Loudness control.
8. Pitch control.
9. Voice quality.

Ling (1976, 1989) noted the consistency in speech errors in respiration, phonation, rate, prosody, and vowel and consonant production. It is Ling's work that has formed the basis for current speech assessment and intervention with D/HH school-age students.

ASSESSMENT OF SPEECH

Assessment of speech can begin in infancy for children who are born deaf and should be continued throughout the student's academic career. After early evaluation of speech skills, many deaf students are proclaimed "oral failures" and never receive quality speech instruction again. Speech has been the area that is most neglected in the rehabilitative process based on the assumption that minimal acoustic cues are available for speech development. Planning and conducting a speech development program with D/HH students requires understanding of speech acoustics and the specific results of hearing evaluation. Although professionals frequently support total communication strategies, they often pay only lip service to speech development unless they are committed to oral education. This is truly a disservice to the deaf student because any use of speech provides clues to communicative partners for improved intelligibility. With systematic speech development programs, many deaf students are capable of significant speech intelligibility. Additionally, knowledge of the phonologic system of English has been shown to facilitate reading competence for both hearing (Lyon, 1994) and hearing-impaired students (Geers and Moog, 1994). Speech intervention is difficult. It requires incredible consistency and creativity and is misunderstood by many professionals working with students with hearing loss. With the increased use of cochlear implants, even greater potential for speech development exists for deaf students.

Assessment of speech at any age should include evaluation of speech intelligibility (discourse, sentence, and word level), word production, syllable production, single phone productions, and underlying prerequisites. Ling (1976, 1989) formulated an organized, comprehensive program for speech assessment. The rationale for using the procedure and specific directions are detailed within the Ling program (Ling, 1976, 1989; Stoker and Ling, 1992).

Assessment precursors to developing a speech program include:

1. Examining the aided or cochlear implant audiogram.
2. Obtaining the best possible amplification or optimal listening devices for the child.
3. Obtaining speech perception test results and programming specifics (for cochlear implant students).
4. Evaluating by using the Ling Five-Sound (or Six-Sound) Test.
5. Using audiometric and Ling Test responses to hypothesize what speech acoustics are audible to the student.
6. Performing phonetic evaluation to determine the repertoire of sound production available to the student.
7. Performing phonologic evaluation to determine the word, phrase, sentence, and conversational production skills of the student.

The first step is careful examination of the audiogram to hypothesize which components of speech fall within the various octave bands paralleling the audiometric frequencies 125 to 8000 Hz. Analysis of the audiogram includes pure-tone frequency specific information, aided responses to pure tones and speech, immittance results, and word recognition. The professional's sensitivity to what is likely to be audible to a student is crucial in developing a speech program for that child. Ling (1989) describes the speech components associated with audiometric frequencies 125 to 8000 Hz. Ling also discusses the concept of the CLEAR zone (conversational level elements in the acoustic range) of speech, which is critical to consider before beginning speech work. The child's hearing levels and the effects of amplification on the various intensity levels of speech received dictate appropriate earmold selection to make all significant components of speech detectable to the child (Ling, 1989, p. 69).

The Ling Five-Sound test is conducted simply by using the "a, u, i, ʃ, s" sounds, which represent the speech range acoustic information represented on the audiogram with the amplification used by the child. The Six-Sound Test adds the "m" sound. The test involves speaking the five or six sounds to the child, requesting a hand raise or spoken imitation of each of the sounds at increasing distances (2, 4, and 8 feet) away from and out of the visual field of the child. This very simple test can be useful in validating the audiometric findings, in checking the hearing aid function, and in the early identification of middle ear pathology. Additionally, it is useful as a hearing test for very young children or multidisabled children who may not respond to pure-tone or speech testing in the more formal situation. Use of this simple test provides information about specific phoneme audibility and the distance the speaker may be from the student while still being audible.

The major stages of speech acquisition described by Ling (1976, 1989) occur at phonetic and phonologic levels. Evaluation of the student's performance is conducted at each level. The phonetic level evaluated via the Phonetic Level Evaluation (Ling, 1976) includes:

1. Vocalization freely and on demand.
2. Suprasegmental patterns (intensity, pitch, duration).
3. Voice control of all vowels and diphthongs.
4. Manner contrasts of consonants with all vowels.
5. Place contrasts of consonants with all vowels.
6. Voicing contrasts of consonants with all vowels.
7. Initial and final consonant blends.

The phonologic evaluation uses the Phonologic Level Evaluation (Ling, 1976) and includes analogous meaningful components:

1. Vocalization as a means of communication.
2. Meaningful voice patterns.
3. Vowel use for word approximation.
4. Voice patterns used with word production.
5. Voice patterns for phrases.
6. Voice patterns for sentences.
7. Intelligible speech with natural voice patterns.

Ling (1989) presents a hierarchy of speech acquisition that must be evaluated before speech program planning. After assessment, a speech development plan is implemented. Ling differentiates between informal learning facilitation, which focuses on speech play for more naturalistic development of speech, and formal teaching with prompted production of specific speech targets. Both emphases are discussed in "Intervention" in this chapter.

Limited attention has been given to evaluating phonologic simplification processes of students with hearing loss. This is a linguistic approach based on the evaluation of whole words. D/HH students' phonologic processes may be evaluated using processes developed for hearing students, such as the *Assessment of Phonological Processes* (Hodson, 1986) or the *Khan-Lewis Phonological Analysis* (Khan and Lewis, 1986).

CHARACTERISTICS OF LANGUAGE

General language learning characteristics have been reported since earliest times; however, it is only within the past 25 years that detailed descriptions of the language systems of school-age students have been compiled. The detailed longitudinal studies of the syntactic system performed by Quigley and associates provided a base for detailed descriptions of other language component use. Language research continues to be hampered by difficulties in research design, subject heterogeneity, and small numbers (Laughton and Jacobs, 1982). Because of communication differences and difficulties, much previous research was conducted by analyzing written rather than interpersonal (spoken or signed) language use. More currently, efforts have been directed toward conversation and narratives (Kretschmer, 1997; Wood and Wood, 1997), school discourse (Kretschmer, 1997), ethnographic inquiry of communication interactions (Maxwell, 1990; Messenheimer-Young and Kretschmer, 1994), cultural aspects (Wilcox and Corwin, 1990), and sign language or sign systems for facilitation of language learning (Coryell and Holcomb, 1997). Additionally, there has been greater use of qualitative and/or single-subjects designs to study, in depth rather than cross-sectionally, the language development of deaf children.

Table 7.1 briefly summarizes the language development of deaf children from a modular perspective of pragmatic, semantic, and morphologic findings. Studies of pragmatic aspects have focused on interactions between children and a small number of adults. Early communicative intents appear to develop in a fashion similar to hearing children, although there may be less use of information-seeking intentional behavior. Register changes for various conversational partners appear to be intact at an early age and continue to be refined. Conversational exchanges are not well developed in spoken language. Reception and expression of clarification or repair during conversational interactions appear to reflect some differences as well.

Semantic development is characterized by well-documented vocabulary deficits that persist into adulthood. Students with hearing loss develop receptive and expressive English vocabulary later and at a slower rate than expected based on chronologic age. Later, they have fewer lexical items and continue to have difficulty with functional word meaning and content words. Some disagreement exists about whether there is delay in onset of semantic relations. Morphologic development suggests a similar sequence of markers, with the exception of present progressive and plural markers for signed English.

The syntactic system has been studied in greater detail. The findings of Quigley and associates (e.g., Russell et al., 1976; Quigley and Paul, 1984) suggest development of the base syntactic structure rules by 10 years of age, although as many as 30 to 40% do not achieve full use of the determiner or auxiliary systems by age 18. As contrasted, hearing students have fairly complete comprehension and production of the base structure of language by 7 or 8 years of age. Deaf students continue to have difficulty with passive structures (instead processing with a subject + verb + object strategy), relative clauses, question forms, conjunctions, and complementation into early adulthood. Pronominalization and negation are acquired in a similar sequence to hearing students but at a much slower rate. Similarities in development of English after development of another language base give support to the English as a Second Language (ESL) issue discussed earlier in this chapter. The relevance here is not to point out differences between hearing and deaf students, but rather to point to the school expectations for English competence that may challenge deaf school-age students. The significance of these findings illustrates the potential for mismatch between the language systems used by deaf and hearing students and the language expectations of the school. More recent language studies of children who are D/HH have integrated earlier work into the study of discourse, narratives, conversation, and teacher instructional style. There is a greater focus on ASL learning, bilingualism, and biculturalism, whereas prior studies focused more on the acquisition of English. The effects of these language formats within the classroom context are relevant in assessment and intervention with students who have hearing loss.

ASSESSMENT OF LANGUAGE

It is clear that the language learning of students who are D/HH is characterized by disruptions in learning across pragmatic, se-

Table 7.1
Language characteristics of deaf children

PRAGMATIC

Interaction between adults/children
    Mothers (hearing) of deaf speak less with atypical intonation; give less verbal praise; use more tutorial strategies (Gross, 1970)
    Mothers are more dominant and use more directives (Weddell-Monig and Lumley, 1980)
    Mothers are more inflexible, controlling, didactic, disapproving (Schlesinger and Meadow, 1972)
    When mothers use language to control a child's behavior, child is less interested in attaining speech as a tool (Beckwith, 1977)
    Mothers may initially engulf child with language stimulation to compensate for hearing loss and inadvertently control the communication actions of the child (Weddell-Monig and Lumley, 1980)

Intents
    Deictic gestures were the most commonly used and first acquired of two categories of gestures used by hearing-impaired children (Feldman, 1975[a])
    Early communicative intents of hearing-impaired children exposed to oral language were similar to normal-hearing (Curtis et al., 1979) children
    No relation of intents to communicative mode were found (Greenberg, 1980)
    Hearing-impaired (signing) children showed less use of heuristic or informative intents (Pien, 1985)

Conversational exchanges
    Use attention-getting statements rather than simple comments about topics to enter conversations (McKirdy and Blank, 1982)
    TDD (Telecommunication Device for Deaf) topic establishment left up to the adult (Johnson and Barton, 1988)
    Difficulty in deciding when to enter a conversation (Brackett and Donnelly, 1982)

Clarification
    Hearing-impaired children tend to repeat rather than revise (Donnelly and Brackett, 1982)
    Differences in responses to requests for clarification; use many nonlinguistic forms of clarification requests (Laughton and Ray, 1982; Laughton, 1992)

Register changes
    Hearing-impaired children can adjust to various registers of parents by 13 months (Blennerhassett, 1984)
    Preschool hearing-impaired children adapt registers to three different adult registers (Small, 1985[b])

SEMANTIC

Vocabulary
    Hearing-impaired children had 0 to 9 words by 18 months compared with 20 to 50 words for hearing children; similar kinds of words; total communication (TC) children had more vocabulary than oral communication (OC) users (Schafer and Lynch, 1980)
    Vocabulary levels of deaf children are far below those of their hearing peers (Simmons, 1962; Cooper and Rosenstein, 1966; DiFrancesca, 1972; Walter, 1978)
    By age 18 years, deaf children have fourth grade reading vocabulary (DiFrancesca, 1972)
    Young deaf children in homes with at least one deaf parent and in which sign was used regularly had vocabularies very similar to those reported for hearing children (Folven et al., 1984/1985)
    Deaf children have fewer lexical items in vocabulary than hearing peers and have a great deal of difficulty with English function words (Odom et al., 1967)
    Deaf children have deficient knowledge of content words (Walter, 1978)
Semantic relations
    Delay in onset of two-word utterances according to some investigators; others disagree; do have same sequence (Goldin-Meadow and Feldman, 1975; Skarakis and Prutting, 1977)
    Frequently select words from appropriate syntactic categories but often choose inappropriate words within those categories (Bochner, 1982)

continued

Table 7.1
Language characteristics of deaf children

Semantic structure heavily weighted toward or even restricted to factors concerned with concrete judgments (Green and Shephard, 1975)

Word associations of deaf subjects resemble those of younger, hearing children (Koplin et al., 1967; Blanton, 1968)

Exhibit differences in semantic organization of words associated with auditory imagery (Tweney et al., 1975)

MORPHOLOGIC

Similar sequence to hearing with reverse development of "-ing" and "-s" (Gilman and Raffin, 1975; Raffin et al., 1978)

Similar sequence to hearing with less differentiation in subject form class and slightly advanced acquisition of structures leading to negative sentence structure

Development of morpheme structure was significantly below that of their hearing peers at 8 years of age but had leveled off by the seventh grade level, suggesting that the deaf students were operating without optimal memory processes during the crucial educational years (Wilbur, 1987)

---

[a]Feldman H. The development of a lexicon by deaf children of hearing parents, or there's more to language than meets the ear. Unpublished doctoral dissertation, University of Pennsylvania, College Park, 1975.

[b]Small A. Negotiating conversation: interactions of a hearing impaired child with her adult communication partners in language therapy. Unpublished doctoral dissertation, University of Cincinnati, 1985.

mantic, syntactic, and morphologic components when language (English language) is viewed from a modularity perspective. More recently, interactionist models of language acquisition and assessment have been discussed for children with hearing loss (Yoshinaga-Itano, 1997). Suggestions for intervention flow from the more current work in discourse and narratives—the major focus of school language use.

Assessment of D/HH students' language functioning is clearly within the purview of the speech-language pathologist, who must be knowledgeable about expected language acquisition during the school-age years for hearing students. (For excellent information about school-age language learning of hearing students, see Bernstein and Tiegerman, 1993; Ripich and Creaghead, 1994; Wallach and Butler, 1994; Nelson, 1998; Nippold, 1998) The language performance of deaf students has been an area of concern since the origins of their education many centuries ago. More recent assessment has centered around the use of naturalistic language sample analysis and the development of language tests where none existed previously. Analysis procedures were detailed by Kretschmer and Kretschmer (1978, 1988, 1989) and others (Thompson et al., 1987). Although early as-

sessment approaches paralleled the structured or naturalistic approaches used for teaching, more recent attempts have moved toward integrated approaches (Yoshinaga-Itano, 1997; Kretschmer, 1997; Wood and Wood, 1997). Recent language assessment has seen more integration of pragmatic, semantic, syntactic, and morphologic systems of D/HH students. Additionally, a series of tests similar to those used for hearing students have emerged (Moog and Geers, 1980, 1985). These tools strip away context (i.e., they are referred to as context stripping tools) and therefore must supplement rather than substitute for assessment in authentic contexts. Assessment must occur in a context that is similar to the classroom contexts where the student uses language.

A comprehensive assessment of language must include multiple contexts in which the child uses language (including teacher language, the curriculum, the classroom discourse, learning formats) as well as a complete description of the student's language system (discourse, narration, and pragmatic, semantic, morphologic, syntactic, phonologic domains) and sign system used (if relevant). School inclusion children with hearing loss are similar to hearing students with language learning disruptions in that they tend to develop first as communicative language users, trying to satisfy basic intents; they then emerge into metalinguistic language users, using language to learn. Some D/HH students never move successfully into the metalinguistic domain. The "pragmatics revolution" of the 1980s (Duchan, 1988) had a significant effect on language assessment. Much of what we know about language and how it is used has come from observing children using language in naturalistic settings. The teacher, speech-language pathologist, or audiologist must understand normal language acquisition and school language expectations to assess the language use, content, and form of students with hearing loss. Some major assessment questions that should be posed are:

1. What is the student's primary language (English, ASL, or a Pidgin form)?
2 . How does the student use language to communicate in a variety of contexts?
3. What strategies does the student use to learn language and to use language to learn?
4. What are the regularities in the child's language performance?
5. What are the areas that need further development?

Answers to the assessment questions may be obtained by:

1. Description of the student's language system in multiple contexts (with particular emphasis on discourse and narration).
2. Description of the language contexts in which the student uses language (school).
3. Expansion of the sampled contexts with information gleaned via language tests (if necessary for school requirements).

Many tests are available to sample parts of the language system of hearing students. Few tests exist that were designed specifically for the D/HH student. A list of language tests appropriate for D/HH students with indication of those developed specifically for this population can be found in Laughton and Hasenstab (1993). Caution is recommended in the administration of tests because of (1) the ample documentation of poor performance by D/HH students on all types of standardized tests, (2) the decontextualized nature of such tests (Laughton and Ray, 1982; Ray, 1989), and (3) the limited educational planning value of such tests.. To perform successfully on most tests, a student must be metalinguistic (i.e., capable of analyzing and reflecting on language).

Factors to consider in test administration are:

1. Rate of stimuli input and response (timed, untimed).
2. Type of input and expected response.
3. Testing conditions (distractions—visual, auditory, linguistic).
4. Directions that are clear, unambiguous, and language appropriate.
5. Context that is communicative or decontextualized.

The language assessment procedures described here are appropriate for students using primarily oral or total communication instruction, and there will be no specific differentiation. Coding of information for students using simultaneously signed and spoken language can follow the convention described by Johnson (1988), in which all of the language and nonlinguistic information is recorded and the modality is indicated by S (speech), I (sign), or C (combined). Recoding English language tests into ASL is problematic because two completely different languages are involved.

Naturalistic settings

For many years, low structured observation has remained a favored method for the study of language of both hearing and hearing-impaired students. Low structured observation occurs in natural social contexts with familiar people. It is relaxed and allows the child more choice in selecting the topics. The assumption is that nonobtrusive sampling will yield the most representative language sample, unlike language tests or structured elicitation techniques (Lund and Duchan, 1983). This is especially relevant in light of research that shows that adults (teachers) can manage conversations to bring about more productive language productions from deaf children (Wood and Wood, 1984, 1997). Some structures such as requests may be more effectively elicited via structured elicitation techniques when such a structure does not spontaneously occur in a low structured situation (Lund and Duchan, 1988).

Curriculum-based assessment (CBA) procedures provide a naturalistic approach for school setting assessments appropriate for school-age students with hearing loss. This method focuses on assessment of the school language contexts and the student's language system before moving into intervention and literacy. The language of instruction involves learning to read, write, and talk about language as well as using language to learn how to perform activities to learn about other information. CBA focuses on how oral and written skills required by the curriculum contrast with the skills and strategies exhibited by the student (Nelson, 1989). The expected skills for future acquisition and modification in curricular expectations are a part of this type of evaluation so it leads directly to instruction. During language evaluation, the examiner is concerned with the child as a language user within the communication world.

Historically, language assessment of D/HH students was accomplished rather informally by their teachers because few tests other than informal, teacher-constructed tests were available. However, during the 1980s, with the advent of a return to language sampling in naturalistic settings and global analysis of the language used in a variety of settings by professionals working with hearing children, these formats became more popular with students with hearing loss as well. Also, several language tests were developed to address specifically the concerns about testing these children. Included among the tests developed are several tests similar to those in batteries for hearing children and several innovative models designed to address the needs of children with hearing loss specifically (Moog and Geers, 1980, 1985; deVilliers, 1988).

Language sample procedures

The practice of language or discourse sample analysis continues to be a popular way to provide a picture of language functioning necessary for planning subsequent language intervention. Evaluation for school-age students has become more discourse-focused. The structures necessary in school are narratives (written, signed, or spoken), description, problem-solving, explanation, instruction-giving, and persuasion (Kretschmer, 1997). Lund and Duchan (1988) proposed a "child-centered pragmatics framework" for analyzing language samples. This process involves reorganization of semantic, morphologic, and syntactic analysis into a pragmatic-focused perspective that includes sense-making, functionalism, and fine-tuning.

Sense-making describes the child's sense of an event (event analysis) and reflects on the student's understanding of common events rather than specific language knowledge. Included in event analysis are scripts of action (e.g., events such as trips to the zoo) and frames of discourse events (talking events such as conversations about a zoo trip). Analysis procedures could include:

1. Identifying the beginning and end of events.
2. Determining the child's idea of an event frame.
3. Identifying the tightness of the frame.
4. Determining the compatibility between partners.
5. Identifying successful contexts and turns.

Functionalism interprets what communicators want to achieve via their communication (i.e., their intentions). This analysis includes:

1. Participant's agenda or what each wants to achieve.
2. Formulation of intents (speech acts).
3. Execution of intents and agenda.

Fine-tuning involves the sensitivity of the communicative partners to each others' comprehension and includes:

1. Contingency analysis.
2. Interaction mode analysis (directiveness/nurturance; motherese).

This type of procedure can be modified for classroom discourse and used effectively for students with hearing loss.

The language sample analysis procedure provides examples of language functioning in several settings. The sampling procedure is helpful in observing the child's move from one linguistic phase to another. Language samples from naturalistic or more structured school settings provide the data. Ongoing samples provide reliability data, that is, whether any single sample is representative of the student's language use and the impact of context variations. The number of utterances necessary for language sample analysis is relative to the language learning level and context (Lund and Duchan, 1988). Whereas 50 utterances have traditionally been considered to be appropriate, we know clinically that young hearing-impaired children may not generate 50 utterances within several settings. With older students the 50 utterances may be obtained easily, but more utterances will reflect flexibility (or lack of flexibility) as well as changes within the utterances contingent on pragmatic demands. For example, single-word utterances may be common when the examiner asks consecutive questions of the child, but longer utterances may occur when a child is engaged in event description or narratives (Wood and Wood, 1997). The specific utterances and the number selected for the analysis should reveal the strengths of the language system. Further discussion of language sample procedures is available from Lund and Duchan (1988). The most preferred language elicitation procedures for preschool-age through adult are informal conversation followed by imperatives and "WH" questions (e.g., What? Where? Who?) for elementary and secondary school-age students (Atkins and Cartwright, 1982). Children's language is richer in content, syntax, and ideas when unstructured elicitation procedures are used; however, there are times when getting the conversation started necessitates specific elicitation.

Specific elicitation tasks

A variety of tasks have been critiqued for use in obtaining language samples. The authors have found the following to be effective:

1. Spontaneous interaction (free play or interaction, conversation) can be productive. With younger children, making puppets "talk," identifying the characters, and beginning action with dialogue have been helpful. With older students, discussion of school or age-related topics is generally more productive. There are many students who do not communicate freely with a stranger in this type of setting, so a teacher or peer may elicit a more representative sample.
2. Elicited interaction may be necessary for students who are somewhat reluctant to communicate. Enticing the student to provide instruction in how to play a game often yields a rich language sample.
3. Specific set-ups, such as role-playing with peers, can be productive as well. A creative example includes a situation in which students were directed to talk with each other about their favorite snack foods while they watched television. Their conversations were audiotaped using an unobtrusive flat microphone taped to the corner of the table (Schober-Peterson D. The conversational performance of low achieving and normally achieving third grade children. Unpublished doctoral dissertation, University of Illinois, Champaign, Illinois, 1988).
4. Other contexts include story-telling or use of a Viewmaster; the clinician directs the child to describe a frame and then tries to guess which one is being described.
5. Requesting that the older school-age student give directions from where he or she is to their home or another location provides a valuable sample.
6. Describing a movie not seen by the examiner is also a good sampling strategy for older school-age students.
7. Deep testing for structures that do not appear in the sample can be done by patterning, sentence completion, inter-

views, questions for information, retells, pretend situations, games, or even language test formats.

The authors have found the following to be most helpful in eliciting a language sample.

1. Make it real communication.
2. Sabotage the environment if necessary.
3. Avoid playing "20 Questions," or single-word answers will be the product.
4. Do not anticipate the child's behavior, wants, or responses (i.e., do not preempt the child).
5. If possible, let someone else interact with the child while the examiner makes notes and observes.
6. Slow the pace, contribute to the conversation with narrative episodes including complex, embedded utterances rather than frequent repair, simple grammar, and numerous questions (Wood and Wood, 1997).
7. Audiotape and/or videotape the interaction; even consider leaving the room briefly while the videotape continues.

Mean length of utterance (MLU), Brown's Stage, and type-token ratio

A morphologic MLU is computed and serves as the entree to the analysis system. Procedures for computing MLU are available from Chapman (1981). Brown's Stage is determined via both MLU and qualitative descriptors rather than MLU alone, which often inflates the Brown's Stage determination. For example, a child who has plateaued developmentally at Brown's Stage II may have a higher MLU than the expected 2.0 to 2.5 with limited development of morphologic markers (pluralization, present progressive) and determiners. Based on MLU alone, the child would qualify for Brown's Stage III but is clearly still at Brown's Stage II qualitatively. A slight modification in morphologic acquisition has been observed with hearing-impaired students using Seeing Essential English (Raffin, 1976; Raffin et al., 1978). The difference observed was

that plural and past tense were apparent before the present progressive marker.

Type-token ratio information is also helpful in adding to the total language functioning picture. Although this procedure has been criticized as a research instrument because of variability related to sample size, it can provide helpful clinical data about the student's flexibility in use of lexical items and linguistic categories. For a further description of this measure, see Miller, 1981 and Hess et al., 1986.

Further analysis of language performance can be obtained through the use of some of the tests developed specifically for students with hearing loss or those modified for use by these students.

PSYCHOEDUCATIONAL ASSESSMENT

Psychoeducational assessment for children with hearing loss may be necessary to determine eligibility for services, to make appropriate decisions for placement, and to establish educational and (re)habilitative objectives. The area of psychoeducational assessment for school-age children with significant hearing loss has received less attention than identification of their language and communicative function. Nevertheless, the psychoeducational domain reflects the impact of the hearing loss on learning within the environment in which these children are expected to compete. In some states, unlike the eligibility requirements for other disability conditions requiring special education, the only requirements for students with hearing loss include audiometric evaluation, otologic evaluation, and minimal assessment of basic academic skills, expressive and receptive communication abilities, and a statement about social/emotional adjustment for developing the individualized education program. A psychological evaluation using instruments appropriate for D/HH students is recommended but not required in some states (Georgia Department of Education Regulations and Procedures, November 1, 1988). Speech and language evaluations occur at least annually for D/HH students, but comprehensive psychoeducational assessment may never occur during a student's school years. This state of affairs continues to present a major challenge for personnel charged with education planning. Horror stories of deaf individuals mislabeled as mentally retarded or emotionally disturbed continue even in these times. Additionally, many students with hearing loss remain underserved because of a lack of comprehensive assessment.

Psychoeducational testing of school-age children often is divided arbitrarily into two areas: assessment of cognitive abilities and assessment of academic performance or achievement. Tests of cognitive ability theoretically tap a child's learning potential, learning style, and problem-solving strategies. Tests of academic performance are designed to determine how well a child performs in areas such as reading, math, general information, and other content subjects. Achievement represents the knowledge and experience that a child has accumulated. Cognitive areas represent the presumed learning potential or capabilities of a child.

Psychoeducational assessment of children with hearing loss

The purposes for assessment of children who are D/HH are the same as for others:

1. To provide baseline information and feedback about progress.
2. To identify the student's strengths and weaknesses.
3. To provide an appropriate educational program with modifications as needed.

The major areas of assessment include cognitive, communicative, achievement, and social-emotional functioning (Heller, 1990). Communicative assessment has been discussed previously. Additional psychoeducational assessment should minimally include measures and behavior samples of:

1. Nonverbal and verbal cognitive functioning or learning abilities.
2. Achievement in reading, writing, math, and when possible other content academic areas.

   a. Reading—see Laughton (1988).
   b. Writing—see Conway (1988).
3. Information-processing performance.
4. Psychosocial characteristics.

In the past, psychological assessment of children with hearing loss was criticized for (1) failure to ensure that the child comprehended the language and concepts used in psychological tests, (2) use of tests standardized on hearing children only, and (3) use of evaluators with limited familiarity with the language and behaviors of students who are D/HH (Elliott et al., 1987). The reader is referred to reviews of appropriate tests for this population (Elliott et al., 1987; Simeonsson, 1987; Bradley-Johnson and Evans, 1991). These concerns continue to be of major interest to professionals within the discipline, because these students often fail to receive comprehensive assessment.

Psychological testing is affected by situational variables, measurement errors associated with test instruments, the personality of the evaluator and the student, and the heterogeneity across individuals with hearing loss (Elliott et al., 1987). Differences among D/HH individuals that are critical and must be considered in assessment include their language, culture, communication mode, interpreter needs, comprehension of the language used by the examiner, familiarity with test instructions, and prior test-taking experiences. Testing assumes the ability to understand and communicate using the English language. Many psychological and achievement tests use complex syntax, idiomatic expressions, and awkward sentences that are not in common usage in informal spoken or signed interpersonal communication. Deaf individuals may not have the English competencies required to deal with this type of language use. They may have experience with spoken English, signed English, ASL, or some modified version of each language. Therefore, they could be expected to be very different in their comprehension of the language used in tests.

Cultural differences are expected across deaf populations as well. Many psychologists testing deaf students are unfamiliar with the diverse cultural aspects influencing testing of these students. These differences may include expectations of the assessment, appropriateness of discussing personal matters, role interaction with hearing people, and how to deal with unclear communication.

Many deaf individuals require an interpreter when the examiner is unable to sign for himself or herself. Few professionals evaluating deaf individuals are fluent in ASL or other English sign systems. There are no magic solutions when an interpreter is used, and questionable practices may occur. According to many psychometrists, conceptual signing used by most interpreters to get across the message may provide too many clues to the examinee. The interpreter used for psychological testing should be trained in psychology and testing as well as sign language (Sullivan and Vernon, 1979). Even when signing for himself or herself, the examiner must continuously check to be sure the student has understood the language used.

The complexities of testing are not necessarily reduced during evaluation of auditory-oral students. Many are intelligible only to professionals trained to recognize the phonetic and phonologic speech characteristics of deaf students. Even when students are intelligible, their comprehension of spoken language cannot be assumed to be intact. The typical psychological evaluator in public schools has had limited experience with deaf students using oral or simultaneous spoken and signed communication.

The psychological tests most commonly used to evaluate students with hearing loss have not changed dramatically since the early 1970s (Levine, 1974; Gibbins, 1989). The WISC-R and WISC-III Performance Scales, the Leiter, the WAIS-R, and the Hiskey-Nebraska continue to be used most frequently. The only one of these tests that included children with hearing loss in the original standardization sample is the Hiskey-Nebraska, which was developed specifically for deaf students. Questions about the generalizability of this test were

raised many years ago (Watson and Goldgar, 1985). The WISC-R and WISC-III do have hearing-impaired norms for the Performance Scale (Anderson and Sisco, 1977); however, they were developed after the fact rather than including these students in the original standardization sample. The Nonverbal Scale of the Kaufman Assessment Battery for Children (K-ABC) follows the above four tests in popularity for use with hearing-impaired students (Gibbins, 1989). Because of its ease of administration, motivation for children, and nonverbal subtest scoring, it became more popular during the 1990s.

Despite the clear statement in the original legislation, PL 94-142 requiring competent evaluators to measure the psychological abilities of students with hearing loss, few professionals are trained or experienced with these children. Of particular concern is the typical school psychologist who performs testing of students who are D/HH within public schools. Gibbins (1989) examined the practices of professionals providing such services. The professionals described themselves as school psychologists, clinical psychologists, administrators, educational diagnosticians, and learning specialists. Eighty percent of the group indicated that their involvement with testing students who were D/HH was only part-time, with the majority of their time dedicated to the evaluation of hearing children (Gibbins, 1989). Improvement of the quality of psychological services is unlikely to occur with school psychologists who have limited experience and lack specialized training for testing this population and who work primarily in regular educational settings that serve these students in special classes or in the continuum of mainstream settings (Gibbins, 1989).

A comprehensive assessment, although critical for educational planning, is not easily accomplished with D/HH students. The interdependence of language and cognition presents difficulty in assessing cognitive function without using language (Orr et al., 1987). Performance tests minimize the use of language but generally require that instructions be given using language. Being certain that students understand the task to be performed becomes complex. The Performance Scale of the WISC-R and WISC-III can be useful in providing an estimate of the student's general nonverbal problem-solving but provides little information about the individual's verbal abilities when the Verbal Scale of the test is not administered, as is often the case.

Psychoeducational assessment of D/HH students must be accomplished within a context that provides meaningful information for educational planning. Most standardized testing is decontextualized, requiring the examinee to ignore the very guidelines they follow in interpersonal communication (Laughton and Ray, 1982; Ray, 1989). Students are removed from their usual surroundings and asked to interact with test stimuli in a structured manner that is disconnected from their world knowledge. Such assessments lack authenticity. Additionally, tests are often timed without direct notification to the student during the testing. These typical test conditions are likely to be unfamiliar to D/HH students who are less "test-wise" than many other school-age students (Ray, 1989). The examiner is cautioned in psychoeducational testing with students with hearing loss with respect to the use of:

1. Verbal tests that measure language rather than intelligence, psychosocial behavior, aptitude, or interest (Vernon, 1976; Zieziula, 1982).
2. Modifications in administration of tests including pantomime (Graham and Shapiro, 1963), visual aids (Reed, 1970), and practice items (Ray, 1976).
3. Oral communication and hearing aids, considering the adverse effect of poor speech skills on understanding (Ross, 1990).
4. Signed communication, considering the variable competencies of the student and the examiner.
5. Lack of validity of timed tests with timed responses (Zieziula, 1982). For hearing children, a timed test establishes an attention set that moves them efficiently through accurate responses (Vernon,

1976); students who are deaf typically try to finish quickly at the expense of accuracy. Such a difference in response to being timed is one of a multiplicity of subtle yet substantial performance factors that inexperienced test administrators may fail to consider.
6. Group testing, because of the attention to test directions and reading level required for understanding directions (Sullivan and Vernon, 1979; Levine, 1981; Zieziula, 1982).
7. Personality assessment that may tend to identify psychological subgroups in view of the language and communication issues presented earlier.

IMPLICATIONS

The implications of early detection of hearing loss and optimal amplification or cochlear implants for students who are D/HH and who develop auditory skills allowing them to function primarily in an auditory environment are that these children then may experience the assessment and intervention services available to any hearing student with a disability. However, students whose speech is not highly intelligible to examiners with general special education backgrounds or whose primary language is conveyed through a signed format (English or ASL) may not receive the comprehensive assessment and subsequent intervention guaranteed by the legislation developed for individuals with disabilities. Although the primary focus of this chapter is directed to significantly hearing-impaired students, the reader is cautioned to be sure that all students with hearing loss, irrespective of severity or relative success of the habilitation, are entitled to a comprehensive assessment before development and initiation of their habilitative programs and periodically through their school years. Therefore, many of the tests and procedures will be applicable to all school-age students who are D/HH. Despite successful rehabilitation, hearing loss is likely to interfere with communication in some interactions that occur daily. Thus, it is likely that all students with hearing loss will need some degree of intervention. Ongoing assessment provides parents and professionals with a fund of new information to expand and alter the child's rehabilitative program to enhance development.

Intervention

The intervention phase of the rehabilitative process follows analysis of the contexts and the repertoire of tools available to the school-age student to apply to these contexts. The long-term goal is that the child with hearing loss will become an independent adult.

Short-term goals include:

1. Well-adjusted parents;
2. A child with a good self-concept;
3. Reduction of the impact of the auditory deficit through amplification, cochlear implants, and/or auditory learning;
4. A child with cognitive skills commensurate with chronologic age;
5. A child with language skills to meet communicative and cognitive needs;
6. A child with speech to express language (Boothroyd, 1988); and/or
7. A child with signs to express language (if this is the selected communication option).

An effective rehabilitation management model includes these components:

1. Parental management: assisting parents in developing the skills to accept, teach, and advocate for their child.
2. Audiologic management: hearing testing, hearing aids and retesting, responsibility for cochlear implants, hearing conservation.
3. Auditory management: establishing a program for development of auditory learning.
4. Cognitive/linguistic management: developing a world schema with a symbolic system to represent the schema.
5. Speech management: developing the auditory, motor, acoustic, phonetic, and phonologic aspects of spoken language.
6. Educational management: developing the learning skills and modification of the learning contexts to facilitate learning across the curriculum.
7. Social and emotional management: developing a perspective that enables active participation in the social environment with a healthy self-concept (Boothroyd, 1988; Brackett, 1997).

Rather than differentiating the rehabilitative process from the education of D/HH students, the focus in intervention is to incorporate both into an integrated model. The history of educating deaf students is rich but marked by controversy. Education for D/HH students in the United States predates special education for other disability groups. The land grants for establishment of state universities also established schools for the deaf. Education of deaf students in the United States began in Hartford, Connecticut, with the establishment of the American Asylum for the Deaf and Dumb (later changed to the American School for the Deaf) in 1817. This program used the language of signs as the primary means of communication. Soon after, the establishment of the Clarke School for the Deaf in Northampton, Massachusetts, provided the option of an oral education for deaf students. To this date, disagreements continue regarding preferred methodology for communication and education of D/HH students. These children and their families are not homogeneous; they have different needs and therefore require different plans for habilitation.

Moores (1991) updated the school placement revolution, documenting the changes in the school-age hearing-impaired population from the 1980s to early 1990s. He noted that fewer students were deaf (had profound losses) and that logically more children were being taught via auditory/oral-only instruction (39% of the school-age population). Simultaneous instruction using signs and speech was used with 60% of the population, with all other modes (sign only, cued speech, other) used with 1% of the population. Moores further summarized the demographics, stating that "the population of children we are serving is becoming less white and less black, less deaf, more oral and younger" (Moores, 1991, p. 307). This was, of course, reflected in educational and rehabilitative practice. In 1986, the Executive Board of the Council on Education of the Deaf (CED) affirmed the principles central to PL 94-142 to provide individualized instruction and services to D/HH students of school-age, noting that "no single method of instruction and/or communication (oral or total communication) or educational setting can best serve the needs of all such children" (Northcott, 1990, p. 3). The school placement trends continued through the late 1990s and into 2000, with the major impact of greater use of cochlear implants with younger children resulting in higher language achievers and more oral communication educational sites being sought.

A significant aspect of the school placement revolution was that the predominance of children with hearing loss are schooled within the public day mainstream or inclusive settings. The students at residential schools for the deaf continue to be the minority. Intervention at the beginning of the new century then must focus on the changes brought about through this placement revolution. Public school personnel must take very seriously their roles as case managers to implement all the communicative, educational, and other services that children with hearing loss are entitled to for them to become contributing members of the mainstream, multicultural community.

Ross (1990, p. ix) describes the context for intervention for D/HH students that continues to be relevant: "The core of any management program of the mainstreamed hearing-impaired child must be the regular classroom. It is the classroom teacher who is faced with the child for most of the school day." The changing map from primarily residential to primarily inclusive educational contexts has brought both new

challenges and old dilemmas. The old dilemmas involved methodology (sign language or speech or combined instructional approaches), lack of a research database, appropriate school placement, community of Deaf or deaf individuals, early identification, and intervention. The current challenges involve methodology, use of technology, multicultural identity, language (ASL, English), individualization based on differences, and availability of educational services based on commonalties.

Alexander Graham Bell taught deaf students to see it, say it, write it, refine it, read it, and think it (1873). As Northcott (1990) notes, the master teachers, Fitzgerald (1949), Buell (1934), and Groht (1958), each added a significant dimension to the art and science of teaching students who are D/HH. Contemporary teachers and scholars such as Kretschmer and Kretschmer (1978, 1988, 1989), L.W. Kretschmer (1997), R.E. Kretschmer (1997), R.R. Kretschmer (1997), Wood and Wood (1997), Yoshinga-Itano (1997), Moog and Geers (1980, 1985), and Luetke-Stahlman and Luckner (1991) have interwoven the insights from the past with the findings of the present to facilitate more effectively the integration of D/HH students into the school community.

A primary purpose of intervention with school-age D/HH students is to facilitate successful academic performance. Such success hinges on the ability to meet the requirements (comprehension and performance) for school language use. D/HH children must learn to move beyond the social and need fulfillment aspects of interpersonal communication into the realm of academic survival and enlightenment through communication using both spoken and written English formats. In one form or another, the spoken or written English language forms the foundation of the educational career for all students. Unless the linguistic rule systems are developed and used, the child will be unable to meet successfully the educational challenges of today's schools. Assessment by itself is incomplete. It should be seen as an initial step in an intervention program and an integral part of ongoing habilitation. To provide an optimal learning environment for children with hearing loss, assessment and educational practice must be bound intimately.

All students need effective communicative language development and metalinguistic instructional strategies to succeed in school. The role of the rehabilitative case manager is to define and locate for each child all the services he or she needs and to assist in integration of those services for the child's benefit. Intervention in language, speech, sign language, and academic areas may be necessary. The key principle that guides intervention with school-age students with hearing loss is integration or interfacing of services. Speech and language therapy from the speech-language pathologist, language development from the teacher of the deaf, and academic instruction from the mainstream classroom teacher will be of limited value without a clearly defined effort by all to integrate these services. Armed with all of the assessment data discussed previously in this chapter, the team should construct a map of services, grounded in ongoing assessment, that guides the student from the tenets of auditory learning to the process of communication (be it a spoken or signed language) through experiential and semantic expansion, toward the ultimate goal of sufficient language facility for academic success. The student is likely to need speech therapy and language therapy but may also need occupational, physical, or psychological therapy, counseling, and/or learning disabilities remediation. Just as curriculum-based assessment (CBA) has become a focus for identifying language needs for school-age students, comprehensive curriculum-based intervention that includes all aspects of school must be developed for the student who is D/HH to learn and realize his or her potential. Specific intervention in language (interpersonal and written), audition, speech, and academic areas becomes the domain of the speech-language pathologist, rehabilitative audiologist, and educator of D/HH students in concert with classroom teachers. Each member of this team bears responsibility for effective integration of services and for the individual components of speech, language, and academics. A brief guide to each follows.

SPEECH INTERVENTION

As Northcott (1990) observed, the 1978 legislation dealing with human rights identified speaking and listening along with reading, mathematics, and written communication as rights to which each child (including the students who are deaf) in the U.S. public schools is entitled. Legislation continues to support the right to comprehensive speech and language assessment and intervention services for all school-age students with hearing loss.

Facilitating intelligible speech production has been a goal since the beginning of education of D/HH students. Success has not always been realized with significantly hearing-impaired students. However, dedication to speech development and consistent strategies based on current technology have not always been a part of the speech development program. Some degree of residual hearing, amplified early, has been a consistent prerequisite for intelligible speech development.

Although speech development strategies were laid out in detail in Haycock's (1972) primer on speech methods for the deaf, it was later with the development of Ling's (1976, 1989) methodology (Stoker and Ling, 1992) that we began to see the specifics of audiologic testing information and appropriate amplification selection brought together with known speech acoustic information to become manageable for interventionists. Speech-language pathologists recognize that speech development with D/HH children is far from synonymous with traditional articulation therapy used with hearing students, although the newer theories of phonologic processes became more relevant to speech development with all of these students.

Intervention in speech commences at the level of breakdown identified through speech assessment (phonetic and phonologic). Ling (1976, 1989) described the phonetic intervention model as consisting of a hierarchy, beginning with the development of suprasegmentals (intensity, duration, and frequency), continuing through vowel and diphthong development, and moving to consonant and consonant cluster development. The phonologic aspect of intervention continues the process in development of words, sentences, and longer chunks of meaningful language. The phonetic and phonologic intervention is implemented by informal learning or formal teaching strategies, depending on the age of the child and on how long the hearing impairment has affected the child's learning (Ling, 1989; Stoker and Ling, 1992). A well laid out curriculum is available for developing the phonetic component through formal teaching, including:

1. Production of speech sounds.
2. Combination of consonants and vowels into syllables.
3. Production of syllables rapidly and automatically.
4. Alternation of syllable pairs automatically.

As soon as a child is able to produce syllables automatically, it is appropriate to add the semantic or meaning component to the production. This is followed by development of words and longer spoken contexts or the phonologic component of speech development. All speech-language pathologists responsible for students with hearing loss should have the Ling materials available for use. Curricula such as the Clarke School for the Deaf Speech Development Curriculum (1995) details the sequence of spoken language development.

Treatment approaches based on elimination of phonologic simplification processes should also be a part of speech intervention. (See Edwards and Shriberg, 1983; Hodson and Paden, 1991; Bernthal and Bankson, 1998.) Specific speech intervention programs have been developed for students who have had cochlear implants, but the Ling methodology continues to be the foundation of many of these programs. The differences are likely to be that with the new processed speech ("hearing system") provided by the cochlear implant, children may not follow

exactly the hierarchy proposed by Ling in vowel and consonant development. Administration of the entire Phonetic Level Evaluation may be necessary, and targets selected for intervention may be more varied. It is likely that most other procedures and strategies proposed by Ling will maintain. More instances of "sound preferences" have been observed with children who have cochlear implants; the children become enchanted with a specific sound, rehearse it, and overuse it. The benefits of an auditory-verbal approach (Pollack et al., 1997), a methodology that has been most successful with children with residual hearing, are becoming more well-known in the successful application with students with cochlear implants. The development of specific intervention programs and the application of auditory approaches for children with cochlear implants are also underway (Tye-Murray, 1992).

LANGUAGE INTERVENTION

Historically, language development/teaching of students who are D/HH has had a rich, colorful past, with remnants of the fabric shaping current teaching methodology. The analytic/synthetic methodologies have been reinterpreted into the structured/naturalistic contexts for language learning. The counterpart to the Groht and Fitzgerald teaching approaches evolved into a metalinguistic/pragmatic/semantic focus. Current models of language intervention draw heavily on the child language acquisition literature of hearing children.

Intervention in language follows a similar sequence as language intervention with hearing students. After a comprehensive analysis, the language goals across all domains are developed and implemented within the school context. For more detailed discussion of school language intervention objectives and strategies, the reader is directed to the following references for school-age language intervention with hearing students: Bloom and Lahey, 1978; Ripich and Spinelli, 1985; Simon, 1985a,b; Lahey, 1988; Wallach and Miller, 1988; Nelson, 1989, 1998; Bernstein and Tiegerman, 1993; Ripich and Creaghead,

1994; Wallach and Butler, 1994; Paul, 1995; Nippold, 1998. The following references are excellent resources for language intervention with D/HH students: Kretschmer and Kretschmer, 1978, 1988, 1989; Texas Developmental Language Centered Curriculum for Hearing-Impaired Children, 1978; Quigley and Kretschmer, 1982; McAnally et al., 1987; Kretschmer, 1989, 1997; Paul and Quigley, 1990; and Luetke-Stahlman and Luckner, 1991. Selection of language targets and strategies should be based on the language needs identified through each student's language assessment. The process is one of determining developmental level, determining school expectations, and then designing intervention that matches the student's capabilities with the school expectations.

EDUCATIONAL INTERVENTION

The array of educational interventions available to the student who is D/HH, such as note-takers, captioning, and interpreters, is discussed elsewhere in this text. However, an area of concern that bears mention here as follow-up to the discussion of psychoeducational assessment is the issue of educational intervention with respect to reading, math, spelling, and the basic skills required for learning the content of school subjects. Custom has dictated that the teacher of the student who is D/HH teach all content areas that cannot be learned readily in the mainstream setting. The inclusion model has seen the teacher of D/HH students collaborate in the classroom with the regular education teacher. The need for collaboration and/or consultation with other professionals, such as reading or learning disabilities specialists, should not be overlooked in the intervention phase of the process. Although not always experienced with D/HH students, these professionals have much to offer in program planning and implementation.

ADDITIONAL LEARNING DIFFICULTIES

There will be instances with multidisabled D/HH students in which the need for learning disabilities services is as great or greater than the need for services for hearing loss. The simultaneous occurrence of additional disabling conditions within the D/HH population presents an additional complication to the task of rehabilitating and educating these children. All the major etiologies of deafness (e.g., prematurity, meningitis, Rh incompatibility, rubella, cytomegalovirus) and inherited deafness may be associated with other disabling conditions (Moores, 1987, 1991; Vemon and Andrews, 1990). Because of additional conditions, as many as 25% of D/HH students are considered to have multidisabilities. There is disagreement over the definitions, precluding specific incidence counts; however, mental retardation, visual impairments, as well as learning and behavioral disabilities frequently occur with hearing loss, making educational planning a complex venture (Moores, 1987). The current operational plan in special education for hearing students is to group these students within a "mildly disabled" rubric, although protests from some teachers suggest there are differences in learning styles among these children. The "learning disabled hearing impaired student" (Laughton, 1989, p. 70) has been discussed with no consensus about the characteristics demonstrated by children with this phenomenon. Many children with hearing loss present additional challenges to professionals engaged in assessment and intervention, requiring multidimensional, interdisciplinary teams working in unison to provide the services necessary. Identification, assessment, and the development of intervention programs for such children are underway (Powers and Elliott, 1990; Elliott and Powers, 1992; Laughton, 1992).

A Look Into the Future

A significant revolution in education of D/HH students occurred in the shift from the residential school as primary service provider to the local school system with strong parental involvement. The effects of this shift are seen as we enter the new century. Increased responsibilities have shifted to local school personnel—responsibilities that include enculturation and rehabilitation. Technology, especially cochlear implants, has produced another culture of deaf children to enter into the matrix of rehabilitative services. Despite roles that may conflict, it is critical that rehabilitative services be integrated for the benefit of the D/HH student. That mission is the responsibility and challenge of those of us who are responsible for choreographing the rehabilitative process.

REFERENCES

Adams M, Bertram B. Background knowledge and reading comprehension. Reading education report no. 13 (ERIC document reproduction service no. ED 181 431). Urbana, IL: University of Illinois, 1980.

Anderson R. Role of the reader's schema in comprehension, learning, and memory. In: Singer H, Ruddell R, eds. Theoretical models and processes of reading. 3rd ed. Newark, DE: International Reading Association, 1985:372–384.

Anderson R, Sisco F. Standardization of the WISC-R performance scale for deaf children. Office of Demographic Studies, Gallaudet College, series T, no. 1. Washington, DC: Gallaudet Press, 1977.

Aslin R, Pisoni D. Some developmental processes in speech perception. In: Yeni-Komshian GH, Kavanaugh J, Ferguson C, eds. Child phonology. New York: Academic Press, 1980;2.

Atkins C, Cartwright L. Preferred language elicitation procedures used in five age categories. ASHA 1982;22: 321–323.

Bahrick L, Pickens J. Classification of bimodal English and Spanish language passages by infants. Infant Behav Dev 1988;11:277–296.

Beckwith L. Relationships between infants' vocalizations and their mothers' behaviors. Merrill-Palmer Quart 1977; 17:211–226.

Bell AG. The Sanders reader. Washington, DC: Alexander Graham Bell Association for the Deaf, 1873.

Bernstein DK, Tiegerman E. Language and communication disorders in children. 3rd ed. New York: Macmillan, 1993.

Bernthal J, Bankson N. Articulation and phonological disorders. 4th ed. Boston: Allyn and Bacon, 1998.

Bever TG. The cognitive basis for linguistic structures. In: Hayes JR, ed. Cognition and the development of language. New York: John Wiley & Sons, 1970.

Bjorklund DF, Harnishfeger KK. The evaluation of inhibition mechanisms and their role in human cognition and behavior. In: Dempster FN, Brainerd CJ, eds. Interference and inhibition in cognition. San Diego: Academic Press, 1995.

Blanton RL. Language learning and performance in the deaf. In: Rosenberg S, Koplin JH, eds. Developments in applied psycholinguistics research. New York: Macmillan, 1968.

Blennerhassett L. Communicative styles of a 13 month-old hearing impaired child and her parents. Volta Rev 1984; 86:217–228.

Bloom L, Lahey M. Language development and language disorders. New York: John Wiley & Sons, 1978.

Bochner JH. English in the deaf population. In: Sims DG, Walter G, Whitehead RL, eds. Deafness and communication: assessment and training. Baltimore: Williams & Wilkins, 1982:107–123.

Boothroyd A. Hearing impairments in young children. Washington, DC: Alexander Graham Bell Association for the Deaf, 1988.

Boothroyd A. Assessment of speech perception capacity in profoundly deaf children. Am J Otol 1991;12(Suppl): 67–72.

Brackett D. Intervention for children with hearing impairment in general education settings. Lang Speech Hear Serv School 1997;28:355–361.

Brackett D, Donnelly J. Hearing impaired adolescents' judgments of appropriate conversational entry point. Paper presented to the meeting of the American Speech-Language-Hearing Association, Toronto, 1982.

Bradley-Johnson S, Evans LD. Psychoeducational assessment of hearing-impaired students. Austin, TX: Pro-Ed, 1991.

Bruner J. On knowing: essays for the left hand. Cambridge: Belnap Press of Harvard University Press, 1962.

Buell EM. A companion of the Barry five slate system and the Fitzgerald key. Washington, DC: The Volta Bureau, 1934.

Coryell J, Holcomb J. The use of sign language and sign systems in facilitating the language acquisition and communication of deaf students. Lang Speech Hear Serv Schools 1997;28:384–394.

Chapman R. Exploring children's communicative intents. In: Miller JF, ed. Assessing language production in children: experimental procedures. Baltimore: University Park Press, 1981.

Clark GM, Cowan RS, Dowell RC. Cochlear implants for infants and children: advances. San Diego: Singular Publishing Group, 1997.

Clarke School for the Deaf. Speech development improvement: curriculum services. Northampton, MA: Clarke School for the Deaf, 1995.

Conway DF. Assessing the writing abilities of hearing-impaired children. J Acad Rehabil Audiol 1988;21(Monogr Suppl):151–172.

Cooper R, Rosenstein J. Language acquisition of deaf children. Volta Rev 1966;68:58–67.

Cowan RS, Blamey PJ, Sarant JZ, et al. Perception of sentences, words and speech features by profoundly hearing-impaired children using a multichannel electrotactile speech processor. J Acoust Soc Am 1990;87:1374–1384.

Cowan RS, Brown C, Whitford LA, et al. Speech perception in children using the advanced SPEAK speech processing strategy. In: Clark GM, Cowan RS, eds. International Cochlear Implant Speech and Hearing Symposium, 1994. Ann Otol Rhinol Laryngol 1995;89(Suppl 166):318–321.

Curtis S, Prutting C, Lowell E. Pragmatic and semantic development in young children with impaired hearing. J Speech Hear Res 1979;22:534–552.

Dawson PW, Blamey PH, Rowland LC, et al. Cochlear implants in children, adolescents and prelinguistically deaf adults: speech perception. J Speech Hear Res 1992;34: 1–7.

DeCasper A, Fifer W. Of human bonding—newborns prefer their mothers' voices. Science 1980;208:1174–1176.

Dempster FN. Resistance to interference: developmental changes in basic processing mechanisms. In: Howe ML, Pasnak R, eds. Emerging themes in cognitive development. New York: Springer-Verlag, 1993a;1.

Dempster FN. The rise and fall of the inhibitory mechanisms. Toward a unified theory of cognitive development and aging. Dev Rev 1993b;12:45–47.

DeVilliers PA. Assessing English syntax in hearing-impaired children: eliciting productions pragmatically motivated situations. J Acad Rehabil Audiol 1988;21(Monogr Suppl):41–71.

Diamond A. Frontal lobe involvement in cognitive changes during the first year of life. In: Givson KR, Peterson AC, eds. Brain maturation and cognitive development: comparative and cross cultural perspectives. New York: de Gruyter, 1991.

DiFrancesca S. Academic achievement results of a national testing program for hearing-impaired students—United States, spring 1971 (series D, no. 9). Washington, DC: Gallaudet College, Office of Demographic Studies, 1972.

Donnelly J, Brackett D. Conversational skills of hearing impaired adolescents: a simulated TV interview. Paper presented at the meeting of the American Speech-Language-Hearing Association, Toronto, 1982.

Dowell RC, Clark GM. Cochlear implants in children—unlimited potential? Aust J Audiol 1994;15:10.

Dowell RC, Blamey PJ, Clark GM. Potential and limitations of cochlear implants in children. Ann Otol Rhinol Laryngol 1995;(Suppl 166):324–327.

Duchan JF. Assessing communication of hearing-impaired children: influences from pragmatics. J Acad Rehabil Audiol 1988;21:(Monogr Suppl):19–40.

Durkin D. What is the value of new interest in reading comprehension? Lang Arts 1981;58:23–43.

Edwards ML, Shriberg LD. Phonology: applications in communicative disorders. San Diego: College-Hill Press, 1983.

Elliott R, Powers A. Identification and assessment of hearing impaired students with mild additional disabilities. Tuscaloosa, AL: The University of Alabama, 1992.

Elliott H, Glass L, Evans JW. Mental health assessment of deaf clients. Boston: Little Brown, 1987.

Erber NP. Auditory training. Washington, DC: AG Bell Association for the Deaf, 1982.

Fitzgerald E. Straight language for the deaf: a system of instruction for deaf children. Washington, DC: The Volta Bureau, 1949.

Flavell JH. The developmental psychology of Jean Piaget. Princeton, NJ: Van Norstrand, 1963.

Folven RJ, Bonvillian JD, Orlansky MD. Communicative gestures and early sign language acquisition. First Lang 1984/1985;5:129–144.

Geers AE, Moog JS. Effectiveness of cochlear implants and tactile aids for deaf children. Volta Rev 1994;96: 1–231.

Georgia Department of Education. Regulations and procedures for special education. Georgia Department of Education, Atlanta, 1988.

Gibbins S. The provision of school psychological assessment services for the hearing impaired: a national survey. Volta Rev 1989;91:95–103.

Gilman L, Raffin M. Acquisition of common morphemes by hearing impaired children exposed to the Seeing Essential English sign system. Paper presented at the annual meeting of the American Speech and Hearing Association, Washington, DC, 1975.

Goldin-Meadow S, Feldman H. The creation of communication system: a study of deaf children of hearing parents. Paper presented to the Society for Research in Child Development, Denver, Colorado, 1975.

Graham E, Shapiro E. Use of the performance scale of the WISC with the deaf child. J Consult Psychol 1963;17: 396–398.

Green W, Shephard D. The semantic structure in deaf children. J Commun Disord 1975;8:357–365.

Greenberg M. Social interactions between deaf preschoolers

and their mothers: the effects of communication method and communication competence. Dev Psychol 1980;16: 465–474.

Groht MA. Natural language for deaf children. Washington, DC: The Volta Bureau, 1958.

Gross R. Language used by mothers of deaf children and mothers of hearing children. Am Ann Deaf 1970;115: 93–96.

Guilford JP. Creativity and learning. In: Lindsley DB, Lundsdaine AA, eds. Brain functions. Berkeley, CA: University of California Press, 1967;4.

Hanley CN. Factorial analysis of speech perception. J Speech Hear Disord 1956;21:76–87.

Hasenstab S, Laughton J. Remediation of children with auditory learning disorders. In: Roeser R, Downs M, eds. Auditory disorders in school children. New York: Thieme-Stratton, 1995.

Haycock GS. The teaching of speech. Washington, DC: The Volta Bureau, 1972.

Heller PJ. Psycho-educational assessment. In: Ross M, ed. Hearing-impaired children in the mainstream. Parkton, MD: York, 1990.

Hess JC, Sefton K, Landry R. Sample size and type-token ratios for oral language of preschool children. J Speech Hear Res 1986;29:129–134.

Hirsh IJ. Information processing in input channels for speech and language: the significance of the serial order of stimuli. In: Millikan CH, Darley FL, eds. Brain mechanisms underlying speech and language. New York: Grune and Stratton, 1967.

Hodson B. The assessment of phonological process—revised. Austin, TX: Pro-Ed, 1986.

Hodson BW, Paden EP. Targeting intelligible speech: a phonological approach to remediation. Austin, TX: Pro-ed, 1991.

Hudgins CV, Numbers F. An investigation of the intelligibility of the speech of the deaf. Genet Psychol Monogr 1942;25:289–392.

Hunt JMCV. Intelligence and experience. New York: Ronald Press, 1961.

Johnson HA. A sociolinguistic assessment scheme for the total communication student. J Acad Rehabil Audiol 1988; 21(Monogr Suppl):101–127.

Johnson H, Barton L. TDD conversations: a context for language sampling and analysis. Am Ann Deaf 1988;133: 19–24.

Kannapell B. Personal reflections: current issues of language and communication among deaf people. In: Garretson M, ed. Eyes, hands, and voices: communication issues among deaf people. Silver Spring, MD: National Association of the Deaf, 1990:65–69.

Kaplan HI, Sadlock BJ. Synopsis of psychiatry. Baltimore, MD: Williams & Wilkins, 1991.

Kendler TS. Levels of cognitive development. Manchester, NJ: Lawrence Erlbrum, 1995.

Khan L, Lewis N. Khan-Lewis phonological analysis. American Guidance Service, Circle Pines, MN, 1986.

Koch C, Davis JL. Large-scale neuronal theories of the brain. Cambridge: MIT Press, 1994.

Koplin JH, Odom PB, Blanton RL, et al. Word association test performance of deaf students. J Speech Hear Res 1967;10:126–132.

Kretschmer LW. Introduction to clinical forum. Lang Speech Hear Serv Schools 1997;28:344–347.

Kretschmer RE. Educational considerations for at-risk/marginal students who are deaf or hard-of-hearing. Lang Speech Hear Serv Schools 1997;28:395–406.

Kretschmer RR. Issues in the development of school and interpersonal discourse for children who have hearing loss. Lang Speech Hear Serv Schools 1997;28:374–383.

Kretschmer RR, Kretschmer LW. Language development and intervention with the hearing impaired. Baltimore: University Park Press, 1978.

Kretschmer RR, Kretschmer LW. Communication competence and assessment. J Acad Rehabil Audiol 1988;21 (Monograph Suppl):5–17.

Kretschmer RR, Kretschmer LW. Communication competence: impact of the pragmatics revolution on education of hearing impaired individuals. Topics Lang Disord 1989; 9:1–16.

Lahey M. Language disorders and language development. New York: Macmillan, 1988.

Laughton J. Perspectives on the assessment of reading. J Acad Rehabil Audiol 1988;21(Monograph Suppl):129–150.

Laughton J. The learning disabled, hearing impaired student: reality, myth, or overextension? Topics Lang Disord 1989;9:70–79.

Laughton J. Identification of hearing impaired children at risk for mild additional disabilities impacting on learning. In: Elliott R, Powers A, eds. Identification and assessment of hearing impaired students with mild additional disabilities. Tuscaloosa, AL: University of Alabama, 1992.

Laughton J, Hasenstab S. The language learning process. Rockville, MD: Aspen, 1986.

Laughton J, Hasenstab M. Assessment and intervention with school age hearing-impaired children. In: Alpiner JG, McCarthy PA, eds. Rehabilitative audiology: children and adults. 2nd ed. Baltimore: Williams & Wilkins, 1993.

Laughton J, Jacobs JF. A model for research methodology in language acquisition and hearing impairment. In: Hoemann H, Wilbur R, eds. Interpersonal communication and deaf people monograph. Washington, DC: Gallaudet College, 1982;5:57–101.

Laughton J, Ray S. Pragmatic violations in language assessment. Presented at the 2nd annual Special Education Conference, Baton Rouge, Louisiana, 1982.

Levine E. The ecology of early deafness. In: Guides to fashioning environments and psychological assessments. New York: Columbia University Press, 1981.

Levine ES. The psychology of deafness. New York: Columbia University Press, 1974.

Lieberman P. The biology and evolution of language. Cambridge: Harvard University Press, 1984.

Ling D. Speech and the hearing-impaired child: theory and practice. Washington, DC: Alexander Graham Bell Association for the Deaf, 1976.

Ling D. Foundations of spoken language for hearing-impaired children. Washington, DC: Alexander Graham Bell Association for the Deaf, 1989.

Luetke-Stahlman B, Luckner J. Effectively educating students with hearing impairments. New York: Longman, 1991.

Lund N, Duchan J. Assessing children's language in naturalistic contexts. 1st ed. Englewood Cliffs, NJ: Prentice-Hall, 1983.

Lund N, Duchan J. Assessing children's language in naturalistic contexts. 2nd ed. Englewood Cliffs, NJ: Prentice-Hall, 1988.

Lyon GR, ed. Frames of reference for the assessment of learning disabilities: new views on measurement issues. Baltimore: Paul H. Brookes, 1994.

Markides A. Type of pure tone audiogram configuration and speech intelligibility. J Br Assoc Teach Deaf 1980;4: 125–129.

Maxwell M. The authenticity of ethnographic research. J Child Commun Disord 1990;13:1–12.

McAnally PL, Rose S, Quigley SP. Language learning practices with deaf children. San Diego: College-Hill Press, 1987.

McKirdy L, Blank M. Dialogue in deaf and hearing preschoolers. J Speech Hear Res 1982;25:487–499.

McLoughlin JA, Lewis RB. Assessing special students. Columbus, OH: Merrill, 1990.

Messenheimer-Young T, Kretschmer RR. "Can I play?": a hearing impaired preschooler's request to access maintained social interaction. Volta Rev 1994;96:5–18.

Miller J. Assessing language production in children. Baltimore: University Park Press, 1981.

Miyamoto RT, Kirk KI, Todd SL, et al. Speech perception skills of children with multichannel cochlear implants or hearing aids. Ann Otol Rhinol Laryngol 1994;9(Suppl 4):334–337.

Moog JS, Geers AE. Grammatical analysis of elicited language complex sentence level. St. Louis: Central Institute for the Deaf, 1980.

Moog JS, Geers AE. Grammatical analysis of elicited language simple sentence level. St. Louis: Central Institute for the Deaf, 1985.

Moores D. Educating the deaf: psychology, principles, and practices. 3rd ed. Boston: Houghton Mifflin, 1987.

Moores D. The school placement revolution. Am Ann Deaf 1991;136:307–308.

Nelson K. Language in cognitive development. Melbourne, Australia: Cambridge University Press, 1996.

Nelson N. Curriculum-based language assessment and intervention. ASHA 1989,20.170–184.

Nelson N. Childhood language disorders in context: infancy through adolescence. 2nd ed. Boston: Allyn and Bacon, 1998.

Nippold M. Later language development. Boston: College-Hill Press, 1988.

Nippold M. Later language development: the school-age and adolescent years. 2nd ed. Austin, TX: Pro-Ed, 1998.

Northcott WH. Mainstreaming roots and wings. In: Ross M, ed. Hearing-impaired children in the mainstream. Parkton, MD: York Press, 1990.

Odom P, Blanton R, Nunnally J. Some 'cloze' technique studies of language capability in the deaf. J Speech Hear Res 1967;10:816–827.

Orr FC, DeMatteo A, Heller B, et al., eds. Mental health assessment of deaf clients. Boston: Little, Brown, 1987:93–106.

Osberger MJ, Miyamoto RT, Zimmerman-Phillips S, et al. Independent evaluation of the speech perception abilities of children with the Nucleus 22-channel cochlear implant system. Ear Hear 1991;12(Suppl 4):66–80.

Paul R. Language disorders from infancy through adolescence. St. Louis: Mosby, 1995.

Paul PV, Quigley SR. Education and deafness. White Plains, NY: Longman, 1990.

Pearson PD. The effect of background knowledge on young children's comprehension of implicit and explicit information. Urbana, IL: University of Illinois Center for the Study of Reading, 1979.

Pearson PD, Johnson D. Teaching reading comprehension. New York: Holt, Rinehardt and Winston, 1978.

Piaget J. The origin of intelligence in children. New York: Norton and Company, 1952.

Piaget J. The construction of reality in the child. New York: Basic Books, 1954.

Piavio A. Imaginary and verbal processes. New York: Holt, Rinehart and Winston, 1971.

Pien D. The development of language functions in deaf infants of hearing parents. In: Martin D, ed. Cognition, education, and deafness. Washington, DC: Gallaudet College Press, 1985;2:30–34.

Pollack D, Goldberg D, Caleffe-Schenck N. Educational audiology for the limited-hearing infant and preschooler. 3rd ed. Springfield, IL: Charles C. Thomas, 1997.

Powers A, Elliott R. Preparation of students who serve hearing-impaired students with additional mild handicaps. Teach Educ Special Educ 1990;13:200–202.

Quigley SP, Kretschmer RE. The education of deaf children. Baltimore: University Park Press, 1982.

Quigley SP, Paul PV. Language and deafness. San Diego: College-Hill Press, 1984.

Raffin M. The acquisition of inflectional morphemes by deaf children using Seeing Essential English. Doctoral dissertation, University of Iowa, 1976.

Raffin M, Davis J, Gilman L. Morphological acquisition of deaf children. J Speech Hear Res 1978;2:387–400.

Ray S. An adaptation of the WISC-R for the deaf. Sulphur, OK: Steven Ray Publishing, 1976.

Ray S. Context and the psychoeducational assessment of hearing impaired children. Topics Lang Disord 1989;9:33–44.

Reed M. Deaf and partially hearing children. In: Mittler P, ed. The psychological assessment of mental and physical handicap. London: Menthen, 1970.

Rees NS. A talent for language. J Commun Disord 1972;5:132–141.

Ripich DN, Creaghead N, eds. School discourse problems. 2nd ed. San Diego: Singular, 1994.

Ripich DN, Spinelli FM, eds. School discourse problems. San Diego: College-Hill Press, 1985.

Ross M. Hearing-impaired children in the mainstream. Parkton, MD: York Press, 1990.

Russell WK, Quigley SP, Power DJ. Linguistics and deaf children: transformational syntax and its applications. Washington, DC: Alexander Graham Bell Association for the Deaf, 1976.

Salvia J, Ysseldyke J. Assessment in special and remedial education. Boston: Houghton Mifflin, 1988.

Schafer D, Lynch J. Emergent language of six prelingually deaf children. Teach Deaf 1980;5:94–111.

Schlesinger H, Meadow K. Sounds and sign. Berkeley: University of California Press, 1972.

Simeonsson RJ. Assessment of hearing-impaired children. Psychological and developmental assessment of special children. Boston: Allyn and Bacon, 1987.

Simmons A. A comparison of the type-token ratio of spoken and written language of deaf children. Volta Rev 1962; 64:417–421.

Simon CS. Communication skills and classroom success: assessment of language-learning disabled students. San Diego: College-Hill Press, 1985a.

Simon CS. Communication skills and classroom success: therapy methodologies for language learning disabled students. San Diego: College Hill Press, 1985b.

Skarakis E, Prutting C. Early communication: semantic functions and communicative intentions in the communication of the preschool child with impaired hearing. Am Ann Deaf 1977;122:382–391.

Smith BE, Goodman KS, Meredith R. Language and thinking in the schools. 2nd ed. New York: Holt, Rinehart and Winston, 1976.

Solomon LN, Webster JC, Curtis JF. A factorial study of speech perception. J Speech Hear Res 1960;3:101–107.

Spence MJ, DeCasper AJ. Prenatal experience with low frequency, maternal voice sounds influences neonatal perception of maternal voice samples. Infant Behav Dev 1987;10:133–142.

Staller SJ, Dowell RC, Beiter AL, et al. Perceptual abilities of children with the Nucleus 22-Channel cochlear implant. Ear Hear 1991;12(Suppl 4):34–47.

Sternberg RJ. Testing intelligence without IQ tests. Phi Delta Kappan 1984;66:694–698.

Stoker R, Ling D. Speech production in hearing-impaired children and youth: theory and practice. Volta Rev 1992; 94:1–168.

Strong M, Prinz P. A study of the relationship between American Sign Language and English literacy. J Deaf Studies Deaf Educ 1997;2:37–46.

Sullivan R, Vernon M. Psychological assessment of hearing-impaired children. School Psychol Digest 1979;8:217–290.

Texas Education Agency. A developmental language centered curriculum for hearing impaired children. Austin, TX: Texas Education Agency, 1978.

Thompson M, Biro P, Vethivelu S, et al. Language assessment of hearing-impaired school age children. Seattle, WA: University of Washington Press, 1987.

Tweney RD, Hoemann HW, Andrews CE. Semantic organization in deaf and hearing subjects. J Psycholing Res 1975;4:61–73.

Tye-Murray N. Cochlear implants and children: a handbook for parents, teachers, and speech and hearing professionals. Washington, DC: Alexander Graham Bell Association for the Deaf, 1992.

Tye-Murray N, Fryauf-Bertschy H. Auditory training. In: Tye-Murray N, ed. Cochlear implants and children: a handbook for parents, teachers and speech and hearing professionals. Washington, DC: A.G. Bell Association for the Deaf, 1992.

Tyler R. Speech perception by children. In: Tyler R, ed. Cochlear implants: audiological foundations. San Diego, CA: Singular, 1993.

Valletutti PH, Dummett L. Cognitive development—a functional approach. San Diego: Singular, 1992.

Vernon M. Psychologic evaluation of hearing-impaired children. In: Lloyd L, ed. Communication, assessment, and intervention strategies. Baltimore: University Park Press, 1976:195–223.

Vernon M, Andrews J. The psychology of deafness. New York: Longman, 1990.

Vygotsky LS. Thought and language. Cambridge: MIT Press, 1934.

Vygotsky LS. Thought and language. New York: Wiley, 1962.

Wood D, Wood H. Communicating with children who are deaf: pitfalls and possibilities. Lang Speech Hear Serv Schools 1997;28:348–354.

Wallach GP, Butler K. Language learning disabilities in school-age children and adolescents. New York: Merrill, 1994.

Wallach GP, Miller L. Language intervention and academic success. San Diego: College-Hill Press, 1988.

Walter G. Lexical abilities of hearing and hearing-impaired children. Am Ann Deaf 1978;123:976–982.

Watson BU, Goldgar DE. A note on the use of the Hiskey-Nebraska test of learning aptitude with deaf children. ASHA 1985;16:53–57.

Weddell-Monig J, Lumley JM. Child deafness and mother-child interactions. Child Dev 1980;51:766–774.

Wilbur RB. American Sign Language: linguistic and applied dimensions. San Diego: College Hill Press, 1987.

Wilcox S, Corwin J. The enculturation of BoMee: looking at the work through deaf eyes. J Child Commun Disord 1990;13:63–72.

Witkin BR. Auditory perception: implications for language

development. Lang Speech Hear Serv Schools 1971;4: 31–52.

Witkin BR, Butler KG, Whalen TE. Auditory processing in children: two studies of component features. Lang Speech Hear Serv Schools 1977;8:140–154.

Wood D, Wood H. An experimental evaluation of five styles of teacher conversation on the learning of hearing impaired children. J Child Psychiat 1984;25:45–62.

Wood D, Wood H. Who are deaf: pitfalls and possibilities. Lang Speech Hear Serv Schools 1997;28:348–354.

Ying E. Speech and language assessment: communication evaluation. In: Ross M, ed. Hearing-impaired children in the mainstream. Parkton, MD: York Press, 1990.

Yoshinaga-Itano C. The challenge of assessing language in children with hearing loss. Lang Speech Hear Schools 1997;28:362–373.

Zieziula F. Assessment of hearing-impaired people. A guide for selecting psychological, educational, and vocational tests. Washington, DC: Gallaudet University Press, 1982.

CHAPTER

8

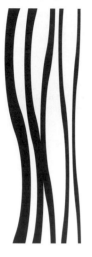

Management of Hearing in the Educational Setting

Cheryl DeConde Johnson, Ed.D.

Access to information is absolutely essential to learning. The reduction of input created by hearing loss begins a spiraling effect that manifests itself in increasingly complex ways as a child grows. The barriers created by hearing loss and the implications for children are generally known. These are portrayed in Figure 8.1. Although the issues related to hearing impairment are recognized in the professions of audiology, communication disorders, and deaf education, they remain imbedded in controversy. In addition, hearing professionals have not done a good job imparting knowledge of hearing loss outside their own professional circles. The necessary level of awareness and proactivity among general educators to affect sufficiently the auditory management and instructional process or the regular school environment in which most children with hearing loss are now educated remains inadequate. As a result, children continue to suffer avoidable consequences of their hearing losses. The problems are exacerbated by dwindling resources, insufficient supports, and inadequate services. Despite research, federal regulations, and best practice standards, the management of children with hearing loss in schools and other learning environments continues to be in crisis.

Whereas the golden age of special education is in the past, the basic provisions delineated in the original Public Law 94-142, and expanded through several reauthorizations, continue to guide services to children with disabilities. (See Appendix 8.1 for current IDEA definitions pertaining to hearing loss and audiology.) Children with hearing loss have been supported through this law in a substantial way, yet hearing professionals have not been able to use the structure provided by the law to ensure that the necessary supports and services are provided for all children with hearing loss. Audiologists and other hearing professionals continue to face hurdles when recommending services, appropriate acoustic spaces, auditory devices, and other assistive technologies. The emphasis on inclusion (e.g., education in the regular classroom) has further affected the roles of deaf education teachers and other supporting service providers and subsequently how services are delivered. Table 8.1 illustrates the increase in children educated in regular classrooms over the past 10 years. With these changes, proper auditory management (e.g., use of appropriate hearing instrumentation, auditory skill development and communication repair strategizing, listening environment management, and understanding of accommodations within the learning environment and modifications of the instructional process) is paramount. A systemic change in how hearing professionals deliver services is necessary to promote more participation in general education, so that these professionals may be more effective in advocacy for the necessary and advocacy services to which children with hearing loss are entitled.

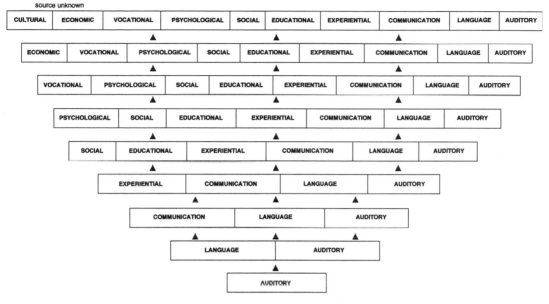

Figure 8.1. The spiraling effects of deafness.

Table 8.1
Percentage of children with hearing impairments served in different educational environments under IDEA, Part B.

Year	Regular Class	Resource Room	Separate Class	Public-Separate Facility	Private-Separate Facility	Public Residential Facility	Private-Residential Facility	Home-Hospital Environment
1985–1986	20%	22.4%	32.6%	9%	3.3%	11%	1.2%	.3%
1994 1995	35%	19%	28.5%	3.8%	9%	9.2%	1%	2%

Source: U.S. Department of Education. Nineteenth Annual Report to Congress on the Implementation of the Individuals with Disabilities Education Act, Appendix A, Table AB8, 1998.

What We Have Learned in the Past Decade: Foundations for the Future

To examine management of hearing, it is helpful to consider some of the broader issues affecting children with hearing loss. A look back at educational management of childhood hearing loss reveals a relatively short history. The 1960s produced the beginning of the real focus on education and management of children with hearing loss in schools; this was in part spurred by the rubella epidemic. The research of the past 10 years further grounded what was known about the effects of hearing loss and provided significant new evidence to guide practices.

When reviewing major research on the educational implications of childhood hearing loss, a trend emerges with each passing decade that focuses on the issues associated with lesser degrees of hearing loss. Whereas the 1960s centered around the needs of children with more severe and profound losses, the 1970s were influenced by Davis' work (Davis, 1977) on children who were hard-of-hearing. The 1980s were significant for the research on unilateral hearing, loss led by Bess (Bess, 1982, 1985; Bess and Tharpe, 1984, 1986; Bess et al., 1986a,b) and Matkin (Oyler et al., 1987, 1988). The 1990s generated evidence on the effects of minimal hearing loss (Crandell, 1993; Downs, 1995; Edwards, 1996; Bess et al., 1998) and long-term effects of otitis media (Gravel and Wallace, 1992, 1995, 1998; Gravel and Nozza, 1997). The 1990s also provided the first scientific evidence of the critical implications of early identification and intervention of hearing loss (Apuzzo and Yoshinaga-Itano, 1995; Yoshinaga-Itano, 1998; Yoshinaga-Itano et al., 1998). The findings of these research efforts underlie many of the basic foundations that guide hearing management practices today. The effects of this evidence and other relevant research of the 1990s are summarized in the following discussion of the critical issues affecting the management of hearing in educational settings.

IMPORTANCE OF HEARING FOR LEARNING FOR ALL CHILDREN

Hearing begins a chain of events that proceeds from sensation of sound to perception and then comprehension. The response begins with formulation of thought, followed by production in a spoken, written, or active form. Perhaps the most significant realization has been the critical role that hearing plays in learning for all children. Brain imaging studies have been particularly enlightening, as a variety of brain activities related to audition have been observed and studied (Hynd et al., 1990, 1991; Merzenich and Jenkins, 1995). In turn, this capability has led to an increased understanding of the neural plasticity of the brain, a change from the former notion that the brain was more or less hard-wired by puberty and therefore unable to undergo significant physical or chemical changes.

Much of communication is based on spoken language. Classrooms are auditory-verbal environments in which listening is often the primary modality used to gain input for learning (Flexer, 1995). Hearing loss of any degree, hearing levels that fluctuate between normal and abnormal such as those associated with otitis media, and central auditory processing problems all can produce wide-ranging effects for the development of speech, language, and later reading and writing. Tallal and Merzenich (Tallal, 1980; Tallal and Stark, 1981; Tallal et al.,

1985, 1996; Merzneich et al., 1996) and others (Bornstein and Musiek, 1984, 1992; Pinheiro and Musiek, 1985) have studied these problems in children with auditory and language learning problems and have found that many of them exhibit difficulties with temporal order processes which affects their ability to distinguish between consonant sounds. Tallal et al. (1996) found that by slowing down the production of consonant sounds through specific skill drills, children could improve their temporal processing for these sounds, resulting in better understanding of the sounds in words and subsequent improvements in the comprehension of speech.

Although hearing is important for learning for all children, there are those for whom access to information through hearing is not possible or is so grossly inadequate that the information heard is insufficient for learning. The use of a visual sign system, whether English-based or American Sign Language (ASL), must be used to provide access to spoken communication. The need for signs and/or other visual cues (speechreading, captioning, written notes, cues) must be considered for children who are deaf and to supplement audition for those who rely primarily on their hearing.

Acoustic accessibility

Acoustic accessibility is access to spoken and auditory input without interference from noise, reverberation, and the problems created by distance listening. Access for children is particularly crucial due to less-well developed language and communication systems that are often present in at-risk children (e.g., young children, children with language problems, and children with auditory problems). Accessibility of the acoustic nature has been overlooked in most of the disability legislation (e.g., 504, Americans with Disabilities Act [ADA], Individuals with Disabilities Education Act [IDEA]). However, recent interest in classroom acoustics has stemmed from continued reports of poor speech intelligibility (Flexer et al., 1990; Elliot, 1992; Crandell, 1991, 1993; Crandell and Smaldino, 1994), the improvements in children's performance with sound field amplification (Sarff, 1981; Jones et al., 1989; Flexer et al., 1990, 1993; Zabel, 1993), and complaints from teachers regarding excessively loud ventilation systems and voice fatigue (Allen, 1995).

For children with auditory problems, noise, excessive reverberation, and distance from the speaker multiply the effects of the hearing loss and create additional barriers to learning. Several early studies provided data on the effects of these variables on speech perception for subjects with both normal hearing and impaired hearing (Crum D. The effects of noise, reverberation, and speaker-to-listener distance on speech understanding. Unpublished doctoral dissertation. Northwestern University, Evanston, IL, 1974; Nebelek and Pickett, 1974; Finitzo-Hieber and Tillman, 1978; Dirks et al., 1982; Nebelek and Nebelek, 1985; Crandell and Bess, 1986). All these studies demonstrated that speech perception or recognition decreased as a function of distance from the speaker or under decreased signal-to-noise ratio conditions. In all situations, the effects were more substantial for individuals with impaired hearing than those with normal hearing. This problem has been exacerbated by the inclusion movement that has resulted in most children with special needs receiving their instruction in regular classrooms. The steady increase in the number of students identified with learning disabilities each year may in part be a result of the problems associated with the instructional conditions of the regular classroom, including poor acoustics.

Hearing versus listening

The Japanese language does not have a word for "listening"; hearing connotes both meanings. However, in the English language, the word "listening" is used to convey attention *to* sound, whereas "hearing" conveys detection *of* sound. This subtle difference has become important because of the need for children to be able to detect sounds and attend to them. Phrases such as "Look and Listen" and "Hearing—Listening—Learning" are commonly used with refer-

ence to children's hearing needs to make this important distinction.

Audibility versus intelligibility

Like hearing and listening, the concepts of audibility and intelligibility have distinct meanings. Audibility refers to the sensation of sound, whereas intelligibility refers to the understanding of sound. It is essential for parents, teachers, and other individuals who work with deaf and hard-of-hearing students to understand the differences between these meanings. Milder degrees of hearing loss including those associated with otitis media, losses of high or low frequencies, and unilateral losses—often result in inconsistent auditory behavior. Because the auditory behaviors are heavily influenced by such factors as the acoustic environment, communication techniques, cognitive and attention abilities, and motivation, children may appear to hear and understand only some of the time. This inconsistency is often interpreted as a behavior, social, or learning problem rather than one resulting from inadequate hearing. Common examples of this problem occur when students are overlooked or reprimanded for behaviors such as not attending, responding inappropriately, or completing incorrect assignments that were a result of hearing loss. Without knowledge of common problems associated with various hearing disorders, these behaviors may wrongfully be dismissed or otherwise misconstrued. The increased awareness and emphasis of the implications associated with mild hearing loss of the past decade have especially heightened this issue's importance.

Incidental hearing and listening

Children with hearing loss or other auditory problems frequently miss out on conversation and information that is not part of their direct, active communication. The result is that children often miss out on verbal exchanges that carry important information as well as the nuances of communication interactions, language pragmatics, and idiomatic expressions. Additional problems may be exhibited, including inappropriate behavior or interactions that in turn can lead to social problems.

Due to these language voids, specific instruction needs to be included in programming for children with auditory problems. This instruction includes the following:

- Pragmatics: strategies for using language, strategies for choosing words/phrases to convey the correct meaning.
- Communication repair: strategies to make your intentions known, strategies for correcting miscommunications.
- Idiomatic expressions: multiple meanings of words; common expressions in the English language.

In addition to these issues, it is critical that as much of the incidental language occurring in classrooms, extracurricular activities, social situations, and family conversations be accessible. It may frequently be necessary to repeat what has been said and who said it for the child or student. Teachers should be instructed on proper classroom listening management techniques to minimize this problem in formal instructional activities.

Assistive listening and communication devices often exacerbate the problem by purposefully limiting input from sound sources other than the primary talker. Accordingly, these devices must be used judiciously. FM systems should be set up to allow for environmental input whenever the child or student is capable of sorting the multiple inputs.

Finally, for young children, redundancy and repetition are paramount. Because of the degradation of the auditory system, access to information frequently, in a variety of modes, with a variety of words, and reinforced through experiences will make learning happen.

INCIDENCE OF HEARING LOSS

In 1998, studies by Niskar et al. and Bess et al. were published that suggested that the incidence of hearing loss in school-age children is substantially higher than previously recognized. Problems that have plagued comparisons of prevalence studies include variations in screening methods and definitions of hearing loss. Table 8.2 summarizes some of the prevalence studies reported over the past several years.

Niskar's group reported data from the Centers for Disease Control's (CDC) Third National Health and Nutrition Examination Survey. The purpose of the study was to describe the prevalence of hearing loss and sociodemographic characteristics among children in the United States. The study used a national population-based cross-sectional survey, an interview, and an audiometric screening test to obtain data on 6166 children aged 6 to 19 years of age. Data were collected between 1988 and 1994. The study reported hearing loss as defined by audiometric thresholds of at least 16 dB hearing levels based on low-frequency (500, 1000, 2000 Hz) and high-frequency (3000, 4000, 6000 Hz) pure-tone averages. The results indicated that 14.9% of children had either low-frequency or high-frequency hearing loss, 7.1% had low-frequency hearing loss (5.6% were unilateral, 1.5% were bilateral), 12.7% had high-frequency hearing loss (9.6% unilateral, 3.1% bilateral), and 4.9% had both low- and high-frequency hearing loss.

On the interviews, 3.7% of all children were reported to have had an earache within the previous week of testing and 1.6% reported having tubes. However, because neither otoscopic inspections nor tympanometry was performed, only children who exhibited draining ears at the time of screening were eliminated from the sample. Some observations made by the authors include:

- More children exhibited high-frequency hearing loss (12.7%) than low-frequency hearing loss (7.1%).
- Unilateral hearing loss is more prevalent than bilateral hearing loss.
- Most hearing loss (4.7% of low-frequency loss and 8.1% of high-frequency loss) was unilateral or slight (16 to 25 dB).
- The prevalence of high-frequency hearing loss was higher in males (15.9%) than females (10.3%) for the 12- to 19-year-old

Table 8.2
Reported prevalences of hearing loss in school-age children

Prevalence	Definition	Source
33%	Failure to respond to 10 dB to 6 of 14 test frequencies (250–8000 Hz, combined ears)	Sarff (1981)
3%	16 dB or greater average in either ear, unilateral, or high-frequency loss	Ross et al. (1991)
5.9% (2nd grade) 11.3% (8th grade) 12% (12th grade)	Hearing thresholds above 25 dB HL on at least 1 of 6 frequencies (2000, 4000, and 8000 Hz, combined ears)	Montgomery and Fujikawa (1992)
2.4%	Bilateral SNHL ($\geq$20 dB PTA): 0.35% Unilateral SNHL ($\geq$35 dB PTA): 0.15% High frequency SNHL (PTA $\geq$): 0.06% Chronic conductive (bilateral or unilateral): 0.05% HL <20 dB HL: 1.8%	Colorado Department of Education (1994)
14.9%	16 dB low- or high-frequency average loss	Niskar et al. (1998)
4.9%	16 dB low- and high-frequency average loss	
11.3%	Bilateral SNHL (20–40 dB): 1% Unilateral SNHL ($\geq$20 dB): 3% HF SNHL ($>$25 dB at 2 or more frequencies above 2K, one or both ears): 1.4% Total minimal HL: 5.4% Conductive HL: 3.4% All other degrees of HL: 2.5% TOTAL HL: 11.3%	Bess et al. (1988)

group; there was no significant difference in the 6- to 11-year-old group.

- Children from low-income families had greater high-frequency hearing loss (16.3%) than either children from middle-income (12.7%) or high-income (7.9%) families.
- Ethnic differences had some effect on prevalence of high-frequency hearing loss.

Bess et al. (1998) designed their study to investigate the prevalence of minimal sensorineural hearing loss in school-age children and its relationship with educational performance. Their final data were based on 1218 students in third, sixth, and

ninth grades in the Nashville Public Schools. The areas assessed included hearing, educational performance, and functional status (physical, emotional, and social dimensions). Minimal sensorineural hearing loss was defined as:

- A unilateral hearing loss of 20 dB HL pure-tone average (500, 1000, and 2000 Hz) with normal hearing (15 dB HL) in the good ear.
- A bilateral sensorineural hearing loss of pure-tone averages between 20 and 40 dB HL with average air-bone gaps of no more than 10 dB at 1000, 2000, and 4000 Hz.

• A high-frequency hearing loss of thresholds greater than 25 dB HL at two or more frequencies above 2000 Hz (i.e., 3000, 4000, 6000, 8000 Hz) in one or both ears with average air-bone gaps of no more than 10 dB at 3000 and 4000 Hz.

Audiologic assessment included tympanometry and air conduction pure-tone thresholds at 500 Hz through 8000 Hz (including 3000 and 6000 Hz). Bone conduction thresholds were also obtained if hearing loss was present. Other children with hearing loss who did not fit the minimal sensorineural categories were categorized as either "conductive" or "other" for all other hearing losses.

The prevalence findings reported by Bess's group are included in Table 8.2. The total reported prevalence of hearing loss was 11.3%, with 5.4% exhibiting minimal sensorineural hearing loss. These figures present a slightly different picture of minimal sensorineural hearing loss than the Centers for Disease Control (CDC) study. Again, due to the sampling and reporting differences, comparisons are difficult. For example, the CDC study reported the prevalence of a 26 dB HL or greater unilateral hearing loss at 1.7% (low-frequency PTA group which has an average of 500, 1000, and 2000 Hz), whereas Bess's group reported a unilateral prevalence of a 20 dB HL or greater (average of 500, 1000, and 2000 Hz) of 3%. Even consideration of the difference between the 20 and 26 dB levels does not appear to account for the discrepancy. The high-frequency hearing loss data sampling is more similar yet still yields very different findings. Bess's group found 1.4% of their sample to have an average high-frequency hearing loss greater than 25 dB HL in one or both ears; the CDC study reported 3% had an average hearing loss greater that 26 dB HL in at least one ear. Both studies do report an increased incidence in high-frequency hearing loss with age.

The variability of prevalence data reported in the literature confirms the need for consistent national standards for school hearing identification programs. Although the evidence exists that hearing loss in children is no longer a low-incidence problem, the inconsistencies reported continue to interfere with a clear definition of the population and the subsequent management of children with hearing loss.

EARLY IDENTIFICATION OF HEARING LOSS

At birth, newborns can recognize their mothers' voices, an indication of the early language learning that occurs during fetal development. Hearing continues to develop, and within the first months of life infants are listening and using auditory cues to connect to their environment and the people in it. In the few short months following birth, infants attend to the suprasegmental features of speech learning to differentiate between speech and nonspeech sounds as well as male and female voices. By 6 months of age, the brain is sufficiently wired from listening to speech for acquisition of language to proceed. Without access to sound, infants must make this connection through visual and tactile modalities, senses that may be less well developed at birth but that have the potential to open the same doors to learning. Fortunately, children with hearing loss finally have the opportunity to have these same experiences.

Evidence now exists that unequivocally demonstrates the positive effects of early identification, stimulation of hearing, and intervention (Apuzzo and Yoshinaga-Itano, 1995; Yoshinaga-Itano, 1998; Yoshinaga-Itano et al., 1998). These researchers identified 6 months as the critical age for identification of hearing loss and initiation of intervention for children with hearing loss to have the opportunity for a normal progression of language functioning. Furthermore, these investigators found that children with all degrees of hearing loss evidenced similar language development if diagnosed and enrolled in intervention programs by 6 months of age. This important research should be the final evidence necessary to support a mandate for newborn hearing screening programs across the nation.

Babies in appropriate early intervention

programs not only experience the important benefits of hearing stimulation described earlier, but also experience knowledgeable parents and enriched language environments. For babies whose parents have chosen audition as part of their child's communication, auditory management is part of their daily routine, providing the opportunity to maximize hearing through the same mother-child interaction rituals that normal-hearing babies enjoy.

Schools are just beginning to have experience with these children, who are now entering the education system with normal to near-normal skills. In fact, some children are no longer qualifying for special education services because they do not have the necessary deficits to meet eligibility requirements. However, they do require auditory management of their environment, proper functioning amplification, and consistent access to all communication or they will quickly fall behind.

EFFECTS OF HEARING LOSS

Effects of minimal hearing loss

The effects of minimal hearing loss in the 16 to 20 dB HL range as identified in the CDC study (Niskar et al., 1998) are difficult to sort out and indeed are even subject to test-retest reliability factors. Whereas a minimal hearing loss of 16 to 20 dB HL might further complicate other existing learning problems, it is unlikely that a significant, direct, causal relationship can be determined that would warrant 504 (Section 504 of the Rehabilitation Act of 1974) or special education services based on the hearing condition alone. Although the CDC study reported that 14.9% of school-age children exhibited some type of hearing loss, it is unlikely that the majority of these children would experience any educational side effects. Furthermore, considering that the prevalence of an average pure-tone bilateral hearing loss (at 500, 1000, 2000 Hz) of 26 dB or greater was 0.4% and a unilateral loss of this same degree was 1.7%, it is probable that even the majority of the 4.9% who were reported as exhibiting a low-frequency and high-frequency hearing loss

(16 dB HL) would not be apt to exhibit significant learning problems directly associated with their hearing loss.

In summary, although the CDC data reported the prevalence of various hearing levels, they did not provide specific evidence to support the conclusion that all these children exhibited associated educational, communicative, or other behavioral sequelae. However, the children who have hearing loss (20 dB), whether unilateral or bilateral, low-frequency or high-frequency, do need attention as confirmed by Bess et al. (1998).

Bess et al. (1998) evaluated educational performance by reviewing the records of all students to obtain scores on the Comprehensive Test of Basic Skills, 4th edition, and to determine if the students were retained for any grade. These data were the basis for comparisons between children with minimal sensorineural hearing loss and normal-hearing control subjects. Additionally, for all children who met the minimal sensorineural hearing loss criteria, teachers completed the Screening Instrument for Educational Risk (SIFTER) (Anderson, 1989) (see Appendix 8.2) and the Revised Behavior Problem Checklist (Quay and Peterson, 1987). These instruments were also completed by teachers on a random sample of normal-hearing children.

Functional status was determined by the 10 areas (emotional feelings, schoolwork, social support, stress, family, self-assessment, behavior, energy, getting along with others, overall health) of the COOP Adolescent Chart Method (COOP) (Nelson et al., 1996). All sixth and ninth grade students were given this quick screening measure that required the student to select a response on a 1 to 5 scale best representing their perception of their own function in each of the 10 areas.

The sequelae of minimal sensorineural hearing loss reported in this study represent some of the most disconcerting evidence to date for the educational, social, and behavioral risks of this group. Although the authors recommend caution when interpreting the data due to a variety of study limitations, the issues raised are significant and deserve attention. Based on the findings, the following observations for children with minimal sensorineural hearing loss were reported:

- Third grade children with minimal sensorineural hearing loss exhibited greater difficulties in the Comprehensive Test of Basic Skills reading subtests of vocabulary, total reading, language mechanics, basic battery, word analysis, spelling, and science; for grades six and nine, no significant differences were identified.
- SIFTER results showed that children with minimal sensorineural hearing loss consistently scored more poorly than their normal-hearing peers; considering failure and marginal categories, 66% experienced difficulty in academics, 48% in attention, and 79% in communication. More than 33% were in the failure category for all three areas.
- No significant differences on the Revised Behavior Problem Checklist were identified.
- The average retention rate (repeating one or more grades) for all children was 37%.
- Functional status, as reported by the COOP, identified dysfunction in 9 of 10 areas for sixth and ninth graders. For sixth graders, the energy domain was statistically significant; for ninth graders, the areas of stress and behavior were statistically significant.

Two other studies that considered minimal hearing loss should be mentioned. Crandell (1993) studied the effects of noise on minimal hearing loss, and Johnson et al. (1997b) investigated the effects of minimal high-frequency hearing loss on speech recognition in children. In Crandell's work, the children with minimal hearing loss performed significantly poorer on sentence recognition tasks presented at five signal-to-noise ratios from +6 dB to −6 dB than the control group of children with normal hearing sensitivity. Furthermore, he found that the difference in performance between the two groups increased as the signal-to-noise ratio worsened. Johnson et al. assessed con-

sonant and vowel identification in children with minimal high-frequency hearing loss (pure-tone thresholds > 20 dB at 2000 Hz and above) in both quiet and noise conditions. They reported that for consonants, the children with minimal high-frequency hearing loss did poorer than their hearing counterparts in quiet, but that the groups did not differ in the noise condition, and that the two groups of children did not differ on the vowel recognition tasks.

Children with minimal hearing loss are in a precarious position on the continuum of profound deafness to normal hearing. Most of them respond to auditory stimuli, have reasonable speech articulation, and have intact language abilities; therefore, they are able to communicate well enough to "fool" their teachers and parents. The problems they experience are often so subtle that they are manifested as inattention, social immaturity, or poor phonetic readers. To manage these children with minimal hearing losses properly, additional detailed studies (although difficult and time-consuming to undertake) need to be conducted to study further the implications associated with hearing loss. In addition, awareness needs to continue, both within audiology and the rest of the educational community, so that these problems may be recognized, understood, and accommodated.

Long-term effects of otitis media

Although the immediate effects of otitis media have been described (Teele et al., 1980; Klein, 1986; Shurin et al., 1986; Todd, 1986), as have some long-term effects (Holm and Kunze, 1969; Howie, 1979; Feagans, 1986; Menyuk, 1986), it has not been until recently that extensive longitudinal data have been available that tracked the development of infants and toddlers with early histories of otitis media (Teele et al., 1984, 1990; Friel-Patti and Finitzo, 1990; Roberts et al., 1991, 1997; Gravel and Wallace, 1992, 1995; Grievink et al., 1993; Gravel and Nozza, 1997; Roberts and Wallace, 1997; Mody et al., 1998). Gravel and colleagues have perhaps made the most significant recent contributions from their studies at the Albert Einstein College of Medicine, Bronx, New York. Through analysis of cohort data, they have reported on speech recognition, speech perception, language development, and learning behavior (Gravel and Wallace, 1998). Some of their conclusions include:

- Multiple factors affect the development of children with early histories of otitis media (age at onset, number and duration of episodes, degree and duration of hearing loss, medical and surgical intervention, family history, cognitive and other developmental disabilities, socioeconomic status, home environment, parent language, attendance at day care) (Gravel and Wallace, 1998).
- Delays may be present on standardized measures of emerging language; "normal language" skills were present at school age on global, standardized language measures (Gravel and Wallace, 1998).
- Subtle perception and production deficits exist; 9-year-olds with a history of chronic otitis media performed more poorly than did 9-year-olds without such a history on speech perception memory tasks and temporal ordering judgments (Mody et al., 1998).
- Higher-order auditory processing problems are present that affect prereading/reading, auditory memory, discourse and narrative production, attention and behavior, and selective listening. These problems are thought to be a product of the low redundancy of the speech message caused by the intermittent hearing loss often associated with chronic otitis media (Gravel and Wallace, 1998).

These recent findings support the earlier work reported by Feagans (1986), Holm and Kunze (1969), Howie (1979), and Menyuk (1986) in which the long-term effects of early chronic otitis media on speech and language skills were also described. Menyuk reported that although overall problems in the comprehension and production of language were found in younger children, the analysis of 7-year-olds indicated differences only in lexical production, production of morphologic markers, and production of more sophisticated sentence structures. She determined that the difficulties in speech perception and production tasks were due to their early inability to hear specific acoustic characteristics of speech sounds. These problems resulted in difficulty categorizing speech sounds and producing morphologic markers. Feagans (1986), investigating later discourse and narrative skills of a day care population, cited the attentional process (thought to be critical for mediating language) as one of the primary long-term effects of early chronic otitis media.

Gravel and Wallace (1998) summarize the issues of the long-term effects of early otitis media in a sequential model reprinted in Figure 8.2. Management of these children during the critical periods of early language development is critical to minimizing these potential long-term problems. Children who are at greater risk for otitis media are more likely to incur the adverse effects and should therefore be monitored closely. In addition to monitoring the ear and hearing status, management should include minimizing background noise, increasing the children's attention to sound, promoting language learning, and making speech louder and clearer (Roberts and Wallace, 1997).

ASSESSMENT

Speech perception assessment

During the past decade, speech perception has achieved heightened interest due to its relationship with hearing instrument advancements and the desire to demonstrate amplification benefits. For children, cochlear implants have especially contributed to this effort due to the need to use more sensitive measures for mapping and tracking auditory skill development. Even with this momentum, speech perception tests remain poorly understood and underutilized.

Mendel et al. (1997) identified the following purposes of speech perception tests:

- To provide a measure of how well listeners understand speech.

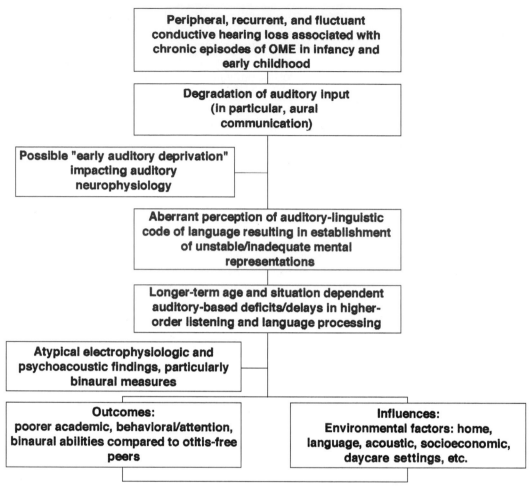

Figure 8.2. A model of the potential effects of the hearing loss accompanying OME on child development. (Reprinted with permission from Gravel JS, Wallace IF. In: Bess F, ed. Children with hearing impairment: Contemporary trends. Nashville, TN: Bill Wilkerson Press, 1998:217.)

- To reflect the degree of communication handicap created by the hearing loss.
- To provide information for planning and managing auditory (re)habilitation.
- To monitor listeners' performance throughout the therapeutic process.
- To assess the success of different types of medical and surgical treatments.
- To monitor subjects' performance in research paradigms.
- To classify the degree and type of hearing loss.
- To be used as a baseline measure for other test procedures.
- To be used in various forms of research (p. 3).

They further defined the following terminology often used to describe speech perception testing:

- Intelligibility: the degree of clarity with which an utterance is understood by the average listener.
- Articulation: the repeatability of the nonmeaningful parts of speech, such as nonsense syllables, used when plotting an articulation or performance-intensity function.
- Discrimination: the process of distinguishing among speech sounds or words by differentiating them as same or different.
- Recognition/identification: the recogni-

tion or establishment of a particular sound or word (i.e., the ability to repeat the stimulus item) (p. 4).

When assessing speech perception in children, the following variables should be considered (Kirk et al., 1997):

- Internal variables: vocabulary and language competency, chronologic age, and cognitive status.
- External variables: appropriate response task, use of reinforcement, and memory load.
- Methodologic variables: taped versus monitored-live-voice presentation, open-set versus closed-set tests, and task domain in closed-set test construction (unrestricted and restricted task domains).

All the above parameters—purpose for assessment, type of assessment to use, and individual assessment variables—are critical considerations when determining appropriate speech perception evaluations for children. Some speech perception tests that are designed for children are included in Appendix 8.3.

Functional hearing assessment

According to IDEA Section 34CFR300.6, Assistive Technology Service, audiologists in education settings are required to assess functional hearing abilities of children with hearing loss. The purpose of this assessment is to be able to determine how children perform in their typical environments (there may be several) and how assistive technologies benefit them. With the parameters described previously for speech perception in mind, audiologists can develop and identify the functional aspects of children's hearing that are necessary to determine what each child is capable of perceiving through audition and how well the hearing potential is being used. The discrepancy between these two performances should be the basis for the auditory habilitation goals and provide a cross-check for the appropriateness of the hearing instrumentation that is used.

Every effort should be made to provide functional speech perception data that reflect listening in a variety of situations. The Functional Listening Evaluation (Johnson and VonAlmen, 1993), located in Appendix 8.4, was designed to assess listening ability at the recognition/identification level under eight listening conditions: auditory only and auditory-visual in close/quiet, close/noise, distant/quiet, and distant/noise. Sentences material is recommended whenever possible so that the stimuli more closely approximates the discourse encountered in the child's classroom. The results of the listening paradigm can be analyzed to consider the effects of each variable (e.g., noise, distance, visual input) on the student's performance. The data can be used as evidence to provide classroom teachers, other staff members, and parents with information that is more predictive of how a student might perform under the real listening conditions of the instructional environment. It can also be given to evaluate the effectiveness of various hearing instrumentation to demonstrate effects on listening performance.

TECHNOLOGY FOR HEARING

Technology continues to make significant gains, providing children with hearing loss with better access, and in some cases new opportunities, to participate in auditory communication. As a result, hearing instruments should be considered for all children who have hearing loss until the need for a device can be ruled out.

In the past decade, the hearing instrument market has seen tremendous growth in programmable devices using multiple channels, multiple microphones, and digital signal processing in their quest to improve audibility and, particularly, the ability to hear speech in noise. Although these improvements have enhanced hearing in noise, they still do not provide sufficient amplification for children in the listening and learning environment of the school. Assistive listening devices are necessary to improve the signal-to-noise ratio in the classroom. Cochlear implants and other specialized devices provide additional amplification alternatives

Table 8.3
Hearing instrument options for children

Personal Devices	Assistive Listening Devices
Hearing aids	Personal FM
Cochlear implants	FM-auditory trainer
Bone conduction and bone-anchored hearing aids	Walkman-style FM
Specialized hearing devices	Classroom sound field FM system
TransSonic/ImpaCT	Personal sound field FM system
EMILY	3-D Induction Mat system
TACTAID	Induction Loop
TRILL	Infrared system
Universal amplifiers	

for children. The array of hearing instrumentation is summarized in Table 8.3.

FM

The most widely used assistive listening technology is FM, frequency modulated transmission of the auditory signal from a microphone to a receiver. The receiver may be connected to an individual hearing aid via a hardwired or wireless boot, be built into the hearing aid, or the transmission may occur through the aid's telecoil within a magnetic field created by a teleloop worn individually or set up around the perimeter of the classroom area. The use of this type of FM, known as personal FM because it works in conjunction with the individual's hearing aid, has increased dramatically since the recent introduction of behind-the-ear FM systems. The advantage to this type of system is that it uses the sophisticated hearing aid technology of the higher-tech circuitry hearing aids. Traditional body-worn FM-auditory trainer devices are mostly linear amplifiers and do not provide the standard of amplification now available in hearing aids.

The even more recent introduction of behind-the-ear "auditory trainers," or FM systems, that allow for interchangeable frequency channels brings the entire amplification system to the ear. The FM-auditory trainer may now provide multiple circuitry options that with the more natural ear level microphone position, will result in superior amplification. With a few exceptions, behind-the-ear FM should replace the traditional body-worn devices.

Walkman-style FM systems are frequently used with individuals who do not require hearing aids but who need the improvement in audibility afforded by FM signal transmission. These body-worn assistive listening devices provide this signal-to-noise advantage with limited output capabilities. This system has been popular with students who do not wear hearing aids, such as those with mild hearing losses including unilateral and high-frequency configurations, fluctuating losses due to otitis media, and central auditory processing disorders. Another application has been for speech-language therapy or other special education instruction that is conducted within the regular classroom. The use of FM minimizes the effects of interfering classroom noise, permitting the students to attend and hear the instructor more clearly.

OTHER ASSISTIVE LISTENING DEVICES

Traditional hardwire induction systems that loop the perimeter of the classroom have been available for many years. Although inexpensive, signal strength and consistency are dependent on the hearing aid telecoil strength and positioning, problems that have minimized their use. Another type of induction system is called the 3-D Induction Mat (Oval Window Audio, Nederland, CO). In this option, the signal from the teacher's microphone is transmitted to a large induction system contained in a mat that is placed under carpeting in the classroom or area to be amplified. The signal is accessed via the child's hearing aid telecoil. Because of the unique properties of the mat, the position of the telecoil, which usually must be horizontal, can be in any dimension; hence the name 3-D (three dimensional). This system provides such a strong signal that it functions well with most hearing aid telecoils. The system is particularly practical with preschool-age children for whom it eliminates the cumbersome body-worn apparatus and cords.

Infrared systems transmit sound via beams of infrared light. The transmitter sends the signal to a receiver, usually a head-worn device, which contains the infrared-sensitive receiving diode. Some systems also interface with the hearing aid through the telecoil or direct audio input. Infrared systems have not been used with children in classrooms due to the interference in signal transmission that occurs from any physical barrier such as bodies or walls. They are more suitable for television, the theater, and religious services.

Classroom amplification systems

The growth of classroom amplification or sound field systems reflects the growing recognition of the important role that hearing plays in learning for all children. These amplification systems consist of a teacher-worn transmitter and speakers placed strategically around the classroom. This configuration allows the teacher's voice to be disbursed equally throughout the classroom, so that all students have equal access to a clear auditory signal even when the teacher's back is to the class and when there is excessive noise from heating/ventilating systems or other noise sources causing poor classroom acoustics. Although these systems benefit all students, Crandell et al. (1995) identified the following groups of at-risk listeners who would benefit from classroom amplification:

- Children younger than 13 years of age.
- Children who have conductive hearing loss.
- Children who have articulation disorders.
- Children who have language disorders.

- Children who have learning disabilities.
- Children who are nonnative English speakers.
- Children with central auditory processing deficits.
- Children with minimal sensorineural hearing losses.
- Children with unilateral hearing losses.

In addition, children with hearing loss, with or without hearing aids, may use these systems as an option to personal FM amplification or as primary amplification when social, cosmetic, or behavior issues are present. Although not the optimum choice for amplification for children with significant hearing loss, audibility is improved.

The potentially large market for classroom amplification systems has resulted in a variety of systems from which to choose. The old adage, "You get what you pay for," applies here. When purchasing systems, careful consideration should be given to the quality of the sound system, number of speakers, ease of use, microphone options, ease of installation, frequency transmission/channel interference, and durability. Likewise, the physical classroom environment and classroom communication characteristics must be analyzed. Some classrooms may have such poor acoustics because of excessively loud heating/ventilation systems or excessive reverberation that classroom amplification systems may actually exacerbate the acoustic problem. When evaluating the communication environment of the classroom, consideration should be given to occupied room noise levels, instructional format, placement in the classroom for the targeted students, teacher's voice intensity and clarity, the use of media, teacher motivation, compatibility of amplification devices worn by other students, and potential FM interference sources.

Personal classroom amplification systems are the newest variation of sound field FM. These systems have a speaker housed in a compact case that sit on the student's desk. They have been particularly beneficial for students who have cochlear implants who are unable to use personal FM and for students who receive their instruction in multiple classrooms. The close proximity of the speaker to the student results in a better signal-to-noise ratio than the conventional classroom systems.

In addition to improving the signal-to-noise ratio within the classroom, additional benefits of classroom amplification include few maintenance problems because no equipment is worn by the student, reduced voice fatigue for the teacher, and reasonable cost. Overwhelming evidence to support the use of classroom amplification with all students has been reported (Sarff et al., 1981; Crandell and Bess, 1987; Flexer, 1989; Crandell and Smaldino, 1992).

Cochlear implants

Recent advancements in cochlear implant technology have led to improvements in signal processing, miniaturization of the speech processors, and increased options with more manufacturers. Additionally, the number of children with implants is growing quickly as more parents seek implants for their children and as more otologists perform the procedure. Cochlear implants now offer the best hearing advantage for children with profound, and even some severe, hearing losses who do not receive sufficient benefit from hearing aids; whose parents desire maximum auditory function for oral communication; and who meet the candidacy requirements. Pediatric candidacy criteria include profound sensorineural hearing loss in both ears, age of at least 18 months, demonstrated lack or plateau of auditory skill development, no medical contraindications, high motivation and appropriate expectations of family and child (when old enough), and placement in an educational program that emphasizes development of auditory skills after the implant has been fitted (Colorado Cochlear Implant Consortium, 1997). Individual centers may consider additional factors related to the amount of residual hearing, age of the child, length of deafness, availability of appropriate educational options, communication methodology, cognitive status, and parent commitment.

The nonsurgical part of the implantation procedure continues to have some problems that need to be resolved before the process can work smoothly. Specifically, there is often confusion between the roles of the implant centers and the educational programs these children attend. The primary issue relates to the responsibility for the additional speech therapy and auditory training once the implant occurs. Another issue is the use of sign language after implantation. Some centers require that children stop signing following implantation so that they are forced to rely on and develop their auditory skills. Open communication between the programs (school and implant center) is an essential step in evaluating candidacy, developing realistic expectations for the child, and providing postimplant intervention. See Chapter 15 for comprehensive information on Cochlear implants.

Specialized devices

Specialized auditory and tactile devices have been designed to improve audibility and access to auditory information for children with profound hearing losses. These include the TranSonic and the recently introduced ImpaCT (which replaces the TranSonic) by AVR Sonnovation, Eden Prarie, MN. These devices shift high-frequency energy to corresponding low-frequency energy in real time to retain as much of the relative spectral information as possible. For children with no measurable high-frequency hearing, this shift provides input to additional auditory information for environmental sounds and speech perception. The EMILY (Somerville, MA) is a digital signal processor that enhances sounds at the frequencies of 1000 and 2000 Hz to provide additional resonance for improvement of the quality of acoustic signals. The TACTAID (Audiologic Engineering) and the TRILL (AVR Sonnovation) are devices that code acoustic energy and convert it to vibrotactile signals that are received on the skin.

Bone conduction and bone-anchored hearing devices are available for individuals with atretic ears or other ear pathologies that prohibit the use of traditional hearing aid fittings. The Bone Anchored Hearing Aid

(BAHA) (Nobel Biocare USA, Inc., West-mont, IL), just recently approved for use in the United States by the Food and Drug Administration, is a bone conduction hearing aid anchored into an abutment implanted in the mastoid bone behind the ear. Vibrations are transferred from the hearing aid through the abutment in the bone to stimulate the cochlea. The device eliminates a headband or other head retainer necessary to keep traditional bone conduction devices in place. Bone conduction device users usually have normal cochlear potential and therefore have excellent speech perception capabilities.

Determining and selecting the appropriate hearing instrument

Hearing instruments should be considered for all children who have a hearing loss until the need for a device can be ruled out. The process for choosing the best hearing instrument for a child is not simple. Table 8.4 summarizes the various considerations when evaluating amplification options for children. Hearing and other related considerations should reflect the child's needs based on auditory sensitivity and functional performance;

age; neurologic, processing, and cognitive abilities; motivation; and self-esteem. The physical listening environment of the child both at school and outside of school is important as well as analysis of the communication variables encountered in these environments.

Regular classroom-inclusive environments, in which most students with hearing loss are now educated, often have multiple simultaneous learning activities. The activity level, combined with 25 to 30 students, may pose very different amplification needs than self-contained or resource classrooms where there are fewer students and more teacher control of the environment. The advantages of sophisticated, multimemory, programmable hearing aids may provide excellent reception in quiet situations and some lecture classes, but not where there is noise from other activities or from poor acoustics. For almost all learning environments, the use of FM is required to overcome the signal-to-noise problems that exist. Therefore, compatibility with the school FM systems becomes another necessary consideration. Audiologists are learning that choosing a device requires a part-

Table 8.4
Considerations for selecting hearing instruments

Hearing Loss Variables	Physical Environment	Communication Environment
Degree of loss	Internal	Occupied room noise levels
Configuration of loss	Room sizes and shapes	Number of occupants
Bilateral versus unilateral	Ambient noise levels	Instructional format (lecture,
High-frequency hearing ability	Reverberation	discussion, team teaching)
Fluctuating hearing levels	External	Distance from speaker
Distance listening abilities	Outside of room noises:	Speaker's voice intensity and
Speech recognition skills	duration and intensity	clarity
Auditory processing abilities	Other environments	Use of media (audio, video,
Hearing and comprehension	(outside, home, car,	computers, movies)
ability in noise	daycare, work)	Lighting
Language competence		Teacher motivation
Attention and listening fatigue		Amplification devices used by
Directionality skills		other students in the
Speechreading skills		classroom
Motivation to use amplification		Potential FM interference
Self-esteem		sources
Age of user		
Craniofacial variances		
Other disabilities		

Adapted from Johnson, DeConde C. Amplification in inclusive classrooms. J Edu Audiol 1998;6:33–44.

nership between the dispensing audiologist and the educational audiologist or deaf education teacher and the parent so that all the issues can be evaluated properly before a final determination is made. Together, all these considerations must guide the selection process. Once the instruments are fitted, a "functional" assessment that evaluates the effectiveness of the devices in the child's environment should be conducted.

In addition to fitting hearing instruments, a training program for the parent and student should be scheduled as well as one with the teacher. Children, their parents, and teachers need to be comfortable with the operational aspects of the devices, be able to perform basic trouble-shooting procedures, and know the behavioral expectations for the child with amplification. These responsibilities are often best shared between the dispensing audiologist and the school audiologist.

Efficacy of amplification is also an issue with children in schools. As the number of amplification options have increased, so has the cost brought on by the technological developments and advancements. Tools such as the Listening Inventories for Education (LIFE) (Anderson and Smaldino, 1998) provide the audiologist with a mechanism for documenting benefit of amplification as measured by both the classroom teacher and the student. Evidence such as this is often necessary to justify certain types of instrumentation that otherwise may not be considered for a student.

PERFORMANCE OF AMPLIFICATION DEVICES

One of the primary issues in auditory management for children is to ensure proper fitting and functioning of hearing devices. Once a device is selected for a student, it must be fit with the necessary verification procedures including real ear analysis. Fitting may require fine-tuning over several weeks as the child's behavior is observed or, for older children, as hearing and listening skills are assessed.

Poor-functioning amplification worn by children in schools is a long-standing problem (Gaeth and Lounsbury, 1966; Zink,

1972; Kemker et al., 1979; Elfenbein et al., 1988; Potts and Greenwood, 1983) that continues. Recent evidence from the Colorado study (Johnson, 1998) fuels the concerns of inclusionary practices for children with hearing loss who do not consistently hear well in school due to improper functioning or absent amplification.

In Colorado, a study was undertaken to evaluate the condition and functioning of student's hearing aids and FM systems. Because Colorado prides itself in providing educational audiology services to children in all school districts, it was hypothesized that with the availability of these services, improved functioning of amplification would be evident. In the survey, school-based educational audiologists were asked to conduct unannounced, detailed checks of student's hearing aids and/or FM amplification systems. All students were checked during a 2-week period. For devices that were not satisfactory, the audiologists reported the problem(s) based on the following categories: aid not worn, problem or defective aid, battery condition, earmold condition, or FM condition. Each of the main categories included subcategories for more specific identification of the problem. Surveys were completed by 23 of 42 administrative units representing 611 students. A total of 950 hearing aids and 212 FM systems were worn by these 611 students. The condition and performance of the devices were then analyzed using the Statistical Package for the Social Sciences (SPSS) (1993). The results are reported in Tables 8.5 to 8.12.

Table 8.5 reports the findings of the overall performance of right ear and left ear hearing aids as well as the FM systems. In addition to these individual conditions, the results show that 73.4% of students had at least one of their devices in satisfactory condition, whereas only 56.8% had all prescribed devices functioning. Table 8.6 breaks down the performance by service delivery. The sources of the hearing aid problems found are identified in Table 8.7, the reasons for the FM problems in Table 8.8, and the earmold problems in Table 8.9. The

Table 8.5
The Colorado survey: overall performance and condition of hearing aids and FM systems

	Number of Units	Percent Satisfactory Condition/Performance
Hearing aid, right ear	478	64.6%
Hearing aid, left ear	472	60.8%
FM	212	75.9%
Right or left ear hearing aid or FM		73.4%
All prescribed amplification		56.6%

Reprinted with permission from Johnson, DeConde C. Amplification in inclusive classrooms. J Educ Audiol 1998;6:33–44.

Table 8.6
The Colorado survey: performance and condition of hearing aids and FM systems according to service delivery mode

Service Delivery Mode	Number of Students	% of Students With Satisfactory Hearing Aid Condition and Performance, Right ear	% of Students With Satisfactory Hearing Aid Condition and Performance, Left ear	% of Students With Satisfactory Performance of FM	% of Students With Satisfactory Condition and Performance of either Right or Left Ear Hearing Aid or FM
No IEP	68	56.1	46.4	85.7	57.4
Consultive	114	60.5	57.3	69.6	64.9
Itinerant	173	69.9	73.8	66.7	76.1
Resource	85	74.6	64.9	80.5	85.8
Self-contained	171	61.2	53.6	82.9	78.9

Reprinted with permission from Johnson, DeConde C. Amplification in inclusive classrooms. J Educ Audiol 1998;6:33–44.

frequency of hearing aid/FM checks are reported in Tables 8.10 and 8.11 which illustrates the effect of frequency of hearing aid/FM checks on performance. Table 8.12 reports the individuals responsible for administering the hearing aid/FM checks.

A number of interesting observations can be made from the data analysis. These include:

• Only 56.8% of students had all devices (as prescribed) working satisfactorily (Table 8.5).
• When considering the number of students who had at least one of their hearing aids or their FM system working satisfactorily, generally the more intense the delivery system, the higher the probability that their amplification functioned properly (Table 8.6). The exception was hearing

aids in self-contained classrooms. It could be postulated that the children in the self-contained classrooms tended to have greater degrees of hearing loss so that they benefited less from hearing aids, or that these children tended to rely more on manual communication than audition.
• For all service delivery modes except itinerant, the FM systems functioned better than the student's hearing aids (Tables 8.5 and 8.6).
• The frequency of hearing aid or FM monitoring did not predict satisfactory performance (Table 8.11). When analyzing the type of hearing aid problems, 79.6% were minor ones ("other" and "battery" categories) that could be addressed by a teacher, technician, or nurse (Table 8.7); 59.6% of the problems were due to students not having their aid(s) on because

Table 8.7
The Colorado survey: reported sources of hearing aid problems

Hearing Aid Problems (n = 354)	% of Responses
Other	59.6
Left at home	28.2
Refuses to wear	19.8
Lost	4.6
In pocket	4.3
Turned off	1.8
Sensitive ear	1.0
Battery	18.3
Weak/dead batter	15.0
No battery	2.5
Battery compartment	.8
Defective hearing aid	15.5
In for repair	6.6
Distortion	2.3
Volume control	2.3
No output	2.0
Intermittent	1.3
Low gain	1.0
Case	3.3
Excessive dirt	2.3
Wet	0.5
Loose hook	0.3
Cracked case	0.3
Unknown	3.3

Reprinted with permission from Johnson, DeConde C. Amplification in inclusive classrooms. J Educ Audiol 1998;6:33–44.

their instrument(s) was at home, lost, in their pocket, or the student refused to wear it. These findings suggest a need to assess whether the hearing aids were fitted appropriately, whether the student had fully adjusted to them, or whether there were other issues affecting the student's desire to wear hearing aids.

• Students with amplification who did not have individualized education programs (IEPs) had the greatest number of nonsatisfactory ratings (Table 8.6).

What do these data mean relative to the school's responsibility for proper functioning of hearing devices? Based on satisfactory condition and functioning, the data clearly would support the use of FM assistive devices over hearing aids, when appropriate. The findings also continue to support

the need for aggressive amplification monitoring and daily amplification checks to achieve a higher rate of amplification performance. However, the data also suggest that more scrutiny be given to the decisions of who should wear hearing aids, the type of amplification, and the training that goes along with using the devices. Often, hearing aids are fitted on the sole basis of the presence of a hearing loss without careful analysis of the student's listening environment, communication needs, and motivation to use amplification. Furthermore, few audiologists provide the crucial support services of hearing aid orientation, adjustment, and auditory (re)habilitation, although the training of these skills is essential to the successful fitting of amplification.

Whereas educational audiologists may not be able to ensure that a high number of instruments are in satisfactory condition on a given day, it is important to look at audiologic management responsibilities beyond those that are quantified in a survey such as this. Studies should also focus on the quality of instrumentation and services that are

Table 8.8
The Colorado survey: reported sources of FM problems

FM Problem (N = 39)	% of Responses
Defective	51.3
Battery	10.3
Interference	2.6
Other	35.9

Reprinted with permission from Johnson, DeConde C. Amplification in inclusive classrooms. J Educ Audiol 1998;6:33–44.

Table 8.9
The Colorado survey: reported sources of earmold problems

Earmold Problem (N = 35)	% of Responses
Dirty	31.4
Poor tubing	28.6
Poor fit	25.7
Lost	5.7
Plugged	5.7
Damaged	2.9

Reprinted with permission from Johnson, DeConde C. Amplification in inclusive classrooms. J Educ Audiol 1998;6:33–44.

Table 8.10
The Colorado survey: frequency
of hearing aid/FM check

Daily "supposedly" daily	20.4%
Daily and weekly	10.8%
Daily and monthly	5.4%
2 to 3 times/week	1.9%
Weekly	16%
Weekly and monthly	2.4%
Monthly	6.9%
2 to 3 times/year	3.7%
Depends on student	32.5%

Reprinted with permission from Johnson, DeConde C. Amplification in inclusive classrooms. J Educ Audiol 1998;6:33–44.

Table 8.11
The Colorado survey: performance and condition
of hearing aid/FM according to frequency of check

Frequency of Check	Right Hearing Aid % Satisfactory	Left Hearing Aid % Satisfactory	FM
Daily	66%	65.5%	78.4%
Weekly	64.1%	63.2%	71.1%
Monthly	61.3%	68.8%	100%
Other	64.1%	54.9%	78.4%

Reprinted with permission from Johnson, DeConde C. Amplification in inclusive classrooms. J Educ Audiol 1998;6:33–44.

Table 8.12
The Colorado survey: person responsible
for administering hearing aid/FM check

Teacher of hearing-impaired	35.8%
Audiologist	32.3%
Educational Interpreter	12%
Classroom teacher	8.7%
Speech-language pathologist	7.3%
Nurse	0.7%
Other	3.1%

Reprinted with permission from Johnson, DeConde C. Amplification in inclusive classrooms. J Educ Audiol 1998;6:33–44.

available and the role of educational audiologists as part of the educational team.

THE ROLE OF FAMILIES

The involvement of parents in the educational program for their children has dramatically increased over the past decade. Parents, by law, have to be an integral part of the individualized family service plan (IFSP) or IEP development process to determine needs, services, and educational goals for their children. Schools continue to struggle to balance the desires of parents with their legal obligation, available resources, and the recommendations of professionals. Schools must also deal with the uninvolved parents who do not, or are unable to, support their children's learning. The best relationship is a partnership built on trust, with common goals that are focused on the child and have the family's support.

Parent support is absolutely essential for proper auditory management. Parents have the responsibility of providing consistently working hearing instruments for their children to ensure appropriate auditory input. They must also be committed to the therapies and interventions that support auditory development; to do so parents must be involved in the development of the services so that they are aligned with their expectations and priorities. It is also often helpful for parents to understand how current goals fit into the larger spectrum of skills that will become future targets. The Listening Development Profile (Johnson et al., 1997a) shown in Appendix 8.5 can be used to provide parents (and therapists) with a continuum of developmental outcomes from which to track the development of listening skills.

THE EDUCATIONAL AUDIOLOGIST: ROLES AND RESPONSIBILITIES

Educational audiology as a specialty has gained respect and recognition as a primary factor in auditory management for children in schools. The distinction between audiology as practiced in the school setting versus audiology practiced in other settings is important. The school setting requires specific knowledge of the associated educational implications of various hearing losses, of the various amplification options, of the possible accommodations and modifications required because of the hearing loss, consultation skills to collaborate with teachers for both deaf/hard-of-hearing and regular education, and knowledge about specific treatments and intervention programs. The educational audiologist is often the one consistent professional throughout the child's school career. The specific roles and responsibilities of audiologists who work in schools were suggested by the American Speech-Language-Hearing Association (ASHA) (1993) and are listed in Table 8.13. These responsibilities vary greatly among states and among school districts within states, as do the number of educational audiologists in schools to provide the services. In the Nineteenth Annual Report to Congress on the Implementation of IDEA (1998), the U.S. Department of Education reported that there were 969 audiologists serving children in the schools during the 1994–1995 school year. If audiologists were hired at the ASHA recommended ratio of 1 audiologist for every 12,000 students (ASHA, 1993), 3771 audiologists would be needed in the schools (based on the reported preschool to 12th grade enrollment of 45,252,928 students).

Because most children with hearing loss are educated in regular classrooms, students are often spread over a number of schools within a district. They often have less contact with a teacher of the deaf or hard-of-hearing than in the past and increasingly rely on the instruction and support of the regular classroom teacher. In many schools, the educational audiologist has evolved as the advocate for issues related to hearing loss for these children and for hearing issues for all students. Now more than ever before, good auditory management programs have to be established if these children are going to have appropriate opportunities to learn in these environments.

Auditory Management: Challenges and Opportunities Ahead

Children with all levels of hearing loss have unique auditory needs, whether hearing is considered their primary mode of input or whether it supplements a more visual language and communication system. Research

has shown repeatedly that the effects of even the mildest hearing loss go beyond hearing and listening. The often-used chart developed by Anderson and Matkin (1991) summarizing the psychosocial and educational sequelae of the various degrees of hearing losses is shown in Appendix 8.6. Because these problems stem from hearing loss, auditory management is one of the most critical services needed by a child. Audiologists remain challenged by this problem and must be prepared to advocate aggressively for all these children.

THE AUDITORY MANAGEMENT FOURSOME

There are four areas that comprise auditory management for children with hearing loss. These are hearing instrumentation, auditory skill development and communication repair strategizing, listening environment management, and instructional accommodations and modifications (Fig. 8.3).

Much has been learned about each of these four areas so that for the most part the knowledge and the tools to deal with them exist. Unfortunately, the questions that arise for families related to their child's hearing loss and the answers to them often present more like a complex web than a straight path. Consequently, it is critical that parents have someone who assists them with sorting through the tangle of issues, opinions, and facts to arrive at a reasonable course for their individual situation. This individual may be another parent, an advocate, an audiologist, or another professional. It is often very difficult, and not always prudent, to separate auditory needs from other associated issues. Therefore, auditory management must always be considered within the larger perspective of the child, the child's family, and their priorities and may often take a back seat to other more immediate needs. The fact that some parents are not able, or not willing, to follow through on the audiologist's instructions is a common problem when parents are not part of the goal or IEP development process. In the end, the key to optimizing outcomes for a child may actually be in how well all of the hearing issues

Table 8.13
Roles and responsibilities of the educational audiologist

Provide community leadership to ensure that all infants, toddlers, and youth with impaired hearing are promptly identified, evaluated, and provided with appropriate intervention services

Collaborate with community resources to develop and implement a high-risk registry, newborn screening, and follow-up

Coordinate hearing screening programs for preschool and school-aged children

Train audiometric technicians or other appropriate personnel to screen for hearing loss

Perform comprehensive, educationally relevant hearing evaluations

Access central auditory function

Make appropriate medical, educational, and community referrals

Interpret audiologic assessment results for other school personnel

Assist in program placement as a member of the educational team to make specific recommendations for auditory and communication needs

Provide in-service training on hearing and hearing impairments and their implications to school personnel, children, and parents

Educate about noise exposure and hearing loss prevention

Make recommendations about the use of hearing aids, cochlear implants, group and classroom amplification, and assistive listening devices

Ensure the proper fit and functioning of hearing aids and other auditory devices

Analyze classroom noise and acoustics and make recommendations for improving the listening environment

Manage the use and calibration of audiometric equipment

Collaborate with school, parents, teachers, special support personnel, and relevant community agencies and professionals to ensure delivery of appropriate services

Make recommendations for assistive devices (radio/television, telephone, alerting, convenience) for students who are deaf and hard-of-hearing

Provide services, including home programming if appropriate, in the areas of speechreading, listening, communication strategies, use and care of amplification (including cochlear implants), and self-management of hearing needs

Adapted from American Speech-Language-Hearing Association. Guidelines for audiology services in the schools. ASHA 1993;35(suppl 10):24–32.

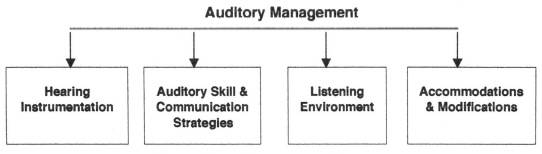

Figure 8.3. The auditory management foursome.

are managed within the family. Given this broader perspective and understanding, the remaining discussion will focus on the four areas of auditory management.

Hearing instrumentation

The first step in auditory management is fitting proper hearing instrumentation. Most hearing losses must be managed through amplification. As a rule of thumb, all children with hearing loss should be considered candidates for amplification until otherwise ruled out. Although surgical and medical procedures may improve hearing for certain etiologies and problems, most hearing loss is due to pathology causing permanent, sensorineural impairment. Once the hearing loss is recognized and defined, habilitation must begin with the fitting of the best hearing instruments available. Amplification variables that must be considered were discussed earlier and are summarized in Table 8.13. The challenge for audiologists will continue to be balancing the best available technology with the financial constraints imposed by insurance and other health-care provider programs. Cochlear implants further add to the continuum of options and should be considered for children who derive little benefit from conventional amplification and whose parents desire audition as their child's primary communication mode.

The provision of hearing instruments is only the first step to audition. Supports and programs must be in place to ensure that the amplification is fitted, used properly, and working consistently. Regular monitoring must occur on a daily basis to check for hearing instrumentation problems. When hearing aid or other amplification problems arise, there must be audiologic problem-solving resources for parents and school staff members so that the issues can be resolved.

Auditory skill development and communication strategies

Once access to auditory input is accomplished, a course of therapy to teach and enhance speech perception and auditory skill development must begin. When children have developed language and cognitive skills, they are also able to learn strategies to aid in their communication skills. Most children will never be successful hearing aid users and auditory learners without the supports and services to develop these skills. Therefore, the dispensing audiologist must work very closely with a team that includes the educational audiologist, speech-language pathologist, or teacher responsible for auditory skill development, and the parents.

IFSP or IEP goals for hearing instrument use and listening development are necessary for every child. For infants, listening development activities should be immediately fully integrated into the child's daily routine

so that audition may develop naturally, similar to hearing infants. For toddlers and preschool children, the addition of therapy for specific auditory skill development is usually needed to teach or practice skills that require more sophisticated auditory perception. For school-age children, auditory training may continue depending on the individual needs of the student. There are commercially available auditory curricula that can assist the therapist and family in designing goals and activities that are appropriate for the child. Some include assessment tools for placement within the curriculum (see Appendix 8.3 for a list of selected programs). Any therapy program that isolates auditory skills should always teach through language-based activities that are embedded in a context that is relevant and functional for the child. This context is necessary if the child is expected to use the skills as part of day-to-day communication repertoire.

Many children with hearing loss do not use their speech because of fear they will fail to communicate. Other children may use their speech but give up when they are not understood. Communication repair strategies are taught through practicing communication skills and may begin as early as preschool. These strategies are best taught through activities that are already part of the child's experience base. An example of early communication repair occurs when children cannot express what they want because their speech is not intelligible. To make their needs known, children will show their parents what they want. Parents, teachers, and therapists can demonstrate repair strategies as problems occur or by teaching children through more formal programs such as reported by Elfenbein (1992), and Tye-Murray (1994).

The listening environment

The listening environments of classrooms, homes, restaurants, and recreational centers present some of the most significant challenges to audiologists and others who work with students with hearing loss. Assistive listening devices, when available, are the only auditory accommodation that improves communication problems created by poor acoustics and speaker distance. The reader is referred to Chapter 16 for an in-depth presentation of assistive devices. Acoustic accessibility and other issues related to the importance of hearing for learning are critical and were discussed earlier in this chapter. The essential problem is that distance reduces speech to inaudible levels either by virtue of the distance itself or in combination with the other acoustic factors. A vicious cycle develops for children with hearing loss. They listen through the filter created by their hearing impairment that is then further degraded by poor acoustic conditions. Hearing aids, by amplifying all sounds, often increase the hearing and listening difficulties rather than improve them. These students then exert extra effort to try to hear and listen in the classroom, which results in greater fatigue. Students who are fatigued experience greater hearing and listening problems.

After years of discussion, classroom acoustics have finally assumed a prominent position as they relate to the hearing needs of all students. The United States Architectural and Transportation Barriers Compliance Board, otherwise known as the Access Board, is considering a course of action that includes developing technical standards for classroom acoustics (Architectural and Transportation Barriers Compliance Board, 1998). This Board monitors compliance with the ADA, which has regulatory authority through the Departments of Justice and Transportation. Unfortunately, the regulations will only affect new construction and remodeling. However, attention to this problem by the Access Board should result in a significant increase in awareness of the problems associated with poor classroom acoustics.

Noise and reverberation are the most significant factors affecting classroom acoustics. Since the heating, ventilating, and air conditioning systems (HVAC) industry standards are based on auditory annoyance rather than speech intelligibility, the noise generated by HVAC systems leaves speech inaudible for many children with hearing loss and unintel-

ligible for most of the others. When the noise generated from within the classroom from children talking and moving in their chairs is multiplied with the reverberation of these sounds when there are no acoustic treatments, the result is auditory chaos. Further noise infiltrates the classroom from open windows and hallway doors, causing additional intermittent distractions. The research studies of the 1970s and 1980s mentioned earlier in this chapter confirm the effects of noise, reverberation, and speaker distance on speech intelligibility for both normal-hearing and impaired-hearing listeners.

To manage poor classroom acoustics, audiologists, teachers, and parents must be strong advocates for acoustic modifications and assistive listening devices. ASHA (1995) recommended the following standards: (1) unoccupied classroom noise levels not exceed 30 dB(A) or a room criteria (RC) curve of 20 dB, (2) reverberation time limits of 0.4 seconds, and (3) classroom minimum signal-to-noise ratios of +15 dB. The Educational Audiology Association (Anderson, 1997) recommended unoccupied classroom noise levels in the range of 30 to 35 dB(A), reverberation times in the range of 0.4 to 0.6 seconds, and signal-to-noise ratios of +10 to +15 dB; for children with hearing loss, a 0.4 reverberation time and a +15 dB signal-to-noise ratio were recommended. Once the Access Board recommendations are published, they should provide additional justification, especially for classes in which children with hearing loss are educated. With inclusion, these children are in classes throughout school districts. The audiologist will need to have their sound level meters and reverberation formulas in hand to see how classrooms measure up. Whereas poor classroom acoustics may lend further justification for personal assistive amplification devices, the use of sound field systems should be judicious. The introduction of a classroom amplification system may further add to the speech perception problems if reverberation levels are high. Other accommodations for improving classroom acoustics are identified in Appendix 8.7.

Communication characteristics between the child and teachers, peers, and others also need to be managed. As soon as students are able, they should express their own communication needs to their teachers and classmates. They should be encouraged to participate in classroom in-services, which are conducted at the beginning of each school year, to prepare the class for having a student with hearing problems among them. Some of these communication strategies are included in Appendix 8.7. They should be discussed with the student and the teacher. Modification of these strategies and the use of other appropriate strategies for outside, in noisy restaurants and other public places, and at home should also be discussed with the student. An important goal of auditory management for listening environments needs to be awareness, knowledge of the effects of hearing loss, and the resulting communication problems created by various listening environments.

ACCOMMODATIONS AND MODIFICATIONS

Accommodations are changes made in the learning process to provide students with access to information and an equal opportunity to demonstrate knowledge and skills without affecting learning outcomes. Examples include special seating, use of an assistive listening device, use of a note-taker, visual supplements, study guides and preteaching, peer partners, adjusted pace of instruction, repetition of ideas, and reduced language level. Modifications are changes made in the instructional level, content, or performance criteria. Examples include reducing the difficulty of the material, shortened assignments, alternative assignments, and an alternative grading system. A document such as the checklist in Appendix 8.8, IEP Checklist: Recommended Accommodations and Modifications for Students with Hearing Impairment, is useful for determining these services.

As mentioned, auditory management includes understanding one's own hearing needs and the ability to self-manage them. Students should participate in the deter-

mination of their own accommodations by middle or junior high school. Modifications will continue to require the input of the student's teachers, as these should also be incorporated into IEP goals. Because self-awareness and self-advocacy are so important, every IEP should contain goals in these areas. There are also several excellent programs that have been developed to teach students about their hearing loss. These are included in Appendix 8.3. There are also two workbooks, now out of print (previously published by Gallaudet University Press), that were excellent resources for this purpose: *Ear Gear* for elementary-age children and *Wired for Sound* for older children. It is worth the effort to try to locate copies.

In summary, auditory management is a fourfold process: hearing instrumentation, auditory skill development and communication strategies, listening environment management, and instructional accommodations and modifications. All four areas should always be considered and included in the child's IEP. Sample IEP goals that promote independent use of amplification, development of auditory skills, development of compensatory strategies, knowledge of hearing loss and its implications, and self-advocacy are included in Appendix 8.9. The Listening Development Profile shown in Appendix 8.5 may also serve as the basis for the development of auditory management goals for the IEP.

Other contributing factors

To manage hearing effectively, consideration must be given to other factors that can have a tremendous effect on the success of any child. The degree to which a child is able to hear is based primarily on the physical characteristics of the hearing loss. However, the ability of the child to learn to use his or her hearing is affected by many factors. Although some skills can be taught and trained, the degree of success is usually dependent on the child's innate ability to learn, the interference of other disabilities, his or her command of language, and parent support. Another important element is one's motivation to learn. Understanding the benefits of what can be learned and experiencing the effects of a strong self-concept are powerful tools in motivating students. Goals and activities should always be functional and relevant to the needs and abilities of the student and should include the support of the parents. In addition, they should be designed to permit the student to experience the success of achievement.

GETTING CHILDREN PREPARED FOR LEARNING

For the first time there is optimism for the future education of deaf and hard-of-hearing children. If hearing loss is identified at birth, if proper amplification is provided, and if appropriate intervention is begun, children should have the opportunity to begin preschool at age 3 with language and communication skills at or near those of their hearing peers. If children enter school with this level of skill, schools will be challenged to ensure that these children have not fallen behind by the time they are ready to enter kindergarten as well as in subsequent years. Supportive families and environments are also critical elements in this quest, but with proper early intervention support, the chances for success are better than ever before.

Early identification and early intervention capitalize on the natural learning process enjoyed by all children. However, a major key for children who will develop and use their auditory skills will be good auditory management. As one of the first steps, this includes selecting and fitting appropriate hearing aids, followed by consistent monitoring and follow-up to ensure that the initial fitting remains appropriate based on both functional performance and electroacoustic/real ear measures. At these earliest stages of auditory management, the communication between the parents, the early interventionist, and the audiologist must be frank and frequent and under an aura of mutual trust.

TO SEE A CHALLENGE IS TO HAVE AN OPPORTUNITY

Children with all levels of hearing loss have unique auditory needs whether hearing is considered their primary mode of input or whether it supplements a more visual language and communication system. As research continues to identify and explore the problems associated with even the very mildest of hearing impairments, audiologists must be prepared to advocate aggressively for all these children so that their abilities are not minimized by avoidable consequences. The challenges will always be present. Whether they be increasing awareness, keeping up with technology, finding funding for new and better hearing instrumentation, finding better methods for educating children who are deaf and hard-of-hearing, creating acoustically sound classrooms, or finding better ways to involve families, there will always be issues requiring attention. The real challenge is to turn each one into an opportunity to create a better future for deaf and hard-of-hearing children. It can be done.

REFERENCES

Allen L. The effect sound field amplification has on teacher vocal abuse problems. Paper presented at the Educational Audiology Association Summer Conference, Lake Lure, North Carolina, June 1995.

American Speech-Language-Hearing Association. Guidelines for audiology services in the schools. ASHA 1993; 35(Suppl 10):24–32.

American Speech-Language-Hearing Association. Acoustics in education settings. ASHA 1995;37(Suppl 14):15–19.

Anderson K. Screening instrument for targeting educational risk in children (SIFTER). Tampa, FL: Educational Audiology Association, 1989.

Anderson K. The sound of learning. Am School Board J 1997;October:26–28.

Anderson KL, Smaldino J. Listening Inventories for Education (L.I.F.E.). Tampa, FL: Educational Audiology Association, 1998.

Anderson KL, Matkin ND. Relationship of degree of longterm hearing loss to psychosocial impact and educational needs. In: KL Anderson. Hearing conservation in the public schools revisited. Semin Hear 1991:12: 361–363.

Apuzzo M, Yoshinaga-Itano C. Early identification of infants with significant hearing loss and the Minnesota Child Development Inventory. Semin Hear 1995;16: 124–139.

Architectural and Transportation Barriers Compliance Board. Petition for rulemaking: request for information on acoustics. Fed Reg 1998;(63)104:29679–29686.

Bench J, Kowal A, Bamford J. The BKB (Bamford-Kowal-Bench) sentence lists for parially-hearing children. British J of Aud 1979;13:108–112.

Bess FH. Children with unilateral hearing loss. J Acad Rehabil Audiol 1982;15:131–144.

Bess FH. The minimally hearing-impaired child. Ear Hear 1985;6:43–47.

Bess FH, Tharpe AM. Unilateral hearing impairment in children. Pediatrics 1984;74:206–216.

Bess FH, Tharpe AM. An introduction to unilateral sensorineural hearing loss in children. Ear Hear 1986;7:3–13.

Bess FH, Klee T, Culbertson JL. Identification, assessment and management of children with unilateral sensorineural hearing loss. Ear Hear 1986a;7:43–51.

Bess FH, Tharpe AM, Gilber A. Auditory performance of children with unilateral sensorineural hearing loss. Ear Hear 1986b;7:20–26.

Bess FH, Dodd-Murphy J, Parker R. Children with minimal sensorineural hearing loss: prevalence, educational performance, and functional status. Ear Hear 1998;19: 339–354.

Bornstein SP, Musiek FE. Implications of temporal processing for children with learning and language problems. In: Beasley D, ed. Contemporary issues in audition. San Diego: College-Hill Press, 1984:25–65.

Bornstein SP, Musiek FE. Recognition of distorted speech in children with and without learning problems. J Am Acad Audiol 1992;3:22–32.

Colorado Cochlear Implant Consortium. Pediatric cochlear implant fact sheet. Denver: CCIC, 1997.

Colorado Department of Education. Survey of students with hearing impairment. Denver: The Colorado Department of Education, 1994.

Colorado Department of Education. Central auditory processing disorders: A team approach to screening, identification, assessment & intervention practices. Denver: The Colorado Department of Education, 1997.

Colorado Department of Education. Suggested annual goals and short term objects relating to audiology needs. Denver: The Colorado Department of Education, 1998.

Comprehensive Test of Basic Skills. 4th ed. MacMillan/McGraw-Hill. Monterey, CA: CTB, 1993.

Craig WN. Craig lipreading inventory: Word recognition. Englewood, CO: Resource Point, 1992.

Crandell C. The effects of classroom acoustics on children with normal hearing: implications for intervention strategies. Educ Audiol Monogr 1991;2:18–38.

Crandell C. Speech recognition on noise by children with minimal degrees of sensorineural hearing loss. Ear Hear 1993;14:210–216.

Crandell C, Bess F. Speech recognition of children in a "typical" classroom. Am J Audiol 1986;1:16–18.

Crandell C, Bess F. Sound-field amplification in the classroom setting. ASHA 1987;29:87.

Crandell C, Smaldino J. Sound-field amplification in the classroom. Am J Audiol 1992;1:16–18.

Crandell C, Smaldino J. An update of classroom acoustics for children with hearing impairment. Volta Rev 1994; 6:18–25.

Crandell C, Smaldino J. The effects of noise on the speech perception of non-native English children. Am J Audiol 1996;5:47–51.

Crandell C, Smaldino J, Flexer C. Speech perception in specific populations. In: Crandell C, Smaldino J, Flexer C, eds. Sound-field amplification: theory and practical applications. San Diego: Singular, 1995.

Davis J, ed. Our forgotten children: hard of hearing pupils in the schools. Minneapolis: Audio Visual Library Service, University of Minnesota, 1977.

Dirks D, Morgan D, Dubno J. A procedure for quantifying the effects of noise on speech recognition. J Speech Hear Disord 1982;47:114–122.

Downs MP. Contribution of mild hearing loss to auditory language learning problems. In: Roesser RJ, Downs MP, eds. Auditory disorders in school children. New York: Thieme Medical Publishers, 1995.

Edwards C. Auditory intervention for children with mild auditory deficits. In: Bess FH, Gravel JS, Tharpe AM, eds. Amplification for children with auditory deficits. Nashville, TN: Bill Wilkerson Center Press, 1996.

Elfenbein JL. Coping with communication breakdown—a program of strategy development for children who have hearing losses. Am J Audiol 1992;1:25–29.

Elfenbein JL, Bentler RA, Davis JM, et al. Status of school children's hearing aids relative to monitoring practices. Ear Hear 1988;9:212–217

Elliot L. Effects of noise and perception of speech by children and certain handicapped individuals. Sound Vibrat 1992;December:9–14.

Elliot L, Katz D. Development of a new children's test of speech discrimination (Technical Manual). St. Louis, MO: Auditec, 1980.

Feagans L. Otitis media: a model for long term effects with implications for intervention. In Kavanagh J, ed. Otitis media and child development. Parkton, MD: York, 1986.

Finitzo-Hieber T, Gerling IJ, Matkin ND, Cherow-Skalka E. A sound effects recogniton test for the pediatric audiological evaluation. Ear Hear 1980;1(5):271–276.

Finitzo-Hieber T, Tillman R. Room acoustic effects on monosyllabic word discrimination ability for normal and hearing-impaired children. J Speech Hear Res 1978;21: 440–458.

Flexer C. Turn on sound: an odyssey of sound field amplification. Educ Audiol Assoc Newsletter 1989;5:6.

Flexer C. Rationale for the use of sound-field FM amplification systems in classrooms. In: Crandell C, Smaldino J, Flexer C, eds. Sound-field amplification: theory and practical applications. San Diego: Singular, 1995

Flexer C, Millin J, Brown L. Children with developmental disabilities: the effects of sound filed amplification in word identification. Lang Speech Hear Serv Schools 1990;21:177–182.

Flexer C, Richards C, Blue C. Soundfield amplification for regular kindergarten and first grade classrooms: a longitudinal study of fluctuating hearing loss and pupil performance. Paper presented at the American Academy of Audiology Annual Convention, Phoenix, Arizona, April 1993.

Friel-Patti S, Finitzo T. Language learning in a prospective study of otitis media with effusion in the first two years of life. J Speech Hear Res 1990;33:188–194.

Gaeth JH, Lounsbury E. Hearing aids and children in elementary schools. J Speech Hear Dis 1966;31:283–289.

Gravel JS, Nozza RJ. Hearing loss among children with OME. In: Roberts J, Wallace I, Henderson F, eds. Otitis media in young children. Baltimore: Paul H. Brookes, 1997.

Gravel JS, Wallace IF. Listening and language at four years of age: effects of early otitis media. J Speech Hear Res 1992;35:588–595.

Gravel JS, Wallace IF. Early otitis media, auditory abilities and educational risk. Am J Speech Lang Pathol 1995; 4:89–94.

Gravel JS, Wallace IF. Audiological management of otitis media with effusion. In: Bess F, ed. Children with auditory disabilities: proceedings of the fourth international symposium on childhood deafness. Nashville, TN: Bill Wilkerson Press, 1998.

Grievink E, Peters S, van Bon W, et al. The effects of early bilateral otitis media with effusion on language ability: a prospective cohort study. J Speech Hear Res 1993;36: 1004–1012.

Haskins H. A phonetically balanced test of speech discrimination for children. Unpublished master's thesis. Northwestern University, Evanston, IL, 1949.

Holm VA, Kunze LK. Effect of chronic otitis media on language and speech development. Pediatrics 1969;43:833–839.

Howie VM. (1979). Developmental sequelae of chronic otitis media: the effect of early onset of otitis media on educational achievement. Int J Pediatr Otorhinolaryngol 1979;1:151–155.

Hynd GW, Semrud-Clikeman M, Lorys AR, et al. Brain morphology in developmental dyslexia and attention deficit disorder/hyperactivity. Arch Neurol 1990;47:916–919.

Hynd GW, Semrud-Clikeman M, Lyytinen H. Brain imaging in learning disabilities. In: Obrzut JE, Hynd GW, eds. Neuropsychological foundations of learning disabilities. San Diego: Academic Press, 1991:475–511.

Jerger S, Jerger J. The Pediatric Sentence Intelligibility test (PSI). St. Louis: Auditec, 1984.

Johnson, DeConde C. Amplification in inclusive classrooms. J Educ Audiol 1998;6:33–44.

Johnson, DeConde C, VonAlmen P. The functional listening evaluation. 1993. In: Johnson CD, Benson PV, Seaton J. Educational audiology handbook Appendix 4-C. San Diego: Singular, 1997.

Johnson, DeConde C, Benson PV, Seaton J. Educational audiology handbook. San Diego: Singular, 1997a.

Johnson CD, Owens L. Common children's phrases. In: CD Johnson, et al. Educational audiology handbook. San Diego: Singular, 1997;Appendix 15F:488–489.

Johnson CE, Stein R, Broadway A, et al. "Minimal" high-frequency hearing loss and school-aged children: speech recognition in a classroom. Lang Speech Hear Serv School 1997b;28:77–85.

Jones J, Berg F, Viehweg S. Listening of kindergarten students under close, distant, and sound field FM amplification conditions. Educ Audiol Assoc 1989;1:56–65.

Kalikow D, Stevens K, Elliott L. Development of a test of speech intelligibility in noise using sentence material with controlled word predictability. J Acoust Society Am 1977;61:1337–1351.

Kemker FJ, McConnell F, Logn SA, et al. A field study of children's hearing aids in a school environment. Lang Speech Hear Serv 1979;10:47–53.

Kirk K, Diefendorf A, Pisoni DB, et al. Assessing speech perception in children. In: Lucks Mendel L, Danhauer J, eds. Audiological evaluation and management and speech perception assessment. San Diego: Singular, 1997.

Klein J. Risk factors for otitis media in children. In Kavanagh J, ed. Otitis media and child development. Parkton, MD: York, 1986.

Mendel Lucks L, Danhauer J. Historical review of speech perception assessment. In: Lucks Mendel L, Danhauer J, eds. Audiological evaluation and management and speech perception assessment. San Diego: Singular, 1997.

Menyuk P. Predicting speech and language problems with persistent otitis media. In: Kavanagh J, ed. Otitis media and child development. Parkton, MD: York, 1986.

Merzenich NM, Jenkins WM. (1995). Cortical plasticity, learning, and learning dysfunction. In: Julez B, Kovacs I, eds. Maturational windows and adult cortical plasticity proceedings. New York: Addison-Wesley, 1995;22:247–272.

Merzenich NM, Jenkins WM, Johnston P, et al. Temporal processing deficits of language-learning impaired children ameliorated by training. Science 1996;271:77–80.

Mody M, Schwartz R, Gravel J, et al. Speech perception and verbal memory in children with otitis media. In: Lim D, Bluestone C, Casselbrant M, Klein K, Ogra P. Recent advances in otitis media: proceedings of the Sixth International Symposium, Toronto: BC Decker, 1996;339–342.

Montegomery J, Fujikawa S. Hearing thresholds of students in the second, eighth, and twelfth grades. Lang Speech Hear Serv Sch 1992;23:61–63.

Moog JS, Kozal VJ, Geers AE. Grammatical analysis of elicited language pre-sentence level. St. Louis, MO: Central Institute for the Deaf, 1983.

Moog JS, Geers AE. Early speech perception test for profoundly hearing impaired children. St. Louis, MO: Central Institute for the Deaf, 1990.

Nebelek A, Nebelek I. Room acoustics and speech perception. In Katz J, ed. Handbook of clinical audiology. 3rd ed. Baltimore: Williams & Wilkins, 1985.

Nebelek A, Pickett J. Reception of consonants in a classroom as affected by monaural and binaural listening, noise, reverberation, and hearing aids. J Acoust Soc Am 1974;56: 628–639.

Nelson EC, Wasson JH, Johnson D, et al. Dartmouth COOP functional health assessment charts: brief measures for clinical practice. In: Spilker B, ed. Quality of life and pharmacoeconomics in clinical trials. 2nd ed. Philadelphia: Lippincott-Raven, 1996:161–168.

Niskar AS, Kieszak S, Holmes A, et al. Prevalence of hearing loss among children 6 to 19 years of age: the third national health and nutrition examination survey. JAMA 1998;279:1071–1075.

Oyler RF, Oyler AL, Matkin ND. Warning: a unilateral hearing loss may be detrimental to a child's academic career. Hear J 1987;9:18–22.

Oyler RF, Oyler AL, Matkin ND. Unilateral hearing loss: demographics and educational impact. Lang Speech Hear Serv Schools 1988;19:201–210.

Potts PL, Greenwood J. Hearing aid monitoring: Are we looking and listening enough? Lang Speech Hear Serv Sch 1983;14:157–163.

Pinheiro ML, Musiek FE. Sequencing and temporal ordering in the auditory system. In: Pinheiro ML, Musiek FE, eds. Assessment of central auditory dysfunction: foundations and clinical correlates. Baltimore: Williams & Wilkins, 1985:219–238.

Quay HC, Peterson DR. Manual for the revised behavior problem checklist. Coral Gables, FL: University of Miami, 1987.

Robbins AM, Renshaw JJ, Berry SW. Evaluating Meaningful auditory integration in profoundly hearing impaired children. American J Otology 1991;12(Suppl): 144–150.

Robbins AM, Renshaw JJ, Osberger MJ. Common Phrases Test. Indianapolis. In: Indiana University School of Medicine, 1995.

Roberts JE, Wallace IF. Language and otitis media. In: Roberts J, Wallace I, Henderson F, eds. Otitis media in young children. Baltimore: Paul H. Brookes, 1997.

Roberts JE, Burchinal MR, Davis BP, et al. Otitis media in early childhood and later language. J Speech Hear Res 1991;34:1158–1168.

Ross M, Lerman J. A picture identification test for hearing impaired children. J Speech Hear Res 1979;13:44–53.

Ross M, Brackett D, Maxon AB. Assessment and management of mainstreamed hearing-impaired children. Austin: Pro-ed. 1991, 3.

Sarff L. An innovative use of free-field amplification in classrooms. In: Roesser R, Downs M, eds. Auditory disorders in school children. New York: Thieme-Stratton, 1981:263–272.

Sarff L, Ray H, Bagwell C. Why not amplification in every classroom? Hear Aid J 1981;34:11.

Shurin P, Johnson C, Wegman D. Medical aspects of diagnosis and prevention of otitis media. In: Kavanagh J, ed. Otitis media and child development. Parkton, MD: York, 1986.

Tallal P. Auditory temporal perception, phonics and reading disabilities in children. Brain Lang 1980;9:192–198.

Tallal P, Stark R. Speech acoustic-cue discrimination abilities of normally developing and language impaired children. J Acoust Soc Am 1981;69:568–578.

Tallal P, Stark R, Mellits D. Identification of language-impaired children on the basis of rapid perception and production skills. Brain Lang 1985;25:314–322.

Tallal P, Miller S, Bedi G, et al. Language comprehension in language-learning impaired children improved with acoustically modified speech. Science 1996;271:81–84.

Teele D, Klein J, Rosner B. Epidemiology of otitis media in children. Ann Otol Rhinol Laryngol 1980;89:5–6.

Teele D, Klein J, Rosner B. Otitis media with effusion in the first three years of life and development of speech and language. Pediatrics 1984;74:282–287.

Teele D, Klein J, Chase C, et al. The Greater Boston Otitis Media Study Group. Otitis media in infancy and intellectual ability, school achievement, speech and language at age 7 years. J Infect Dis 1990;162:685–694.

Todd NW. High risk populations for otitis media. In: Kavanagh J, ed. Otitis media and child development. Parkton, MD: York, 1986.

Tye-Murray N (ed.). Let's converse! A how to guide to develop and expand the conversational skills of children and teenagers who are hearing impaired. Washington, DC: Alexander Graham Bell Association.

U.S. Department of Education. Nineteenth annual report to Congress on the implementation of the Individuals with Disabilities Education Act. Washington, DC: U.S. Government Printing Office, 1998:A-175.

Yoshinaga-Itano C. Factors predictive of successful outcomes of deaf and hard of hearing children of hearing parents. Paper presented at the National Symposium on Infant Hearing, Denver, Colorado, July, 1998.

Yoshinaga-Itano C, Sedey A, Coulter D, et al. Language of early- and later-identified children with hearing loss. Pediatrics 1998;102:1161–1171.

Zabel H, Tabor M. Effects of classroom amplification on spelling performance of elementary school children. Educ Audiol Monogr 1993;3:5–9.

Zink CD. Hearing aids children wear: A longitudinal study of performance. Volta Rev 1972;74:41–51.

| APPENDIX **8.1** | *IDEA: Definitions Pertaining to Hearing Loss and Audiology* |

IDEA-Part B
Definition of Audiology (34CFR300. 24(b)1)

(i)   Identification of children with hearing loss;

(ii) Determination of the range, nature, and degree of hearing loss, including referral for medical or other professional attention for the habilitation of hearing;

(iii) Provision of habilitation activities, such as language habilitation, auditory training, speechreading, (lipreading), hearing evaluation, and speech conservation;

(iv) Creation and administration of programs for prevention of hearing loss;

(v)   Counseling and guidance of pupils, parents, and teachers regarding hearing loss;

(vi) Determination of the child's need for group and individual amplification, selecting and fitting an appropriate aid, and evaluating the effectiveness of amplification.

IDEA-Part C Definition of Audiology (34CFR303.12(d))

(i)   Identification of children with impairments, using at risk criteria and appropriate audiological screening techniques;

(ii) Determination of the range, nature, and degree of hearing loss and communication functions, by use of audiologic evaluation procedures;

(iii) Referral for medical and other services necessary for the habilitation or rehabilitation of children with auditory impairment;

(iv) Provision of auditory training, aural rehabilitation, speechreading and listening device orientation and training, and other services;

(v)   Provision of services for the prevention of hearing loss; and

(vi) Determination of the child's need for individual amplification, including selecting, fitting, and dispensing of appropriate listening and vibrotactile devices, and evaluating the effectiveness of those devices.

IDEA-Part B Proper Functioning of Hearing Aids (34CFR300.303)

Each public agency shall ensure that the hearing aids worn in school by children with hearing impairment, including deafness, are functioning properly.

IDEA-Part B & Part C: Assistive Technology
(34CFR300.5–6; 34CFR303.12)

Assistive technology devices and services are necessary if a child with a disability requires the device and services in order to receive a free and appropriate education (FAPE); the public agency must ensure that they are made available.

"Assistive technology device" means any item, piece of equipment, or product system, whether acquired commercially off the shelf, modified, or customized, that is used to increase, maintain, or improve the functional capabilities of children with disabilities.

"Assistive technology service" means any service that directly assists a child with a disability in the selection, acquisition, or use of an assistive technology device. The term includes

(a) The evaluation of the needs of a child with a disability, including a functional evaluation of the child in the child's customary environment;

(b) Purchasing, leasing, or otherwise providing for the acquisition of assistive technology devices by children with disabilities;

(c) Selecting, designing, fitting, customizing, adapting, applying, retaining, repairing, or replacing assistive technology devices;

(d) Coordinating and using other therapies, interventions, or services with assistive technology devices, such as those associated with existing education and rehabilitation plans and programs;

(e) Training or technical assistance for a child with a disability or, if appropriate, that child's family; and

(f) Training or technical assistance for professionals (including individuals providing education or rehabilitation services), employers, or other individuals who provide services to, employ, or are otherwise substantially involved in the major life functions of children with disabilities.

Definitions: IDEA-Part B (34CFR300.7(b))

[2] "Deaf-blindness" means concomitant hearing and visual impairments, the combination of which causes such severe communication and other developmental and educational problems that they cannot be accommodated in special education programs solely for children with deafness or children with blindness.

[3] "Deafness" means a hearing impairment that is so severe that the child is impaired in processing linguistic information through hearing, with or without amplification, that adversely affects a child's educational performance.

[5] "Hearing impairment" means an impairment in hearing, whether permanent or fluctuating, that adversely affects a child's educational performance but that is not included under the definition in this section.

S.I.F.T.E.R.—SAMPLE

SCREENING INSTRUMENT FOR TARGETING EDUCATIONAL RISK

By Karen L. Anderson, Ed.S., CCC-A

STUDENT _____   TEACHER _____   GRADE _____

DATE COMPLETED _____   SCHOOL _____   DISTRICT _____

The above child is suspect for hearing problems which may or may not be affecting his/her school performance. This rating scale has been designed to sift out students who are educationally at risk possibly as a result of hearing problems.

Based on your knowledge from observations of this student, circle the number best representing his/her behavior. After answering the questions, please record any comments about the student in the space provided on the reverse side.

1.	What is your estimate of the student's class standing in comparison of that of his/her classmates?	UPPER 5	4	MIDDLE 3	2	LOWER 1			
2.	How does the student's achievement compare to your estimation of his/her potential?	EQUAL 5	4	LOWER 3	2	MUCH LOWER 1	ACADEMICS	☐	
3.	What is the student's reading level, reading ability group or reading readiness group in the classroom (e.g., a student with average reading ability performs in the middle group)?	UPPER 5	4	MIDDLE 3	2	LOWER 1			
4.	How distractible is the student in comparison to his/her classmates?	NOT VERY 5	4	AVERAGE 3	2	VERY 1			
5.	What is the student's attention span in comparison to that of his/her classmates?	LONGER 5	4	AVERAGE 3	2	SHORTER 1	ATTENTION	☐	
6.	How often does the student hesitate or become confused when responding to oral directions (e.g., "Turn to page . . .")?	NEVER 5	4	OCCASIONALLY 3	2	FREQUENTLY 1			
7.	How does the student's comprehension compare to the average understanding ability of his/her classmates?	ABOVE 5	4	AVERAGE 3	2	BELOW 1			
8.	How does the student's vocabulary and word usage skills compare with those of other students in his/her age group?	ABOVE 5	4	AVERAGE 3	2	BELOW 1	COMMUNICATION	☐	
9.	How proficient is the student at telling a story or relating happenings from home when compared to classmates?	ABOVE 5	4	AVERAGE 3	2	BELOW 1			
10.	How often does the student volunteer information to class discussions or in answers to teacher questions?	FREQUENTLY 5	4	OCCASIONALLY 3	2	NEVER 1			
11.	With what frequency does the student complete his/her class and homework assignments within the time allocated?	ALWAYS 5	4	USUALLY 3	2	SELDOM 1	CLASS PARTICIPATION	☐	
12.	After instruction, does the student have difficulty starting to work (looks at other students working or asks for help)?	NEVER 5	4	OCCASIONALLY 3	2	FREQUENTLY 1			
13.	Does the student demonstrate any behaviors that seem unusual or inappropriate when compared to other students?	NEVER 5	4	OCCASIONALLY 3	2	FREQUENTLY 1			
14.	Does the student become frustrated easily, sometimes to the point of losing emotional control?	NEVER 5	4	OCCASIONALLY 3	2	FREQUENTLY 1	SCHOOL BEHAVIOR	☐	
15.	In general, how would you rank the student's relationship with peers (ability to get along with others)?	GOOD 5	4	AVERAGE 3	2	POOR 1			

Copyright © 1989 by Karen Anderson

TEACHER COMMENTS

Has this child repeated a grade, had frequent absences or experienced health problems (including ear infections and colds)? Has the student received, or is he/she now receiving, special support services? Does the child have any other health problems that may be pertinent to his/her educational functioning?

The S.I.F.T.E.R. is a SCREENING TOOL ONLY

Any student failing this screening in a content area as determined on the scoring grid below should be considered for further assessment, depending on his/her individual needs as per school district criteria. For example, failing in the Academics area suggests an educational assessment, in the Communication area a speech-language assessment, and in the School Behavior area an assessment by a psychologist or a social worker. Failing in the Attention and/or Class Participation area in combination with other areas may suggest an evaluation by an educational audiologist. Children placed in the marginal area are at risk for failing and should be monitored or considered for assessment depending upon additional information.

SCORING

Sum the responses to the three questions in each content area and record in the appropriate box on the reverse side and under Total Score below. Place an **X** on the number that corresponds most closely with the content area score (e.g., if a teacher circled 3, 4 and 2 for the questions in the Academics area, an **X** would be placed on the number 9 across from the Academics content area). Connect the **X**'s to make a profile.

CONTENT AREA	TOTAL SCORE	PASS						MARGINAL		FAIL				
ACADEMICS		15	14	13	12	11	10	9	8	7	6	5	4	3
ATTENTION		15	14	13	12	11	10 9		8	7	6	5	4	3
COMMUNICATION		15	14	13		12	11	10	9	8	7	6 5	4	3
CLASS PARTICIPATION		15	14	13	12 11	10	9	8		7	6	5	4	3
SOCIAL BEHAVIOR		15	14	13	12	11	10	9	8	7	6	5	4	3

ᵒFrom Anderson KL. Screening instrument for targeting educational risk in children (SIFTER). 1989. Reprinted with permission from the Educational Audiology Association, 4319 Ehrlich Road, Tampa, FL 33624.

APPENDIX
8.3 *Auditory Management Resources*

Common Speech Perception Tests for Children

Words
  Word Intelligibility for Picture Identification (WIPI)—Ross and Lerman, 1979
  Northwestern University-Children's Perception of Speech (NU-CHIPS)—Elliott and Katz, 1980
  PBK-50 Word List—Haskins, 1949
  Grammatical Analysis Elicited Language-Modified Single Word Task—Moog et al., 1983
  Early Speech Perception Test (ESP), standard and low-verbal versions—Moog and Geers, 1990
Phrases
  The Common Phrases Test—Robbins et al., 1995
  Common Children's Phrases—Johnson and Owens, 1997
Sentences
  Bamford-Kowal-Bench Sentences (BKB)—Bench et al., 1979
  Pediatric Sentence Inventory—Jerger and Jerger, 1984
  Speech Intelligibility in Noise sentences (SPIN)—Kalilkow et al., 1977
Other
  Sound Effects Recognition Test (SERT)—Finitzo-Hieber et al., 1980
  Meaningful Auditory Integration Scale (MAIS)—Robbins et al., 1991
  Craig Lipreading Inventory—Craig, 1992

Auditory Curricula

Auditory Skills Curriculum (1976)
  Foreworks
  Box 82289
  Portland, OR 97282
  503-653-2614
Developmental Approach to Successful Listening (DASL) II (1992)
  Resource Point
  61 Inverness Drive East, Suite 200
  Englewood, CO 80112-9726
  800-688-8788
The SKI-HI Model: A Resource Manual for Family-Centered, Home-Based Programming
    for Infants, Toddlers, and Pre-School-Aged Children with Hearing Impairment (1993)
  SKI*HI Institute
  Department of Communication Disorders
  Utah State University
  Logan, UT 84322-1900
Parent-Infant Communication (4th Edition, 1998)
  Infant Hearing Resource
  Hearing & Speech Institute
  3515 SW Veterans Hospital Road
  Portland, OR 97201
  503-228-6479

SPICE: Speech Perception Instructional Curriculum and Evaluation (1996)
Central Institute for the Deaf
818 S. Euclid Avenue
St. Louis, MO 63110
314-977-0133
Let's Converse: A how-to guide to develop and expand the conversational skills of children
and teenagers who are hearing impaired (1994) N. Tye-Murray.
Alexander Graham Bell Association for the Deaf and Hard of Hearing
3417 Volta Place NW
Washington, DC 20007-2778
202–337–5220

Hearing Awareness Programs

HIP Magazine
1563 Solano Ave, #137
Berkeley, CA 94707

KIP-Knowledge is Power
Audiological & Education HI Services Department
Attn: KIP
Mississippi Bend Area Education Agency
729-21st St.
Bettendorf, IA 52722-5096

Self-Advocacy for Students who are Deaf and Hard of Hearing
Kristina M. English
Pro-Ed
8700 Shoal Creek Boulevard
Austin, TX 78757-9965
512-451-3246

APPENDIX 8.4 *The Functional Listening Evaluation*[b]

Cheryl DeConde Johnson
Weld County School District 6, Greeley, Co

Peggy Von Almen
Utah State University

Purpose of the Functional Listening Evaluation

The purpose of this evaluation is to determine how a student's listening abilities are affected by noise, distance, and visual input. It is designed to simulate the student's listening ability in a situation that is more representative of his or her actual listening environment than the sound booth. This protocol is based on a listening paradigm suggested by Ying (1990) and Ross et al. (1991).

Materials Needed

Cassette tape recorder
Sound level meter (can be purchased inexpensively from Radio Shack)

Noise tape (Multi-talker babble—can be purchased from Auditec, St. Louis, MO)
Tripod or stand to hold sound level matter (optional)
Sentence/word lists for scoring
Tape measure or yard stick
Masking take or marker (optional)

Environment for Testing

Use the student's classroom during a time when it is empty; if this is not possible choose a room that most closely simulates the size, ambient noise level, and floor and wall surfaces of the student's classroom.

Physical Set-up of Test Environment

Close: Noise and examiner are 3 feet in front of the student (Diagram A).
Distant: Noise remains 3 feet in front of the student; examiner moves back to a distance of 15 feet from the student (Diagram B).

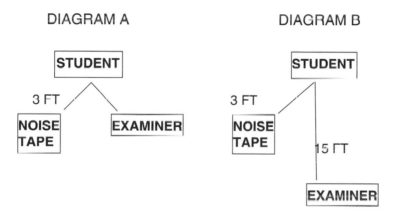

For ease these distances can be marked with masking tape on the floor; be sure that the markers are from the student's ear to the examiner's mouth.

Types of Evaluation Materials

Whenever possible sentence material should be used since it is more like speech encountered in the classroom. However, due to age and limited language and memory abilities of some students, it may be necessary to use single words. In selecting either sentence or word materials caution should be used to ensure that the vocabulary and sentence structure are appropriate for the student's language ability. When the student has poor speech intelligibility, it may be necessary to use materials which allow picture-pointing responses.

Possible Sentence Materials:	BLAIR Sentences	WIPI Sentences
	SPIN Sentences (older students)	BKB Sentences
	PSI Sentences	
Possible Word Lists:	PB-K	NU-CHIPS
	WIPI	

In most cases there will not be enough lists for the entire protocol (8 lists are needed). When selecting lists to repeat, try to use lists which were more difficult for the student.

Presentation Levels

Speech: Monitor with sound level meter so that speech averages 75 dBA at 1 foot from the examiner's mouth.

Noise: Set with sound level meter so that noise, which is 3 feet from the student, averages 60 dBA at the student's ear.

This will result in a signal-to-noise ratio of $+3$ dB in the close condition. The signal-to-noise ratio in the distant condition will vary depending upon the acoustics of the room, but it will be approximately -5 dB.

Presentation Protocol

The evaluation should be conducted in the student's typical hearing mode. If hearing aids are usually worn at school, they should also be worn during the evaluation. This protocol can also be used to demonstrate the improved listening ability with FM amplification.

Eight sentence or word lists should be presented in the following order, as indicated by the numbers on the scoring matrix:

1.	AUDITORY-VISUAL	CLOSE	QUIET
2.	AUDITORY	CLOSE	QUIET
3.	AUDITORY-VISUAL	CLOSE	NOISE
4.	AUDITORY	CLOSE	NOISE
5.	AUDITORY-VISUAL	DISTANT	NOISE
6.	AUDITORY	DISTANT	NOISE
7.	AUDITORY	DISTANT	QUIET
8.	AUDITORY-VISUAL	DISTANT	QUIET

This order was selected to present easier tasks at the beginning and end of the protocol.

The examiner should present the speech materials at a normal, but not slow, rate. The student should repeat the test stimuli or point to the appropriate picture, as dictated by the material used.

It will take approximately 30 minutes to set up and administer the test protocol if sentences are used as the stimulus. If words are used, the protocol will take about 20 minutes.

Scoring

Scoring should be done using the protocol established for the selected test materials. All scores should be reported in percent correct.

Variations in Protocol

This protocol is based on the listening situation in a typical classroom. For an individual student, it may be useful to modify this protocol to account for variations in the level and source of noise, classroom size, typical listening distances for the student, or other factors. In order to accommodate these variations, the following modifications should be considered:

1. Placement of noise/tape recorder.
2. Distance of examiner from student for the distant condition.
3. Level of noise.
4. Order of presentation.

Any modifications of the typical protocol should be noted on the test form.

Interpretation

In order to interpret the effects of noise, distance, and visual input for the individual student, the conditions can be compared on the Interpretation Matrix. These scores can be used to determine educational modifications which would be beneficial for the student. They can also be shared with the student's parents and teachers to help them understand their student's listening abilities and needs.

Scores may be affected by different speakers, rate of speaking, attention of the listener, or status of amplification. As long as variables are kept constant throughout the evaluation, comparisons can be made.

REFERENCES

Ross M, Brackett D, Maxon A. Communication assessment. In: Assessment and management of mainstreamed hearing-impaired children. Austin, Tx: Pro-Ed, 1991:113–127.

Ying E. Speech and language assessment: communication evaluation. In: Ross M, ed. Hearing-impaired children in the mainstream. Parkton, MD: York, 1990;45–60.

FUNCTIONAL LISTENING EVALUATION
Cheryl DeConde Johnson & Peggy VonAlmen, 1993.

NAME: _____   DATE: _____

EXAMINER: _____   AGE/DOB: _____

AUDIOMETRIC RESULTS

HEARING SENSITIVITY: PURE TONE AVE: RIGHT EAR ____ LEFT EAR ____

WORD RECOGNITION: RIGHT EAR ____ % @ ____ dBHL LEFT EAR ____ % @ ____ dBHL

SOUND FIELD: ____ AIDED ____ UNAIDED

QUIET ____ % @ ____ dBHL

NOISE ____ % @ ____ dBHL @ ____ S/N

FUNCTIONAL LISTENING EVALUATION CONDITIONS

AMPLIFICATION: ____ NONE ____ HEARING AIDS ____ FM ____ SOUND FIELD

____ OTHER

CLASSROOM AMBIENT NOISE LEVEL: ____ dBA

ASSESSMENT MATERIAL: SENTENCES ____ WORDS ____

MODIFICATION IN PROTOCOL:

FUNCTIONAL LISTENING MATRIX SCORES

	CLOSE/QUIET	CLOSE/NOISE	DISTANT/QUIET	DISTANT/NOISE
AUDITORY-VISUAL	1	3	8	5
AUDITORY	2	4	7	6

INTERPRETATION MATRIX

NOISE

	QUIET	NOISE
CLOSE-AUD	2	4
CLOSE-AUD/VIS	1	3
DISTANT-AUD	7	6
DISTANT-AUD/VIS	8	5

Average of above scores: ____ % QUIET   ____ % NOISE

	QUIET-AUD	QUIET-AUD/VIS	NOISE-AUD	NOISE-AUD/VIS

DISTANCE

	CLOSE	DISTANT
	2	7
	1	8
	4	6
	3	5

____ % CLOSE   ____ % DISTANT

VISUAL INPUT

	AUD-VIS	AUD
CLOSE-QUIET	1	2
CLOSE-NOISE	3	4
DISTANT-NOISE	5	6
DISTANT-QUIET	8	7

____ % AUD/VIS   ____ % AUD

INTERPRETATION AND RECOMMENDATIONS

[b]From Johnson DeConde C, VonAlmen P. Appendix 4-C pp 336–339. Reprinted with permission from Johnson DeConde C, Benson PV, Seaton JB. Educational audiology handbook. San Diego: Singular, 1997.

APPENDIX 8.5

*Listening Development Profile*c

Listening Development Profile

Name _____ DOB _____ Ages @ ID _____

Age @ beginning intervention _____Age @ initial amplification _____   Type/Model _____

Amplification:

Date														
Unaided AI														
Aided AI														
Hrs/day of HA use														
ALD used/ freq of use														

Rating: 1 = skill introduced   Mode: AVQ = auditory-visual/quiet
2 = skill emerging   AQ = auditory/quiet
3 = skill in progress   AVN = auditory-visual/noise
4 = skill established   AN = auditory/noise

Stage 1: Beginning Listener

STUDENT OUTCOMES	PERFORMANCE INDICATORS	RATING: MODE/DATE			
		1	2	3	4
• increases auditory detection/ awareness	• can differentiate the presence or absence of sound				
	• responds to sounds around the home, e.g., doorbell, telephone (response may be voluntary or involuntary)				
	• responds to people's voices				
	• increases time on listening task				
• directs attention to sound (auditory localization)	• turns head in response to sound				
	• turns directly to sound source				
• increases linguistic interaction	• parents use appropriate communication strategies (turntaking, eye contact, child initiated conversation)				
	• child begins to demonstrate age appropriate conversation behavior				
• increases auditory attention	• child indicates desire to wear hearing aids, amplification device & demonstrates a listening attitude				

Stage 2 - Intermediate Listener

• identifies when amplifica- tion is not working	• child reports that equipment is not working without prompting				
• demonstrates benefit of listening	• student enjoys listening tasks, initiates desire to hear				
	• startled response (loud sounds)				
• responds to loud/quiet sounds	• says "huh" or looks puzzled (quiet sounds)				
	• demonstrates use of appropriate loud vs quiet sound				
• responds to fast/slow sounds	• moves appropriately to speed of sound				
	• demonstrates fast & slow through vocalizations				
• responds to high/low sounds	• matches pitch of voice				
	• demonstrates high & low through vocalizations				

• understands rhythm of songs	• follows rhythmic patterns of songs				
• understands words in songs	• performs action, i.e., demonstrates understanding of words				
• increases linguistic interaction	• uses more complex sentence forms and vocabulary				
	• discriminates words with similar speech sounds (bat vs pat)				
	• uses language for a variety of purposes				
	• uses appropriate intonation patterns				

Stage 3: Advanced Listener

• participates in groups -listens in groups -uses appropriate language & conversation rules	• takes turns				
	• uses appropriate clarification strategies for misunderstood messages				
	• uses discussion to complete assignments				
	• uses phrases appropriately for content				
• increases awareness of pronunciation of words, phrases, sound & symbol connections	• asks for auditory representation or repetition of words so that he/she can internalize auditory images (modeling)				
• increases use of words/ concepts in various contexts	• discriminates/self corrects between correct & incorrect productions				
• increases responsibility for understanding oral messages	• follows multi-step instructions				
	• more frequent interactions with teachers, peers				
	• reduce frequency of conversation repair ("huh," "what," "I didn't understand")				
• begins to troubleshoot amplification systems	• reports dead battery or static sounds, intermittency, spill over of signal, clogged mold				
• advocates for services	• asks teacher to check transmitter using appropriate language				

Stage 4: Sophisticated Listener/Communicator

• demonstrates knowledge of audiograms	• explains audiograms in terms of degree and configuration (shape)				
• knowledge of various types of amplification & assistive devices (HA, ALD, TDD, captioner, phone)	• discuss characteristics of various hearing aids, cochlear implants & assistive devices				
	• demonstrates appropriate use of ALD, TDD, captioner, phone				
• uses amplification equipment appropriately	• reports malfunctioning equipment & conducts basic troubleshooting				
• increases awareness of communication/listening environment & appropriate accommodations	• requests appropriate physical accommodations (seating, sound system, etc.)				
	• requests appropriate support services (interpreter, captioning, written materials, notetaker)				
• utilizes professionals & agencies appropriately (audiology, ENT, SLP, inter-preter, relay systems, voca-tional rehabilitation, etc.)	• identifies roles of professionals & community agencies				
	• uses professionals & community services appropriately				
• able to educate others about hearing loss & its implications	• selects target audience for presentation on hearing & communication				
	• does presentation to peers, other schools				
	• explains listening needs in work situations				

cAdapted from Rizak ZR. The development of successful listening 1994. Reprinted with permission from Johnson De-Conde C, Bensen PV, Seaten JB. Educational audiology handbook. San Diego: Singular, 1997.

Degree of Hearing Loss Based on modified pure tone average (500–4000 HZ)	Possible Effect of Hearing Loss on the Understanding of Language & Speech	Possible Psychosocial Impact of Hearing Loss	Potential Educational Needs and Programs
NORMAL HEARING −10–+15 dB HL	Children have better hearing sensitivity than the accepted normal range for adults. A child with hearing sensitivity in the −10 to +15 dB range will detect the complete speech signal even at soft conversation levels. However, good hearing does not guarantee good ability to discriminate speech in the presence of background noise.		
MINIMAL (BORDERLINE) 16–25 dB HL	May have difficulty hearing faint or distant speech. At 15 dB student can miss up to 10% of speech signal when teacher is at a distance greater than 3 feet and when the classroom is noisy, especially in the elementary grades when verbal instruction predominates	May be unaware of subtle conversational cues which could cause child to be viewed as inappropriate or awkward. May miss portions of fast-paced peer interactions which could begin to have an impact on socialization and self-concept. May have immature behavior. Child may be more fatigued than classmates due to listening effort needed.	May benefit from mild gain/low MPO hearing aid or personal FM system dependent on loss configuration. Would benefit from soundfield amplification if classroom is noisy and/or reverberant. Favorable seating. May need attention to vocabulary or speech, especially with recurrent otitis media history. Appropriate medical management necessary for conductive losses. Teacher requires inservice on impact of hearing loss on language development and learning.
MILD 26–40 dB HL	At 30 dB can miss 25–40% of speech signal. The degree of difficulty experienced in school will depend upon the noise level in classroom, distance from teacher and the configuration of the hearing loss. Without amplification the child with 35–40 dB loss may miss at least 50% of class discussions, especially when voices are faint or speaker is not in line of vision. Will miss consonants, especially when a high frequency hearing loss is present.	Barriers beginning to build with negative impact on self-esteem as child is accused of "hearing when he or she wants to," "daydreaming," or "not paying attention." Child begins to lose ability for selective hearing, and has increasing difficulty suppressing background noise which makes the learning environment stressful. Child is more fatigued than classmates due to listening effort needed.	Will benefit from a hearing aid and use of a personal FM or soundfield FM system in the classroom. Needs favorable seating and lighting. Refer to special education for language evaluation and educational follow-up. Needs auditory skill building. May need attention to vocabulary and language development, articulation or speech reading and/or special support in reading. May need help with self esteem. Teacher inservice required.
MODERATE 41–55 dB HL	Understands conversational speech at a distance of 3–5 feet (face-to-face) only if structure and vocabulary controlled. Without amplification the amount of speech signal missed can be 50% to 75% with 40 dB loss and 80% to 100% with 50 dB loss. Is likely to have delayed or defective syntax, limited vocabulary, imperfect speech production and an atonal voice quality.	Often with this degree of hearing loss, communication is significantly affected, and socialization with peers with normal hearing becomes increasingly difficult. With full time use of hearing aids/FM systems child may be judged as a less competent learner. There is an increasing impact on self-esteem.	Refer to special education for language evaluation and for educational follow-up. Amplification is essential (hearing aids and FM system). Special education support may be needed, especially for primary children. Attention to oral language development, reading and written language. Auditory skill development and speech therapy usually needed. Teacher inservice required.

Degree of Hearing Loss	Possible Effect of Hearing Loss on the Understanding of Language & Speech	Possible Psychosocial Impact of Hearing Loss	Potential Educational Needs and Programs
MODERATE TO SEVERE 56–70 dB HL	Without amplification, conversation must be very loud to be understood. A 55 dB loss can cause child to miss up to 100% of speech information. Will have marked difficulty in school situations requiring verbal communication in both one-to-one and group situations. Delayed language, syntax, reduced speech intelligibility and atonal voice quality likely.	Full-time use of hearing aids/FM systems may result in child being judged by both peers and adults as a less competent learner, resulting in poorer self-concept, social maturity and contributing to a sense of rejection. Inservice to address these attitudes may be helpful.	Full-time use of amplification is essential. Will need resource teacher or special class depending on magnitude of language delay. May require special help in all language skills, language based academic subjects, vocabulary, grammar, pragmatics as well as reading and writing. Probably needs assistance to expand experiential language base. Inservice of mainstream teachers required.
SEVERE 71–90 dB HL	Without amplification may hear loud voices about one foot from ear. When amplified optimally, children with hearing ability of 90 dB or better should be able to identify environmental sounds and detect all the sounds of speech. If loss is of prelingual onset, oral language and speech may not develop spontaneously or will be severely delayed. If hearing loss is of recent onset speech is likely to deteriorate with quality becoming atonal.	Child may prefer other children with hearing impairments as friends and playmates. This may further isolate the child from the mainstream; however, these peer relationships may foster improved self-concept and a sense of cultural identity.	May need full-time special aural/oral program for with emphasis on all auditory language skills, speechreading, concept development and speech. As loss approaches 80–90 dB, may benefit from a Total Communication approach, especially in the early language learning years. Individual hearing aid/personal FM system essential. Need to monitor effectiveness of communication modality. Participation in regular classes as much as beneficial to student. Inservice of mainstream teachers essential.
PROFOUND 91 dB HL or more	Aware of vibrations more than tonal pattern. Many rely on vision rather than hearing as primary avenue for communication and learning. Detection of speech sounds dependent upon loss of configuration and use of amplification. Speech and language will not develop spontaneously and are likely to deteriorate rapidly if hearing loss is of recent onset.	Depending on auditory/oral competence, peer use of sign language, parental attitude, etc., child may or may not increasingly prefer association with the deaf culture.	May need special program for deaf children with emphasis on all language skills and academic areas. Program needs specialized supervision and comprehensive support services. Early use of amplification likely to help if part of an intensive training program. May be cochlear implant or vibrotactile aid candidate. Requires continual appraisal of needs in regard to communication and learning mode. Part-time in regular classes as much as beneficial to student.
UNILATERAL One normal hearing ear and one ear with at least a permanent mild hearing loss	May have difficulty hearing faint or distant speech. Usually has difficulty localizing sounds and voices. Unilateral listener will have greater difficulty understanding speech when environment is noisy and/or reverberant. Difficulty detecting or understanding soft speech from side of bad ear, especially in a group discussion.	Child may be accused of selective hearing due to discrepancies in speech understanding in quiet versus noise. Child will be more fatigued in classroom setting due to greater effort needed to listen. May appear inattentive or frustrated. Behavior problems sometimes evident.	May benefit from personal FM or soundfield FM system in classroom. CROS hearing aid may be of benefit in quiet settings. Needs favorable seating and lighting. Student is at risk for educational difficulties. Educational monitoring warranted with support services provided as soon as difficulties appear. Teacher inservice is beneficial.

NOTE: All children with hearing loss require periodic audiologic evaluation, rigorous monitoring of amplification and regular monitoring of communication skills. All children with hearing loss (especially conductive) need appropriate medical attention in conjunction with educational programming.

REFERENCES

Olsen, W. O., Hawkins, D. B., VanTassell, D. J. (1987). Representatives of the Longterm Spectrum of Speech. *Ear & Hearing*, Supplement 8, pp. 100–108.

Mueller, H. G. & Killion, M. C. (1990). An easy method for calculating the articulation index. *The Hearing Journal*, 43, 9, pp. 14–22.

Hasenstab, M. S. (1987). *Language Learning and Otitis Media*, College Hill Press, Boston, MA.

Developed by Karen L. Anderson, Ed.S & Noel D. Matkin, Ph.D (1991)

Adapted from: Bernero, R. J. & Bothwell, H. (1966). Relationship of Hearing Impairment to Educational Needs. Illinois Department of Public Health & Office of Superintendent of Public Instruction.

Peer Review by Members of the Educational Audiology Association, Winter 1991.

APPENDIX
8.7 *Improving Classroom Acoustics[e]*

High noise levels and excessive reverberation of sound in classrooms create educational barriers for children by diminishing their ability to hear and subsequently learn. The following considerations and suggestions specifically target solutions to these problems.

Physical Characteristics of Classroom Design

- Classroom placement within the building should be away from high noise areas such as the gym, cafeteria, and music rooms
- Windows that open should be away from busy streets and playground areas
- Heating, air conditioning and ventilation systems should not exceed a noise level of 35 dBA
- Walls should be permanent—no moveable partitions
- Disproportionately long or circular shaped rooms should be avoided
- Signal-to-noise ratio for teacher's voice should be at least +10 dB; for classrooms with children who are deaf/hard-of-hearing, a +15 dB S/N ratio should be maintained
- Reverberation in the range of 0.4–0.6 sec; for classrooms with children who are deaf/hard-of-hearing
- Reverbation should not exceed 0.4 sec

Adaptations to Improve Acoustics for Classrooms

- Carpet or cork flooring
- Rubber tips on chair legs or desk if carpet is not available
- Drapes for windows and walls
- Cork board for bulletin boards
- Bookshelves as room dividers to create a quiet classroom area
- Cushions in place of chairs
- Mobile bulletin boards position at an angle (not parallel) to walls to reduce reverbation
- Landscaping with trees and burms to reduce outside noise
- Louvered shutters for outside window covers
- Door to hallways closed to reduce noise
- Suspended acoustic tile
- Visual features of classrooms should insure adequate lighting and reduction of reflective surfaces

Classroom Communication Strategies to Enhance Hearing and Listening

Many classroom teachers' management styles naturally incorporate the strategies identified below. The most critical aspect of these strategies is to promote student hearing and access to information.

STRATEGY	BENEFIT
Special seating near teacher or speaker with full face-to-face view	Provides louder, less reverberant signal Provides advantage of visual instruction aides Provides access to visual spoken language Helps maintain attention and interest to tasks

Obtain student's attention through touch or verbal use of name

Train students to "look and listen"

Check student's comprehension of verbal information

Quiet study areas that are free from visual distractions may be helpful

Monitor student for fatigue and length of attending time, providing breaks when necessary

Use of a personal FM system, a classroom amplification system or other assistive listening device

S = state the topic to be discussed

P = pace your conversation at a moderate speed with occasional pauses to permit comprehension

E = enunciate clearly, without exaggerated lip movements

E = enthusiastically communicate, using body language and natural gestures

CH = check comprehension before changing topics

Prepares child for listening

Student will usually comprchend better if watching person who is speaking

Determines student's level of understanding information

Identifies information that needs to be restated

Verifies when student is ready to move on to new material

Helps to minimize problems with auditory and visual distractions, improving concentration and productivity

Permits student to have "down time" and then redirect attention

Improves signal-to-noise level of teacher's voice to provide louder, less reverberant signal

Helps maintain student attention and interest to task

Distributes teacher's voice evenly throughout room (classroom amplification)

Decreases teacher voice fatigue (classroom amplification)

Mnemonic device highlighting basic strategies for dealing with attending, memory, and receptive language deficits

---

*e*Adapted from Central auditory processing disorders: a team approach to screening, assessment and intervention practices. The Colorado Department of Education, 1997.

APPENDIX 8.8 *IEP Checklist: Recommended Accommodations and Modifications for Students with Hearing Impairment[f]*

Name:_____   Date: _____

Amplification Options

_____ Personal hearing device (hearing aid, cochlear implant, tactile device)
_____ Personal FM system (hearing aid + FM)
_____ FM system/auditory trainer (without personal hearing aid)
_____ Walkman-style FM system
_____ Sound-field FM system

Assistive Devices

_____ TDD
_____ TV captioner
_____ Other _____

Communication Accommodations

_____ Specialized seating arrangements:
_____
_____ Obtain student's attention prior to speaking
_____ Reduce auditory distractions (background noise)
_____ Reduce visual distractions
_____ Enhance speechreading conditions (avoid hands in front of face, mustaches well-trimmed, no gum chewing)
_____ Present information in simple, structured, sequential manner
_____ Clearly enunciate speech
_____ Allow extra time for processing information
_____ Repeat or rephrase information when necessary
_____ Frequently check for understanding
_____ Educational interpreter (ASL, signed English, cued speech, oral)

Physical Environment Accommodations

_____ Noise reduction (carpet & other sound absorption materials)
_____ Specialized lighting
_____ Room design modifications
_____ Flashing fire alarm

Instructional Accommodations

_____ Use of visual supplements (overheads, chalkboard, charts, vocabulary lists, lecture outlines)
_____ Captioning or scripts for television, videos, movies, filmstrips
_____ Buddy system for notes, extra explanations/directions
_____ Check for understanding of information
_____ Down time/break from listening
_____ Extra time to complete assignments
_____ Step-by-step directions
_____ Tutor
_____ Note-taker

Curricular Modifications

_____ Modify reading assignments (shorten length, adapt or eliminate phonics assignments)
_____ Modify written assignments (shorten length, adjust evaluation criteria)
_____ Pretutor vocabulary
_____ Provide supplemental materials to reinforce concepts
_____ Provide extra practice
_____ Alternative curriculum

Evaluation Modifications

_____ Reduce quantity of tests
_____ Use alternative tests
_____ Provide reading assistance with tests
_____ Allow extra time
_____ Other modifications:_____

Other Needs/Considerations

_____ Supplemental instruction (speech, language, pragmatic skills, auditory, speechreading skills)
_____ Counseling
_____ Sign language instruction
_____ Vocational services
_____ Family supports
_____ Deaf/hard-of-hearing role models
_____ Recreational/social opportunities
_____ Financial assistance
_____ Transition service

---

[f]Reprinted with permission from Johnson DeConde C, Benson PV, Seaton JB. Educational audiology handbook. San Diego: Singular, 1997.

APPENDIX

8.9 *Suggested Annual Goals and Short-Term Objectives Relating to Audiology Needs*[g]

The following goals and their accompanying objectives were developed to be used with students with hearing impairment when developing IEPs. The goals represent developmentally based skills which students should acquire to maximize their residual hearing. These goals and objectives should be used as basic guidelines and be expanded as needed for each student. Every student with hearing impairment should have audiology goals on their IEP until competency or maximal potential has been reached.

ANNUAL GOALS

Independent use of amplification

Develop and improve auditory skills

Demonstrate appropriate compensatory strategies related to hearing impairment

Knowledge of hearing loss and its implications

Advocate appropriately for hearing-related needs

Annual Goals and Short-Term Objectives

GOAL 1

The student will demonstrate independent use of amplification (hearing aids, cochlear implants, FM device, or other system).

OBJECTIVES

1. The student will arrive at school wearing properly functioning amplification _____ out of _____ times as measured by daily checks.
2. The student will be able to correctly insert and remove amplification _____ out of _____ times as measured by observation.
3. The student will monitor his/her own amplification function (batteries, volume settings, cleaning of earmolds) _____ out of _____ times as measured by observation or checklist.
4. The student will notify appropriate personnel when amplification is not functioning properly _____ out of _____ times as measured by observation.
5. The student will demonstrate basic knowledge, use and/or care of assistive listening device utilized in his/her academic settings, _____ out of _____ times as measured by demonstration or observation.
6. The student will be responsible for the use of his/her FM system in all appropriate education situations _____ out of _____ times as measured by observation.

GOAL 2

The student will develop or improve his/her auditory skills.

OBJECTIVES

1. The student will develop/improve sound awareness skills _____ out of _____ times across a variety of settings (quiet, noise, close, distant, with and without visual clues, familiar, unfamiliar) as measured by an auditory curriculum.[h]
2. The student will develop/improve suprasegmental listening skills (pitch, duration, intensity, rate etc.) _____ out of _____ times across a variety of settings as measured by an auditory curriculum.
3. The student will develop/improve vowel discrimination and identification across a variety of settings as measured by an auditory curriculum.
4. The student will auditorially discriminate his/her name _____ out of _____ times across a variety of settings as measured by observation or a teacher made test.
5. The student will develop/improve consonant discrimination and identification _____ out of _____ times across a variety of settings as measured by an auditory curriculum.
6. The student will develop/improve auditory comprehension skills by following _____ out of _____ step directions across a variety of settings as measured by an auditory curriculum.
7. The student will discriminate common phrases _____ out of _____ times across a variety of settings as measured by an auditory curriculum.
8. The student will identify familiar language patterns _____ out of _____ times across a variety of settings as measured by an auditory curriculum.
9. The student will increase his/her ability to answer questions following auditorially presented information _____ out of _____ times as measured by observation or teacher made test.

GOAL

The student will demonstrate appropriate compensatory strategies (accommodations and modifications).

OBJECTIVES

1. The student will explain his/her need for preferential seating _____ out of _____ times as measured by informal evaluation.
2. The student will independently choose or request to sit in an appropriate seat _____ out of _____ times as measured by observation and teacher feedback.
3. The student will ask for repetition/clarifications _____ out of _____ times as measured by observation and teacher feedback.
4. The student will utilize available clues (visual, contextual, lipreading, etc.) to aid in comprehension _____ out of _____ times as measured by observation and teacher feedback.

GOAL 4

The student will demonstrate knowledge of his/her hearing loss and resulting needs.

OBJECTIVES

1. The student will describe the type, amount and cause of his/her hearing loss _____ out of _____ times as measured by informal evaluation.
2. The student will demonstrate an understanding of the benefits/limitations of amplification as they relate to his/her own hearing loss _____ out of _____ times as measured by informal evaluation.

GOAL 5

The student will advocate appropriately for his/her needs.

OBJECTIVES

1. The student will inform teachers of his/her hearing loss and resulting needs _____ out of _____ times as measured by teacher feedback and observation.
2. The student will request appropriate visual and or supplementary materials as needed (copy of notes, film script, captioning, lecture outline. . . .) _____ out of _____ times as measured by teacher feedback and observations.
3. The student will demonstrate and make use of appropriate technology (TTY, captioner, Relay COLORADO, etc.) _____ out of _____ times as measured by teacher feedback, observations, and/or informal evaluations.

ᵍFrom Colorado Department of Education. Colorado school audiology resource handbook.

ʰThe Development Approach to Successful Listening (DASL) or the Auditory Skills Curriculum are examples of curricula that include a variety of subskills for each of these objectives areas that are measurable in a variety of settings.

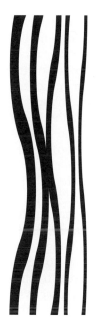

9

Family Counseling for Children With Hearing Loss

Patricia B. Kricos, Ph.D.

Overview of Family-Centered Counseling

DEFINITION OF FAMILY-CENTERED COUNSELING

Over the past two decades, there has been a gradual shift in the conception of early intervention, from services provided directly to the child with special needs to services provided to the child's family. The underlying rationale for this shift in philosophy was that children's functioning can be maximized by intervention that aims to improve the effectiveness of their families (Mahoney et al., 1990). One of the major influences underlying this transformation was a considerable body of research regarding families of children with special needs. One set of findings showed clearly that the presence of a child with special needs often disrupts family functioning, which in turn can lead to a decrease in parental effectiveness (Mahoney et al., 1990). Concerns in this regard for families of children with hearing impairment have been expressed by a number of authors (Goss, 1970; Moses and Van Hecke-Wulatin, 1981; Jamieson, 1995; Waxman et al., 1996). A second set of research findings delineated the effects of family effectiveness on the developmental functioning of young children with special needs (Bodner-Johnson, 1986; Warren and Hasenstab, 1986; Dunst et al., 1997). Implementation of Public Laws 99-457 and 102-119, both of which emphasize a family-centered philosophy for early intervention, has resulted in substantial changes in how services are delivered to children and their families (Roush and McWilliam, 1994; Romer and Umbreit, 1998). Family-focused services are defined as those practices that include families in the decision-making process for all aspects of intervention services; are guided by the families' priorities for goals and services; encompass services for the entire family, not just the child; and respect families' preferences for their level of participation in the intervention program (Murphy et al., 1995). The contemporary model of parent-professional relationships is based on the tenet that families are the most important influence on children's development, and that the lives of both families and children are enhanced when interventionists acknowledge, support, and collaborate with the family systems in which children live.

Mahoney et al. (1990) suggest a number of ways in which family-focused intervention activities can be provided. These include (1) systems engagement in which the family is provided with information about laws, parental rights, and community services; (2) information regarding the child's particular handicapping condition, including intervention services and prognosis; (3) instructional activities for home stimulation of the child; (4) personal and family assistance, including counseling and social activities designed to help families cope more effectively; and (5) resource assistance to help families to obtain financial, medical, respite, and other resources.

Winton and Bailey (1994) describe several themes underlying approaches to intervention with families of children who are handicapped. One of these themes is family empowerment and equal partnerships with professionals. Implicit in this theme is that the family's resources and strengths should be capitalized on and incorporated into the intervention program and that families should be involved in the decision process as intervention is planned and implemented. Over the past two decades there has been a tremendous change in the perceived role of parents and professionals in the intervention process. Parental involvement used to mean that the parents assumed a relatively passive role by complying with the recommendations of the professional. Family involvement then evolved to the inclusion of parents as partners in their child's program, with the parents being consulted regarding intervention priorities and serving as cotherapists. The most current approach to family involvement revolves around the concept of family empowerment, with intervention goals and strategies guided by parental input (Trivette et al., 1990).

CHARACTERISTICS OF FAMILY-ORIENTED COUNSELING

The concept of parents having an active role in their child's intervention program in itself is not new. Simmons-Martin (Simmons-Martin and Rossi, 1990) and Pollack (1985), for example, espoused an active role for parents in their pioneering work with infants with hearing loss. In the 1990s, however, a major shift occurred from viewing parents as being more than just involved with their child's intervention program, but rather actually in control of it. Earlier models of parent involvement were based on the parents being fairly passive recipients of the professional's expertise. The role of the parent was primarily to implement the home training program designed by the professional. The contemporary model of parent involvement is based on collaboration between the professional and the parents, with the parents ultimately viewed as the "experts" responsible for decision-making for their child (Bagnato and Dunst, 1998). In this model of collaboration, it is understood that professionals have as much to learn from families as the families have to learn from professionals. Some major characteristics of family-centered practices are summarized in Table 9.1.

The shift in the family's role in the intervention process has necessitated changes in the ways professionals approach families. Rather than providing information to families, the professional's role has shifted to acquiring information from families about their needs, strengths, resources, and intervention priorities. This is not in any way to suggest that intervention and counseling goals are left solely to the parents' preference, but rather that the professional is viewed less as the expert and more as a partner, with families and professionals joining in a collaborative effort to facilitate the child's development (Winton and Bailey, 1990, 1994).

Trivette et al. (1990) noted that other shifts in thinking are necessary for provision of quality family-centered intervention and counseling. The professional will need to rethink the concept that families need to be fixed or changed somehow; instead, professionals need to seek out and capitalize on the positive aspects of family functioning. Rather than trying to solve problems confronting a family, the professional's role should be viewed as enabling and empowering families to master problem areas in their lives.

Several studies have been conducted to determine the viewpoints of parents regard-

Table 9.1
Characteristics of family-centered intervention

Includes families in all aspects of decision-making, planning, evaluation, and service delivery

Shares responsibility for the child's intervention with the parents

Provides for the needs of the whole family and not just the child

Is guided by families' priorities for goals and services

Offers and respects families' choices regarding the level of their participation in the child's intervention program

Provides for the family's counseling and intervention needs on a proactive basis

Has strengthening of family functioning as a primary goal of services

Encourages and facilitates parent-to-parent networking and support

Identifies and capitalizes on family's strengths

Respects families' unique characteristics and methods of coping

Provides honest, unbiased, and complete information to parents so that the parents can make informed decisions

---

ing their counseling and education needs. Summers et al. (1990) polled parents and early intervention specialists to determine priorities for program services. The most frequently mentioned theme was the need for sensitivity to families. Participants cited the need for professionals to be supportive of families' emotional needs, to be accepting and nonjudgmental, and to conduct all interactions in an unhurried atmosphere. They also mentioned the need for acknowledgment of the family as the ultimate decision-maker, for clear communication between parent and professional, for enhanced social support for families, and for acknowledgment of the diversity among families.

Interviews of parents of young children with special needs by Able-Boone et al. (1990) yielded similar suggestions. In addition, these parents emphasized their desire to become knowledgeable about their children's needs and about available services. The parents stressed the importance of being informed decision-makers in their children's intervention program and recommended that professionals avoid imposing goals and home programs on parents.

A study by Bernstein and Barta (1988) was designed specifically to obtain input from parents of children who are hearing-impaired regarding their parent education and counseling needs and to compare parents' goals with those of professionals. Their results indicated considerable agree-

ment between parents and professionals but highlighted the perception by parents that they wished to have more opportunity to inform the professional of their own needs as parents of children who are hearing-impaired.

RATIONALE FOR FAMILY-CENTERED COUNSELING

Bailey et al. (1986) reviewed a number of studies that documented the benefits of family-focused intervention for young handicapped children. These positive effects include improved teaching skills of the parents, improved behavior of the child as a result of the parents' enhanced teaching skills, improved caregiver-child interactions, successful parent training of spouses, increased participation of siblings in the child's intervention program, and a reduction in stress experienced by parents. More recently, Romer and Umbreit (1998) showed in their research that a high degree of family satisfaction is associated with a family-centered model of services, and a low degree of satisfaction is associated with social services that are not based on a family-centered model.

Carney and Moeller's (1998) review of the literature concerning treatment efficacy for children with hearing loss included several studies indicating a large amount of maternal stress in mothers of children who are hearing-impaired, which ultimately had an effect on family functioning and child development. Carney and Moeller review a number of studies that demonstrate the value of family counseling early in the intervention process for improving the child's achievement socially, emotionally, and even academically. Thus, along with auditory perceptual, language, academic, and speech goals, Carney and Moeller suggest that treatment goals may be directed to establishing appropriate family understanding and acceptance of hearing loss and to reducing family stress as the child develops to improve the child's overall adjustment.

Mahoney et al. (1998) reviewed four early intervention evaluation studies that provide compelling evidence of the effectiveness of early intervention services for at-risk children and children with disabilities. Little, if any, support for the child-focused, directive teaching model was found. In contrast, family-centered intervention characterized by parent-professional collaboration, responding to the families' needs and priorities, and other family support endeavors was effective in enhancing children's development if the intervention activities encouraged parents to engage in more responsive interactions with their children. According to Mahoney and his coauthors, the effectiveness of family intervention is determined not just by involving parents in the intervention program nor by simply responding to parents' needs and priorities, but additionally by encouraging and supporting parents to engage in highly responsive interactions with their children.

Of particular concern for professionals who work with families of children with hearing impairment is the almost uniform finding in various research studies that hearing mothers of children who are deaf are more directive, more controlling, and less responsive with their children than are mothers of hearing children (Waxman et al., 1996). Jamieson (1995) provides an extensive review of research in this area. It is well documented that cognitive, linguistic, social, and emotional development are significantly affected by the quality and quantity of caregiver-child interactions (Waxman et

al., 1996). Because there is clear evidence that early caregiver-child interactions form the cornerstone of language and cognitive development, these aberrant patterns of mother-child interaction should be of grave concern to professionals responsible for designing effective intervention programs for young children with hearing impairment. For young children with hearing loss, it has been demonstrated in longitudinal research at Gallaudet University that support services offered to parents are likely to result in positive mother-child interaction and in less stress for both mothers and fathers (Mac-Turk et al., 1993; Meadow-Orlans and Sass-Lehrer, 1995).

GOALS OF FAMILY-CENTERED COUNSELING AND INTERVENTION

Given the mandates by PL99-457 and 102-119 for dramatically increased family involvement in intervention services for young children with handicaps, as well as the increasing awareness of the importance of the family to the child's overall development, the goals of parent counseling need to be considered within a family-centered context. The following parent counseling goals are presented, adapted from Bromwich (1978), Dunst and Trivette (1990), and Winton and Bailey (1990, 1994), all of whom are renown for their work in early intervention within a family focus:

1. To promote positive child, parent, and family functioning.
2. To help family members appraise their problems and needs.
3. To base parent counseling and other forms of intervention on family-identified needs and priorities.
4. To reduce stress and anxiety associated with parenting a child who is hearing-impaired.
5. To identify family strengths and unique resources.
6. To define means of using the family's strengths and resources within the intervention program.
7. To ensure the availability and use of

formal and informal social network resources and service systems for meeting family needs.

8. To promote family members' sense of confidence and to reinforce the parent's perception of being the primary agent responsible for the child's intervention program and overall development.

9. To promote family's abilities to acquire and use competencies and skills necessary for optimal family functioning.

10. To assess the nature of parent-child interaction and to see ways to make interactions more reciprocal and mutually satisfying.

How a Child's Hearing Loss Affects Families

McKellin (1995), an anthropologist associated with the University of British Columbia and also the parent of a child with severe to profound hearing loss, has pointed out that although it is individuals, not families, who incur hearing loss, the impact of a child's hearing loss is nevertheless experienced by the entire family. McKellin argues for consideration of the numerous ways in which a child with hearing loss will affect the family, and the ways in which the family will influence the child's development.

INITIAL REACTIONS

The emotional reactions that may be experienced by parents of children with hearing impairment are similar to the reactions of individuals who have lost a loved one through death. Although in reality the parents have not "lost" their child, they nevertheless may feel as if they have lost the hopes, dreams, and aspirations they once held for the child. Thus, they may experience grief as intense and acute as if they had lost the child through death. It is important that professionals respond to grieving family members in a manner that will facilitate their ultimate acceptance of the hearing loss. When the grieving process is facilitated properly, parents and other family members may be better able to participate in the collaborative intervention program for their child (DeConde Johnson, 1994; Van Hecke, 1994; Luterman, 1996; Shipley, 1997).

The stages of grief experienced by parents of children who are hearing-impaired parallel the sequences of grieving described by Kubler-Ross (1969) for the dying patient. These include denial, anger, bargaining, depression, and ultimately acceptance. Each of these, in addition to the frequently observed reaction of guilt, will be discussed separately.

Denial is usually one of the first reactions to any major loss and, as Kubler Ross (1969) points out, may serve as an emotional buffer that allows the grieving person time to absorb the impact of the loss and to mobilize inner strengths to deal with it. Deafness is relatively easy to deny because it is invisible, and parents may deny the diagnosis of the child's hearing loss in a number of ways. They may reject the diagnosis of deafness, taking the child to a number of different professionals and clinics, in essence "shopping" for a more palatable professional opinion. They may accept the diagnosis but reject its permanence, expressing hopes that the child will eventually outgrow the condition or be cured of it. The impact of the diagnosis may be rejected, with parents appearing unperturbed in the face of a severe disability. These latter parents often appear to be "ideal" parents to clinicians because of their seemingly positive attitudes; yet, ultimate acceptance of the child's impairment demands confrontation with the significant impact of the child's hearing loss on almost all aspects of communicative and academic development. Parents in the denial stage may appear to clinicians to be blocking efforts to initiate the intervention program. However, it should be remembered that this initial reaction to the diagnosis of deafness may provide a time for parents to search for inner strength and to accumulate information. The goal for clinicians during this stage of grieving is to find ways of not merely tolerating parental denial but accepting it, while still offering, to the best of their abilities, the services the child needs. Unfortunately, parents who appear to be denying their child's hearing impairment are often viewed by clinicians as foolish and stubborn, when they should be viewed as loving parents who, for the time being, cannot accept the professional's diagnosis of such a severe disability in their child.

The parents of newly diagnosed children may experience guilt, which can be manifested in several ways. Some parents may express the feeling that something they did caused their child's hearing loss. Even more difficult to respond to are the parents who believe that their child's impairment is punishment for a prior sin or simply because they are not "good" people and therefore do not deserve an unimpaired child. The professional must recognize feelings of guilt as a natural process, not a psychopathology, and respond to them as such. If not condemned or responded to as foolishness, guilt will run its course and cease on its own (Moses and Van Hecke-Wulatin, 1981).

Feelings of anger mark the second reaction in Kubler-Ross's (1969) stages of mourning. The parents, no longer denying the diagnosis, may be left with feelings of inner rage, which are often expressed toward family, friends, and professionals. As difficult as it may be to depersonalize the anger expressed to them in various ways, clinicians must attempt to understand the parent's anger as a normal reaction to loss and as an indication of at least partial acceptance of the child's disability. The clinician confronted with an angry parent must understand that the parent's anger is not necessarily a personal reaction to the clinician or to the rehabilitation program, and the clinician must avoid responding to the parent in a negative manner. Likewise, the angry parent's spouse and/or family should be counseled to ensure understanding, acceptance, and handling of the parent's frustrations.

The third stage in Kubler-Ross's (1969) grieving cycle is bargaining. In this stage the parent may bargain with clinicians, health professionals, family, God, and/or themselves. Bargaining parents, for example, may vow openly or surreptitiously to do everything requested of them by the child's clinician, and often beyond, in return for which amelioration of the child's disorder is expected. On the surface, unflagging dedication to the child's needs appears to be a commendable quality, but it might also serve as a signal that the parent is engaged in unrealistic bargaining. Although bargaining may be helpful to the parent in that it offers a little more time for resolution of the loss, long periods of bargaining may not be healthy for either the parent or the child. Eventually the parent's false hopes, which accompany bargaining, will have to be acknowledged and resolved to achieve full acceptance of the hearing loss. In addition, the physical health and emotional security of parents who set unrealistic demands for themselves should be of concern to clinicians because of the eventual negative effect on the child's intervention program.

Depression is the fourth stage of grieving described by Kubler-Ross (1969). The parent no longer denies the loss, no longer feels inner rage toward the loss, and may realize that bargaining attempts have failed to alleviate the problems encountered as a result of the loss. Unfortunately, clinicians may view the parent's subsequent depression as a psychopathology rather than a normal reaction within the grief cycle. A natural, very human response of clinicians who face a depressed parent is to point out that things are really not as bad as the parent views them; that the child, despite a severe impairment, is a beautiful, intelligent, personable, outgoing child; and that in view of this, the parent ought to cheer up. Other clinicians may feel uncomfortable with the parent's depression and may exert great effort to avoid acknowledging the parent's sorrow. Although the clinicians' reactions are understandable, the result may be to make the parent feel worse. In essence, the depressed parent's response to the clinician's well-meaning attempts to downplay the significance of the loss may be to view himself or herself as inadequate in coping with the child's problem. Thus, a vicious cycle may be set up in which the depressed parent may feel even more depressed. One of the best responses that clinicians can make to the depressed parent may be nonverbal consolation. Simply touching a parent's hand or shoulder or just listening quietly and compassionately as the parent expresses inner feelings of depression may be far more effective in helping the depressed parent than verbal attempts to cheer up the parent.

According to Kubler-Ross (1969), acceptance is both the final stage and the ultimate goal of the grieving process and may provide the first evidence that the grief has been resolved. The parent may not necessarily feel happy about his or her predicament, yet the intense feelings of denial, depression, anger, and guilt are no longer present either. The parent of a child with hearing loss may simply accept the situation as the way things are, thus enabling energies and constructive actions to be directed to the child's intervention program.

It is important for clinicians to realize that the grief that accompanies the initial diagnosis of deafness and then is resolved may reappear later. For example, the impact of the child's disability may be cyclically magnified in the parent's eyes at certain predictable occasions. When the child reaches 5 years of age, the parents may realize that this would have been the time for the child to enter a regular kindergarten, had the child not been disabled. Thus, the parent's initial feelings of loss, disappointment, and depression may resurface after seemingly being dormant for a number of years. The loss of a special teacher, the onset of pubescence, the reaching of the typical age of high school graduation as well as the age for living independently, and even the parent's reaching of retirement age may trigger emotional reactions typical of the initial mourning period at the time of diagnosis. Although reactions to these occasions may be more transient than initial reactions, they should be recognized by professionals and responded to in a manner that will facilitate their speedy resolution.

Although from a theoretical viewpoint, these stages seem straightforward, their manifestations may actually not be quite so discernible. Clark (1990, 1994) describes a number of transformations that these emotional reactions may undergo when being

expressed by parents, making it difficult to recognize when the clinician responds only to the surface of clinical exchanges. For example, a parent may have strong feelings of sorrow yet fear to express them because such a reaction might not be acceptable to the clinician and might appear to others as rejection of the child. Instead, the parent may redirect the initial reaction of sorrow, putting aside their feelings of sadness, jumping into the child's rehabilitation program, signing up for three sign language classes, and giving up previously enjoyed recreational activities to make more time for the child with hearing impairment. This type of response is not necessarily negative or counterproductive, unless the parent is repressing the sadness. If parents cannot find an outlet for their repressed feelings of sorrow, their enthusiastic drive will be difficult to maintain. It requires a sensitive clinician to be able to encourage parents to do all that needs to be done for their child, while at the same time providing a supportive environment in which the parents can divulge their innermost feelings regarding the situation in which they now find themselves. The clinician must be alert to any repressed feelings of anxiety or sorrow that the parent may harbor, letting the parent know that the welfare of parents is as much a concern to the clinician as the welfare of the child. Sometimes just asking the parent frankly, "How are you doing with all the demands that are now being put on you? Are you finding time for yourself, to meet your physical and emotional needs?" will let the parent know that the clinician is sensitive, empathetic, concerned, and willing to recognize the strains that are on the parent.

The previous paragraphs have emphasized the importance of recognizing the strong emotional reactions that parents of children who are hearing-impaired may experience. Equally important to recognize, however, is that not all parents will predictably go through these stages exactly as described. The only definitive thing that can be said about the grief patterns of parents of newly diagnosed children with hearing impairment is that the clinician should be cognizant of the range of emotional reactions that may be experienced, should respond in a sensitive, empathetic manner to these reactions as they manifest, and above all should never assume that the parents will progress systematically, step by step, through the classic grieving stages described by Kubler-Ross (1969). The degree to which these emotional reactions will be experienced will likely vary from family to family depending on a number of complex factors. These include personal resources (e.g., personality, coping strategies, attitudes, educational background); social status factors (e.g., age, gender, ethnic background, income); and numerous other variables such as the parent's current marital relationship; degree of support from spouse, other family members, social networks, and service agencies; availability and quality of intervention programs and counselors; and demands on working parents (Kampfe, 1989). From this discussion, it is easy to understand the danger in overgeneralizing the stages of emotional reactions through which parents progress. Whether a parent goes through any of these stages, the manner in which the emotional state is expressed, the degree to which constructive or maladaptive strategies are adopted, and the time frame in which these emotional reactions might be experienced all depend on the complex interactions of these, and likely many more, variables. The professional is cautioned, therefore, to understand the potential range of emotional states that may be experienced at various times by parents, without assuming that each parent will respond in a fully predictable manner. Each parent must be approached as an individual with a unique system of personal resources, social support, and background experiences. Even the mother and father of a particular child can be expected to react to their child's hearing difficulties in significantly different ways because of their unique set of characteristics, experiences, and perceptions.

Luterman (1996) has cautioned that the concept of grief stages has in many respects been oversimplified and overused in its application to counseling individuals with communicative disorders. Indeed, there is some research to indicate that families with children who are hearing-impaired actually cope quite well. In a recent study, for example, Mapp and Hudson (1997) found that parents adjust well and rather quickly to learning that they have a child who is hearing-impaired. These authors suggest that it is likely that the initial diagnosis of hearing loss is accompanied by high levels of stress, but that parents for the most part are able to reduce stress in a short period through the use of various coping strategies. These results are consistent with information obtained by Martin et al. (1987) that 90% of the parents they interviewed had reached the acceptance level of the grieving process by the 12th month after the diagnosis of hearing loss. Similarly, other studies have found that despite the potential for increased stress levels, families with children who are hearing-impaired are not typically dysfunctional families and in fact adjust admirably well to the stressors associated with raising a child with hearing impairment (Henggeler et al., 1990; Fisiloglu and Fisiloglu, 1996).

In this section, it has been emphasized that the emotional responses of parents should be viewed as normal, nonpathologic responses to loss and/or disability. This section will conclude with a caveat, however. Although many parents will experience these stages in response to learning that their child is hearing-impaired and will ultimately resolve their emotional conflicts, achieving acceptance of some form, the clinician must nevertheless be aware that some parents may experience distressful feelings of anxiety and depression for which a sympathetic ear will not be enough. Harvey and Green (1990), for example, describe the psychotherapeutic treatment of a mother who was obsessed with anxiety about her deaf daughter's future. When confronted with a parent who appears to be having recurrent anxieties and fears about the child's status, or with a parent whose depression seems to be interfering with most aspects of the parent's life, the clinician must make an immediate referral to a qualified mental health counselor for resolution of the emotional difficulties. When in doubt as to whether the normal range of emotional reactions is being experienced or there is a more serious psychiatric disturbance, the clinician should assist the parent in setting up a consultation with a mental health professional who can determine whether formal psychotherapeutic intervention is warranted.

NEED FOR INFORMATION

The vast majority of parents of children with hearing impairment are hearing parents, with little or no prior experience with childhood hearing loss (McKellin, 1995; Meadow-Orlans and Sass-Lehrer, 1995). At the same time that parents are coping with powerful emotional reactions such as shock and sorrow, they are also confronted with the need for an abundance of information regarding their child's hearing loss. Terminology from medical, educational, and audiologic professionals must be mastered in a short amount of time. Parents need information about educational and treatment options available for their child and are confronted almost immediately with conflicting opinions regarding medical treatment, sensory devices, mode of communication, and educational placements. The balance that must be struck between giving parents a chance to absorb the diagnosis while at the same time providing them with information requires a sensitive, compassionate professional.

PARENTS

Mothers versus fathers

Research conducted by Meadow-Orlans (1995) suggests that although the levels of stress experienced by mothers and fathers of children with hearing loss are relatively equal, the sources of stress may differ between the two. Sources of stress for the fathers in her study included finding the child less acceptable and more demanding, whereas sources of stress for the mothers revolved around the child's distractibility, the mothers' perceived restriction in their roles, and concerns about their relationships with their husbands. Meadow-Orlans emphasizes

the need for truly individualizing an intervention plan to meet the counseling needs of both parents.

Based on their interviews of mothers and fathers of children who are hearing-impaired, Hadadian and Rose (1991) conclude that the children have far more contact and interaction with their mothers than with their fathers, and that the hearing mothers of deaf children are more actively involved in sign language and communication intervention programs than the fathers. Hadadian and Rose recommend that early intervention programs develop new models that actively enlist the participation of fathers. Likewise, Kampfe et al. (1993) stress the importance of making education, guidance, and counseling available to both parents and significant others so that the process of adjusting to and learning about the child's hearing problems will be facilitated.

Deaf versus hearing parents

Meadow-Orlans and Sass-Lehrer (1995) point out that it would be a mistake to assume that deaf parents respond to the diagnosis of deafness in some uniform manner. Although some deaf parents may greet the diagnosis with relief, others, with their keen knowledge of the problems experienced by deaf individuals in a hearing society, may be devastated. As with all families, deaf parents of deaf children should be approached as having unique strengths and needs.

The concerns that have been expressed regarding aberrant patterns of interactions between mothers and the children who are hearing-impaired seem not to be applicable to deaf children of deaf parents. Waxman et al. (1996) reviewed a number of studies that indicate that deaf mothers use a variety of effective communication strategies to facilitate interactions with their deaf infants. Hearing parents may experience more frustration when attempting to interact and communicate with their children with hearing impairment (Hadadian and Rose, 1991). Interestingly, there is a body of research showing higher educational achievement and more positive social behavior patterns in deaf children of deaf parents, despite the parents' relatively lower educational and occupational status than that of hearing parents (Hadadian and Rose, 1991).

OTHER FAMILY MEMBERS

Research on the effects of a handicapped child on the family has focused primarily on how the child affects the parents. Examination of the effects on other family members has received negligible attention. Research on siblings of children with handicaps other than hearing loss has shown pronounced individual variation among siblings in effects and experiences (Israelite, 1986; Morgan-Redshaw et al., 1990). Some siblings feel that having a handicapped brother or sister has a positive influence on them. Others report a more negative experience, and still others report that the presence of a handicapped child in the family had virtually no effect on their growth and development. Atkins (1994) points out a number of reasons to be concerned about the well-being and adjustment of siblings of children who are hearing-impaired. These include, among others:

1. Their parents, knowingly or unknowingly, being less involved with them because of time demands in meeting the needs of the sibling with the hearing impairment.
2. The parents' fatigue, worry, and preoccupation detracting from a satisfying interaction with the hearing siblings.
3. Inquiries from friends and strangers regarding the child with hearing impairment.
4. A feeling that the sibling who is hearing-impaired is not disciplined by the parents.
5. Possible feelings of guilt and responsibility for the handicap of the child with hearing impairment.
6. Increased responsibilities around the home, including care-taking of the sibling with hearing loss.

Atkins (1987) points out that sibling relationships in any family, regardless of the presence of a child with hearing loss, are influenced by a number of variables, including family size, birth order, gender, roles of various family members, self-perceptions, temperaments, marital harmony, parenting styles, and economic status. For families with children who are hearing-impaired, there will likely be other variables, such as those listed above, affecting family adjustment and sibling relationships.

Israelite (1986) investigated the effects of a child with impaired hearing on the psychological functioning of siblings by comparing 14 siblings of children who are hearing-impaired with 14 siblings of normal-hearing children on self-reported levels of family responsibility, depression, anxiety, and self-concept. Her results revealed two primary differences between the groups, one relating to identity and the other to social self-concept. The siblings of children who are hearing-impaired tended to define themselves not only as individuals in their own right but also as siblings of children who are hearing-impaired, and their social self-concept was lower than that of siblings of normal-hearing children. The two groups performed similarly on measures of family responsibility, depression, anxiety, and self-esteem. Thus, although some differences in psychological functioning were noted, they did not appear to have any pronounced negative effects on the emotional stability or overall adjustment of siblings of children who are hearing-impaired.

Atkins (1987, 1994) points out that we have extremely limited information about the effect of children who are hearing-impaired on their siblings and that intervention programs for children who are hearing-impaired rarely include brothers and sisters. She suggests that sibling programs be designed to meet the needs of the entire family, which is congruous with the current emphasis on family-centered programming. Thus, one of the areas that should be probed when discussing family needs (see next section) should be sibling considerations. Intervention approaches might be offered that include special programs that bring siblings together for practical information about hearing impairment and for sharing experiences, or routine sibling meetings at the same time group parent meetings are held (Luterman, 1994; Rushmer and Schuyler, 1994).

Another often overlooked family member is the grandparent. The emotional reactions described earlier for parents of children who have been newly diagnosed as hearing-impaired are also relevant for grandparents. In fact, they may experience grief for their beloved grandchild and worry about their own child's ability to cope with the added responsibilities of raising a child with hearing impairment. Vadasy et al. (1986) reported that grandparents of handicapped children frequently experience initial feelings of sadness, and to a lesser extent, shock and anger. Most of the grandparents they interviewed reported that they eventually accepted their grandchild's handicap, although almost half of their sample continued to express feelings of sadness long after the initial diagnosis of the child's handicap. Vadasy et al. (1986) describe a grandparent workshop in which participants are offered information about their grandchild's handicap as well as opportunities for sharing concerns and experiences with other grandparents. The authors point out the valuable resources that grandparents can be within a family with a child who has special needs, and advise professionals to look closely at the extended networks of families to appreciate the strengths and contributions of extended family members such as grandparents.

In this section, a perspective on the influence of a child with hearing impairment on family functioning has been provided. As Trivette et al. (1990) point out in an excellent article on family strengths, the goal of intervention should not be viewed so much as provision of needed services by the professional, as much as strengthening the functioning of families so that they will ultimately be less dependent on the professional for help. These authors espouse a shift in intervention services toward enabling and empowering families to meet the needs of their children with handicaps.

Evaluating Family Strengths and Needs

An inherent part of family-centered counseling and service provision is determination of the family's strengths and needs. Part H provisions of PL 99-457 stipulate that the individualized family service plan must contain a written statement of family strengths and needs as they relate to enhancing the development of the infant or toddler with special needs. There is little guidance within the federal law, however, about how to determine the family's strengths and needs. Nevertheless, any intervention plan developed for the child must be considered within the context of the family, who ultimately will implement the plan. The clinician must have a thorough understanding of the functional aspects of family life to plan an intervention program that is relevant, effective, and likely to be carried out within the daily routines of the family. In addition to a thorough evaluation of the competence, problems, and needs of the child with hearing loss (as described in Chapters 6 and 7), it is important to determine each family's unique strengths and needs.

FAMILY NEEDS

One of the major features of Public Law 99-457 is the requirement that initial and ongoing assessments that are part of the early intervention process must include the child's family, with particular emphasis on delineation of the family's needs. Because of their unique characteristics, the needs and strengths of each family will differ. Bailey et al. (1986) list six areas that should be probed to obtain information regarding a family's needs. These areas, with examples relevant to audiology, include: (1) needs for information (e.g., regarding the hearing loss, auditory stimulation activities, care of the sensory device), (2) needs for support (e.g., from parents of other children with hearing loss, from reading materials, from a skilled counselor), (3) explaining the child's hearing problems to others (e.g., family members, friends, strangers), (4) community services (e.g., medical, therapy, day care), (5) financial needs (e.g., for medical treatment of the hearing disorder, sensory devices, audiologic habilitation), and (6) family functioning (e.g., assistance with division of labor, marital counseling).

There are a number of measurement tools available for determining family needs (Roush and McWilliam, 1994). Two well-known inventories are the Family Needs Scale (Dunst et al., 1988) and the Family Needs Survey (Bailey and Simeonsson, 1988). Both tools are parent questionnaires that probe various categories of family needs.

Bernheimer and Keogh (1995) point out that the assessment of families' needs must take into account the parents' beliefs, goals, and values. That is, a family's perception of the problems, their sense of what can be done to solve the problems, and their sense of what is important to be done all must be taken into consideration during counseling and when planning the intervention program. Bernheimer and Keogh suggest that determination of the family's daily routines, through in-depth interviews, will reveal considerable information about the family's priorities, means of adjusting, and needs. Simply asking the parents to describe a typical day, from morning to night, will reflect much about the family's strategies to cope with the demands of raising a child with special needs. Consideration of the daily routines of a family will enable the design of more feasible and practical intervention programs for the child and family, and the counseling process will be facilitated by an understanding of how the family functions.

Summers et al. (1990) used nine consumer focus groups to determine family preferences for gathering information about family strengths and needs. The families consistently indicated a preference for informal methods of gathering information. Informal conversations, rather than the use of forms or formal interview techniques, were preferred by the families. To gain the trust of families and to put them at ease, professionals ought to try to establish a "kitchen table" conversation with the parents, rather than a formal interview, which may be intimidating to parents. The results of Summers et al.'s research suggest that professionals who counsel families who have children with special needs must play the dual role of being knowledgeable, capable, and professional while also being friendly and emotionally responsive.

During interviews with parents to ascertain family needs, the professional must be sensitive to the fact that some families may be more open and candid than others. The clinician must watch for any signs that the family feels uncomfortable with revealing details about their personal lives and situations. If privacy appears to be a family priority, then intrusive questions should be omitted (Brown and Yoshinaga-Itano, 1994). Perhaps as the family gains trust in the collaborative relationship with the professional, there will be more willingness to reveal specific needs for assistance.

Although the needs identified by families should be addressed when possible, the clinician may also target additional goals. The clinician brings a wealth of information regarding hearing loss and audiologic habilitation to the partnership with the parent. For example, the clinician is fully aware of the importance of consistent, full-time use of the child's sensory device and the importance of the parent's interaction style with the child; goals for these areas will likely be a part of the intervention plan. The rationale for selection of these goals should be explained to parents. Of course, as is fundamental to the family-centered counseling philosophy, the parents' goals should receive at least as much priority as clinician-initiated goals.

A final word of caution regarding determination of family needs is that early intervention professionals should not assume that just because parents fail to communicate needs they do not need services. Mahoney and Filer (1996) found in their study of the type and scope of services provided to families in early intervention programs that families with optimal patterns of family functioning were more likely to receive services than were families at risk for dysfunction. Programs must be vigilant to the possibility that some families with immense needs may have limited abilities to express their requirements or negotiate within the early intervention system to obtain the services they need. Mahoney and Filer's findings that families with positive characteristics, who are likely to have relatively fewer needs for support, received the greatest amount of services is a sobering thought that should be kept in mind by all early intervention professionals.

IDENTIFYING AND CAPITALIZING ON FAMILY STRENGTHS

Although identification of family needs is critical for intervention planning, it is equally important to identify and acknowledge family strengths. A focus solely on family needs fails to recognize all of the positive features and coping strategies that each family will bring to the intervention process. Although the emphasis has been on the development and use of scales and questionnaires for identifying family needs, the observant clinician will be able to discern a family's unique strengths and will be able to weave these competencies into the intervention plan. Simply remarking on the family's strengths and features of well-being may boost the family's confidence in addressing their child's needs. The clinician needs to note positive coping strategies exhibited by fathers and mothers. Too often professionals focus on what the parents need to be doing, rather than what they are doing to help their child.

EVALUATION OF PARENT-CHILD INTERACTIONS

A number of authors have expressed concern regarding the detrimental effect that knowledge of a child's hearing handicap may have on the mother's communication style with her child. Goss (1970) was one of the first to delineate striking differences between the verbal behavior of mothers of deaf children and mothers of hearing children. His results suggested that mothers of deaf children are less likely to use verbal praise, to ask for opinions and suggestions, and to

use questions; they are also more likely to show disagreement, tension, and antagonism and to give more suggestions than are mothers of hearing children. Since Goss first published his findings, there have been numerous other studies of parent-child interactions in which concern has been expressed about the communication styles of mothers of children who are hearing-impaired (Meadow et al., 1972; Moses and Van Hecke-Wulatin, 1981; Kricos, 1982). Given these concerns, as well as the assertion by Mahoney et al. (1998) that the responsiveness of parents is a critical determinant of the success of family-centered intervention programs, it is essential that the quality of interactions and the environment that parents provide young children with hearing impairment be evaluated.

Several measures for evaluating the quality of interactions and the environment that parents provide young children with special needs are summarized in Table 9.2. The only measure in Table 9.2 that was designed specifically for parents with children who are hearing-impaired is the Caregiver-Child Interaction Analysis. The authors of this measure espouse a caregiver-child interaction analysis protocol based on videotaping the child and the caregiver during everyday play and communication transactions (Cole and St. Clair-Stokes, 1984; St. Clair-Stokes and Mischook, 1990). Although much of their checklist evaluates the language and conversational behaviors exhibited by the caregiver, an important area for analysis is what these authors refer to as "sensitivity to child." Items included on their checklist for this parameter include handling the child in a positive manner, pacing play and conversation at the child's tempo, following the child's interest at a particular moment, providing stimulation activities and play that are appropriate for the child's age and developmental stage, as well as encouraging and facilitating the child's play with objects and materials.

The use of measures such as these are important for understanding the quality of parent-child interaction and for designing appropriate intervention to facilitate parent-

Table 9.2
Measures of parent-child interactions

Maternal Behavior Rating Scale (Mahoney et al., 1985)	Eighteen maternal behavior items and four child behavior items that are rated on a five-point scale; provides information on maternal pleasure, quantity of stimulation, and control
Teaching Skills Inventory (Rosenberg and Robinson, 1985)	Evaluates areas such as maternal responsiveness and instructional skills as well as child interest
HOME Inventory for Infants and Toddlers (Caldwell and Bradley, 1984)	Checklist format; assesses quality of parent-infant (0–36 months) interaction within six areas: responsivity, acceptance, organization, play materials, parental involvement, and variety of stimulation
Parent Behavior Progression (Bromwich, 1978)	Observation checklist; assesses areas such as parental enjoyment of the child, parental sensitivity/responsiveness, mutuality of interaction, developmental appropriateness of interactions, ability to generate new developmentally appropriate activities independently
Caregiver-Child Interaction Analysis (Cole and St. Clair-Stokes, 1984)	Checklist for evaluating caregiver's language, conversational behaviors, and sensitivity to child

child interaction. This is a critical area to consider because there is evidence that a child's hearing handicap may alter his or her interactive capacities (thus impairing the ability to contribute to mutually enjoyable exchanges with his or her parents) and because there is evidence that parents may alter their interactions with a child who is hearing-impaired. Measures such as those described in this section can provide guidelines for working with individual families.

Despite the availability of several assessment tools, Mahoney et al. (1996) express concern about a number of issues regarding evaluation of parent-child interactions. Care must be taken to ensure that there is sufficient interrater agreement for a particular assessment protocol to assure an acceptable level of reliability. Raters must receive adequate training in the analysis of parent-child interactions in general and in use of the specific protocol. The environment in which the parents are evaluated can have a substantial effect on how parents and children interact. The sterile environment of the clinic may

yield restricted, stilted parent-child interactions that are not indicative of their typical interaction patterns. If the parents are asked to just play with their child, they may seem less directive to the rater than if they are asked to get their child to perform a specific task. The length of observation time may be critical. Assessments that last up to 30 minutes may strain the parent, who more typically interacts with the child for shorter periods throughout the day. Simply knowing that they are being observed can result in parent-child interactions that are not representative of everyday communication. Serious consideration of these and other factors must be given during parent-child interaction assessments to ensure productive outcomes.

Building Strong Relationships With Families

A family-centered approach to counseling and service provision depends on a collaborative relationship between families and professionals. Collaboration, according to

Dunst and Paget (1991), entails a close relationship between families and professionals, one in which there is a high degree of cooperation. To facilitate a collaborative process, clinicians must demonstrate sensitivity to family issues, have exceptional communication abilities, and show a willingness to create a supportive climate in which parents feel valued. Dinnebeil and Rule (1994) used structured interviews of parents, service coordinators, and experts to explore variables that either enhance or detract from collaboration between families and service providers. Tables 9.3 and 9.4 summarize the characteristics and behaviors that were perceived as either productive or counterproductive to forming partnerships with families.

In a follow-up study, Dinnebeil et al. (1996) surveyed both parents and service coordinators to determine the variables that influence collaborative relationships. Their survey results indicated the importance of interpersonal and communication skills for successful collaboration. The effects of the service provider's personality and disposition—such as friendliness, optimism, patience, sincerity, and open-mindedness—were frequently commented on by both parents and service coordinators. The finding of the importance of personality characteristics is consistent with the results of research by McWilliam et al. (1995). These authors found that parents were more satisfied with the efforts of early interventionists when the interventionists were enthusiastic, outgoing, cheerful, and friendly.

In the Dinnebeil et al. (1996) study, a number of communication variables were frequently cited as important for collaboration, including honesty, tact, willingness to listen, responsivity, willingness to share information, and openness to suggestions. A commitment to the value of a family-centered philosophy was also viewed as essential. The service provider's knowledge base and degree of expertise, although viewed as important to the success of a collaborative relationship, was seen as less important than the service provider's interpersonal and communication skills. Similarly, a common theme in comments made by parents in the Summers et al. (1990) study was the need for early intervention professionals to exhibit sensitivity and respect for families.

To build strong relationships with families, practitioners need to scrutinize objectively their own personal attributes and demeanor to

Table 9.3
Behaviors and personal characteristics of case managers that facilitate collaboration

Respect family's attributes
Emphasize family's strengths
Genuine commitment to the value of family-centered early intervention
Prompt and efficient in follow-up
Build rapport
Genuine concern for children
Provide useful information and expertise
Positive attitude toward children and families
Cheerful
Outgoing
Patience
Self-confidence
Honesty and tactfulness
Effective communication and good listening skills
Encourage and support the family
Teamwork skills and leadership abilities
Well-informed

Source. Dinnebeil LA, Rule S. Variables that influence collaboration between parents and service coordinators. J Early Intervent 1994;18:349–361.

Table 9.4
Behaviors and personal characteristics of case managers that impede collaboration

Poor attitude toward parents; coldness, rudeness; patronizing
Inadequate provision of privacy for parents
Lack of concern for parents' self-esteem
Insufficient time to meet with family; rushed approach to meetings
Lack of self-confidence
Withholding information
Emphasis on family's deficiencies
Lack of commitment to family-centered practices; prescribing to families
Paternalistic attitude toward families
Slow or haphazard follow-through in case management
Lack of sensitivity to family schedules

Source: Dinnebeil LA, Rule S. Variables that influence collaboration between parents and service coordinators. J Early Intervent 1994;18:349–361.

ensure superior collaborative skills. According to Dinnebeil et al. (1996), one of the most important ways to build strong relationships with families is simply to acknowledge parents as competent individuals who provide for their family's needs.

Using Effective Listening and Interviewing Techniques

Collaboration with parents will undoubtedly necessitate the use of effective listening and interviewing skills. During the counseling process, there will be numerous occasions, especially at the onset of a case, in which the clinician will want to obtain information regarding the child, the family's strengths and needs, and the family's perspectives on having a child with hearing impairment. Interviewing skills that are necessary include certain personal characteristics that will help establish rapport, formulation of questions that will yield detailed information, and excellent listening skills. How the audiologist responds to comments and questions made by family members can have a significant effect on the collaboration process.

PERSONAL CHARACTERISTICS OF THE FAMILY COUNSELOR

Shipley (1997), in his book on interviewing and counseling for professionals in the communicative disorders field, has pointed out that to perform interviewing and coun-

seling functions well, clinicians must possess certain personal attributes and attitudes. These include spontaneity, flexibility, openness, emotional stability, a genuine interest in people and the belief that they can change, sensitivity, good listening and expressive skills, and expertise in their fields. Respect, empathy, and objectivity are also prerequisites to establish and maintain rapport with family members. According to Clark (1994), the best way to establish rapport with patients is to demonstrate genuine interest and attentiveness to them.

FORMULATION OF QUESTIONS DURING THE COUNSELING PROCESS

The manner in which questions are posed during the interview and/or counseling session can significantly affect the outcome of the session. Wording choices and presentation of the questions can affect how comfortable the interviewee feels during the counseling session and how much detailed and useful information can be obtained by the clinician. Shipley (1997) provides the following suggestions for question-formation:

1. Use clear, concise language, free of technical jargon.
2. Avoid asking multipart questions or several questions at one time.
3. Allow sufficient time for the interviewee to answer the question before asking another.

4. Use open-ended questions that will yield more detailed information than close-ended questions (which often can be answered in a single word). For example, "Please tell me about your child's means of communicating with you," may yield a richer, more detailed answer than, "Does your child use signs to communicate?"
5. Try to word questions in a neutral manner that will not bias the interviewee's answer in any way.

IMPORTANCE OF LISTENING SKILLS

The importance of listening skills to the counseling process cannot be overemphasized. At all times during interactions with families, the clinician must exhibit considerable concentration and focus. Admittedly, this task will be easier on some days than others! To understand fully a family's perspectives, it is essential that the clinician listen attentively to both verbal and nonverbal messages. When professionals show their willingness to listen to parental concerns, families feel more comfortable, cared about, and respected (Meadow-Orlans and Sass-Lehrer, 1995). Shipley (1997) provides a detailed discussion of listening, including a number of suggestions for developing and refining listening skills. He describes four major factors for effective listening: concentration, active participation, comprehension, and objectivity. To concentrate, the counselor needs to prepare the interaction room ahead of time to minimize potential distractions (such as telephones ringing, unrelated papers on the desk, etc.) and to keep constant vigil against thoughts that are unrelated to what the family members may be saying. Similarly, via active participation, the clinician's mind remains alert, flexible, and open during the interview process. By comprehension, Shipley means that the clinician tunes in to verbal, surface messages as well as verbal and nonverbal underlying meanings. For example, the mother who asks for information on the academic achievement of children who are deaf may really be revealing her anxiety about her

daughter's future, rather than requesting a barrage of statistics on the average reading levels of deaf children. Finally, Shipley urges counselors to remain objective during family interactions, not judging the interviewee by imposing their own personal feelings, biases, or viewpoints.

DeConde Johnson (1994) points out that knowing when to listen and when to talk can be difficult. Counselors are often uncomfortable with periods of silence, wanting instead to fill pauses or lulls in the conversation with questions or comments. Many times, however, these periods of silence should be honored, as they may allow the interviewee time to reflect on the issues being discussed and/or to formulate thoughts or ideas that they need to express (Clark, 1994; Shipley, 1997).

RESPONDING TO FAMILIES DURING COUNSELING SESSIONS

Clark (1990) contends that the one attribute that is absolutely essential when responding to families during counseling sessions is honesty. Beyond that, however, there are a number of ways of responding to families' questions and comments. Clark describes the hostile response, the evaluative response, the probing response, and the understanding response to families. The hostile response occurs when the counselor feels threatened, challenged, or frustrated. Every attempt should be made to avoid responding hostilely to families, because this type of response will undermine the counselor's efforts to establish a collaborative relationship with the family and to increase the family's' confidence.

The evaluative response involves the audiologist making a judgment as to the appropriateness of the patient's comments, questions, or behaviors. Like the hostile response, telling family members how they should act or feel is detrimental to the collaborative relationship between the family and the counselor. There may be times when the audiologist will provide advice to the family, but this should always be done in an objective, nondirective way, with consideration of the family's viewpoints kept in mind.

The probing response, according to Clark (1990), is designed to obtain further information or to seek clarification or expansion. Thus, these types of responses can be helpful. However, Clark cautions the audiologist that probing responses should not be used to control the direction of the counseling session, and that family members must not be led into thinking that, with more information, the audiologist will be able to provide solutions.

The most ideal of the responses for building and maintaining strong relationships between the counselor and the family is the understanding response (Clark, 1990). The understanding response is characterized by active or reflective listening (i.e., attempts to reflect back what the audiologist understands to be the patient's viewpoint, concern, or feeling), reassurance, and acceptance. The latter characteristic, acceptance, does not imply agreement or approval of what the patient says or does; rather, it means that the counselor appreciates or understands the patient's words or actions.

A dilemma that may occur during the counseling process is the need for the counselor to use different response types according to the family's needs at a given time. That is, there will be times when families need direct answers and advice, and other times when the counselor should use probing and/or reflective responses to help the family gain insights into their own feelings or should maintain silence and just let the family vent. Likewise, Othmer and Othmer (1994) suggest that skillful interviewers must be flexible in the roles they assume during counseling sessions. At times, the counselor will need to be an empathetic listener who puts the family member at ease and who expresses compassion. At other times, the counselor will need to assume an expert or leader role, providing information and guidance. The challenge is to be flexible in assuming these roles and to monitor continually whether there is an appropriate balance between the empathetic role and the expert role.

Special Counseling Considerations

COUNSELING FAMILIES WITH CHILDREN WHO HAVE MULTIPLE DISABILITIES

According to statistics reviewed by Meadow-Orlans and co-researchers (Meadow-Orlans and Sass-Lehrer, 1995; Meadow-Orlans et al., 1995), the number of children with hearing impairment who have an additional handicapping condition has remained fairly constant over the years at approximately 30%. However, Meadow-Orlans and Sass-Lehrer (1995) point out that there has been an increase since the early 1980s in the proportion of preschoolers who have two or more disabilities beyond deafness. Meadow-Orlans et al. (1995) compared mother-infant interactions and parental stress levels of parents who have children with and without additional handicaps beyond hearing loss. The mother-child interaction behaviors of the mothers with multiply-handicapped infants did not differ from those of mothers whose children had hearing loss and no other conditions. However, the mothers of the multiply-handicapped infants tended to have either very high or very low stress scores. Meadow-Orlans and coauthors attributed this distribution of scores to the fact that mothers of children who have multiple disabilities may experience extremely high degrees of stress or they may deny the severity of the child's problems. The lower degrees of stress could be due to denial of the severity of the child's problems or to the fact that the mothers had been so traumatized by the serious medical ailments of their multihandicapped child that their gratitude for the child's survival might have lessened the degree of the stress they experienced. The higher degrees of stress are not surprising.

The decisions the family must make regarding communication approach and school placement are complicated by additional disabilities. Anxiety about the child's future may be even more pronounced than that experienced by parents whose children have no other conditions. The child with multiple handicaps will probably be seen by a larger number of professionals (e.g., physical therapists, occupational therapists, medical personnel, etc.), creating even greater time demands for the parent, not to mention the greater possibility of conflicting opinions that the parents must reconcile. Based on their experiences at the Kendall Demonstration Elementary School at Gallaudet University, Meadow-Orlans and Sass-Lehrer suggest that in some cases parent support groups might be inadvisable, in that some of the discussions might be too painful for parents whose children have additional handicaps that affect their progression toward the acquisition of communication skills. The need for approaching each family as unique in its outlook, needs, and strengths, as mandated by PL 99-457, is even greater for families with multiply-handicapped children (Meadow-Orlans et al., 1995).

MULTICULTURAL CONSIDERATIONS IN THE COUNSELING PROCESS

In this chapter, the importance of audiologists embracing a family focus to their services has been emphasized. To provide effective, relevant services to families, it will be necessary to take into account the impact of cultural diversity on family functioning and on the counseling process. This need for consideration of cultural diversity is underscored by the rapidly changing demographics in the United States (McGonigel, 1994; Roseberry-McKibbin, 1997). It is estimated that by 2000, 38% of children younger than 18 will be from non-white, non-Anglo families (Hanson et al., 1990). As the country's demographics change, it can be expected that in many areas of the country nearly 50% of all young children will be from cultural and language groups that are different from those of most early intervention professionals. Thus, early interventionists who embrace a family-centered focus will be interacting with families whose values and practices may be quite different from their own.

There are numerous ways in which cultural differences between the family and the audiologist may affect the counseling and

collaboration process. Communicative interactions that are stressed in many early intervention programs for children and parents, such as encouraging the child to maintain eye contact or having the mother sit on the floor and playfully imitate the child's vocalizations, may be in direct conflict with language socialization practices typical of the parents' culture (Crago and Eriks-Brophy, 1993). Home intervention programs or interviews to obtain information may seem to be invasions of privacy to some cultural groups (Meadow-Orlans and Sass-Lehrer, 1995). Families may have cultural mores that view punctuality, rules for initiating and conducting conversations, gender, directness of communication, and family participation quite differently from the professional's culture (Roseberry-McKibbin, 1997). Cultural groups may have significantly different views of medicine and health care, of attitudes toward disabilities and etiologies of disabilities, and of child rearing practices (Harry, 1997). The audiologist's own cultural identity, beliefs, and value systems will influence how he or she interacts with families and works with them to formulate and prioritize intervention goals. Obviously, it will be critical for audiologists who work with families of children who are hearing-impaired to acknowledge and respect different cultural perspectives and to learn how to work effectively with families whose views and practices are quite different from their own.

Unlike the traditional Anglo-American family, which tends to be small, nuclear, and clearly defined in family members' roles, families from other cultural backgrounds may have radically different family structures, with multiple generations living together in a single household, diverse roles among family members, and responsibilities for child care shared by all. This difference alone, coupled perhaps in some cases with the family's limited English proficiency, may necessitate the audiologist's rethinking of how best to serve the family via counseling. Before designing appropriate intervention goals for culturally diverse families, the audiologist needs to address a number of issues. For example, if there are language problems, how might these be circumvented? Who are the members of the child's family? Who is the child's primary caregiver(s)? What are the family's beliefs about disability and causal factors of disability? What is the style of interaction among family members? What are the family's specific child-rearing practices? What are the family's attitudes toward help-seeking, professionals, intervention, health, and healing?

The audiologist needs to determine whether problems that arise during the collaboration process are due to cultural differences. The fact that the professional and the family come from different cultural backgrounds and have different viewpoints on the meaning of disability, parenting styles, and appropriate goals for the child increases the possibility of discord. Harry (1997) argues for the importance of trying to avoid mutual frustration and misunderstanding by the professional being open to learning about the family's underlying beliefs/values and being flexible in reframing intervention goals within the context of these values. Harry points out that admittedly it is time-consuming to have dialogues with families in an effort to learn about their cultural backgrounds, and it may be difficult for clinicians to make concessions on intervention goals. However, the outcome of not making the effort to learn about the family's cultural norms may be alienation between the professional and the family, which of course is not conducive to helping the child. Building on the strengths of the family's cultural influences is one of the keys to success. Practitioners in cross-cultural situations need to learn about the cultural norms of the various communities in which they work, and approach each family with no preconceived notions or judgments and with an attitude of building on the strengths and resources that the family brings to the collaboration process (McGonigel, 1994; Roseberry-McKibbin, 1997).

The results of a survey of African-American parents of children who are hearing-impaired by Jones and Kretschmer (1988) hint that our present models for parent education are ineffective in teaching culturally diverse and/or lower socioeconomic status parents. Although the parents they surveyed reported a high degree of satisfaction with their children's educational program, they also reported being minimally involved with the program and unfamiliar with many of the terms, practices, and methods of teaching children who are hearing-impaired.

Wayman et al. (1990) caution early intervention professionals not to set up a priori expectations of family functioning for various culture groups. They point out that families within specific cultures may or may not reflect characteristics that are considered typical for that culture. Variables such as socioeconomic status, length of residence in the United States, and the degree of cultural identification may have more influence on family beliefs and style than the culture itself. Therefore, an appropriate, culturally sensitive way of approaching families would be to view each family as a unique unit that potentially may be influenced by its culture but not necessarily locked into the culture's standard characteristics.

In the past decade, there have been several articles regarding how counseling and other forms of early intervention might be affected by specific cultures (Maestas and Erickson, 1992; Grant, 1993; Konstantareas and Lampropoulou, 1995; Mapp and Hudson, 1997). If a specific culture's language socialization and family practices are unknown, then it is essential that the audiologist make every effort, in a respectful and diplomatic way, to establish two-way dialogue with the family so that appropriate counseling and intervention can be facilitated (Crago and Eriks-Brophy, 1993). Baird and Peterson (1997) suggest that the early interventionist invite families to share their vision for their child's future as well as their child-rearing goals. Thus, the interventionist can be sensitive to the family's cultural values and child-rearing preferences as the family describes its hopes, dreams, and expectations for the child and the family's role in helping the child to achieve these outcomes.

Challenges to Implementing Family-Centered Counseling

Along with the rewards of collaborating with families of young children with hearing loss, there undoubtedly will be numerous challenges. Knowledge of some of the barriers to implementing family-centered counseling and intervention may be helpful for overcoming these challenges. Indeed, research suggests that many professionals who subscribe to a family-centered philosophy of early intervention fail to practice it (Roush et al., 1991; Mahoney et al., 1998).

FOCUS ON THE CHILD'S NEEDS

The history of early intervention with children who are hearing-impaired has been characterized by a focus on the child's needs, rather than the family's (Meadow-Orlans and Sass-Lehrer, 1995). Results of a recent study by McBride and Petersen (1997) suggest that home-based early interventionists who work with families of children who have disabilities continue to focus almost exclusively on the child with special needs, spending more than half of the duration of intervention sessions directly teaching the child. From observations of early interventionists, it was apparent from this study that there continued to be little emphasis on strengthening or supporting the parent-child relationship.

Rather than teaching the child, audiologists must now understand the complexities of family life and how to strengthen the role of the family in the child's intervention. Treatment plans consisting of goals for the child have to be recast as family intervention plans. It requires some adjustment to discontinue service provision that focuses almost exclusively on the child. Additionally, the skills needed to teach parents to implement an appropriate intervention program for the child are considerably different from those required to implement a program based on the dated therapist-child model. In addition to proficiency with the intervention, specialists who work with families must also have skills for presenting relevant and useful information to parents, coaching, providing positive examples and specific instructions to parents, giving feedback in a useful and positive manner, and evaluating the child's progress in the context of the parent's implementation of the intervention plan (Hester et al., 1995).

TRADITION OF DIRECTIVENESS

Families of children who are deaf or hard-of-hearing traditionally have been prescribed to as far as what the teaching goals and procedures should be (Meadow-Orlans and Sass-Lehrer, 1995). Engaging in collaborative relationships with parents means that the professional has to accept a role that involves less control and directiveness. Families must be encouraged to engage in all aspects of the intervention program, including decision-making. Rather than discussion of the audiologist's concerns and priorities, the focus must be on issues determined by the family. It simply is not enough to have parents involved in the intervention process. To embrace a family-centered, collaborative approach to early intervention means that the professional relinquishes control of the child' program of intervention to the family. The solution, according to Winton and DiVenere (1995), lies in preprofessional preparation, in which students not only read about and discuss family empowerment, but are also given the opportunities to see intervention models in action, in which family expertise is recognized, supported, and nurtured. Most individuals who choose a career in audiology or speech-language pathology do so because of their interest in working in a helping profession. Bailey (1987) points out, however, that early interventionists are often too eager to offer solutions and answers to a families' needs. The task at hand for interventionists, according to Bailey, is to learn to solve problems with families, not for them.

PROFESSIONAL PREPARATION FOR FAMILY-BASED INTERVENTION

Professionals who work with families of children who have special needs require considerable training, knowledge, and skills so that they have the confidence and compe-tence to assist families (Winton and Di-Venere, 1995; Baird and Peterson, 1997; Winton, 1998). They must be knowledge-able regarding family systems, analysis of infant-caregiver interactions, collaborative problem-solving and decision-making, and intradisciplinary collaboration. The preser-vice educational needs of audiologists in the areas of parent counseling, including appro-priate coursework and supervised clinical experience in family-based intervention, will need to be addressed to provide appro-priate services to families with children who are hearing-impaired.

PARENTAL PREFERENCE FOR EXPERT MODEL OF SERVICES

It has been the author's experience on quite a few occasions that some parents actually prefer the "expert" model of counseling and intervention, rather than the family collabo-ration model. That is, some parents may feel so overwhelmed by the child's hearing dif-ficulties that they look to the clinician to be a sort of Annie Sullivan, who will assume full responsibility for the child's instruction and who ultimately will work miracles. This observation was borne out in a survey by McWilliam et al. (1996) of parents of in-fants, toddlers, and preschoolers with dis-abilities and of professionals who work with these families. Many of the therapists who were surveyed mentioned that in many cases families preferred direct service provided to the child by the therapist, rather than con-sultation. The families felt that the consulta-tion model results in the therapist spending less time working directly with the child.

In the author's experience, the best way to overcome the challenge of parents who want to relinquish their role in making de-cisions for the child and in collaborating with the clinician in the child's intervention program is to build up their confidence in their own skills and knowledge of the child. It is not because they are apathetic or lazy that parents prefer the clinician to work di-rectly with the child. Rather, it is more typ-ically because the parent feels ill equipped

to know what should be done and how it should be accomplished. The sensitive clin-ician will take every opportunity to address and bolster the parents' self-efficacy. A fo-cus on the family's strengths will be a tre-mendous help in this regard.

CONFLICTS IN VALUES AND PRIORITIES FOR SERVICE

Implicit in the family empowerment model of early intervention is the concept that the clinician must put his or her own profes-sional agenda aside and instead look to the family to share in the determination of goals and service priorities. Of course, problems will inevitably arise when parents and pro-fessionals disagree about the goals of inter-vention and/or the methods by which these goals will be achieved. Bailey (1987) offers a number of suggestions for either avoiding conflict or resolving it. These include:

1. Use collaborative goal-setting so that parents will be involved in setting goals and thus more likely to follow through on them.
2. Obtain as much information as possible about the family's perspectives, values, needs, and priorities by using question-naires, interviews, and observation.
3. Use negotiation and the consideration of multiple alternatives to attempt to obtain agreement on goals and/or methods when there are obvious differences in values between the professional and the family.
4. Address parent values/behaviors that seem detrimental to the child directly and specifically (having already established a positive relationship with the family will be helpful in these cases).
5. Realize that strong professional beliefs may at certain times have to be sacrificed in favor of collaborative goal-setting.

Bernheimer and Keogh (1995) suggest that the reason parents frequently do not fol-low through on well-designed intervention plans is that the plans do not fit the daily rou-tine of the family and/or are not compatible with the goals, values, and beliefs of the parents. As Minke and Scott (1995) point out, the energy that it would take to struggle with a parent over desired goals and services would be better off spent on finding ways to strengthen the parent-professional relationship and bolster family support. There may be times when the professional simply is not willing to accept a family's priorities and unable through negotiation to reach a satisfactory resolution with the parent regarding differences in values and priorities for service. In these cases, the audiologist might need to determine alternative sources of help for the family and to refer the family, without hostility or resentment, to another service provider.

TIME DEMANDS IN SERVING FAMILIES

It is not uncommon for practitioners in certain settings, particularly those in private practice or hospital settings, to lament their hectic schedules, which often leave little time for audiologic rehabilitation or counseling. The purpose of an article by Tye-Murray et al. (1994) was to describe audiologic rehabilitation and counseling services that are feasible and realistic to offer in busy clinical settings. At Tye-Murray's facility, staff members developed services that are relatively inexpensive, easy to implement, require little of the audiologist's time, and are likely to meet with good client competence. These services include home training programs, a client library, a children's circuit, a family center, and an assistive devices center.

The home training program was designed for children with cochlear implants and their parents. Some of the features of this service are videotapes and audiotapes, workbook activities, computerized activities, daily diaries maintained by the parents, and weekly telephone contact with the audiologist. The client library was organized to include relevant books, periodicals, videos, and audiotapes available for browsing or loan. The appendix to the Tye-Murray et al. (1994) article includes a splendid list of suggested items for the library. The children's circuit consists of learning activities that were placed in the waiting room so that they would be accessible to both pediatric patients and their siblings. The learning activities include picture booklets, sign language flash cards, puzzles, and materials for a sibling pen pal program. The family center was designed to offer a home-like setting to be used for counseling and for demonstration of auditory learning activities in a realistic environment, and the assistive devices center was created to display an array of assistive devices that patients and their families could try.

PERSONALITY CONFLICTS

Schuyler and Rushmer (1987) point out that it would be unreasonable to expect clinicians to be compatible with every family they see. The more self-confident, empathetic, and people-oriented the clinician, the less likely there will be personality conflicts. Almost inevitably, however, there will be families or specific family members to whom the specialist cannot relate and with whom the specialist cannot feel comfortable. When there appears to be tension between the clinician and the family, the clinician must engage in serious introspection to determine his or her contribution, if any, to the breakdown in the relationship. Sometimes a thoughtful examination of the issues will reveal the source of the antagonism and the clinician may be able to resolve it. When there are insurmountable differences between the family and the professional that jeopardize the collaborative relationship, every attempt should be made to assign a different specialist to the family.

Counseling the Child With Hearing Impairment

Much of this chapter has focused on meeting the needs of parents of recently diagnosed children who have hearing impairment. Special note must also be made of the counseling needs of children who are hearing-impaired, particularly adolescents. The onset of adolescence is usually a turbulent period, even for adolescents who are normal-hearing and their parents, with a lack of communication frequently perceived by both parties in parent-child dyads. It is not surprising that these difficulties may be magnified with the existence of a severe communication handicap such as deafness. It is also likely at this time that the parents' original hopes for the child's communication, academic, and social achievements may have depreciated with the realization that little time is left in which to achieve initial expectations.

Several authors have expressed concern regarding the low self-esteem of children who are hearing-impaired (Davis et al., 1986; Loeb and Sarigiani, 1986; Meadow-Orlans, 1990; Atkins, 1994). Davis et al. (1986) conducted an extensive psychoeducational evaluation of 40 children with hearing impairment, ages 5 to 18 years, to determine the effects of hearing loss on intellectual, academic, social, and language behaviors of children. Their results highlighted the heterogeneity of children who are hearing-impaired, with the effects of hearing loss differing from child to child. Half the children in their study expressed concern about their abilities to make friends or to be accepted socially compared with only approximately 15% of hearing children surveyed. Many of the children with hearing loss reported that they were teased by other children, frequently because of their hearing aids; only approximately one-third said that they would be open with their normal-hearing classmates about wearing hearing aids; and many others reported spending most of their time alone. The audiologist who works with children who are hearing-impaired needs to be aware of these opinions when dealing with children so that the issue of hearing aid use is treated sensitively.

Loeb and Sarigiani (1986) reported similar results in their study of the self-perceptions of 250 mainstreamed children between the ages of 8 and 15 years. Their research indicated that children with hearing loss who are in regular classrooms report that they are not popular, that they have a hard time making friends, that they are shy around their peers, and that they do not feel accepted by their families.

In addition to the increased potential for diminished self-concept, some authors have described a high incidence of neuropsychiatric disorders (Hindley et al., 1994) among deaf children and a high incidence of depression among adolescents who are hearing-impaired (Watt and Davis, 1991). The sensitive audiologist will consider this diminished self-concept and possible emotional-behavioral difficulties when interacting with children who are hearing-impaired and their families. There are a number of small but important ways that the audiologist might help nurture a positive self-concept in children. One is to be circumspect about unintended messages we might be sending to children as we interact with them. If we frown, look uncomfortable, or act frustrated or otherwise nonaccepting of their, in many cases, limited communication, we may be inadvertently reinforcing their perceptions of being inferior. If we downplay or ignore their cosmetic concerns about wearing aids or assistive devices, we are disregarding what to them is one of the greatest sources of their social difficulties. By acknowledging their negative feelings about hearing aids and FM devices, while at the time emphasizing the social benefits of these listening aids, the audiologist might gain more trust and respect from the child and ultimately more complicity in use of the hearing aids.

Other ways that the audiologist might help bolster self-esteem might be to take every opportunity to make positive comments about any of the child's strengths (and, of course, all children have strengths in some area of life), to allow children to participate at least to some degree in decisions that concern them, and to encourage families to "accent the positive." Group counseling sessions by a qualified counselor may help both teenagers who are hearing-impaired and their parents adjust to this often confusing period. The importance of attempting to foster positive family climates in families with a child who has hearing impairment to avoid or minimize disruptions of the child's sense of self and autonomy has been emphasized by several authors (Meadow-Orlans, 1990; Marschark, 1993).

Evaluating Audiology Practices for Family-Centeredness

As noted previously, there has been a gradual shift over the past two decades in audiology services for young children with hearing loss, from a clinically oriented therapeutic model (with its focus on the child with hearing loss) to a family-centered collaborative model, in which parents are recognized as full partners in the intervention process and in which the focus is on both child and family needs. Murphy et al. (1995) point out, however, that there is often a gap between an intervention program's stated values and philosophies and its practices. These authors suggest that the lack of clearly stipulated practice indicators constitutes a major barrier to having a bona fide family-centered practice. Even in programs that claim to embrace family-based services, there may be a tendency to continue to try to involve families in the program's goals and activities, rather than recognizing that the program needs to determine how it can involve itself in the families' lives (Crais, 1991).

Murphy et al. (1995) developed the Family-Centered Program Rating Scale (FamPRS) as a means of monitoring a program's progress in implementing family-centered services. The FamPRS is a paper-and-pencil rating scale designed to evaluate programs serving young children with disabilities, aged birth through 5 years, and their families. Items on the FamPRS consist of statements about early intervention program features that are consistent with a collaboration model. The rating scale has parallel forms for parents and staff members. The authors state that average ratings from both forms of the FamPRS (parent and staff versions) can be used as indicators of a program's performance in a number of areas of practice, including:

1. Providing flexibility and innovation in programming (e.g., "The program gives us information on how to meet other families of children with similar needs").
2. Providing and coordinating responsive services (e.g., "Someone on staff can help my family get services from other agencies").
3. Providing individual services and ways of handling complaints (e.g., "There is a comfortable way to work out disagreements between families and staff").
4. Providing appropriate and practical information (e.g., "Staff members help my family see what we are doing well").
5. Providing good communication timing and style (e.g., "Staff members are friendly and easy to talk to").
6. Developing and maintaining comfortable relationships (e.g., "Staff members regularly ask my family about how well the program is doing and what changes we might like to see").
7. Building family-staff collaboration (e.g., "Staff members give my family time to talk about our experiences and things that are important to us").
8. Respecting the family as decision-maker (e.g., "Staff members respect whatever level of involvement my family chooses in making decisions").
9. Respecting the family's expertise and strengths (e.g., "Staff members help my family feel more confident that we are experts on our children").
10. Recognizing the family's need for autonomy (e.g., "Staff members do not try to tell my family what we need or do not need").
11. Building positive expectations (e.g., "Staff members help my family feel we can make a positive difference in our child's life").

Murphy et al. suggest that the FamPRS, beyond its use for program evaluation, can also be used for program planning, staff development, and research.

In addition to the FamPRS, there are a number of other instruments that are useful for evaluating the extent of a program's family-centeredness. These include the Family-Focused Intervention Scale (Mahoney et al., 1990), the FOCAS: Family Orientation of Community and Agency Services (Bailey, 1989), Brass Tacks: A Self-Rating of Family-Focused Practices in Early Intervention, Parts I and II (McWilliam and Winton, 1990), and the Family Support Principles: Checklist for Program Builders and Practitioners (Dunst, 1990). Regardless of which instrument or technique is used, the important point is that audiologists who work with young children should attempt to examine the extent to which parents perceive their early intervention programs as providing family-centered versus child-centered services. Does the intervention program provide services in response to the priorities or needs of families, or does the program provide services based on its own initiatives (Mahoney and Filer, 1996)? An objective way to gain the answer to this question is to poll the families who are served by the program.

Summary

An overview has been presented of the counseling process with families of children who are hearing-impaired. Audiologists will continue to play an important role in reducing the effects of hearing handicap on family functioning and in maximizing the child's chances for successful communication, academic achievement, and life satisfaction. An emphasis in this chapter has been placed on determining and meeting family needs in counseling. This emphasis in no way is meant to suggest that audiologists abdicate their responsibilities in designing intervention programs, leaving goal determination and program implementation solely to parents. Instead, the shift in early intervention, away from child-centered services (which in audiology have traditionally focused on the communication needs of the child) to a more family-centered perspective, may enable each family to capitalize on its strengths in meeting the challenges of raising a child with hearing impairment. Families will continue to look to audiologists for advice, guidance, and service provision, and audiologists will continue to play a key role in meeting the needs of families of children with impaired hearing.

REFERENCES

Able-Boone H, Sandall SR, Frederick LL. An informed, family-centered approach to Public Law 99-457: parental views. Top Early Child Spec Educ 1990;10:100–111.

Atkins DV. Siblings of the hearing impaired: perspectives for parents. Volta Rev 1987;89:32–45.

Atkins DV. Counseling children with hearing loss and their families. In: Clark JG, Martin FN, eds. Effective counseling in audiology: perspectives and practice. Englewood Cliffs, NJ: Prentice-Hall, 1994:116–147.

Bagnato S, Dunst C. Psychoeducational interventions. In: Coffey CE, Brumback RA, eds. Textbook of pediatric neuropsychiatry. Washington DC: American Psychiatric Press, 1998:1465–1478.

Bailey DB. Collaborative goal-setting with families: resolving differences in values and priorities for services. Top Early Child Spec Educ 1987;7:59–71.

Bailey DB. FOCAS: family orientation of community and agency services. Chapel Hill, NC: Frank Porter Graham Child Development Center, University of North Carolina, 1989.

Bailey DB, Simeonsson RJ. Family assessment in early intervention. Columbus, OH: Merrill, 1988.

Bailey DB, Simeonsson RJ, Winton PJ, et al. Family-focused intervention: a functional model for planning, implementing, and evaluating individualized family services in early intervention. J Div Early Child 1986;10:156–169.

Baird S, Peterson J. Seeking a comfortable fit between family-centered philosophy and infant-parent interaction in early intervention: time for a paradigm shift? Top Early Child Spec Educ 1997;17:139–164.

Bernheimer LP, Keogh BK. Weaving interventions into the fabric of everyday life: an approach to family assessment. Top Early Child Spec Educ 1995;15:414–433.

Bernstein ME, Barta L. What do parents want in parent education? Am Ann Deaf 1988;133:235–246.

Bodner-Johnson B. The family environment and achievement of deaf students: a discriminant analysis. Except Child 1986;52:443–449.

Bromwich R. Working with parents and infants: an interactional approach. Austin, TX: Pro-Ed, 1978.

Brown AS, Yoshinaga-Itano C. F.A.M.I.L.Y. assessment: a multidisciplinary evaluation tool. In: Roush J, Matkin ND, eds. Infants and toddlers with hearing loss: family-centered assessment and intervention. Baltimore: York, 1994:133–163.

Caldwell B, Bradley R. Home observation for measurement of the environment. Little Rock: University of Arkansas Press, 1984.

Carney AE, Moeller MP. Treatment efficacy: hearing loss in children. J Speech Lang Hear Res 1998;41(Suppl):61–84.

Clark JG. Emotional response transformations: redirections and projections. ASHA 1990;32:67–68.

Clark JG. Understanding, building, and maintaining relationships with patients. In: Clark JG, Martin FN, eds. Effective counseling in audiology: perspectives and practice. Englewood Cliffs, NJ: Prentice-Hall, 1994:1–18.

Cole EB, St. Clair-Stokes, J. Caregiver-child interactive behaviors: a videotape analysis procedure. Volta Rev 1984;86:200–216.

Crago MB, Eriks-Brophy AA. Feeling right: approaches to a family's culture. Volta Rev 1993;95:123–129.

Crais ER. Moving from "parent involvement" to family-centered services. Am J Speech Lang Pathol 1991;9:5–8.

Davis JM, Elfenbein J, Schum R, et al. Effects of mild and moderate hearing impairments on language, educational, and psychosocial behavior of children. J Speech Hear Dis 1986;51:53–62.

DeConde Johnson C. Educational consultation: talking with parents and school personnel. In: Clark JG, Martin FN, eds. Effective counseling in audiology: perspectives and practice. Englewood Cliffs, NJ: Prentice-Hall, 1994:184–210.

Dinnebeil LA, Rule S. Variables that influence collaboration between parents and service coordinators. J Early Intervent 1994;18:349–361.

Dinnebeil LA, Hale LM, Rule S. A qualitative analysis of parents' and service coordinators' descriptions of variables that influence collaborative relationships. Top Early Child Spec Educ 1996;16:322–347.

Dunst CJ. Family support principles: checklists for program builders and practitioners. Family Systems Intervention Monograph. Morganton, NC: Family, Infant, and Preschool Program, Western Carolina Center 1990;2(5).

Dunst C, Paget K. Parent-professional partnerships and family empowerment. In: Fine M, ed. Collaboration with parents of exceptional children. Brandon, VT: Clinical Psychology, 1991:25–44.

Dunst C, Trivette C. A family systems model of early intervention. In: Powell DP, ed. Parent education and support programs: consequences for children and families. Norwood, NJ: Ablex, 1990:108–116.

Dunst C, Trivette C, Deal A. Enabling and empowering families: principles and guidelines for practice. Cambridge, MA: Brookline Books, 1988.

Dunst C, Trivette C, Jodry W. Influences of social support on children with disabilities and their families. In: Guralnick MJ, ed. The effectiveness of early intervention: directions for second generation research. Baltimore: Paul H. Brookes, 1997:499–522.

Fisiloglu G, Fisiloglu H. Turkish families with deaf and hard of hearing children: a systems approach in assessing family functioning. Am Ann Deaf 1996;141:231–235.

Goss R. Language used by mothers of deaf children and mothers of hearing children. Am Ann Deaf 1970;115: 93–96.

Grant J. Hearing-impaired children from Mexican-American homes. Volta Rev 1993;95:131–135.

Hadadian A, Rose S. An investigation of parents' attitudes and the communication skills of their deaf children. Am Ann Deaf 1991;136:273–277.

Hanson MJ, Lynch EW, Wayman KI. Honoring the cultural diversity of families when gathering data. Top Early Child Spec Educ 1990;10:112–131.

Harry B. Leaning forward or bending over backwards: cultural reciprocity in working with families. J Early Intervent 1997;21:62–72.

Harvey MA, Green CL. Looking into a deaf child's future: a brief treatment approach. Am Ann Deaf 1990;135:364–370.

Henggeler SW, Watson SM, Whelan JP, et al. The adaptation of hearing parents of hearing-impaired youth. Am Ann Deaf 1990;135:211–216.

Hester PP, Kaiser AP, Alpert CL, et al. The generalized effects of training trainers to teach parents to implement milieu teaching. J Early Intervent 1995;20:30–51.

Hindley PA, Hill PD, McGuigan S. Psychiatric disorder in deaf and hearing impaired children and young people: a prevalence study. J Child Psychol Psychiatry 1994;35: 917–934.

Israelite NK. Hearing-impaired children and the psychological functioning of their normal-hearing siblings. Volta Rev 1986;88:47–54.

Jamieson JR. Interactions between mothers and children who are deaf. J Early Intervent 1995;19:108–117.

Jones RC, Kretschmer LW. The attitudes of parents of black hearing-impaired students. Lang Speech Hear Serv Schools 1988;19:41–50.

Kampfe CM. Parental reaction to a child's hearing impairment. Am Ann Deaf 1989;134:255–259.

Kampfe CM, Harrison M, Oettinger T, et al. Parental expectations as a factor in evaluating children for the multichannel cochlear implant. Am Ann Deaf 1993;138: 297–303.

Konstantareas MM, Lampropoulou V. Stress in Greek mothers with deaf children. Am Ann Deaf 1995;140:264–270.

Kricos P. Response of mothers to the nonverbal communication of their hearing-impaired preschoolers. J Acad Rehab Audiol 1982;15:51–69.

Kubler-Ross E. On death and dying. New York: McMillan, 1969.

Loeb R, Sarigiani P. The impact of hearing impairment on self-perceptions of children. Volta Rev 1986;88: 89–100.

Luterman D. The Thayer Lindsley Family-Center Nursery: Emerson College. In: Clark JG, Martin FN, eds. Effective counseling in audiology: perspectives and practice. Englewood Cliffs, NJ: Prentice-Hall, 1994:301–319.

Luterman DM. Counseling persons with communication disorders and their families. 3rd ed. Austin, TX: Pro-Ed, 1996.

MacTurk RH, Meadow-Orlans KP, Koester LS, et al. Social support, motivation, language, and interaction: a longitudinal study of mothers and deaf infants. Am Ann Deaf 1993;138:19–25.

Maestas AG, Erickson JG. Mexican immigrant mothers' beliefs about disabilities. Am J Speech Lang Pathol 1992; 10:5–10.

Mahoney G, Filer J. How responsive is early intervention to the priorities and needs of families? Top Early Child Spec Educ 1996;16:437–457.

Mahoney G, Finger I, Powell A. The relationship of maternal behavioral style on the developmental status of organically impaired mentally retarded infants. Am J Ment Defic 1985;90:296–302.

Mahoney G, O'Sullivan P, Dennebaum J. Maternal perception of early intervention services: a scale for assessing family-focused intervention. Top Early Child Spec Educ 1990;10:1–15.

Mahoney G, Spiker D, Boyce G. Clinical assessments of parent-child interaction: are professionals ready to implement this practice? Top Early Child Spec Educ 1996; 16:26–50.

Mahoney G, Boyce G, Fewell RR, et al. The relationship of parent-child interaction to the effectiveness of early intervention services for at-risk children and children with disabilities. Top Early Child Spec Educ 1998;18:5–17.

Mapp I, Hudson R. Stress and coping among African American and Hispanic parents of deaf children. Am Ann Deaf 1997;142:48–56.

Marschark M. Psychological development of deaf children. New York: Oxford University Press, 1993.

Martin FN, George KA, O'Neal J, et al. Audiologists' and parents' attitudes regarding counseling of families of hearing-impaired children. ASHA 1987;29:27–32.

McBride SL, Peterson C. Home-based intervention with families of children with disabilities: who is doing what? Top Early Child Spec Educ 1997;17:209–233.

McGonigel MJ. The individualized family service plan: philosophy and conceptual framework. In: Clark JG, Martin FN, eds. Effective counseling in audiology: perspectives and practice. Englewood Cliffs, NJ: Prentice-Hall, 1994: 99–113.

McKellin WH. Hearing impaired families: the social ecology of hearing loss. Soc Sci Med 1995;40:1469–1480.

McWilliam P, Winton P. Brass tacks: a self-rating of family-focused practices in early intervention. Chapel Hill, NC: University of North Carolina, 1990.

McWilliam RA, Lang L, Vandiviere P, et al. Satisfaction and struggles: family perceptions of early intervention services. J Early Intervent 1995;19:43–60.

McWilliam RA, Young HJ, Harville K. Therapy services in early intervention: current status, barriers, and recommendations. Top Early Child Spec Educ 1996;16:348–374.

Meadow K, Schlesinger H, Holstein C. The developmental process in deaf preschool children: communication competence and socialization. In: Schlesinger H, Meadow K, eds. Sound and sign: childhood deafness and mental health. Berkeley: University of California Press, 1972:249–259.

Meadow-Orlans KP. Research on developmental aspects of deafness. In: Moores DF, Meadow-Orlans KP, eds. Educational and developmental aspects of deafness. Washington DC: Gallaudet University Press, 1990:283–298.

Meadow-Orlans KP. Sources of stress for mothers and fathers of deaf and hard of hearing infants. Am Ann Deaf 1995;140:352–357.

Meadow-Orlans KP, Sass-Lehrer M. Support services for families with children who are deaf: challenges for professionals. Top Early Child Spec Educ 1995;15:314–334.

Meadow-Orlans KP, Smith-Gray S, Dyssegaard B. Infants who are deaf or hard of hearing, with and without physical/cognitive disabilities. Am Ann Deaf 1995;140:279–286.

Minke KM, Scott MM. Parent-professional relationships in early intervention: a qualitative investigation. Top Early Child Spec Educ 1995;15:335–352.

Morgan-Redshaw M, Wilgosh L, Bibby MA. The parental experiences of mothers of adolescents with hearing impairments. Am Ann Deaf 1990;135:293–298.

Moses KL, Van Hecke-Wulatin M. The socioemotional impact of infant deafness: a counseling model. In: Mencher GT, Gerber, SE, eds. Early management of hearing loss. New York: Grune & Stratton, 1981:243–278.

Murphy DL, Lee IM, Turnbull AP, et al. The family-centered program rating scale: an instrument for program evaluation and change. J Early Intervent 1995;19:24–42.

Othmer E, Othmer S. The clinical interview using DSM-IV. Washington, DC: American Psychiatric Press, 1994.

Pollack D. Educational audiology for the limited-hearing infant and preschooler. Silver Spring, MD: Fellendorf Associates, 1985.

Romer EF, Umbreit J. The effects of family-centered service coordination: a social validity study. J Early Intervent 1998;21:95–110.

Roseberry-McKibbin C. Working with linguistically and culturally diverse clients. In: Shipley KG, ed. Interviewing and counseling in communicative disorders: principles and disorders. Boston, Allyn and Bacon, 1997:151–174.

Rosenberg S, Robinson C. Enhancement of mothers' interactional skills in an infant educational program. Educ Train Ment Retard 1985;20:163–169.

Roush, J, Harrison M, Palsha S. Family-centered early intervention: the perceptions of professionals. Am Ann Deaf 1991;136:360–366.

Roush J, McWilliam RA. Family-centered early intervention: historical, philosophical, and legislative issues. In: Roush J, Matkin ND, eds. Infants and toddlers with hearing loss: family-centered assessment and intervention. Baltimore: York, 1994:3–23.

Rushmer N, Schuyler V. Infant Hearing Resource: Portland, OR. In: Roush J, Matkin ND, eds. Infants and toddlers with hearing loss: family-centered assessment and intervention. Baltimore: York, 1994:277–300.

Schuyler V, Rushmer N. Parent-infant habilitation: a comprehensive approach to working with hearing-impaired infants and toddlers and their families. Portland, OR: Infant Hearing Resource, 1987.

Shipley KG. Interviewing and counseling in communicative disorders: principles and procedures. Boston: Allyn and Bacon, 1997.

Simmons-Martin AA, Rossi KG. Parents and teachers: partners in language development. Washington, DC: Alexander Graham Bell Association for the Deaf, 1990.

St. Clair-Stokes J, Mischook M. Caregiver-child interaction analysis: theory and application. Short course presented at the 1990 biennial international convention of the Alexander Graham Bell Association for the Deaf, Washington DC, July 1990.

Summers JA, Dell'Oliver C, Turnbull AP, et al. Examining the individualized family service plan process: what are family and practitioner preferences? Top Early Child Spec Educ 1990;10:78–92.

Trivette CM, Dunst CJ, Deal AG, et al. Assessing family strengths and family functioning style. Top Early Child Spec Educ 1990;10:16–35.

Tye-Murray N, Witts S, Schum L, et al. Feasible aural rehabilitation services for busy clinical settings. Am J Audiol 1994;3:33–45.

Vadasy PF, Fewell RR, Meyer DJ. Grandparents of children with special needs: insights into their experiences and concerns. J Div Early Child 1986;10:36–45.

Van Hecke ML. Emotional responses to hearing loss. In: Clark JG, Martin FN, eds. Effective counseling in audiology: perspectives and practice. Englewood Cliffs, NJ: Prentice-Hall, 1994:92–115.

Warren C, Hasenstab S. Self-concept of severely to profoundly hearing-impaired children. Volta Rev 1986;88:289–295.

Watt JD, Davis FE. The prevalence of boredom proneness and depression among profoundly deaf residential school adolescents. Am Ann Deaf 1991;136:409–413.

Waxman RP, Spencer PE, Poisson SS. Reciprocity, responsiveness, and timing in interactions between mothers and deaf and hearing children. J Early Intervent 1996;20:341–355.

Wayman KI, Lynch EW, Hanson MJ. Home-based early childhood services: cultural sensitivity in a family systems approach. Top Early Child Spec Educ 1990;10:56–75.

Winton P. Socially valid but difficult to implement: creative solutions needed. J Early Intervent 1998;21:114–117.

Winton PJ, Bailey DB Jr. Early intervention training related to family interviewing. Top Early Child Spec Educ 1990;10:50–62.

Winton PJ, Bailey DB Jr. Becoming family centered: strategies for self-examination. In: Roush J, Matkin ND, eds. Infants and toddlers with hearing loss: family-centered assessment and intervention. Baltimore: York Press, 1994:23–39.

Winton PJ, DiVenere N. Family-professional partnerships in early intervention personnel preparation: guidelines and strategies. Top Early Child Spec Educ 1995;15:296–313.

AUDIOLOGIC REHABILITATION: ADULTS

10

Rehabilitative Evaluation of Hearing-Impaired Adults

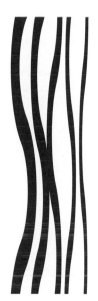

Jerome G. Alpiner, Ph.D., and Ronald L. Schow, Ph.D.

The discovering or labeling of hearing loss often occurs through a screening process such as at a health fair. Health fair screenings lead to audiology referrals and audiometric assessment. Self-referrals and medical referrals also result in an audiology diagnostic workup. A hearing diagnostic assessment in turn may lead to medical treatment or audiologic rehabilitation. If medical restoration is not feasible, amplification is generally the first rehabilitation option considered for persons with loss of hearing.

A rehabilitation evaluation occurs to guide the rehabilitation process after the hearing loss is identified. This evaluation may be a quite simple one or a very complex one in more involved cases. In most instances it involves relatively simple procedures that result in the fitting of hearing aids and/or assistive devices and providing hearing aid orientation (HAO). Hearing aid fitting and orientation are, in fact, the most common forms of audiologic rehabilitation and—if done thoroughly—will serve the needs of most patients. In other cases, the rehabilitation evaluation may be more extensive. The more extensive evaluations often result in amplification and orientation.

Fortunately, there has been significant improvement in instrumentation to help the hearing-impaired. Advanced technology has provided a variety of options, such as hearing aids that are fully digital and/or multichannel. These devices may even be completely in-the-canal. In other cases, persons use personal FM devices, infrared receivers and decoders for watching television, telephone amplifiers of various designs, and even telephones with digital displays. Even with this wonderful new technology, the successful use of hearing with these tools and devices is a very individual matter and cannot be taken for granted. Although many forms of amplification may not require extensive evaluations, we still need consistent methods for evaluation to ensure favorable outcomes.

When something as complex as a cochlear implant is needed, then a much more careful rehabilitation evaluation is required, to be followed with counseling and carefully planned rehabilitation procedures. To summarize, clients needing both simple and complex treatment require evaluation procedures to help in the planning of rehabilitation and the demonstrating of a satisfactory outcome.

Schow and Nerbonne (1996) proposed a model for a rehabilitation evaluation or assessment, which is slightly different but closely aligns with earlier work by an American Speech-Language-Hearing Association (ASHA) (1984) committee and Goldstein and Stephens (1981). This model is outlined in Table 10.1. It is recommended that four major issues be addressed in the assessment. First, communication status should be measured including a full audiogram with word recognition tests, visual skills including lip-reading, and an assessment of overall communication that might include sign language and previous rehabilitation progress. Second, the associated variables in psychological, sociological, vocational, and educational areas should be measured. Third,

Table 10.1
Audiologic rehabilitation model (enter through diagnostic identification process)[a]

Areas	ASHA	Sub-Areas
Assessment (CARA)		
Communication status	I-A, B	Auditory
		Visual
		Language
		Manual
		Communication strategies
		Previous rehabilitation
		Overall
Associated variables	II-B	Psychological
		Sociologic
		Vocational
		Educational
Related conditions		Mobility
		Upper limb
		Audiologic pathology
Attitude	II-D	Type I
		Type II
		Type III
		Type IV
Management (PACO)		
Psychosocial/counseling	II-A, B, D	Interpretation
		Information
		Counseling/guidance
		Acceptance
		Understanding
		Expectation
Amplification (instrumental)	I-C	Hearing aid fitting
		Cochlear implants
		Assistive devices
		Assistive listening
		Alerting/warning
		Tactile
		Communication
		Instruction/orientation
Communication training	II-B, C; II-A, V)	Goals
		Philosophy
		Tactics
		Skill-building
Overall coordination (ancillary)	II-B, C, E; III-C, IV	Vocational
		Educational
		Social work
		Medicine

[a]This model is consistent with the Goldstein and Stephens (1981) model and the ASHA position statement on definition of and competencies for audiologic rehabilitation (ASHA, 1984). The numbers and letters in parentheses refer to the ASHA statement as related to the areas listed.

related conditions such as mobility, upper limb status, and audiologic pathologies like tinnitus should be considered. Finally, the attitude on a four-point scale from positive to negative should be evaluated.

In most cases, the primary emphasis begins in looking at communication status, and the audiologist has various tools to do this. In assessing and evaluating communication, we may first consider hearing impairment as measured with an audiogram. Impairment refers to the difficulty or loss of hearing as measured by pure-tone and speech thresholds. Second, the primary effect of the loss on everyday communication needs to be examined (according to the World Health Organization [WHO, 1980] this is called disability). One way to infer conclusions about everyday communication is with formal tests of word recognition and speechreading, which will be discussed later in this chapter. These primary difficulties with communication can also often be measured with self-assessment questionnaires.

World Health Organization (WHO, 1997) issued a new draft of its earlier scheme and the terms *activity* and *participation* now have replaced *disability* and *handicap*. The original terms are still used here due to their familiarity and because they remain meaningful and some transition in usage will be required. Unfortunately in the United States, when hearing loss has an effect on earning a living, it is referred to as a hearing disability (AAO, 1979). In European countries the effect on jobs is called a hearing handicap (WHO, 1980; Stephens and Hetu, 1991).

Evaluation of the effects of hearing impairment in diverse communication situations (primary effect) and in various types of psychosocial and school/work environments (secondary effects) allows us to better plan and evaluate the effect of audiologic rehabilitation. After remediation by amplification or other strategies, it is helpful to evaluate the restoration of communication function and any resolution in the secondary handicap areas. In this chapter, we recommend that both audiologic procedures and self-report facilitate the evalua-

tion process and that these procedures follow an initial screening and audiometric assessment.

Screening and Audiometric Assessment

SCREENING

For many years there has been a guideline for screening school-age children with immittance and pure-tones. Several recent proposals have been made to facilitate screening of adults as well. All these screening procedures are now contained in one guideline (ASHA, 1997). The purposes for screening are to identify those with hearing disorders who may need medical attention and also to identify those who may have impairment and need nonmedical remediation so that they may receive the help they need. Therefore, a screening protocol should provide checks for medical concerns as well as communication and social/emotional issues related to hearing. Pure-tone impairment testing usually serves as one key item in screening. However, pure-tone screening is not enough by itself and should be incorporated along with other procedures. Case history information and selective use of immittance and/or visual inspection are useful procedures in screening for hearing disorders (Schow, 1991). A screening measure of handicap and/or disability is also important, and in recent years some tools have been proposed for this purpose (Schow and Nerbonne, 1982; Weinstein, 1986; ASHA, 1997).

AUDIOMETRIC ASSESSMENT TEST BATTERY

The initial audiologic test battery usually consists of pure-tone air and bone conduction audiometry, which will indicate the severity and frequency dimensions of hearing loss and whether the type of hearing loss is conductive, sensorineural, or mixed. Immittance may also be helpful for this purpose. Speech audiometry provides information on speech thresholds plus speech recognition at suprathreshold (comfortable hearing) levels. Relevant case history information includes time of onset of hearing loss, etiology, medical data, and general communication problems.

Rehabilitation Evaluation

Following an initial audiologic assessment, the client needing audiologic rehabilitation will require additional testing that may be referred to as the rehabilitation evaluation. As part of this evaluation, consideration should be given to communication difficulties encountered in the client's environment. Psychosocial issues and other handicap concerns also need to be identified. One good way to evaluate the primary disability issues and the secondary handicap issues is with self-assessment questionnaires. Evaluation of speechreading, auditory abilities, and tinnitus also is needed and will be considered in this chapter.

Disability/Handicap/Communication Questionnaires

EARLY EFFORTS

In the 1930s, self-assessment was used to place persons into a category of normal hearing, and this was in turn used to set the first standard for pure-tone thresholds (USPHS, 1938; Noble, 1978). In the 1940s and 1950s, an effort was made to look at social interaction through use of audiologic numeric data. Davis (1948) helped develop this procedure, which was called the Social Adequacy In-dex (SAI). He later reported that it was not effective and stated that more knowledge about the relationship between hearing and understanding connected speech was needed. The Hearing Handicap Scale was developed in the 1960s by High et al. (1964). It was a pioneering effort and the first in a long line of similar questionnaires designed to measure hearing impairment, disability, or handicap (Ewertsen and Birk-Nielsen, 1973; Noble and Atherley, 1970; Schein et al., 1970; Alpiner JG, Chevrette W, Glascoe G, et al. The Denver Scale of Communication Function. Unpublished study, University of Denver, 1974).

CURRENT STATUS

Self-report communication evaluation efforts have generated a variety of evaluation methods. Several of these methods will be discussed in this chapter. A 1980 survey of ASHA audiologists revealed that only 18% were using self-assessment procedures at that time. A survey of ASHA audiologists as of 1990, however, revealed that 33% were by then using such procedures (Schow et al., 1993). Even more audiologists are thought to be using self-report tools in recent years based on more recent surveys. The most used of these, according to the 1990 survey, are shown in Table 10.2.

Dancer and Gener (1999) surveyed members of the Academy of Rehabilitative Audiology, asking them to report those questionnaires that they considered most valid and useful. The most frequently used procedures were the Hearing Handicap Inventory for the Elderly (HHIE or HHIE-S), followed by the Self-Assessment of Communication (SAC), Communication Profile for the Hearing Impaired (CPHI), and the Hearing Handicap Inventory for Adults (HHI-A).

Progress has been made in the area of

Table 10.2
Various self-assessment questionnaires reported as being used by 33% of 469 clinically active ASHA audiologists

Questionnaires	1990 (N = 140)[a]	
	No.	%
HHIE	50	36
HHS	34	24
Denver	32	23
HPI	21	15
SAC/SOAC	19	14
CPHI	14	10
Other	27	9

Adapted from Schow RL, Balsara N, Whitcomb C, et al. Aural rehabilitation by ASHA audiologists: 1980–1990. Am J Audiol 1993;2:28–37.

HHIE, Hearing Handicap Inventory for the Elderly; *HHS,* Hearing Handicap Scale; *Denver,* Denver Scale of Communication Function; *HPI,* Hearing Performance Inventory; *SAC,* Self-Assessment of Communication; *SOAC,* Significant Other Assessment of Communication; *CPHI,* Communication Profile for the Hearing Impaired.

[a]These were the only audiologists who reported use of self-assessment questionnaires among 469 clinically active ASHA audiologists.

self-report procedures; the increasing use of self-assessment instruments by audiologists represents an improvement for both the client and the profession. Table 10.3 shows the varied dimensions that are assessed with various self-assessment questionnaires.

PURPOSES OF SELF-ASSESSMENT

These and other measures that have been developed have a variety of purposes and should be used appropriately. Giolas (1990) suggested that a self-assessment tool can be a valuable part of the audiologist's methods by explaining how an individual feels about hearing loss. He also stated that audiologists could use self-assessment to translate these handicapping effects into procedures for audiologic rehabilitation. Other purposes for self-assessment have also been noted.

Self-assessment is really a form of case history interview, and there are a variety of uses for self-assessment questionnaires. These include screening, initial diagnostic interview and counseling, rehabilitation evaluation, benefit measures, satisfaction, compensation, demographic uses, and others.

Table 10.3
Summary of various aspects assessed in self-assessment questionnaires

	HHIE	HHS	DSCF	HPI	SAC/ SOAC	CPHI	M-A
Speech communication	X	X	X	X	X	X	X
General speech	X		X	X	X	X	X
Home/family			X			X	X
Vocational/work			X	X		X	X
Social	X			X			
Individual or group	X			X			
Special communications	X	X		X	X	X	
With and without visual cues				X			
Adverse conditions		X		X		X	
Telephone/TV/radio		X		X			
Personal reactions	X		X	X	X	X	X
Response to auditory failure				X		X	
Acceptance of self/loss						X	
Hearing aid use							
Effect on activities/use	X						
Discouragement/embarrassment	X					X	
Anger/stress/anxiety	X					X	
Withdrawal/introversion	X					X	
Neuroticism							
Opinion/behavior of others			X	X	X	X	
Family relations							
Work performance							
Societal response							
Nonspeech communication		X		X	X		
Intensity/localization		X		X			
Doorbell/telephone bell							
Warnings in traffic							
Related symptoms					X		
Tinnitus/fluctuations/tolerance				X			

Adapted from Schow RL, Gatehouse S. Fundamental issues in self assessment of hearing. Ear Hear 1990;11:65–165.

HHIE, Hearing Handicap Inventory for the Elderly; *HHS,* Hearing Handicap Scale; *DSCF,* Denver Scale of Communication Function; *HPI,* Hearing Performance Inventory; *SAC,* Self-Assessment of Communication; *SOAC,* Significant Other Assessment of Communication; *CPHI,* Communication Profile for the Hearing Impaired; *M-A,* McCarthy-Alpiner Scale of Hearing Handicap.

Screening

A self-assessment screening questionnaire can alert professionals and the hearing-impaired person to problems due to hearing loss. These questionnaires are frequently used along with case history and pure-tones in screening programs. They can help form the basis for identification of hearing loss and lead to medical and audiologic referrals (Schow et al., 1991; ASHA, 1997).

Diagnostic interview/counseling

If the client is asked to complete a self-report form before the diagnostic evaluation, the audiologist will have information when the person first appears in the clinic. This is particularly helpful when both the client and a significant other complete the forms, because the feelings of both can be evaluated and counseling can be planned accordingly.

Rehabilitation evaluation

When a more extensive evaluation is undertaken, after diagnosis of the hearing loss, self-report can be a very valuable tool. This often involves the use of a longer, more detailed instrument and allows one to look at impairment, disability, and handicap.

Benefit measures/satisfaction

Audiologists are increasingly measuring self-reported improvement after remediation procedures. Most audiologists measure amplification benefits with real-ear measures or sound field functional gain. Several self-report measures have now been devised for a parallel purpose in reporting communication improvement. In addition, ratings of use in hours or satisfaction with hearing aid use have been used to evaluate success in hearing aid fitting (Oja and Schow, 1984; Schow et al., 1991; Brooks, 1989; Smedley, 1990; Gatehouse, 1994, 1997).

Compensation

The major emphasis in compensation has usually been on pure-tone findings, but some recommendations suggest that self-report measures may have a part in this process (Salomon and Parving, 1985).

Demographic and research uses

Self-report has been used in national health interview surveys and for measuring improvement in cochlear implant studies, to indicate two examples.

Screening Tools

Schow and Nerbonne (1982) were among the first to emphasize the need for a screening tool to measure the communication ability of hearing-impaired adults. The SAC and Significant Other Assessment of Communication (SOAC) are 10-item self-assessment screening questionnaires. These items were drawn from longer diagnostic instruments. The forms for SAC and SOAC are found in Attachments 1 and 2 at the end of this book. Items 1 through 6 of the scales assess communication difficulties in various situations and measure disability, whereas items 7 through 10 measure handicap by examining the client's general feelings about the handicap and the individual's perception of the attitudes of others toward hearing. The SOAC contains the same 10 items but with pronoun changes so that a closely associated observer can report on the hearing status of the client. Schow and Nerbonne (1977) had previously developed a multiple form of an assessment questionnaire to measure reports from significant others (staff members at a nursing home). Following the introduction of SAC and SOAC, Ventry and Weinstein (1983) modified a longer instrument they had developed to produce another 10-item screening procedure (HHIE-S). Weinstein (1986) described use of the HHIE-S in a screening protocol for the elderly, and Schow (1991) proposed use of SAC/SOAC in connection with an overall procedure for screening adult and elderly persons. In a recent ASHA document (ASHA, 1997), both the SAC and HHIE-S have been proposed for use. Other screening questionnaires have been developed (Schein et al., 1970; Schow et al., 1990), and audiologists now have several screening self-assessment tools from which to choose.

Intermediate-Length Questionnaires

HEARING HANDICAP SCALE

As noted earlier, the Hearing Handicap Scale (HHS) was one of the first self-assessment questionnaires developed. It has two forms that were standardized. Respondents use a five-point scale. One limitation of the HHS cited by its authors was that the questions are similar and designed to focus on only the softness/loudness aspect of hearing. Psychological, vocational, and other secondary problems caused by hearing loss are not considered. Despite its limitations, the HHS is still a popular tool among audiologists and has been a factor in encouraging additional research. In terms of recent terminology, it would be better to describe what it measures as impairment and disability rather than handicap.

Schow and Tannahill (1977) suggested a categoric method for interpreting HHS results. In this system, scores of 0 to 20% indicate no hearing handicap, 21 to 40% a slight handicap, 41 to 70% a mild-moderate handicap, and 71 to 100% a severe handicap. They found that most candidates for hearing aids or audiologic rehabilitation will have scores of 41% or higher (Table 10.4). This categoric procedure is now being used with several other self-assessment questionnaires.

DENVER SCALE OF COMMUNICATION FUNCTION

The Denver Scale of Communication Function (Alpiner JG, Chevrette W, Glascoe G, et al. The Denver Scale of Communication Function. Unpublished study, University of Denver, 1974) was designed for use with a semantic differential-type continuum for each of 25 statements (Attachment 3). It examines communication function in four categories: family, self, social-vocational, and general communication experience. To encourage "first impression" responses, it was recommended that a time limit of 15 minutes be allowed for clients to complete the scale. Client responses are recorded on a form (Fig. 10.1), so that pretherapy and posttherapy testing compares the client with himself, not his therapy counterparts or any other norms.

A quantified version of the Denver Scale was proposed by Schow and Nerbonne (1980) (Attachment 4). It is called the Quantified Denver Scale (QDS) and was used initially on 50 subjects divided into 3 subgroups. The degree of disability increased as a function of greater pure-tone averages. The subjects with normal hearing had QDS scores from 0 to 15%, those with slight hearing disability had scores of 16 to 30%, and those with mild-moderate disability had scores of 31% or greater.

MCCARTHY-ALPINER SCALE OF HEARING HANDICAP

The McCarthy-Alpiner Scale of Hearing Handicap (M-A Scale) (McCarthy and Alpiner, 1983) assesses effects of adult hearing loss for an individual and also for a family member who completes a parallel form of the scale (Attachment 5). This scale represented a pioneering effort to quantify the feelings of family members of hearing-impaired individuals. The M-A Scale consists of 34 items representing psychological, social, and vocational effects of hearing loss. These items fit the proposed criteria of 0.80 correlation for test-retest at a 2-week interval and also internal consistency reliability of 0.80 or better using Cronbach's alpha method.

Several aspects emerged in connection with development of this scale: (1) the hearing-impaired individual may fail to accept, understand, or deal with hearing problems, whereas the family member is keenly aware

Table 10.4
Categories and associated percentage scores for use in classifying hearing handicap scale performance

Category	Percentage Scores
No handicap	0–20
Slight hearing handicap	21–40
Mild-moderate hearing handicap	41–70
Severe hearing handicap	1–100

From Schow RL, Tannahill C. Hearing handicap scores and categories for subjects with normal and impaired hearing sensitivity. J Am Audiol Soc 1977;3:134–139.

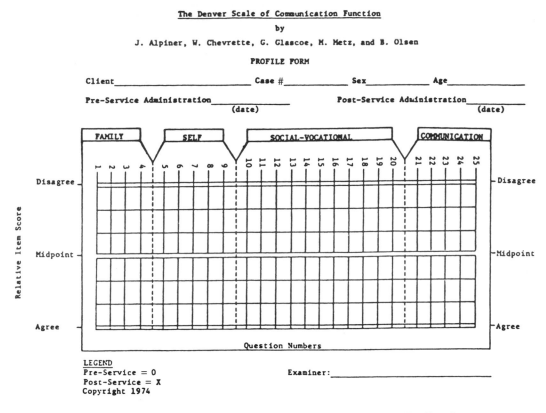

Figure 10.1. Profile form for scoring the Denver Scale of Communication Function.

of the handicapping effects; (2) the family member may be unable to recognize, understand, or deal with the individual's hearing impairment; (3) the two persons may fail to agree on the problem areas; and (4) any combination of the above.

A significant use of this scale relates to the counseling needs of hearing-impaired individuals and family members. It is apparent that any counseling of the hearing-impaired individual should involve the family. With this scale it is possible to determine systematically the attitudes and relationships of family members compared with those of hearing-impaired individuals. Furthermore, family involvement can contribute to a more complete rehabilitation program for hearing-impaired persons.

This scale fulfills at least three objectives (McCarthy and Alpiner, 1983): (1) it provides an index of whether the organic hearing loss has manifested itself as a handicap, (2) it provides diagnostic data to guide the use of rehabilitative and/or hearing aid procedures, and (3) it provides for a detailed analysis of psychological, social, and vocational problem areas.

Other Questionnaires

The HHIE has been used on an adult population, but it is really designed for use with the elderly (see Chapter 13). Another version of the HHIE (Newman et al., 1991) has been proposed for use with adults, the Hearing Handicap Inventory for Adults (HHIA). The test-retest reliability of the HHIA was assessed on a sample of 28 hearing-impaired adults and was found to be r = 0.97. This procedure is useful with adults (Attachment 6).

Diagnostic Tools

Two major diagnostic tools have been developed for use with the hearing impaired. A description of each follows.

HEARING PERFORMANCE INVENTORY

The Hearing Performance Inventory (HPI) was developed to assess hearing performance in everyday communication situations (Giolas et al., 1979). The inventory items were divided into six categories. The basic format of the HPI consists of presenting listeners with everyday situations and asking them to judge their listening performance according to a rating from one to five. The original form of the inventory consisted of 158 items. The HPI has been revised three times into several shorter versions.

The 90-item revised form of the HPI was described by Lamb et al. (1983) and can be administered within 20 minutes. Giolas (1983) states that the revised version can be used in most clinical settings, and the longer form will provide an additional pool of items. In the clinical scoring process, an overall percentage of difficulty is obtained by adding the numeric responses (1 to 5) for all items attempted, dividing by the number of items attempted, and multiplying by 20. Giolas (1983) stated that profiles for one or more of the sections may be generated. A comparable procedure may be followed for each section or for categories within or across sections. The HPI is not generally used in the standard audiologic test battery; rather, its greatest clinical utility is in extensive rehabilitation evaluations.

Weinstein (1984) discussed the advantages of the HPI. It was indicated that the HPI has value as an assessment technique and that the items provide a description of the difficulties experienced in a wide variety of listening situations. Further, the profiles allow a convenient way of displaying responses for a rehabilitation program.

COMMUNICATION PROFILE FOR THE HEARING IMPAIRED (CPHI)

This profile, developed by Demorest and Erdman (1986), is also lengthy and uses 145 items that are divided into 25 scales. These different scales describe the communication performance, communication environment, communication strategies, and personal ad-justment of hearing-impaired adults. Communication is assessed in a variety of environments including social situations, at home, and at work. In addition, attitudes and behavior of others are assessed, as are verbal and nonverbal strategies. Personal adjustment issues include self-acceptance, acceptance of loss, anger, discouragement, stress, withdrawal, and denial. This profile was psychometrically developed through pilot use on 827 active-duty military personnel at Walter Reed Army Medical Center. The CPHI is useful when an extensive rehabilitation evaluation of a client is needed. Because of its psychometric refinement, it is possible to make pretherapy and posttherapy measurements and know when a true change has taken place. Data are available on the Walter Reed population (Demorest and Erdman, 1987) and have since been reinforced by reports from other populations.

Specialized Self-Report Approaches

OPEN-ENDED QUESTIONNAIRES

Stephens (1980) proposed the use of an open-ended questionnaire in evaluating the problems of hearing-impaired patients. In this procedure the questionnaire contains the following statement: "Please make a list of the difficulties which you have as a result of your hearing loss. List these in order of importance, starting with the greatest difficulties. Write down as many as you can think of." He reported on results from the first 500 responses. There were 48% who complained of difficulty with TV/radio, 34% with general conversation, 24% with the doorbell, 23% with group conversation, 23% with speech in noise, and 20% with a telephone ring. Embarrassment was mentioned by 14%, and tinnitus was mentioned by only 8% of respondents. Although conversation problems were not listed as often as TV/radio difficulties, they were listed first about 60% of the time (meaning they were more important), whereas TV/radio was listed first less than 10% of the time. Stephens encouraged use of an open-ended procedure plus one of the more traditional handicap questionnaires along with some measure of personality to look at issues such as extroversion, anxiety, and depression. He examined nearly 200 patients with personality scales and found them to be more introverted and neurotic, with pronounced elevations in the anxiety scale compared with control subjects.

Hearing performance inventory for severe to profound hearing loss

Owens and Raggio (1984) reported the use of the Hearing Performance Inventory for Severe to Profound (HPI-SP) hearing loss. The HPI-SP may be used in connection with hearing aid use, cochlear implants, and vibrotactile use. Kaplan et al. (1990) proposed a similar communication assessment scale for deaf adults.

Hearing Aid Satisfaction, Use, and Benefit Self-Report

SATISFACTION AND USE REPORTS

A variety of reports have appeared to measure the satisfaction levels of hearing aid users. Smedley (1990) provided a summary of these, which indicated that hearing aid users' satisfaction may range from 50 to 90%. In general, less than 20% are highly satisfied, and 10 to 20% tend to be strongly dissatisfied. He compared satisfaction levels on hearing aid, eyeglass, and denture users and found that hearing aid users were the least satisfied (denture, 92% satisfied; eyeglass, 83% satisfied; hearing aid, 71% satisfied).

Several reports on hearing aid use have appeared. Brooks (1989) reported on 758 hearing aid clients' use levels and found that use increases with greater hearing loss and with younger ages. Use drops off dramatically for persons older than 80 years of age. Schow et al. (1991) reported on 680 hearing aid users and found trends similar to those reported by Brooks, except that use levels were greater in the U.S. study (6 to 14 hours) compared with Brooks's study done in the United Kingdom, where hours of use ranged from 4 to 10.

HEARING PROBLEM INVENTORY

Hutton (1980) pioneered the use of a questionnaire to assess dimensions of hearing aid use. This questionnaire, the Hearing Problem Inventory-Atlanta (HPI-A), was used to examine patients' perceptions of their problems and the amount of time the aids were worn. His findings included (1) before and after data from patients receiving initial fittings and (2) before and after data for those receiving replacement fittings.

Older persons reported increased problems and decreased wear time, whereas employed persons had slightly higher problem scores but longer hours of hearing aid use. Before and after data showed larger reductions in self-assessed problems by persons who were receiving their initial fittings compared with experienced hearing aid users. Hearing aid wear time increased for those having their aids longer and as hearing loss increased, but wear time decreased with age of the person. In persons older than 55, there is a decrease in aid wear of roughly 1 hour per day per decade.

HEARING AID PERFORMANCE INVENTORY

The Hearing Aid Performance Inventory (HAPI) is another self-report procedure for measuring hearing aid benefit. It was proposed by Walden et al. (1984). This procedure involves a 64-item questionnaire that was shown to have excellent internal consistency reliability. These authors concluded that the patient's reported benefit received from the hearing aid can be used as one measure of successful hearing aid use in daily life. They identified four types of situations that can be analyzed separately: (1) noisy situations, (2) quiet situations with the speaker in proximity, (3) situations with reduced signal information, and (4) situations with nonspeech stimuli. In general, they found that significantly more benefit was reported with hearing aids in quiet than in noise.

APHAB AND COSI QUESTIONNAIRES

Recently, several additional questionnaires were developed for patient-assessed hearing aid benefit by Cox and associates, including the Profile of Hearing Aid Benefit (PHAB) and the Intelligibility Rating Improvement Scale (IRIS). The PHAB allows estimation of the proportion of time that certain situations presented communication problems, and the IRIS allows estimation of the proportion of speech that can be understood in various situations. Based on use with 42 hearing aid users, the PHAB did not show as much benefit as the IRIS, but it was more sensitive to different listening situations and more like other previous results (Cox et al., 1991). An abbreviated form of the PHAB is now available and is called the APHAB (Cox and Alexander, 1995).

A recent open-ended, self-report form for use with hearing aid users called the Client-Oriented Scale of Improvement (COSI) was developed in Australia and appears to be a promising approach based on initial reports (Dillion et al., 1997). Twelve audiologists compared the COSI with various versions of the HAPI, the HHIE, the PHAB, and several other self-report measures of satisfaction, use, and benefit when fitting hearing aids. They rated the COSI to be more useful and convenient than the other longer self-report tools. Furthermore, it was found to be just as reliable as the longer instruments, even though the COSI was based on only three to five items.

Combined Rehabilitation Evaluation and Postfitting Self-Report

An extremely versatile self-report procedure was recently developed by Gatehouse (1997) for use in the U.K. program of hearing aid fitting and follow-up. This procedure, the Glasgow Hearing Aid Benefit Profile (GHABP), allows for a hearing-impaired person to report on four common situations (TV, one-on-one in quiet, in noise, and listening in a group of people) and up to four items that the person suggests in an open-ended format. The procedure is simple, short, and gleans an extraordinary amount of information on the front and back of a single sheet of paper. First, the person reports how much difficulty they experience in these eight situations without a hearing aid. This is a measure of disability. Second, they report how much this difficulty worries, annoys, or upsets them. This is a measure of handicap. This is an extremely simple way to measure relevant information on disability and handicap for a rehabilitation evaluation. The same form allows measurement after hearing aid fitting in each of these situations for the amount of (1) use time, (2) benefit from that use, (3) residual disability when the hearing aid is used, and (4) satisfaction. This format has much to recommend it, combining as it does the best features of open-ended and standardized short self-reports. It has been modified, with permission, for use with the SAC and SOAC. This allows the use of previous SAC self-report data gathered on several thousand hearing-impaired and normal-hearing persons, so that useful comparisons in the areas of disability and handicap as related to various levels of hearing and various aged persons can be derived. The GHABP seems to have many of the advantages of the COSI because it works toward the major concerns that the person has with his or her hearing, yet it has the advantage that the four common situations to which all persons respond allow comparison with others. The reader is referred to Chapter 11 for a discussion of use of these tools in the hearing aid fitting process.

Evaluation of Speechreading Ability

DEFINITIONS AND CONSIDERATIONS

Speechreading and lipreading are terms that have been used synonymously for many years, although separate definitions have been provided. Prescod (1986) considers the terms as synonymous with meaning "a method of transmitting language by the visible components of oral discourse." Lipreading may be used narrowly to define the process by which a person uses the position and movements of the speaker's lips as cues (Thorn and Thorn, 1989). Speechreading may be used to describe the process by which a person uses many cues to understand ongoing speech. The cues include lipreading, facial expressions of the speaker, the residual hearing of the hearing-impaired person, and grammatical and semantic context (Walden et al., 1977). The speechreading process may include the following components: (1) listening with or without amplification, (2) recognition of gestural cues, (3) awareness of facial expressions, (4) awareness of environmental cues, and (5) vision training (lipreading).

Gagne (1994) defined lipreading as the process whereby visual sensory information is extracted from the articulatory movements available from a talker's lips, jaws, and adjacent facial musculature. Boothroyd (1988) defined speechreading as the process of perceiving spoken language using vision as the sole source of sensory evidence which includes facial expressions as well as environmental and contextual cues. Jeffers and Barley (1981) relate lipreading to a process involving three steps: (1) sensory reception of the motor or movement pattern, (2) perception of the pattern, and (3) association of the pattern with meaningful concepts. The lipreader receives limited visual information and must fill in information not received.

The emphasis on speechreading has diminished in the past few years, probably due to the technological advances in hearing aids. Many professionals believe that amplification eliminates or minimizes the need for visual training. Ross (1982) has stated that there is quite a difference between deaf persons who need the additional assistance of vision much more and "hard-of-hearing" persons who primarily understand communication through the auditory mode. The research in speechreading presents varying results; the implication is that we cannot definitively say one should or should not provide this therapy to clients. The reader is referred to Gagne (1994) who presents significant research information on the topic.

From a traditional point of view, there are two primary speechreading approaches: analytical and synthetic. The analytical approach focuses on the need to visually learn to identify the basic components of speech, that is, phonemes through visemes (distinctive movements seen visually that are associated with speech). Training then proceeds to the recognition of words, phrases, sentences,

and continuous discourse. Considerable time is spent on this process. The end point is for the individual to engage in regular communication. Alpiner (1982) advocated the progressive approach, a synthetic approach. The intent of this approach is to make rehabilitation training more realistic in terms of everyday communication, the way in which normal-hearing people speak and listen. In this approach, vision is only one modality of communication. We add the auditory component (auditory-visual), listening training, repair strategies, environmental cues, client needs, and counseling. Indeed, this approach can be incorporated into the HAO process in which the client interacts with the audiologist. We believe that this approach enables a client to confront more effectively the communication situations in the real world after the hearing aid fitting. This approach helps to ensure that individuals will be given the benefit of the doubt in an effort to provide them with the maximum rehabilitation tools for improved communication ability. It also helps to minimize the frequently asked question, "Is speechreading ability learned or innate?"

Gagne (1994) states that the goal of perceptual training is to optimize one's overall receptive communication skills during interactive verbal communication. He further suggests that only individuals with a hearing loss who do not display optimal speech perception skills should be considered for speechreading perception training programs. The task for the rehabilitative audiologist, therefore, is to determine who should receive speechreading instruction regardless of philosophy. We believe that the judgment of the audiologist is very much based not only on academic knowledge of the subject, but also on extensive hands-on experience. Realizing that there are differing ways to perform audiologic rehabilitation and different tools to use, we present a general overview of speechreading evaluation.

LIPREADING TESTS

O'Neill and Oyer (1981) provided several reasons for the use of lipreading tests:

1. They are useful in the measurement of basic lipreading ability.
2. They can be used as instruments to measure the effects of lipreading training. Although one cannot always be certain of all the factors that bring about improvement, many persons will increase their skills as a result of practice.
3. They can be used in proper placement of individuals within a training program. For diagnostic purposes, it is necessary to categorize the acoustically handicapped as excellent, average, or poor lipreaders.
4. They can be used to help decide which teaching (rehabilitative) methods, or combination of methods, are most appropriate.

It is important for the client to have normal or corrected vision to see the visual stimuli appropriately (Thorn and Thorn, 1989). Hipskind (1996) discussed optimal conditions for presentation of visual stimuli. Live, face-to-face presentations should be conducted carefully with optimal consideration for distance (5 to 10 feet), lighting (no shadows), and viewing angle (0 to 45°). Video presentations should take into account similar considerations.

Hipskind also outlined possible limitations of lipreading tests: (1) absence of accompanying auditory cues, (2) unnatural and limited gestures, (3) unnatural and inappropriate facial expressions, (4) nonfunctional sentences, (5) use of a single speaker, (6) scored as an identification task rather than as a person's ability to perceive thoughts visually, (7) no differentiation between skilled and unskilled lipreaders, and (8) poor predictors of lipreading success. A variety of lipreading tests are available, and the choice of which measuring instrument to use will probably be made according to the personal preference of the rehabilitative audiologist. Whether the test will be presented live or by some media mode, and whether sound will be used, will also be at the audiologist's discretion. Jeffers and Barley (1981) indicated that live presentations tend to yield better scores than a video presentation. However, there are limitations to either manner of presentation. Live presentation requires considerable practice on the part of the audiologist (to prevent smiling, overenunciation, etc.). Items should be presented in as true-to-life a manner as possible, because this is the way in which we receive communication in the everyday environment.

Table 10.5 shows the percentage of respondents within groups of 140 (1980) and 77 (1990) who use various tests for evaluating speechreading abilities. These were the only audiologists who reported speechreading tests among 371 (1980) and 479

Table 10.5
Various tests used for evaluating speechreading

Test Used	1980 (N = 140)		1990 (N = 77)[a]	
	N	(%)	N	(%)
Utley	83	59	39	51
Informal	36	26	25	33
Barley	21	15	18	23
Self made	30	21	14	18
Modification of std	14	10	7	9
Keaster	6	4	3	4
Other	11	8	7	9

[a]These were the only audiologists who reported speechreading tests used among 371 (1980) and 469 (1990) clinically active ASHA audiologists.

Source: Adapted from Schow RL, Balsara N, Whitcomb C, and Smedley TC. Aural rehabilitation by ASHA audiologists: 1980–1990. Accepted by the American Journal of Audiology (1993).

(1990) clinically active ASHA audiologists (Schow et al., 1993).

The Denver Quick Test of Lipreading Ability (Alpiner JG, Chevrette W, Glascoe G, et al. The Denver Scale of Communication Function. Unpublished study, University of Denver, 1974) (Table 10.6) is composed of 20 common, everyday expressions, and scored on the basis of the thought or idea of the sentence. Each sentence has a value of 5%. The Quick Test was administered live, without voice, to 40 hearing-impaired adults. Results were compared with the Utley Sentence test, presented live, without voice. Correlation between the two tests was 0.90, indicating good intertest reliability.

MODELS FOR TEST USE

Erber (1977) proposed a conceptual model which may be used for the evaluation of lipreading. Although this model is designed for children, it may have clinical application for adults. This system previously has been used for auditory tasks. A simple matrix (Fig. 10.2) summarizes the variety of

Table 10.6
Denver quick test of upreading ability[a]

1. Good morning.
2. How old are you?
3. I live in (state of residence).
4. I only have one dollar.
5. There is somebody at the door.
6. Is that all?
7. Where are you going?
8. Let's have a coffee break.
9. Park your car in the lot.
10. What is your address?
11. May I help you?
12. I feel fine.
13. It is time for dinner.
14. Turn right at the corner.
15. Are you ready to order?
16. Is this charge or cash?
17. What time is it?
18. I have a headache.
19. How about going out tonight?
20. Please lend me 50 cents.

[a]Devised at the University of Denver Speech and Hearing Center.

the different types of speech stimuli that can be used: speech elements, syllables, words, phrases, sentences, and connected discourse. Four response tasks are used in this matrix: detection, discrimination, recognition, and comprehension. Each box in Figure 10.2 describes the interaction between a particular type of visual speech stimulus and a specific manner of response. Detection is the ability to respond differently to the presence or absence of speech movements. Visual detection of articulatory movements should re-sult in the individual's orientation to the speaker's mouth for gaining more visual information and indicating the presence of postdental consonants in certain vowel contexts. Discrimination requires a same-different response for the ability to perceive similarities and differences between two or more speech samples. Recognition is the ability to reproduce a visual speech stimulus by naming or identifying it in some way. Comprehension is the ability to understand the meaning of speech stimuli within an individual's language ability. The information obtained from the use of this procedure may help in planning audiologic rehabilitation.

Another application was suggested by Dodds and Harford (1968), who used the Utley test as part of a hearing aid evaluation. This test was used to evaluate how well clients understand sentences under visual and auditory-visual conditions. In this study, Form A of the Utley Sentence Test was presented unaided, and Form B was presented with auditory-visual cues. The latter condition resulted in greater understanding of the stimuli material.

REPAIR STRATEGIES

Marzolf et al. (1998) compared the effects of two repair strategies on speechreading of words and sentences: repetition and paraphrasing. Interest in repair strategies for audiologic rehabilitation has increased in recent years. Subjects for this study consisted of 20 college-aged adults ranging in age from 19 to 26 years. All had normal hearing and normal or corrected-for-normal vision.

	Speech Elements	Syllables	Words	Phrases	Sentences	Connected Discourse
Detection						
Discrimination						
Recognition						
Comprehension						

Figure 10.2. A lipreading skills matrix for hearing-impaired children. The child's visual speech perception abilities are evaluated at each level of stimulus/response complexity. These measures are used to specify goals for instruction in visual communication (Erber, 1977).

The stimuli were word and sentence lists on videotapes selected by previous studies from Gagne and Wylie (1989) and Tye-Murray et al. (1990). Testing was done individually in a sound-treated booth. All subjects sat 36 inches from a 19-inch video monitor. The tapes were presented in a visual only modality. Subjects attempted to repeat test items verbatim after the first presentation. When a correct response was given, the video was advanced to the next test item. Following incorrect responses, subjects viewed a repair strategy and the test item was repeated. For the sentence items, a correct response consisted of repeating the basic meaning of the item. Results suggested that both repeat and paraphrase re-pair strategies are moderately effective in facilitating speech perception visually. The repeat strategy appeared to be more helpful in the visual perception of sentences, whereas paraphrasing provided slightly more improvement when words are the form of stimuli being perceived. Overall, the repeat strategy produced significantly greater gains in speechreading for both stimulus types combined. The researchers recommend additional research using a combined audiovisual perceptual condition with hearing-impaired subjects to address the issue further. This concept of repair strategy seems to lend itself to a more "real life" communication approach. Communication between individuals is not simply, "I say it one time," and "You understand it the first time." Even normal-hearing persons need to engage in, "Please repeat it, I didn't get it." Perhaps we need to modify our thinking regarding lipreading so that a repair strategy is a proper technique to help our clients hear and understand everyday conversation.

Everyday Speech and Bisensory Evaluation

Traditional pure-tone and speech-hearing tests do not provide much information about a patient's ability to hear the many levels of real-world speech (Martin, 1996). Martin also comments that many clients have complex speech-perception problems: loss of sensitivity, significant distortion, inability to process rapidly spoken speech, intolerance of loud sounds, and years of living without adequate amplification. Martin presents a practical way to conduct a multilevel speech test. He presents a short list (10 items) of monosyllabic words at each level between the patient's SRT and speech UCL. Presentation levels are in 10-dB increments. The tests can be presented with a speech audiometer. Results can indicate the client's word-recognition ability in a narrow range of intensities. Martin states, "I believe that hearing deteriorates in stages. In the early stage of hearing loss, the patient's pure-tone hearing sensitivity may accurately reflect the person's ability to hear and understand speech. However, as the auditory system continues to deteriorate with age, the relationship between sensitivity and fine word recognition diverges until the patient is able to hear and understand only loud, clear, slowly spoken speech. Classic hearing tests do not show us this deterioration of word understanding ability." When a patient complains that speech is not understood, it is appropriate to compare real-ear targets with multilevel speech tests for any adjustments that may be needed.

Word recognition is very much related to hearing aid fittings because many clients state that they hear but do not understand. We may say that the new hearing aid technology will help reduce the problem; we also may say that auditory training can help, although many audiologists do not say that. Stach (1998) has provided some interesting comments about this topic in a *Hearing Journal* article. He reflects on a question about the use of word recognition testing. The question is, "Why do word recognition testing?" The response is, "I have been amazed at how many times audiologists and graduate students do not know when word recognition scores are abnormal. Physicians and residents are no better. Someone, somewhere teaches them that a word recognition score of 70% or less is abnormal. I don't know where that comes from. Do we teach them that?" In addition, Stach addresses the issue of the usefulness of word recognition testing. He cites three main points:

1. First, we should not expect much from these measures in terms of helping to understand a patient's ability to hear and understand speech at suprathreshold levels. It is just too simple a measure, and the score is dictated primarily by the relationship between degree and configuration of hearing loss and the level at which testing is performed. Thus, from the perspective of helping to understand a patient's communication disorder, its usefulness can be considered marginal at best.
2. Second, word-recognition testing is most useful when the results are abnormal or poorer than would be expected from the degree and configuration of the hearing loss. In such cases, of course, the poorer-than-expected performance is diagnostically useful as an indication of retrocochlear disorder. Thus, word recognition can be useful.
3. Third, if shortcuts are taken and the testing is not carried out effectively, then it will never be known if the results are normal or abnormal. If the test results cannot be determined as normal or abnormal, then the practitioner might as well not bother performing the test.

Obviously, the practitioner needs to know the communication function of his or her clients relative to word discrimination accuracy. For example, the client with a significant high-frequency hearing loss who is listening to the weather person on the radio hears a temperature of 50° but may not know whether the temperature is 50 or 60° because /f/ and /s/ may sound alike. Further, the typical comment from many clients is, "I hear you but I don't understand all of the words."

We now consider bisensory evaluation. Sometimes lipreading tests are administered in the visual-only condition. It is assumed that clients who score well in the visual-only modality have less difficulty understanding communication and should have fewer concomitant difficulties often associated with hearing loss. However, it is thought that testing in a visual-only condition is not sufficiently comprehensive for most purposes. Assessment should generally include a bisensory evaluation, allowing the client to use both visual and auditory modalities. The significant work of Binnie (1973) indicated that auditory-visual scores might suggest how individuals receive person-to-person speech in general conversation situations. Because this is the general mode of communication for most people, the information would be useful to the clinician in planning a realistic remediation program.

Bisensory approaches are very helpful in determining how well clients perform with hearing aids. In this approach to lipreading evaluation, test materials can be presented both in a quiet condition and in the presence of different background noises, which often create major difficulties for the hearing-impaired adult. The Hearing in Noise Test (HINT) for the measurement of speech reception thresholds in quiet and in noise (Nilsson et al., 1994) is a tool used to determine how well clients do in both aided and unaided conditions at periodic time intervals (e.g., 30 days, 3 months, etc.). Numerous clients state that they seem to do well in one-to-one, quiet environmental situations but simply cannot understand what is being said when there is background noise. Binnie (1973) demonstrated the benefits of the bisensory approach. He states that the level at which the best auditory-visual score is

Table 10.7
Effect of auditory presentations at various sensation levels

Sensation Level of Presentation[a]	Auditory Sensorineural Loss Cases					Mean Scores for Normals
	1	2	3	4	5	
			%		%	
0	30	22	20	46	42	21
8	64	40	46	86	38	59
16	74	62	60	90	54	80
24	84	84	78	94	36	94

Reprinted by permission from Binnie CA. Bi-sensory articulation functions for normal hearing and sensorineural hearing loss patients. J Acad Rehabil Audiol 1973;6:43–53, copyright 1973, *Journal of the Academy of Rehabilitative Audiology.*
[a]Re: Sound field SRT.

Table 10.8
Effect of audio-visual presentations at various sensation levels

Sensation Level of Presentation[a]	Audio-Visual Sensorineural Loss Cases					Mean Scores for Normals
	1	2	3	4	5	
			%			%
−20	22	14	12	8	18	23
0	66	58	46	76	72	57
8	70	76	68	84	84	85
16	88	82	86	98	74	94

Reprinted by permission from Binnie CA. Bi-sensory articulation functions for normal hearing and sensorineural hearing loss patients. J Acad Rehabil Audiol 1973;6:45–53, copyright 1973, *Journal of the Academy of Rehabilitative Audiology.*
[a]Re: Sound field SRT.

obtained may serve as the starting point for audiologic rehabilitation. The data in Tables 10.7 and 10.8 show the effects of auditory and auditory-visual presentations at various sensation levels. With a combined sensory modality presentation, the contribution of visual speech cues to auditory-visual speech perception increases as the speech-to-noise ratio decreases. That is, as noise increases with respect to speech, the visual modality plays a greater role in the individual's understanding of speech. The use of audition and vision results in higher scores than when either audition or lipreading is used alone.

The research cited emphasizes the need to evaluate lipreading through a bisensory approach. Because most persons perceive speech in this way, it would appear to be a realistic consideration. The work of Binnie et al. (1974) provides substantive data for bisensory assessment. They studied 16 con-

sonants in which 5 distinct homophenous categories were apparent:

1. Bilabials: /p, b, m/
2. Labiodentals: /f, v/
3. Interdentals: /θ, ʒ/
4. Rounded labials: /f, ʒ/
5. Linguals: /s, z, t, d, n, k, g/

Stimuli were presented in auditory, auditory-visual, auditory in quiet, and visual-only conditions. Signal-to-noise (S/N) ratios used for auditory and auditory-visual conditions were −18 dB, −12dB, and −6dB using a broad-band masking noise. The results of their study demonstrated that identification of consonants under noise conditions improved significantly with vision. The auditory-visual condition approaches the results of materials presented in quiet. The visual-only condition indicates the difficul-

Table 10.9
Results of stimuli presentations under auditory, auditory-visual, auditory in outlet, and visual only conditions

Condition	Correct Response
	(%)
Auditory	
S/N ratio: −18	6
S/N ratio: −12	34
S/N ratio: −6	54
Auditory-visual	
S/N ratio: −18	47.7
S/N ratio: −12	83.5
S/N ratio: −6	88.7
Auditory in quiet	95
Visual only (overall)	43.2

Reprinted by permission from Binnie CA, Montgomery AA, Jackson PL. Auditory and visual contributions to the perception of consonants. J Speech Hear Res 1974;17:619–630, copyright 1974, *Journal of Speech and Hearing Research.*

S/N, signal-to-noise.

ties posed when relying on this modality. Table 10.9 summarizes their results.

Walden et al. (1974) found that hearing-impaired adults were able to distinguish visually within the Woodward and Barber (1960) consonant categories. These consonant categories are as follows:

1. Bilabial: /p, b, m/
2. Rounded labial: /m, w, r/
3. Labiodental: /f, v/
4. Nonlabial: /t, d, n, θ, ʒ, ʃ, h, ɡ, ʃ, z, k, n, ʒ, g/

Brannon (1961) indicates that words of less visibility are harder to lipread than words of greater visibility. He suggests that a synthetic approach to lipreading, in which additional clues are provided, is more effective for developing lipreading ability. Erber (1975) suggests that evaluation of each client's auditory-visual perception of speech can be helpful, because most hearing-impaired clients typically receive speech through both auditory and visual modalities during everyday communication. This means they usually watch the speaker's mouth and face to maximize perception of speech information.

The research of Preminger et al. (1998) provides additional information to be considered in bisensory approaches. Their experiments established which parts of the face are important for distinguishing the five consonant visemes in the four vowel contexts in the speech of the test talker. Some of the results indicated that visibility of the tongue and teeth was only necessary to identify /t/ and /k/ in the /u/ vowel context. The results of the speaker indicate that the visibility of the tongue and teeth appears to be of limited importance in visual speech perception. Visibility of the lips was important; however, the visemes /p/ and /f/ could still be identified with greater than 96% accuracy in the /a/ and /i/ vowel contexts when the lips were blocked from view. They conclude that areas of the face other than the mouth are important during speechreading. Keeping this information in mind, auditory-visual evaluation in the clinic can give the audiologist a better estimate of the client's ability to communicate socially.

Real-life situations demand that hearing-impaired individuals understand continuous speech discourse. Clinical experience has shown that clients can perceive differences in sounds according to homophenous categories. More difficulty is encountered in understanding what is said on a day-to-day basis at work, at home, and in a variety of social situations. Clients often indicated that they experience little difficulty recognizing sound in isolated categories in therapy. Their attempts to follow general conversation in the outside environment, however, are frustrating because the rate of the typical speaker may be either too fast or too slow or enunciation may be poor.

Evaluation of Auditory Recognition

Sims (1985) has indicated that criteria for selecting clients for auditory training are difficult to find in the literature. Rubenstein and Boothroyd (1987) state that audiologists disagree about the value of formal auditory training with adventitiously hearing-impaired adults. Some of the problems associated with research in this area may be due to controlling variables of stimulus materials and the time-consuming nature of these studies. Studies have been reported that do indicate improvement as a result of auditory training. As further efforts are made in better understanding of auditory training, it appears that audiologists should continue with such endeavors because there is some evidence that improvement occurs.

Oyer and Frankmann (1975) indicated that the primary areas of concern regarding the need for auditory training are (1) confusions among various sounds due to the condition of the sensorineural hearing mechanism, (2) adjustment problems in the use of amplification systems due to recruitment problems, and (3) adjustment problems due to amplification because of speech sounding unnatural (hearing aids are not precise replacements for abnormally functioning ears). Poor auditory recognition may result from sensorineural impairment. The individual with a conductive hearing loss is not usually confronted with this difficulty, because the etiology of the impairment is in the outer or middle ear. Once speech has been made sufficiently loud, it can be understood.

Owens (1978) analyzed consonant errors of hearing-impaired subjects and showed that 14 consonants caused most of the difficulty in consonant recognition. This study constitutes (1) a summary of auditory consonant recognition errors in a multiple-choice word format for persons with sensorineural hearing loss and (2) a consideration of implications for remediation. Items for this study consisted of a battery of consonant-vowel-consonant words. The initial-position consonants show lower error probabilities than their counterparts in the final position. Place errors were the most frequent, but manner errors also were noted frequently. Substitutions tended to be the same over a wider range of pure-tone configurations. Therefore, only in a few instances would the type of configuration of a given subject be of any special help in predicting those consonants that are particularly difficult to recognize. This study demonstrated that auditory recognition of consonants can be improved by training. Visual recognition errors of persons with normal hearing were consistent among consonants within visual groups. An approach directed at enhancing or sharpening consonant recognition per se may contribute substantially to speech perception ability.

Another aspect of consonants as they relate to speech perception is frequency of their occurrence in everyday speech. The consonants /j, n, w, r, h, l, m/ are the most easily recognized auditorily by hearing-impaired persons. The consonants /t, d, s, k, z/, on the other hand, provide auditory and visual difficulty. The /s/ emerges as the most troublesome in speech perception. Along with /s/ is the cognate /z/ with /k/ close behind. Owens (1978) proposed that it might be helpful to devote part of aural rehabilitation to direct auditory training work with consonants. A variety of stimulus materials exists to ascertain an individual's recognition ability, but there is no agreement on which is best. The stimuli are presented at a level above the speech reception threshold at which the client indicates that speech sounds are comfortable. Words and sentences are used for auditory recognition testing.

AUDITORY RECOGNITION TESTS

We recommend that the audiologist evaluate the client's confusion with individual sounds and general speech discourse for the purpose of planning auditory training. Some confusions may be assessed with the monosyllabic words used in speech recognition testing. We can opt to indicate sound errors and whether a word was correctly identified. From List 1 of the 8 Northwestern University Word Test Number 6 (Tillman and Carhart, 1966), the following four words, for example, can be used: bean, burn, knock, and moon. Hypothetical responses might be bean, bird, dock, mood. While scoring, we may note that /d/ is confused with /n/. Therapy could be planned to emphasize the auditory differences between the two sounds. Recognition of word tests, already a part of the audiologic assessment battery, may be used. The same purpose can be accomplished with any recognition test used in an audiologic test battery. The first five of these are tests developed for use with children. This indicates that much auditory training is done with children, but such materials can also be used with adults when language age or difficulty level requires the use of easier material.

For more intensive discrimination testing between consonants, the Larson Sound Discrimination Test (Fig 10.3) is recommended. The California Consonant Test (CCT) also allows for the identification of auditory recognition errors. List 1 of the CCT is found in Attachment 7.

In addition to assessment of individual phonemes through the auditory modality, it also is recommended that evaluation of ability to perceive continuous discourse be made. This procedure may be helpful in determining a client's auditory function with additional contextual information. The CID Everyday Speech Sentences (Davis and Silverman, 1970) is available for this purpose. These sentences are suggested for evaluation, because they represent a sample of American speech of high face validity. The 10-sentence lists are presented in Attachment 8).

As indicated by Davis and Silverman (1970), certain important characteristics exist for these sentences:

1. The vocabulary is appropriate for adults.
2. The words appear with high frequency in one or more of the well-known word counts of the English language.
3. Proper names and proper nouns are not used.
4. Common, nonslang, idioms and contractions are used freely.
5. Phonetic loading and "tongue-twisting" are avoided.
6. Redundancy is high.
7. The level of abstraction is low.
8. Grammatical structure varies freely.
9. Sentence length varies.
10. Different sentence forms are used, including declarative, interrogative, imperative, and falling interrogative.

In addition to evaluating recognition ability for both individual phonemes and con-

tinuous speech discourse, the audiologist must consider any tolerance problems affecting hearing-impaired adults. The ability to tolerate auditory stimuli at comfortable levels has significance for those clients using or needing amplification. In evaluating recognition ability, the test materials should be presented in an auditory-only condition, without the use of visual cues. Emphasis in this phase of the evaluation is on assessment of the auditory modality only.

SUMMARY

Results of these evaluation procedures enable the audiologist to make some rehabilitative judgments regarding specific auditory communication deficits of the client. However, these should be seen as part of a broader effort. Oyer (1968) indicated that in a majority of cases, auditory training will not stand alone as a method of rehabilitating the hearing-impaired individual. It is part of a broad conceptual framework encompassing the entirety of audiologic rehabilitation.

Tinnitus Evaluation

The National Center for Health Statistics (1980) indicates that tinnitus is a common complaint. The Center reports that 32% of the population reports some form of tinnitus. According to Axelsson and Ringdahl (1989), tinnitus is uncomfortable for both the patient and the counseling physician. The reason cited is that in most cases, there is no successful treatment to eliminate tinnitus. We have experience with hundreds of veterans in VA medical centers who have described the problem of "noises" in their ears and the frustrations that have resulted from tinnitus: "I have difficulty sleeping at night," "The noises make me nervous," "I have difficulty hearing my family," "What can I do about this problem?" In some cases, clients have requested appointments because of tinnitus, not hearing loss. There are a variety of techniques now being emphasized to help minimize the problem of tinnitus, and Chapter 12 of this text covers tinnitus in greater detail.

Name_____

Date_____

Score: (Errors)

With Aid

Without Aid

Directions to be Given the Listener: Draw a line through the words that are pronounced to you from each box.

Box 1	f and ch	Box 2	l and z	Box 3	l and n	Box 4	d and n	Box 5	m and l
few	chew	lip	zip	lame	name	dot	not	mine	line
fin	chin	loan	zone	light	night	die	nigh	mast	last
filed	child	dale	daze	loan	known	deed	need	moan	loan
calf	catch	mail	maze	pail	pain	ode	own	name	nail
four	chore	hail	haze	rail	rain	did	din	home	hole

Box 6	b and m	Box 7	l and v	Box 8	k and g	Box 9	p and b	Box 10	m and v
bill	mill	lane	vane	coal	goal	pin	bin	mice	vice
boast	most	lie	vie	came	game	pie	by	ham	have
bake	make	lace	vase	coat	goat	pole	bowl	glum	glove
robe	roam	lull	love	luck	lug	cap	cap	mine	vine
tab	tam	rail	rave	rack	rag	rope	robe	mile	vile

Box 11	n and v	Box 12	sh and f	Box 13	f and k	Box 14	f and b	Box 15	s and sh
nice	vice	show	foe	fit	kit	fun	bun	lease	leash
nurse	verse	shore	fore	four	core	fig	big	sew	show
nine	vine	shade	fade	find	kind	cuff	cub	sigh	shy
loans	loaves	cash	calf	cliff	click	call	cab	sap	ship
lean	leave	leash	leaf	laugh	lack	graph	grab	save	shave

Box 16	p and f	Box 17	s and z	Box 18	v and f	Box 19	ch and sh	Box 20	b and d
pour	four	ice	eyes	five	fife	chop	shop	bid	did
pile	file	seal	zeal	vase	face	chair	share	big	dig
par	far	bus	buzz	leave	leaf	watch	wash	buy	die
cap	call	lice	lies	view	few	catch	cash	rob	rod
cup	cuff	juice	Jews	loaves	loafs	cheap	sheep	robe	rode

Box 21	d and g	Box 22	t and p	Box 23	l and s	Box 24	b and v	Box 25	v and z
doe	go	tail	pail	fine	sign	bet	vet	live	lies
date	gate	cat	cap	flat	slat	dub	dove	have	has
drove	grove	cut	cup	cuff	cuss	base	vase	rave	raise
bud	bug	tar	par	knife	nice	bigger	vigor	view	zoo
dad	gag	toll	pole	lift	list	robe	rove	wives	wise

Box 26	th and f	Box 27	t and th	Box 28	k and t	Box 29	k and p	Box 30	m and n
thin	fin	tie	thigh	kick	tick	pike	pipe	mine	nine
thirst	first	tin	thin	kite	tight	cat	pat	new	knew
three	free	trill	thrill	code	toad	crock	crop	time	tine
thought	fought	mit	myth	shirk	shirt	cry	pry	dime	dine
thrill	frill	pat	path	park	part	coal	pole	dumb	done

Box 31	Word Endings		Box 32	th and s	Box 33	th and v
store	stores	stored	thumb	sum	than	van
will	wills	willed	truth	truce	thy	vie
start	starts	started	path	pass	that	vat
cough	coughs	coughed	thing	sing	thine	vine
cap	caps	capped	thank	sank	loathes	loaves

Figure 10.3. Larson School Discrimination Test. (Reprinted by permission from Sanders DA. Aural rehabilitation. Bloomington, IN: Indiana University Press, 1950.)

Overall Test Battery

Information acquired from the audiologic test battery serves as a guide to planning remediation. Client input is also important because an estimate of the problem may provide a starting point for remediation. Although information obtained from the client is subjective, therapy based on individual problems can be initiated, avoiding a generalized remediation approach. As noted previously, we also recommend sequencing treatment depending on attitude types (see Tables 10.1 and 10.10). Although the sequencing is related to hearing aid attitudes, it appears that the attitude types may also apply to overall audiologic rehabilitation:

1. Attitude Type I—this implies that the patient has a strongly positive attitude toward hearing aids and audiologic care.
2. Attitude Type II—this implies that there is an essentially positive attitude toward hearing aids and audiologic rehabilitation.
3. Attitude Type III—this implies a fundamentally negative attitude, although there exists a shred of cooperative intent.
4. Attitude Type IV—tis implies a small group who reject hearing aids and the audiologic rehabilitation process. A total discharge from the rehabilitation process is likely, but a last ditch effort may be attempted. The authors of this chapter believe that patience is a great virtue in this helping profession.

AMAR—A Comprehensive Screening Scale: Self-Assessment, Auditory, Visual

Limited resources are available in a screening format that assess hearing handicap, visual ability, and auditory aptitude. Alpiner and Garstecki (1996) report that measures of skills related to the communication competence of hearing-impaired individuals have been given low priority in many clinical settings. Lesner (1990) speculates that possible reasons for this situation include a lack of awareness of assessment tools, time constraints in ENT clinical practices, and limited funding sources for audiologic rehabilitation. Alpiner et al. (1991) developed a multipurpose screening scale: the Alpiner-Meline Aural Rehabilitation (AMAR) Screening Scale (Attachment 9). To measure hearing handicap, nine items were selected from the M-A Scale (1983), five items were chosen from the Denver Quick Test of Lipreading Ability (Alpiner, 1978), and six word-pair items were selected from the Larson Sound Discrimination Test (Sanders, 1950). Percentile ranks for scoring purposes were established. It was determined that individuals who scored within the 85th percentile or higher for the number of errors could be identified as those with absolute need for aural rehabilitation. "Absolute needs" patients are defined as individuals who demonstrate significant difficulties in using resources, coping skills, and auditory/visual information to optimum benefit. The percentile range for "questionable needs" for rehabilitation is from the 70th to the 84th percentile. These individuals demonstrate moderate difficulty. Clients who fall into the range from the 1st to 69th percentile would be unlikely to need audiologic rehabilitation. The AMAR scale allows the identification of problems quickly and efficiently.

Steele and Britten (1998) further investigated the AMAR scale as it related to audiologic rehabilitation in older adults. Their study used 22 subjects residing in a semiindependent living center. Subjects ranged in age from 76 to 97 years with a mean age of 85.9 years. Fourteen subjects had mild hearing loss (less than 40 dB HL) in the better ear. Eight subjects had moderate hearing loss (greater than 40 dB HL) in the better ear. Average PTA for mild hearing loss subjects was 23 dB, and average PTA for the moderate losses was 54 dB. Eight subjects wore hearing aids. All subjects were screened using the AMAR scale. Pure-tone thresholds were obtained for the frequencies 500 to 8000 Hz; otoscopic examinations were also completed. In addition, a mental status questionnaire (MSQ) (Attachment 10) was administered to screen for cognitive deficits (Khan et al., 1960).

Although there is no statistically significant correlation between PTAs and AMAR scores, the authors believe that the two events are related. Although some of the subjects reported few difficulties during the AMAR screening, observations made during the aural rehabilitation sessions that followed indicated that there were difficulties that some of the subjects were experiencing for which they were unaware or refused to report. Furthermore, the fact that there was a significant difference between the AMAR scores for the mild hearing loss group compared with the moderate hearing loss group suggests that audiologic rehabilitation screening for older adults may be sensitive in showing a rehabilitation need for the moderate loss group. This may be due to the fact that many subjects in the mild hearing loss group do not believe or understand that they have a significant loss of hearing.

Additional Evaluation Considerations

Alpiner et al. (1995) developed a clinical trial protocol for Food and Drug Administration (FDA) approval of a new Completely-in-the-Canal (CIC) hearing aid model (CIC/FT). The study was done for an electronics manufacturer. Ten claims were investigated, eight of which may be applicable for audiologic rehabilitation. These items were designed specifically for client input (i.e., their feelings toward the new CIC model). Thirteen subjects participated in this investigation. Subjects were selected from HEAR NOW's pool of eligible candidates (see Chapter 1). All subjects were new hearing aid users with symmetric mild to moderately severe sensorineural hearing loss. Following a complete audiologic evaluation, ear impressions were taken, binaural hearing aids were ordered, and subjects were scheduled for hearing aid fittings in 2 weeks. The hearing aids were manufactured according to specific computer matrices.

The eight evaluative procedures used were as follows:

1. Subjects will demonstrate improvement both in quiet and in noise in the aided versus unaided condition, as measured by the Speech in Quiet/in Noise Test modified from the HINT TEST (Attachment 11) (administered pre and post hearing aid fitting).
2. The hearing aids will fit comfortably, as determined by the Hearing Aid Comfort Scale (Attachment 12) (administered post fitting only).
3. Communication (including visual/auditory skills) will improve, as determined by the AMAR scale (Attachment) (administered pre and post hearing aid fitting) (Attachment 9).
4. Feedback will be minimized with the CIC/FT, as determined by the Presence of Feedback Scale (Attachment 13) (administered post hearing aid fitting only).
5. Sound quality will be acceptable, as determined by the Sound Quality Measurement Scale (Attachment 14) (administered post hearing aid fitting only).
6. The CIC/FT will be inconspicuous to the user, as determined by the Cosmetic Assessment Scale (Attachment 15) (administered post hearing aid fitting only).
7. The CIC/FT will serve as a masker to minimize tinnitus, as determined by the Tinnitus Questionnaire (Attachment 16) (administered post hearing aid fitting only).
8. Subject expectations will be fulfilled with the CIC/FT, as determined by the Fulfillment of Expectations Questionnaire (see Chapter 1) (administered pre and post hearing aid fitting).

RESULTS

Thirty days after the hearing aid fittings, subjects returned for posttesting measurements:

1. The Speech in Quiet/in Noise test was administered under the following conditions: (a) in quiet (at 40 dB HL) unaided

Table 10.10
Recommended evaluation and remediation components

Procedure	Rationale
1. Screening (pure tones at 25 dB, SAC/SOAC, selective use of visual inspection, immittance)	1. Quick screen to identify potential hearing problems of medical or disability/handicap nature.
2. Audiologic assessment (pure-tone and speech audiometry)	2. Determination of type and severity of hearing loss, contribution of results to physician's diagnosis. Information on determining tolerance and recognition abilities.

3. Rehabilitation evaluation
  a. Communication evaluation
	3. Rehabilitation
	  a. Client and family member evaluation of communication.

(1) Selection of Assessment Tool as appropriate	(1) Evaluation of specific problem areas in communication situations. (2) Additional evaluation of personality and unstructured reports on communication.
(2) Denver Quick Test of Lipreading or other appropriate test	(3) Assessment of client's ability to understand visual communication. (Should be administered under visual and auditory-visual conditions.)

(3) Auditory discrimination testing:
      (a) NU Auditory Word Tests
      (b) CID Everyday Sentences
      (c) California Consonant Test
	(4) Assessment of client's ability to recognize phonemes and assessment of recognition ability of everyday speech discourse through the auditory modality.

(4) Alpiner-Meline Aural Rehabilitation Screening Scale
  b. Associated variables evaluation
	(5) Initial screen.
	
	  b. Psychological social, vocational, and educational aspects.

c. Related conditions
    (1) Tinnitus Questionnaire
    (2) Other conditions
  d. Attitude evaluation
	c. Conditions
	    (1) To determine if tinnitus poses communication problem.
	
	  d. Assign attitude as type I, II, III, IV.

4. Remediation
  a. Counseling/psychosocial issues
	4. Remediation
	  a. Synthesis of all evaluative information and counseling efforts to assist a client to achieve as near normal communication function as possible.

b. Amplification/assistive devices	b. Determination if amplification is necessary to minimize the auditory deficit. Orientation/adjustment.
c. Communication plan of remediation	c. Speechreading and communication strategies
d. Overall coordination	d. Working cooperatively with other medical, counseling, school, and vocational professionals

and aided, (b) in noise at 0 dB (S/N) ratio, and (c) in noise at -3 dB (S/N) ratio. Based on nonparametric sign test results, significant improvement was noted in quiet and in both S/N conditions.

2. The Hearing Aid Comfort Scale indicated that 45% of subjects could wear their hearing aids all day with no problem, 40% could wear their hearing aids all day but they felt stuffy in the ears, and 15% had to remove their aids after several hours due to discomfort.

3. The AMAR scale consisted of four parts: self assessment, visual aptitude, auditory aptitude, and total scale. Statistically significant improvement was noted in all areas except auditory only.

4. The Feedback Scale indicated that 60% of subjects experienced no feedback, 25% seldom experienced feedback, 10% occasionally, and 5% frequently.

5. Sound quality was reported to be natural by 75% of subjects, 15% reported a tinny or sharp quality, and 10% reported the hearing aids to sound hollow.

6. Client feelings regarding cosmetic appearance of the hearing aids revealed that 55% of subjects felt that their hearing aids were not visible by others, 30% felt the aids were slightly visible, and 15% felt the aids were noticeable.

7. The Tinnitus Questionnaire indicated a significant reduction in perception of tinnitus by all subjects.

8. The majority of subjects had 10 of the 12 expectations fulfilled, as determined by the Expectation Questionnaire. Only one subject was disappointed regarding his expectation levels.

Although the subject sample is small in this clinical claims study, the information reported by the respondents appears to be very useful for audiologists in planning audiologic rehabilitation. We believe that direct client input sometimes can be more useful than lengthy assessment procedures, especially when we consider one client at a time. Not all clients fit into standardized procedures. Albeit, additional research can be definitive regarding all these issues.

Summary

There is no one approach to rehabilitation. The test battery presented in Table 10.10 is recommended as a guideline for sequencing the audiologic rehabilitation process. Audiologists now have a wide choice of tools from which to select for rehabilitation. Regardless of approaches used, it is the client with hearing loss who becomes the major concern for proper and efficient hearing help. With new technological advances, it will be interesting to learn about relationships that may exist between audiologic rehabilitation and the "new" hearing aid options.

REFERENCES

AAO (American Academy of Otolaryngology). Guide for the evaluation of hearing handicap. JAMA 1979;241: 2055–2059.

Alpiner JG. Evaluation of communication function. In: Alpiner JG, ed. Handbook of adult rehabilitative audiology. Baltimore, MD: Williams and Wilkins, 1982.

Alpiner JG. Handbook of adult rehabilitative audiology. Baltimore, MD: Williams and Wilkins, 1978.

Alpiner JG, Garstecki DC. Audiologic rehabilitation for adults: assessment & management. In: Schow RL, Nerbonne MA, eds. Introduction to aural rehabilitation. Austin, TX: Pro-Ed, 1989.

Alpiner JG, Hansen EM, Dinner MB, et al. Project CIC/FT pilot study. Hearing aid clinical trials project. Denver: HEAR NOW, 1995.

Alpiner JG, Meline NC, Cotton AD. An aural rehabilitation screening scale: self assessment, auditory aptitude, and visual aptitude. J Acad Rehab Audiol 1991;24: 75–83.

ASHA (American Speech-Language-Hearing Association) Definition of and competencies for aural rehabilitation. A report from the committee on rehabilitative audiology. ASHA 1984;26:37–41.

ASHA. Guidelines for audiologic screening. American Speech-Language-Hearing Association Panel on Audiologic Assessment, 1997. Rockville, MD.

Axelsson A, Ringdahl A. Tinnitus—a study of its prevalence and characteristics. Br J Audiol 1989;23:53–62.

Binnie CA. Bi-sensory articulation functions for normal hearing and sensorineural hearing loss patients. J Acad Rehabil Audiol 1973;6:43–53.

Binnie CA, Montgomery AA, Jackson PL. Auditory and visual contributions to the perception of consonants. J Speech Hear Res 1974;17:619–630.

Boothroyd A. Linguistic factors in speechreading. In: De Filippo CL, Sims DG, eds. New reflections on speechreading (monograph). Volta Rev 1988;90(5): 77–87.

Brannon C. Speechreading of various speech materials. J Speech Hear Dis 1961:348–354.

Brooks DN. The effect of attitude on benefit obtained from hearing aids. Br Soc Audiol 1989;23:3–11.

Cox RM, Alexander GC. The abbreviated profile of hearing aid benefit. Ear Hear 1995;16:176–186.

Cox RM, Gilmore C, Alexander GC. Comparison of two questionnaires for patient-assessed hearing aid benefit. J Am Acad Audiol 1991;2:134–145.

Dancer J, Gener J. Survey on the use of adult hearing assessment scales. Hear Rev 1999;6:26–35.

Davis H. The articulation area and the social adequacy index for hearing. Laryngoscope 1948;58:761–778.

Davis H, Silverman SR. Hearing and deafness. New York: Holt, Rinehart and Winston, 1970.

Demorest ME, Erdman SA. Scale composition and item analysis of the communication profile for the hearing impaired. J. Speech Hear Res 1986;29:515–535.

Demorest ME, Erdman SA. Development of the communication profile for the hearing impaired. J Speech Hear Disord 1987;52:129–142.

Dillion H, James A, Ginis J. Client oriented scale of improvement (COSI) and its relationship to several other measures of benefit and satisfaction provided by hearing aids. J Am Acad Audiol 1997;8:27–43.

Dodds E, Harford E. Application of a lipreading test in a hearing aid evaluation. J Speech Hear Dis 1968;33:167–173.

Erber NP. Auditory-visual perception of speech. J Speech Hear Dis 1975;40:481–492.

Erber NP. Developing materials for lipreading evaluation and instruction. Volta Rev 1977;79:35–42.

Ewertsen H, Birk-Nielsen H. Social hearing handicap index: social handicap in relation to hearing impairment. Audiology 1973;12:180–187.

Gagne J-P. Visual and audiovisual speech perception training: basic and applied research needs. In: Gagne J-P, Tye-Murray N, eds. Research in audiological rehabilitation: current trends and future directions. J Acad Rehab Audiol Monogr Suppl 1994;27:133–159.

Gagne J-P, Wyllie KA. Relative effectiveness of three repair strategies on the visual-identification of misperceived words. Ear Hear 1989;10:368–374.

Gatehouse S. Components and determinants of hearing aid benefit. Ear Hear 1994;15:30–49.

Gatehouse S. The Glasgow hearing aid benefit profile: a client-centered scale for the assessment of auditory disability, handicap and hearing aid benefit. Presented at the annual meeting of the American Academy of Rehabilitative Audiology, Montreal, 1997.

Giolas TG. The self-assessment approach in audiology. Audiology 1983;3:157–171.

Giolas TG. The measurement of hearing handicap revisited: a 20-year perspective. Ear Hear 1990;11:28–58.

Giolas TG, Owens E, Lamb SH, et al. Hearing performance inventory. J Speech Hear Dis 1979;44:169–195.

Goldstein DP, Stephens SDG. Audiological rehabilitation: management model I. Audiology 1981;20:432–452.

High WS, Fairbanks G, Glorig A. Scale for self-assessment of hearing handicap. J Speech Hear Dis 1964;29:215–230.

Hipskind NM. Visual stimuli in communication. In: Schow RL, Nerbonne MA, eds. Introduction to aural rehabilitation. Boston: Allyn and Bacon, 1996.

Hutton CL. Responses to a hearing problem inventory. J Acad Rehab Audiol 1980;13:133–154.

Jeffers J, Barley M. Speechreading (lipreading). Springfield, IL: Charles C. Thomas, 1981.

Kaplan H, Bally S, Brandt FD. Communication strategies, attitudes, and difficulties in the prelingually deaf population. ASHA Convention Program 1990:116.

Khan R, Goldfarb A, Pollack M, et al. Brief objective measures for the determination of mental status in the aged. Am J Psychiatry 1960;117:326–338.

Lamb SH, Owens E, Schubert ED. The revised form of the hearing performance inventory. Ear Hear 1983;4:152–159.

Lesner S. Are hearing handicap scales really necessary? Presented at the American Academy of Audiology National Convention, New Orleans, 1990.

Martin RL. Evaluate word understanding with multilevel speech tests. Hear J 1996;49:43–44.

Marzolf CA, Stewart M, Nerbonne MA, et al. Effects of two repair strategies on speechreading of words and sentences. J Am Acad Audiol 1998;9:165–171.

McCarthy PA, Alpiner JG. An assessment scale of hearing handicap for use in family counseling. J Acad Rehab Audiol 1983;16:256–270.

National Center for Health Statistics. Basic data on hearing levels of adults 25–74, United States, 1971–75. Vital and Health Statistics Publication, Series II, No. 215. U.S. Government Printing Office Washington, DC. (1980).

Newman CW, Weinstein BE, Jacobson GP, et al. Test-retest reliability of the Hearing Handicap Inventory for Adults. Ear Hear 1991;12:355–357.

Nilsson MJ, Soli SD, Sullivan JA. Development of the hearing in noise test for the measurement of speech reception thresholds in quiet and in noise. J Acoust Soc Am 1994; 95:1085–1099.

Noble W. Assessment of impaired hearing: a critique and a new method. New York: Academic Press, 1978.

Noble WG, Atherley GRC. The Hearing Measurement Scale: a questionnaire for the assessment of auditory disability. J Audiol Res 1970;10:229–250.

Oja G, Schow RL. Hearing aid evaluation based on measures of benefit, use, and satisfaction. Ear Hear 1984;5:77–86.

O'Neill JJ, Oyer HJ. Visual communication for the hard of hearing. Englewood Cliffs, NJ: Prentice-Hall, 1981.

Owens E. Consonant errors and remediation in sensorineural hearing loss. J Speech Hear Dis 1978;43:331–347.

Owens E, Raggio MW. Hearing performance inventory for severe to profound hearing loss. San Francisco: University of California, 1984.

Oyer HJ. Auditory training—significance and usage for children and adults. In: Alpiner JG, ed. Proceedings of the Institute on Aural Rehabilitation, University of Denver, 1968.

Oyer HJ, Frankmann JP. The aural rehabilitation process. New York: Holt, Rinehart and Winston, 1975.

Prescod SV. A standard dictionary of audiology. Santa Monica: Vanguard Institutional, 1986.

Preminger JE, Lin Hwei-Lin, Payen M, Levitt H. Selective visual masking in speechreading. J Speech Hear Dis 41, 564–575(1998).

Ross M. Hard of hearing children in regular schools. Englewood Cliffs, NJ: Prentice Hall, 1982.

Rubenstein A, Boothroyd A. Effect of two approaches to auditory training on speech recognition by hearing-impaired adults. J Speech Hear Res 1987;30:153–160.

Salomon G, Parving A. Hearing disability and communication handicap for compensation purposes based on self-assessment and audiometric testing. Audiology 1985;24:135–145.

Sanders DA. Aural rehabilitation. Bloomington, IN: Indiana University Press, 1950.

Schein J, Gentile J, Haase K. Development and evaluation of an expanded hearing loss scale questionnaire. Series 2, no. 37. Washington, DC: USDHEW: National Center for Health Statistics, 1970.

Schow RL. Considerations in selecting and validating an adult/elderly hearing screening protocol. Ear Hear 1991; 12:337–348.

Schow RL, Gatehouse S. Fundamental issues in self-assessment of hearing. Ear Hear 1990;11:65–165.

Schow RL, Nerbonne MA. Assessment of hearing handicap by nursing home residents and staff. J Rehabil Audiol 1977;10:2–12.

Schow RL, Nerbonne MA. Communication screening profile: use with elderly clients. Ear Hear 1982;3:135–147.

Schow RL, Nerbonne MA. Introduction to audiologic rehabilitation. Boston: Allyn and Bacon, 1996.

Schow RL, Tannahill C. Hearing handicap scores and categories for subjects with normal and impaired hearing sensitivity. J Am Audiol Soc 1977;3:134–139.

Schow RL, Reese L, Smedley TC. Hearing screening in a dental setting using self assessment. Ear Hear 1990;11 (Suppl):28–40.

Schow RL, Smedley TC, Brockett J, et al. Hearing aid referral strategies based on screening of adults. Hear J 1991; 44:30–43.

Schow RL, Balsara N, Whitcomb C, et al. Aural rehabilitation by ASHA audiologists: 1980–1990. Am J Audiol 1993;2:28–37.

Sims DG, Visual auditory training for adults. In: Katz J, ed. The handbook of clinical audiology. Baltimore, MD: Williams and Wilkins (1985).

Smedley TC. Self-assessed satisfaction levels in elderly hearing aid, eyeglass, and denture wearers. Ear Hear 1990;11(Suppl):41–47.

Stach BA. Word-recognition testing: why not do it well. Hear J 1998;51:10–16.

Steele H, Britten F. Aural rehabilitation screening with older adults. Presented at the Kansas Speech and Hearing Association Annual Convention, Kansas City, Kansas, 1998.

Stephens SDG. Evaluating the problems of the hearing impaired. Audiology 1980;19:205–220.

Stephens D, Hetu R. Impairment, disability and handicap in audiology: towards a consensus. Audiology 1991;30: 185–200.

Thorn F, Thorn S. Speechreading with reduced vision: a problem of aging. Optic Soc Am 1989;6:491–499.

Tillman TW, Carhart R. An expanded test for speech discrimination utilizing CNC monosyllabic words. Northwestern University auditory test no. 5. Technical report, SAM-TR-66–55. Brooks Air Force Base, TX: USAF School of Aerospace Medicine, 1966.

Tye-Murray N, Purdy S, Woodworth G, Tyler RS. The effect of repair strategies on the visual identification of sentences. J Speech Hear Dis 1990;55:621–627.

USPHS (United States Public Health Service). Preliminary analysis of audiometric data in relation to clinical history of impaired hearing. The national health survey, hearing study series. Bulletin 2. Washington, DC: Public Health Service, 1938.

Ventry IM, Weinstein BE. Identification of elderly persons with hearing problems. ASHA 1983;25:37–41.

Walden BE, Prosek RA, Montgomery AA, et al. Effects of training on the visual recognition of consonants. J Speech Hear 1977;20:130–145.

Walden BE, Demorest ME, Hepler EH. Self-report approach to assessing benefit derived from amplification. J Speech Hear Res 1984;9:91–109.

Weinstein BE. A review of hearing handicap scales. Audiology 1984;9:91–109.

Weinstein BE. Validity of a screening protocol for identifying elderly people with hearing problems. ASHA 1986; 28:41–46.

WHO (World Health Organization). International classification of impairments, disabilities, and handicaps: a manual of classification relating to the consequences of disease. Geneva: WHO, 1980:25–43.

Woodward MF, Barber CG. Phoneme perception in lipreading. J Speech Hear Res 1960;3:212–222.

World Health Organization ICIDH-2: International Classification of impairments, activities, and participation. A manual of dimensions of disablement and functioning. Beta-1 draft for field trials. Geneva: World Health Organization, 1997

CHAPTER

11

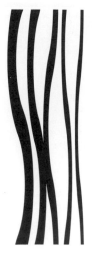

Hearing Aid Selection and Assessment

Catherine V. Palmer, Ph.D., and H. Gustav Mueller, Ph.D.

Introduction

This chapter is meant as an introduction to the process of fitting hearing aids to adult patients. For the student planning to participate in fitting hearing aids, he or she will need more detailed information and should refer to a variety of more comprehensive texts dealing with hearing aids (e.g., Mueller et al., 1992; Studebaker and Hochberg, 1993; Valente, 1994, in press). The student of hearing aids will find that continuing education is the most critical aspect of education related to hearing aids, because technology and fitting strategies are changing rapidly as a result of improved technology transfer from other disciplines and auditory research. The information in this chapter should allow the clinician involved in an aural rehabilitation program to assess the appropriateness of a hearing aid fitting and to assess what one can expect for a given hearing aid fit to a particular individual. Knowing what one can expect from the hearing aid is critical when planning audiologic rehabilitation that may involve listening strategies, speechreading, etc.

The hearing aid should be thought of as a tool in the rehabilitative process. The rehabilitative audiologist must understand the tool and its limitations for any particular individual. At a minimum, it would seem practical to define the audibility produced by the current hearing aids so the rehabilita-

tive specialist knows what he or she is working with auditorily. For instance, if the hearing loss and hearing aid technology used precludes any audibility beyond 2000 Hz, then one would not want to spend a great deal of time practicing discriminating high-frequency sounds. One would better spend time working with repair strategies and speechreading to enhance communication performance.

The hearing aid is the tool that not only allows many individuals to receive audible sound, it is the tool that allows individuals to couple to the world of assistive technology. Although assistive devices are discussed in detail elsewhere in this text, coupling options that must be included on the hearing aid will be discussed in this chapter. Most importantly, the hearing aid fitter must think ahead to the possible assistive technology that the individual will require to communicate and function successfully and the appropriate coupling options must be included on the hearing aid.

The Hearing Aid Candidate and the Impaired Auditory System

CANDIDACY

Who is a candidate for hearing aid use? This seemingly simple question is one of the most important and, unfortunately, one of the most commonly misunderstood issues in the area of hearing aid fitting. Difficulty hearing can be thought of as having three dimensions. First, one may have a sensitivity loss, which implies that once a signal is made audible, the person will function well. Second, the individual may have difficulties in frequency, loudness, and/or temporal resolution due to hearing loss. In this case, the individual will need a return of audibility but may still have difficulty, especially in difficult listening environments. Third, the individual who may or may not have sensitivity and resolution difficulties may have central auditory processing difficulties. This implies a problem with processing the signal even though it may reach the temporal lobe intact. Although central auditory processing difficulties will make understanding sound difficult, we know that an individual cannot possibly use sound if he or she cannot hear it. Therefore, even an individual identified with central auditory processing deficits may benefit from amplification. Because central auditory processing deficits often reveal themselves in the most challenging listening situations (noise and reverberation), various technologies that reduce the contribution of noise and reverberation to the signal should be explored.

An individual is a candidate for personal amplification as soon as communication is affected. When the audiogram is viewed, it is useful to predict the potential handicap of a given hearing impairment by determining what proportion of the entire speech spectrum is audible to the patient. This approach requires a comparison of a patient's audiometric data to the known frequency/intensity distribution of speech. Olsen et al. (1987) published a review that compares many of the various calculations of the speech spectrum data from different studies on an audiogram format. Figure 11.1a illustrates the normal speech levels for men, women, and children based on the work of Pearsons et al. (1977). These average data show the speech spectra to be approximately 45 dB HL at 500 Hz, 30 to 40 dB HL from 1000 to 4000 Hz, and only 20 dB HL for the 6000 Hz range. Figure 11.1b is based on the work of Tyler (1979). This figure shows the intensity range of different types

of speech sounds separated according to the manner of production. Whereas the spectrum illustrated in Figure 11.1a is slightly different from that of Figure 11.1b, both clearly illustrate the reduction in intensity that occurs above 3000 Hz for important speech material.

The relatively low average speech spectra shown for the higher frequencies in Figure 11.1a points out several practical applications regarding hearing aid candidacy and hearing aid fittings. First, individuals with even a 30 to 40 dB impairment at 3000 to 4000 Hz have impaired speech understanding ability. Second, because these frequencies are important for speech intelligibility, it is critical that effective hearing aid gain is available in this region to make the speech signal audible. Finally, because the speech signals in this frequency range are relatively weak, even with amplification, it is often difficult to make these speech signals audible if the person has a severe hearing loss. Therefore, other rehabilitative strategies may be necessary.

When determining hearing aid candidacy (i.e., whether a given hearing loss is handicapping), it is helpful to consider the range of average speech and the typical listening environments experienced by the patient. The data presented in Figure 11.1a represent average speech spectrum levels. Figure 11.2, also from the work of Pearsons et al. (1977), illustrates the variation of the speech spectrum averaged for five female talkers. It can be seen that the range between "casual" and "raised" speech is approximately 15 to 20 dB. As shown in this figure, people who are engaged in conversations using casual-level speech must rely on signals no more than 30 to 35 dB SPL for the frequencies above 2000 Hz (note that these values are SPL and would be less when converted to dB HL for direct comparison to the pure-tone thresholds plotted on an audiogram).

It also is important to consider the intensity of speech relative to background noise in a particular environment. It is well known that background noise has a significant effect on speech understanding and that this effect

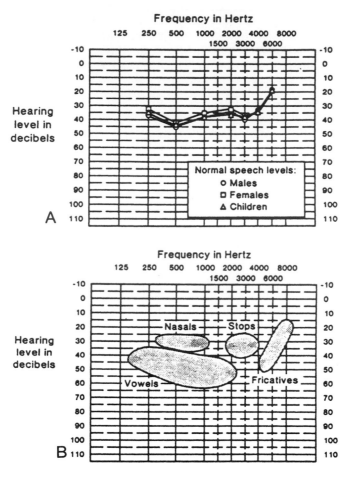

Figure 11.1. Normal speech levels (**A**) and distribution of speech sounds (**B**), both plotted in hearing level on audiogram form. (From Olsen W, Hawkins D, Van Tasell D. Representations of the long-term spectra of speech. Ear Hear 1987;8:1003–1085.)

seems to be more handicapping for the hearing-impaired person than for the normal-hearing person (see Skinner [1988] or Mueller and Hawkins [1990] for review). One factor contributing to the speech-understanding-in-noise problem is that talkers do not typically raise their voices proportionately as the background noise increases. This relationship is shown in Figure 11.3, again taken from the work of Pearsons et al. (1977). As shown in this figure, people normally speak at 55 dB SPL for background noise up to 45 dB SPL; thus, a favorable signal-to-noise ratio (SNR) of at least +10 dB will exist. Hearing-impaired individuals usually do relatively well at a +10 dB SNR if the speech spectrum has been made audible with hearing aids. The regression line in Figure 11.3, how-

ever, clearly illustrates that when the background noise becomes more intense, talkers raise their voices disproportionately. For example, when the background noise is 55 dB, average speech is 61 dB (+6 dB SNR), and when the background noise reaches 65 dB, average speech is only 68 dB (+3 dB SNR). The SNR becomes 0 dB or worse when the background noise exceeds 75 dB. These data help explain the difficulties experienced by hearing-impaired persons and must be considered in hearing aid technology selection and patient counseling.

PATIENT MOTIVATION

After an individual has been identified as a hearing aid candidate based on the degree

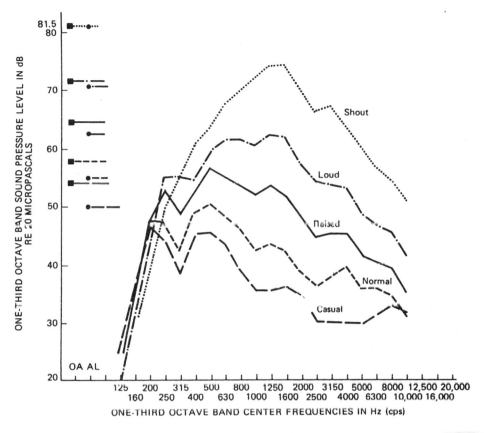

Figure 11.2. Average speech spectra for females measured at 1 m from the talker. (From Pearsons K, Bennett R, Fidell S. Speech levels in various noise environments. Project report on contract 68 01–2466. Washington, DC: Office of Health and Ecological Effects, U.S. Environmental Protection Agency, 1977.)

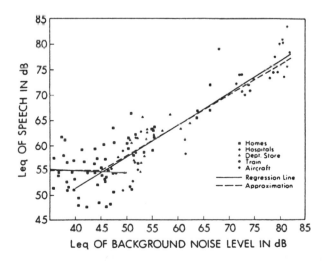

Figure 11.3. Relationship between level of speech as a function of level of background noise for five different environments. (From Pearsons K, Bennett R, Fidell S. Speech levels in various noise environments. Project report on contract 68 01–2466. Washington, DC: Office of Health and Ecological Effects, U.S. Environmental Protection Agency, 1977.)

and nature of the hearing impairment, a second consideration is the motivation of the patient to use hearing aids. Like most other prosthetic devices, hearing aids are a visible indication of a handicap and generally are associated with aging. It is not unexpected, therefore, that many individuals in need of hearing aids postpone the fitting and attempt to convince others that they can "get by" without the use of amplification.

Is it possible that an individual who was not otherwise motivated to try hearing aids could be persuaded to do so by an audiologist? Will this person subsequently use and benefit from hearing aids? To some extent, these questions were answered through research by Mueller and Bender (1988). These authors surveyed 300 new hearing aid users 12 to 14 months after they received hearing aids to determine if the reason that they obtained hearing aids had a long-term effect on hearing aid use or benefit. Mueller and Bender reported that at the time of the original hearing aid fitting, three factors were listed most commonly by the subjects as having a "strong influence" on the decision to obtain hearing aids. These factors were communication problems (reported by 65% of respondents), followed by encouragement from spouse (54%), and direction from a medical professional, usually an audiologist or an otolaryngologist (44%).

After the hearing aid use period of 12 to 14 months, 208 patients responded. Table 11.1 shows the distribution for these respondents for the three main factors. The "X" designator shows what factor(s) each group reported as a strong influence. For example, 43 individuals cited all three factors as a strong influence (Group A), whereas 28 respondents did not consider any of the three factors as a strong influence (Group H). Of primary interest were the responses from the three groups that reported only one of the main factors as a strong influence (Groups D, F, and G). Figure 11.4 shows the use and benefit ratings for these three groups. Seventy-two percent of patients in Group D reported using their hearing aids more than 69% of the average day. This value is substantially larger than the other two groups and is somewhat predictable—one might expect the patients reporting communication difficulty to use their hearing aids the most. When hearing aid benefit is examined, however, Group G (encouragement from professional) has the same percentage of subjects reporting the hearing aid to be "very beneficial" as does Group D. It would appear, therefore, that long-term hearing aid benefit is not necessarily related to self-motivation.

The overall motivation of a patient to use hearing aids clearly is a contributing factor for successful hearing aid use. Fortunately, this factor can be influenced significantly by the advice of medical professionals. Because nearly everyone with a hearing loss benefits from hearing aids, it is clearly important that this fact is related to the patient in a positive manner.

Table 11.1
Distribution for the three most common reasons for obtaining hearing aids

Group No.		Communication Problems	Encouragement From Spouse	Direction From Professional
A	43	×[a]	×	×
B	39	×	×	
C	25	×		×
D	29	×		
E	11		×	×
F	20		×	
G	13			×
H	28			

Source: McCarthy P, Montgomery A, Mueller HG. Decision making in rehabilitative audiology. J Am Acad Audiol 1990;1:23–30.

[a]Factors marked with "×" represent "strong influence" ratings. Subjects were allowed to list more than one factor as a strong influence or no factor as a strong influence.

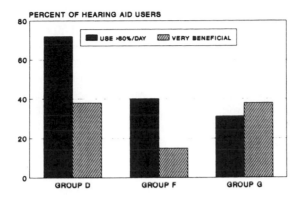

Figure 11.4. Percentage of respondents reporting greater than 60% average hearing aid use per day, and percentage of respondents rating their hearing aids as "very beneficial" for three selected groups. (From McCarthy P, Montgomery A, Mueller H. Decision making in rehabilitative audiology. J Am Acad Audiol 1990;1:23–30.)

GOALS OF AMPLIFICATION

The minimal goals of any hearing aid fitting are to achieve the best possible audibility (ability to hear soft, moderate, and loud sounds) while providing comfort (physical fit and loudness) and excellent sound quality. In addition, the hearing aid must meet the expectations of the patient, which usually include communicating in a variety of situations including communication in background noise. The individual involved in hearing aid fitting also must consider safety—whether this includes hearing from both ears to localize sound or hearing warning signals such as sirens and/or smoke detectors. The hearing aid alone, combined with other devices, or the sole use of other devices when the hearing aid is not being worn (e.g., in the middle of the night) may make up the technology that ensures safety for the individual.

The goals of any hearing aid fitting should be defined carefully by the audiologist through empiric data, patient needs assessment, and patient expectations. These goals should dictate the assessment measures, the technology selected, and the verification and validation measures that will follow hearing aid selection. For instance, if excellent sound quality is desired, then the audiologist either should use a hearing aid that consistently demonstrates excellent sound quality on physical measures or should use sound quality judgment as a verification technique in the fitting.

Currently, four different (not necessarily incompatible) audibility goals are used when selecting and fitting hearing aids. One may desire to return a normal perception of loudness to an individual. This would mean that soft sounds would be judged as soft, moderate sounds judged as moderate, and loud sounds judged as loud after the hearing aid fitting. This is referred to as loudness normalization, and the goal is to apply an acoustic transform to the input signal so that the hearing impaired listener's perceived loudness of an input signal matches the perceived loudness of a normal-hearing listener across frequencies (Cornelisse et al., 1995). A different goal might be to provide loudness equalization where speech is amplified to approximate the MCL contour. The goal of loudness equalization is to apply an acoustic transform to the input signal so that the hearing-impaired listener's perceived loudness of speech is equal across frequency bands. A typical goal for hearing aids with a linear response (same amount of gain regardless of input level) is to make average sounds comfortable and to limit loud sounds before becoming uncomfortable (loudness equalization for moderate input levels). Quiet sounds are not worried about and will generally be inaudible. A final goal that may be set along with any of the above goals is an enhancement of the SNR that is presented to the listener. This implies that either special signal processing is being used to decrease some of what the hearing aid defines as "noise" and/or the microphone of the hearing aid via assistive device coupling is being placed close to the sound source of interest, thus eliminating some of the background noise in the environment that would have reached the hearing aid microphone.

Whatever the hearing aid fitter's goal, hearing aid technology known to at least attempt the particular goal should be selected, and verification and validation strategies designed to evaluate the achievement of the goal should be used. For instance, if a return to normal loudness perception is attempted, then a reasonable verification strategy for an individual would be to play sounds judged as soft, moderate, and loud by normal-hearing individuals and expect soft, moderate, and loud ratings from the hearing aid user.

MATCHING TECHNOLOGY TO THE IMPAIRED SYSTEM

In the past few years, more and more has been learned about the impaired cochlea, which is the primary site of hearing difficulty. The function of outer and inner hair cells have been defined and can be assessed relatively independently from neural function using otoacoustic emission and auditory brainstem response evaluation along with the standard audiometric evaluation. (See Humes, 1991; Killion, 1995; and Moore, 1996 for reviews of the hearing-impaired system and matching technology to various impairments.) More than ever, the clinician is able to evaluate hearing aid technology based on whether a particular processing scheme or technology makes sense in terms of what we know has gone wrong with the impaired auditory system. Table 11.2 provides a summary of Moore's (1996) review of hair cell loss, the resulting problems, and proposed solutions. Although scientists and clinicians alike most likely would argue about the solutions column, this is presented as a way to think about technology and special circuitry. The solutions should directly address the problems resulting from a specific impaired system. These problems may be consistent for all individuals with a particular type of hearing loss or may need to be measured individually.

Data Used in Hearing Aid Selection

The focus of current hearing aid evaluations is on the individual's hearing status (sensi-

Table 11.2
Relating sensorineural hearing loss to hearing aid technology

	Problems	Possible Solutions
Outer hair cell damage produces (≤60 dB HL)	Reduced amplitude of vibration on the basilar membrane in response to weak sounds	Wide dynamic range compression, multiple bands for frequency shaping, multiple channels for audibility
	Reduced sharpness of tuning on the basilar membrane (reduced frequency selectivity), causing greater difficulty in noise	Minimize distortion, increase signal-to-noise ratio (directional mic, ALDs, binaural hearing)
	More linear input-output functions	Compression over a fairly wide range of inputs
Inner hair cell damage produces (≥70 dB HL)	Less efficient transduction of mechanical vibration into neural activity	Directional microphones or ALDs
	Loss of sensitivity	Sufficient gain and then compression output limiting
	Reduced information flow in the auditory nerve	Directional microphones or ALDs
	No transduction of activity at some regions of the basilar membrane, dead spots (extreme cases)	Directional microphones or ALDs, do not "go after" severely impaired thresholds

tivity and ability to understand speech in quiet and noise) and communication needs and demands. Items included in the hearing aid evaluation will fit into one of three categories: information needed to use a particular prescriptive fitting strategy, information needed to select hearing aid features (upfront decisions discussed below), or information needed to complete a posttest after a trial period of hearing aid use. The evaluation may include the individual's perception of sound, perception of communication ability and communication demands, and the physical response of the individual's ear.

PERCEPTION OF SOUND

Hearing ability is usually described as a function of threshold measures and may include threshold of sensitivity as well as threshold of discomfort (Mueller and Bentler, 1994). In other cases, the clinician may want to document the individual's complete range of loudness perception from threshold to right below discomfort. This is commonly referred to as assessing individual loudness growth. Typically narrow band signals are presented in at least two frequency ranges (low and high), and the individual indicates the loudness of each pre-

sentation. After the rating, another tone is presented 2 to 5 dB more intense and another rating is provided by the listener. In this way, the entire dynamic range of the individual is described and can be used in certain hearing aid prescription formulae (Cox, 1994). Figure 11.5 shows an example of the rating sheet that is used by the patient.

Fitting formulae that do not require complete loudness growth data assume that loudness growth can be predicted from threshold of sensitivity and threshold of discomfort data. Further prescriptive formulae that only require threshold of sensitivity rely on predicting threshold of discomfort as well as the rest of the range of loudness perception (Pascoe, 1988). These formulae use average data collected on large groups of individuals. The ranges associated with the average data illustrate that there are individuals for whom the average data will not well describe the dynamic range of hearing. For this reason, if average data are used, the hearing aid fitter should ensure that appropriate verification techniques are used and the hearing aids dispensed have the flexibility to be modified according to individual difference from average. In essence, the clinician must decide how to spend his or her time. If average data are used in the

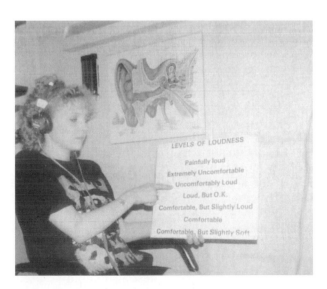

Figure 11.5. Patient using descriptive anchors to rate loudness during unaided loudness discomfort level measurements.

hearing aid selection process, then time must be dedicated to the verification process to account for differences from average (and flexible technology must be used). If individual data are used in the hearing aid selection process, then time potentially is saved in the verification process. Individual data are especially important for patients who will not be able to participate in a cooperative manner in the verification process (e.g., young children, difficult-to-test adults, etc.) and when conventional hearing aids (generally not as flexible as digitally programmable hearing aids) are being dispensed (Valente et al., 1997).

A measure of an individual's word recognition (traditionally the ability to repeat single words in quiet) used to be the hallmark of a hearing aid selection protocol. These tests were used to select among hearing aids and/or select responses within a hearing aid. A variety of data (e.g., from Thornton and Raffin, 1978; Walden et al., 1983) have made it apparent that these are not reliable tests and, perhaps more importantly, that these tests have very little face validity for the typical patient who is complaining that he or she can understand in one-to-one situations in quiet but cannot communicate in noisy, multiple-talker situations. For this reason, the traditional word recognition test does not make a valuable contribution to hearing aid fitting. Some individuals continue to use it to assess whether an individual has particularly poor word recognition in one or both ears in order to assist in decisions related to monaural versus binaural fittings and in terms of encouraging realistic expectations. Certainly, many individuals with poor word recognition receive a great deal of benefit from amplification, so it is difficult to know if a decision not to amplify should be made on the basis of a largely unreliable measure. An individual cannot attempt to comprehend speech if it is not audible, so amplification is the first step. If after appropriate amplification the individual still cannot make use of the signal, then other rehabilitative procedures should be explored. Even individuals with poor word recognition may benefit from audible signals that contribute to feelings of safety and connection to the world around them.

Two measures have been introduced recently that may contribute to the hearing aid selection process. The Speech in Noise (SIN) test (Killion, 1997) and the Hearing in Noise Test (HINT) (Soli and Nilsson, 1994) are both tests that produce an SNR measure. After completing the tests, the clinician knows the SNR required for the individual to perform at a particular criterion level. For instance, with the HINT, the SNR is determined and then plotted on a chart that displays normative values (performance by normal-hearing individuals). This type of test could be used in several ways. First, the test could be administered at a comfortable level in the soundfield for the hearing-impaired listener before hearing aid fitting (this in essence mimics basic amplification without any special signal processing). If the individual's ability under these circumstances reveals similar performance to normal-hearing individuals, then the assumption would be that the individual does not require special circuitry or devices that would enhance SNR. In essence, this individual would be displaying an audibility problem without problems related to frequency and temporal resolution. On the other hand, if the individual needs an enhanced SNR in this condition compared with normal-hearing listeners, then one could assume that this individual has a problem not only with audibility (sensitivity loss), but also with understanding in noise (which may be related to other suprathreshold abilities). This type of result might direct the clinician to special signal processing or device options depending on how much signal-to-noise enhancement was necessary.

Another use for these types of measures might be in setting the parameters of the hearing aid. One might have a set of programmable parameters that would be manipulated until the lowest required SNR was obtained or an SNR similar to a normal-hearing listener's was obtained. This type of test also could be used to compare several types of technology that the hearing aid fitter is not able to select between based on existing empiric data (e.g., one or two of the high-level digital products with various claims regarding performance in noise). These tests provide concrete data for the clinician on which to base various decisions and also have excellent face validity for the typical patient who complains about his or her ability to communication in noisy environments. Others are not as enthusiastic about including this type of test as part of the initial evaluation because they believe the majority of hearing-impaired individuals experience difficulty in noise even after audibility is restored; therefore, they consistently recommend signal-to-noise enhancing options (e.g., directional microphones, assistive devices, etc.). For these individuals, this type of testing may be useful in determining treatment outcomes (improvement of communication in noise, aided versus unaided) or in setting programmable hearing aid responses as opposed to choosing original technology.

PERCEPTION OF COMMUNICATION ABILITY AND COMMUNICATION DEMANDS

The Abbreviated Profile of Hearing Aid Benefit (APHAB) (Cox and Alexander, 1995) is an example of a questionnaire that may be used to assess what types of communication difficulty are currently being experienced by the individual and then can be used as a posttest of benefit once the hearing aid has been worn for a time. The Hearing Handicap Inventory for the Elderly and the Hearing Handicap Inventory for Adults (Ventry and Weinstein, 1982) also can be used to identify if the individual perceives himself or herself as handicapped by the hearing loss; again, the measure can be used as a posttest to see if the handicap is diminished through hearing aid use. These scales and their psychometric properties are discussed in detail elsewhere in this text. The clinician must choose what should be measured about the individual (perception of handicap, perception of ability in various communication situations, etc.) and how the information will be used related to hearing aid selection decisions. Most importantly,

the clinician should be sure to use a scale that allows for readministration after hearing aid use to collect outcome data. It is becoming more and more critical to be able to document the effects of any rehabilitative treatment, and these scales can be a powerful tool in documenting treatment efficacy if they are chosen carefully and have appropriate psychometric data that allow for comparison of pretest and posttest scores or comparison to normative data.

Every individual involved in fitting hearing aids knows that the individual's self-perceived communication needs and expectations of the hearing aid need to be defined before selecting a particular hearing aid. These needs and expectations may affect choices related to style, arrangement (monaural, binaural, special devices), and assistive technology needs. Palmer and Mormer (1997) proposed several clinical forms that assist in organizing this type of interview and patient data collection (Figs. 11.6 and 11.7). The Hearing Demand, Ability, and Needs (HDAN) form takes the clinician and patient through a complete set of auditory demands and identifies what areas the patient has difficulty with regardless of hearing aid condition (on or off). The responses to these items help the clinician select coupling options that may need to be included in the hearing aid in order to work with various assistive technology. Perhaps most importantly, the use of this type of interview and form allows the clinician to provide complete hearing health care and not just hearing aids. This type of interview also helps highlight the variety of situations in which the individual may be having difficulty. Many of these situations may have gone unnoticed by the hearing-impaired individual and his or her family (e.g., hearing the smoke detector) and/or it may have been assumed that there was no readily available solution to these situations. The last column, which asks what is currently being used to compensate in a given situation, may tell a story of dependence on the family members for a variety of listening situations (e.g., hearing the telephone, doorbell, and alarm clock; getting telephone messages). Hearing

Name :

Description of Communication Situation	Communication Problem Is Present...									The Problem Is Due To...					Currently I Compensate By... (describe) Comments
	hearing aid on at home	hearing aid off at home	hearing aid on in travel	hearing aid off in travel	hearing aid on at work/school	hearing aid off at work/school	hearing aid on in dorm	hearing aid off in dorm		Hearing	Angle	Noise	Distance	Visibility	
ALERTING															
Telephone Bell															
Doorbell															
Door Knock															
Dependent (baby, adult)															
Alarm Clock															
Smoke Alarm															
Siren															
Turn Signal Indicator															
Personal Pager															
PERSONAL COMMUNICATION															
Telephone															
TV/Stereo/Radio															
One-to-one (planned)															
One-to-one (unplanned)															
Group															
Large Room															
OTHER COMMUNICATION NEEDS															
(e.g., stethoscope) fill in below															
Athletic Activities															
Extracurricular Activities															

Further Information (e.g., status of hearing aids, telecoil, DAI, communication environment)

Recommendations (HAD/S, communication strategies, environmental manipulation)

Clinician's Initials

Figure 11.6. The Hearing Demand, Ability, and Needs profile. (Reprinted with permission from Palmer C and Mormer E. High performance hearing solutions, Vol. I: counseling, supplement to the *The Hearing Review*, Jan. 1997.)

I am successful in this situation...

Communication Goal (list in order of priority)	Hardly Ever	Occassionally	Half the Time	Most of the Time
1				
2				
3				
4				
5				

C = how the patient functions currently (pre-hearing aid or with old hearing aid)

E = how the patient expects to function post-hearing aid fitting

√ = level of success that the audiologist realistically targets

HA = how the patient actually perceives level of success post-hearing aid fitting

Figure 11.7. The Patient Expectation Worksheet. (Reprinted with permission from Palmer C and Mormer E. High performance hearing solutions, Vol. I: counseling, supplement to *The Hearing Review,* Jan. 1997.)

aids and assistive technology are often tools to independence that make a variety of interfamily relationships more positive.

Although identifying the variety of communication needs that an individual may have appears to be essential to the clinician, defining and then choosing technology that will meet the patient's expectations of the hearing aid treatment may be the most important element to a successful hearing aid fitting. The form presented in Figure 11.7 can be used to capture patient expectations. After completing the HDAN, the patient is aware of the variety of areas in which he or she may need help. In reality, the patient came to the clinic with at least one or two communication areas in which help was needed. The Patient Expectation Worksheet allows the patient to rank the order of the top five expectations he or she has for hearing aid use. These should be very specific and include measurable outcomes. For instance, a patient may indicate that he would like to go an entire evening without his wife complaining about how loud the television sounds. This expectation implies that the patient will be wearing appropriate hearing aids that will make it unnecessary to turn up

the television; however, the patient does not desire "to have hearing aids with appropriate gain for watching television," he desires to have less complaining. This is easy to measure (wife complains or not for 1 week) and brings great satisfaction to both communication partners. The practitioner should have the patient identify several (up to five) expectations and mark on the sheet where he or she is currently functioning and where he or she expects to function after treatment. The clinician also indicates where the patient would be expected to function after treatment. These marks must be in agreement. The patient may have to modify his or her expectations based on degree of hearing loss or willingness to try various technology (e.g., if the patient refuses to attempt binaural listening, he or she should not expect to function as well in noisy situations). We have found this tool to be very powerful in our clinical practice. In essence, if an individual's expectations are met, he or she is very satisfied. Having documentation is useful for counseling purposes and record-keeping related to treatment outcomes. The Client Oriented Scale of Improvement (COSI) (Dillon et al., 1997) is another instrument that deals with patient expectations, but it does not create a premeasure and post-measure; it simply documents the expectations after hearing aid fitting.

PHYSICAL RESPONSE OF THE EAR

Along with the decision regarding collecting individual data related to loudness perception, one must decide whether to collect individual data regarding the acoustic response of the individual ear. An open ear canal has a particular frequency response. This means that some frequencies are passed by the pinna and through the ear canal to the ear drum without amplifying or attenuating the signal, while other frequencies may have some enhancement due to the physical characteristics of the pinna and ear canal (shape, length, eardrum impedance). A frequency area that is amplified is called the resonant frequency of a particular system. The average adult male will have approximately 15 dB of gain at around 2700 Hz. When creating a hearing aid response, the insertion loss due to occluding the ear canal with a hearing aid must be accounted for. In other words, the typical 15 dB of gain at 2700 Hz will be lost once a hearing aid is placed in the ear. How much of this enhancement will be loss will depend on the style of

the hearing aid and placement of the microphone. For instance, almost all of this enhancement is lost in a behind-the-ear (BTE) style of hearing aid, whereas quite a bit of this natural response is maintained in the most deeply inserted completely-in-the-canal (CIC) hearing aids. As with signal perception, whether to measure the individual's real ear unaided response (REUR) and incorporate it into the hearing aid prescriptive formulae is a decision that must be made by the clinician.

The second physical measure that can be applied to the prescriptive formulae is the individual ear's response compared to the response of a 2 cm^3 coupler. The hearing aid fitter and manufacturer of hearing aids must communicate about the hearing aid's response by referring to the response of the hearing aid in a coupler, because the patient's ear is not sent to the manufacturer along with the hearing aid order. The coupler (Fig. 11.8) is constructed to mimic a typical adult male ear fit with a BTE, in-the-ear (ITE), or CIC (separate couplers for each) hearing aid. This means that the amount of volume between the end of the hearing aid and the eardrum is estimated and used in the coupler system. If this estimate is wrong, the response of the hearing aid in the individual's ear will not be accurate. There are av-

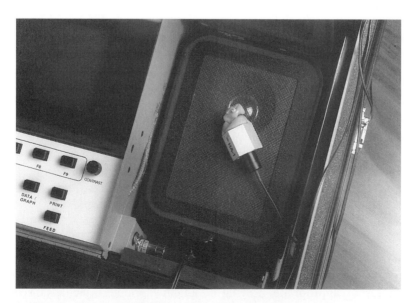

Figure 11.8. ITE hearing aid coupled to an HA-1 coupler set in an open test box.

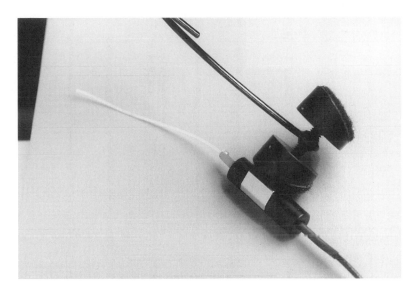

Figure 11.9. A probe-microphone (plastic tube) attached to the assembly that hooks around the pinna during testing.

erage correction factors to use between couplers and average ears, but this will be off by a large margin in some ears. With the use of a test box (Fig. 11.8) and probe microphone system (Fig. 11.9), the hearing aid fitter can measure the individual ear's difference from the standard coupler (real ear to coupler difference [RECD]). A signal is presented through insert earphones or through the individual's personal earmold, and the sound pressure level is measured at the eardrum by using a probe tube microphone. The same signal is presented through the earphone or earmold when connected to the standard coupler. For this measurement, the probe tube microphone is at the end of the coupler. The sound pressure levels in both measurements are subtracted, and the result is RECD. These values can then be used in the hearing aid fitting formulae to correct the prescribed response.

Several authors have discussed the importance of these individual physical measures (Bentler and Pavlovic, 1989; Feigin et al., 1989; Hawkins et al., 1990; Lewis and Stelmachowicz, 1993), and it is evident that they will be more important in some individuals than in others. Nevertheless, it is not possible to determine who will be different from average without taking the measure-

ments. Once again, the decision to collect REUR and/or RECD data comes down to spending measurement time during the selection process or spending the time during the verification process and, most importantly, is dependent on the flexibility of the instruments that will be fit and the ability of the patient to participate in a demanding verification process.

An observation of the size and texture of the pinna and ear canal during the above assessments will assist the hearing aid fitter in a variety of up-front decisions that will be discussed in the next section.

Up-Front Decisions

A great deal of the above data will be used to make the various up-front decisions that are described below. The up-front decisions are all the decisions that must be made before ordering the hearing aid. The decisions are based on clinician experience, patient preference, individual patient assessment, or group empiric data. Table 11.3 provides a list of up-front decisions and how the decisions are made. The clinician who keeps abreast of the most current advances in hearing aid technology will find that these advances usually mean updating the up-

Table 11.3
Up-front decisions in the selection of hearing aids

Up-Front Decisions	How Is the Decision Made?			
	Clinician's Experience	Patient Preference	Empiric Data	Diagnostic Test/ Demonstration
BTE, ITE, ITC, CIC	×	×	×	
CROS, BICROS, MULTICROS (transcranial)	×	×		
Air conduction versus bone conduction	×			×
Frequency transposition	×	×		×
Cochlear implant	×	×	×	×
Implantable	×	×		
Monaural versus binaural	×	×	×	
Microphone type/location	×		×	
Earmold material/type/color	×	×	×	
Earmold length/vent	×		×	
Sound channel	×		×	
Volume control	×	×		
Receiver type			×	
Compression options	×		×	
Telephone use and coupling	×	×		×
Output limiting			×	
Multichannel	×		×	
Ability to fine-tune	×			
Multi-memory	×	×		
Analog versus digital	×	×	×	
Previous experience	×	×	×	
Coupling to ALDs	×			×

front decision list. One finds that certain choices no longer apply and are replaced by others. Although the experienced clinician makes many of these decisions without consciously thinking about them, it would be wise to revise ones' up-front decision list periodically to make sure that patients are receiving the best technology choices based on the complete set of choices available to the clinician. Each decision is described briefly below, and the reader is guided to literature providing more in-depth discussions.

STYLE

A preselection decision that relates directly to the patient's willingness to wear hearing aids is the selection of hearing aid style. Even in the early 1990s, the custom hearing aid (ITE, in-the-canal [ITC]) had replaced the BTE as the standard hearing aid fitting (Mueller, 1992). In the mid-1990s, CIC style was quickly gaining popularity. Figure 11.10 shows various styles of hearing aids. This growth in custom hearing aid sales has been fueled by the demand from the consumer for a smaller, less visible hearing aid. At the same time, the consumer wants excellent technology contained in this small package.

Although the BTE style continues to provide benefits that cannot be achieved in the smaller hearing aids, there are fewer and fewer differences. The ITE styles can now achieve a large amount of amplification. The most amplification will be provided from a BTE hearing aid due to the ability to separate the microphone and receiver to reduce feedback (squealing) sound often associated with high-gain instruments. Directional microphone technology even can be achieved in the ITE styles (full ITE shell). In addition, with digitally programmable hearing aids, the ITE styles are just as electroacoustically flexible as the BTEs be-

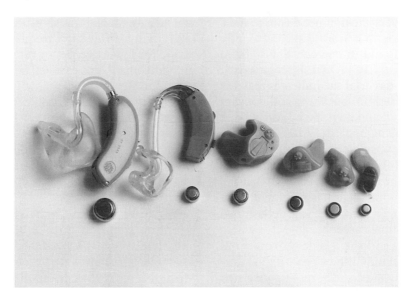

Figure 11.10. Examples of hearing aids. From left to right: large BTE with earmold, small BTE with earmold, full shell ITE, low profile ITE, ITC, and CIC. Appropriate batteries are under each style and illustrate the various battery sizes.

cause the hearing aid no longer needs room for all the controls. Parameters are manipulated via computer. The biggest advantage to the BTE continues to be the ability to couple to various assistive technologies through powerful telecoil circuitry and/or direct audio input (DAI). Both of these technologies are discussed elsewhere in this book.

Although patients often choose an ITE product for cosmetic reasons, depending on hair style, the BTE can be less obvious (coupled to the ear with a clear earmold) than a full ITE. The least conspicuous style is the CIC, which is deeply inserted in the canal and must be removed by pulling on a thin plastic wire. The CIC has several advantages because of its deep placement that include lessening of the occlusion effect (the bothersome quality of the user's own voice when there is a shallow blockage of the ear canal [Killion et al., 1988]), increased sound pressure level due to the decreased volume of air between the receiver (end of the hearing aid) and the eardrum, and increased preservation of the normal ear canal resonance and maintenance of the outer ear effects (e.g., localization) due to the deep placement of the microphone.

When new hearing aid users are allowed to select their hearing aid style, more than 90% will choose an ITE over a BTE (Mueller and Budinger, 1990). It is often possible, however, to convince a given patient that a specific style is "really the best for you" during the prefitting counseling session. This instilled belief probably will be short-lived. Mueller et al. (1991) surveyed a group of people fitted with ITEs and a separate group of individuals fitted with BTEs. The patients had been arbitrarily placed in the ITE or BTE group at the time of their hearing aid fitting. Six months after the hearing aids were given to the patients, they were asked questions about the other style, that is, the style that they were not fitted with. The responses overwhelmingly favored the ITE style. It appears that people fitted with ITE hearing aids continue to favor this style, whereas people fitted with the BTE style believe that they received an inferior product.

Whenever possible, it is best to allow the patient to choose the hearing aid style after being informed regarding the pros and cons of each related to the patient's hearing loss and communication demands. The selection of style may have to be a process. The following case illustrates this process. A young, active woman with mild to moderate bilateral hearing loss comes into the clinic indicating that she has difficulty hearing at work. She is very clear in her desire to have the smallest possible hearing aid and to only wear a hearing aid in one ear. She is fitted with a monaural CIC. When she comes back during the 30-day trial she indicates that this hearing aid is helpful but she is still not succeeding at work and now she is worried that her job may be in jeopardy. After further interview (only possible now that the patient has identified that her difficulties are more serious than she thought), it is found that she is a transcriptionist and has been making a large amount of mistakes. She is determined to continue in this career because it is where her training is and she is able to work from her home. Still unwilling to give up the idea of CIC hearing aids, she agrees to wear two hearing aids. Now she is provided with a hardwired assistive device that plugs into the tape recorder output and provides her with a volume control. She wears the headphones from this system over her two CICs (there is not a feedback problem when covering the ears because of the deep placement of the hearing aids). She now reports that she has gone from making 30 errors per page to 10 errors per page. This is a concrete measurement that she can appreciate. She also recognizes that 10 errors per page is too much and will jeopardize her work. Thus, she is ready to consider that a direct connection between the signal (recorded dictation) and her ears may be the best solution. The most efficient way to do this is to use DAI to binaural BTE hearing aids. She pursued this arrangement and is now almost 100% correct in her transcription and 100% correct in her telephone communication. Her job is secure and she is relaxed. Her hair style makes it impossible to know she uses hearing aids. Her original style choice made it impossible to know she wore hearing aids but it was very evident that she had hearing difficulty because it did not solve her communication problems.

Decisions related to whether the signal will be through air conduction (traditional hearing aids) or bone conduction (a vibrator placed on the mastoid), whether a cochlear implant will be pursued, whether an implantable hearing aid would be desirable, or whether frequency transposition technology (shifting inaudible high-frequency information to the lower-frequency region where the individual has some residual hearing; Davis-Penn and Ross, 1993; Velmans and Marcuson, 1983) might be advisable will largely be related to the type of hearing loss (conductive, sensory, sensorineural), the degree of hearing loss (any usable residual hearing in any region), and patient preference.

ARRANGEMENT

Based on empiric evidence, it is clear that individuals with two aidable ears should wear two hearing aids (Valente, 1982a,b). Most patients will try binaural amplification if the hearing aid fitter starts out with a "binaural attitude," that is, reacting to the idea of fitting only one ear as the exception rather than the rule. The major advantages of binaural hearing include elimination of head shadow, loudness summation, binaural squelch, localization, and wider dynamic range. Each will be reviewed briefly below. There are some reports that aiding one ear may eventually cause a deprivation effect in the unaided ear (e.g., Silman et al., 1984; Silverman and Silman, 1990; Silverman and Emmer, 1993). The hearing aid fitter should fully inform the hearing aid user as to the benefits of binaural amplification and the possible detriments of monaural amplification. Considering that most hearing aid users are allowed a 30-day trial period with the new amplification, it would make sense to create a binaural fitting and allow the individual to try different arrangements within his or her own communication situations.

Elimination of head shadow

Monaural hearing aid fittings may result in attenuation of important high-frequency speech signals by as much as 12 to 16 dB if they originate from the nonaided side of the head. Because these high-frequency speech signals have relatively low intensity (Fig. 11.1a), the head-shadow effect may render them inaudible. With binaural fittings, a talker positioned on either side of the listener is always speaking into a hearing aid microphone, and the head shadow is thereby eliminated.

Loudness summation

Binaural hearing aids allow for the summing of two signals, resulting in binaural thresholds that are approximately 3 dB better than monaural. The summation effect can be several decibels greater than this for suprathreshold levels. Theoretically, therefore, binaural users require less gain from each hearing aid, reducing the chances of exceeding loudness discomfort level (LDL) and reducing the occurrence of acoustic feedback.

Binaural squelch

When speech and noise are presented binaurally, an improvement in SNR over a similar monaural presentation occurs. This SNR improvement is approximately 2 to 3 dB (see Mueller and Hawkins, 1990). For listening situations that are either very easy or very difficult, this improvement may not be very noticeable to the hearing aid user. For listening situations in which the user is understanding only portions of the speech message, a 2 to 3 dB improvement in the SNR can result in a 30 to 40% improvement in speech intelligibility.

Localization

Localization of sound in the horizontal plane is dependent on interaural differences in intensity, time, and phase. A monaural fitting disrupts this relationship and in fact might cause localization to be poorer than if the person were unaided. Binaural hearing aids enhance localization over a monaural fitting.

Wider dynamic range

As previously stated, binaural hearing lowers a person's threshold due to binaural summation. The patient's LDL, however, is not significantly different for a binaural signal than for a monaural one (Hawkins, 1986). The dynamic range, therefore, becomes larger, which is especially helpful for patients with reduced LDLs.

Other advantages of binaural hearing aid

use include improved quality of speech and spatial balance. McCarthy et al. (1990) have reported that patient counseling at the time of hearing aid selection and fitting can have a significant influence on the use of and benefit from binaural hearing aids. Successful binaural fittings can be achieved with individuals who have as much as 30 dB of aided asymmetry.

Contralateral routing of signals

For the individual who has an unaidable hearing loss in one ear and normal hearing or an aidable hearing loss in the other ear, some type of contralateral routing of signal amplification might be the most appropriate hearing aid arrangement. In general, this arrangement is designed to allow the person to have two-sided hearing, although all signals are channeled into a single ear. This arrangement would be a Contralateral Routing of Signal (CROS) hearing aid for the person with normal or near-normal hearing in one ear and an unaidable hearing loss in the other ear (based on pure-tone sensitivity or disproportionate loss in speech recognition ability). For the person with an aidable hearing loss in one ear and an unaidable loss in the other ear, a Bilateral Contralateral Routing of Signals (BI-CROS) arrangement may be most beneficial. A complete discussion of CROS-type amplification can be found in a review by Pollack (1975).

More recently, a new method of CROS stimulation has been discussed (Sullivan, 1988; Valente et al., 1995b). The concept is transcranial amplification provided by a high-gain ITE hearing instrument fitted to an audiometrically dead ear, which provides amplification to the better ear via bone conduction cross-over. This arrangement requires normal or near-normal hearing in the good ear.

MICROPHONE TYPE AND LOCATION

Microphone technology is changing rapidly and is one of the most exciting areas as the new millennium begins (see Valente [1998] for a brief review). Laboratories around the world are experimenting with various microphone arrays to enhance the signal that the listener would like to pick up. Directional microphone technology (in which the listener receives the majority of the signal from wherever the microphone is pointing) was introduced in the 1970s. This type of microphone was available on the BTE style only (because that is the only microphone that would be pointing in front of the listener which is generally where the signal of interest can be found). This technology grew in popularity until it peaked at a 20% market share in the early 1980s. The use of custom (in the ear) products eliminated this option. In addition, although the advantage of directional microphones was clear (Hawkins and Yacullo, 1984), many dispensers worried that there were some communication and/or environmental situations that the user would be in that would be more appropriate for an omnidirectional response (needing to hear all around). Most expert hearing aid fitters and scientists agree that directional microphone technology is the best hearing aid feature available today to improve speech intelligibility. The only better solution is to use a remote microphone that can be placed directly by the sound source and transmit the signal directly to the hearing aid (e.g., an assistive listening device). In the late 1990s, directional microphones are back and better than ever. They can be found on BTE styles and ITE styles (full shell ITEs) because of multiple microphone use (Valente et al., 1995a). Perhaps most importantly, the hearings aids with directional technology and multiple memories allow the user to switch from a directional to an omnidirectional microphone response depending on the listening situation.

ACOUSTIC PROPERTIES

The earmold of the BTE and the shell of the ITE products are the most important and bothersome features of the hearing aid. A good fitting earmold or shell will dictate feedback problems (when amplified sound reaches the microphone and produces a squealing sound), achievable gain without feedback, sound quality of the patient's own voice (Killion et al., 1988), and patient comfort. These features alone will likely dictate success or failure for the patient regardless of the most complex fitting algorithm and hearing aid circuitry. In addition, the plumbing of the earmold or shell (this includes the venting and the sound channel in a BTE) will affect the frequency/gain response of the hearing aid. The hearing aid fitter who understands earmolds will be able to achieve more gain without using electronics and battery power by manipulating the acoustic properties (vent and sound channel length and diameter) of the earmold (Sweetow, 1992; Agnew, 1994). Palmer (1998) provides a simple tutorial that demonstrates the effect of venting and sound channel choices.

In addition, the hearing aid fitter and patient have a variety of colors to choose from for the BTE or ITE shell. Either skin or hair color can be matched depending on the style, or the more adventurous patient may opt for a neon color. There are a range of earmold materials from which to choose, and the student interested in hearing aid fitting would be wise to dedicate time to hands-on training in this area. The Microsonic catalog (Microsonic, 1988) provides a wonderful tutorial for the student of earmolds along with a self-study guide, and Westone, Inc. (1996) supplies a great teaching kit with an excellent video for instruction in this area.

VOLUME CONTROL

Hearing aids using compression technology with a low kneepoint should not require a volume control. In essence, the primary reason for compression technology is to eliminate the need for the user to constantly turn the hearing aid volume up and down. Via compression, quiet signals are supplied with the most amplification and loud signals receive the least or no amplification. In theory, the user should be consistently comfortable and not feel the need to either turn the hearing aid volume up or down. For new users, this is generally the case assuming the hearing aid has been programmed correctly and fine-tuned based on patient preferences after a period of use. For a previous user of linear technology, one often finds that the patient is desperate for a volume control and needs this to feel in control of the hearing aid. Therefore, inclusion of the volume control is now an up-front decision and a feature that may be included for previous hearing aid users.

The lack of need for the volume control is a feature that has opened up hearing aid use for populations in which it was assumed that manipulation of the volume control would pose a problem (e.g., children, some challenging adult populations). Palmer et al. (1998, 1999) reported data related to fitting hearing aids on patients with Alzheimer's disease and concluded that part of the success was due to the fact that the patients did not need to manipulate a volume control. The caregiver (spouse or adult child) inserted the battery and the hearing aid into the individual's ear, and then the hearing aid responded automatically to the listening environment to which the user was exposed.

SIGNAL PROCESSING

The categories from Table 11.3 that include receiver type, compression options, multichannel, multimemory, analog versus digital, output limiting, and ability to fine-tune the instrument all relate to signal processing decisions. With each new fitting algorithm promoted by a manufacturer, there are more and more signal processing decisions to be made. It may be useful for the reader to have a basic understanding of compression technology as opposed to linear technology and then to understand that there are many variations to compression as one manipulates the parameters associated with it (attack time, release time, compression threshold or kneepoint). A complete discussion of various signal processing schemes is not appropriate in this text, and the most important resource for the student of hearing aids is continuing education through journals, conferences, and special workshops because the technology is currently changing every 3 to

6 months. The reader is referred to Dillon (1996), Kuk (1996), and Mueller (1993) for reviews of signal processing.

A linear response implies that a hearing aid fitting is two-dimensional. Although gain may vary as a function or frequency (the person may have more hearing loss in one frequency region compared with another), gain does not vary as a function of input level. Therefore, a moderate amount of gain is used that will not make soft sounds audible, will make moderate sounds comfortable, and will make moderately loud and loud sounds come in at the limits of the hearing aid. Figure 11.11 shows a schematic of this type of response. Compression technology with a low kneepoint (input level at which compression is triggered) produces a three-dimensional hearing aid fitting. This means that gain does not only vary as a function of frequency but also as a function of input level. The compression ratio or ratios will dictate the amount of gain for a given change in input. Figure 11.11 illustrates a wide dynamic range compression hearing aid response for a particular frequency region. The compression can be changed by altering the threshold of compression (kneepoint), providing more than one kneepoint (curvilinear compression), and altering the attack and release time of the compression.

In addition, any of the signal processing described above can be mixed and matched and applied differently as a function of hearing aid channel. A multichannel hearing aid implies that the hearing aid has distinct amplifiers for various frequency regions and, therefore, the compression parameters can be set differently depending on what frequency region is being processed. Channels can number anywhere from 1 to 9 in current hearing aid technology. There are mixed data as to how many channels should be used and how channels should be defined in hearing aids (e.g., Villchur, 1988; Yund and Buckles, 1995).

Further, multimemory technology allows the hearing aid fitter to create two or more distinct ways to hear a signal (e.g., manipulating frequency response, compression parameters, etc.) for the hearing-impaired indi-

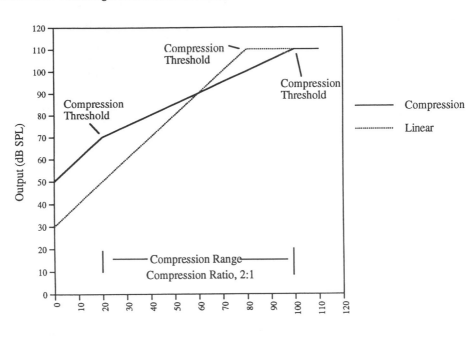

Figure 11.11. Input/output functions for linear and compression signal processing.

vidual. Many applications of multimemory hearing aid fittings seem to be a solution to a less than ideal hearing aid fitting. On the other hand, there are a variety of productive uses for this technology. For instance, the individual experiencing fluctuating hearing loss may have one memory for "better" hearing days and one memory for "poorer" hearing days. Individuals who must communicate with business associates seated next to them while they are driving the car may use a second memory switch located on a remote control to automatically turn off the left hearing aid and turn up the right hearing aid. This, of course, could be done by manipulating each hearing aid individually, but a multimemory configuration with a remote makes the adjustment faster and less conspicuous.

The ability and means to fine-tune a hearing aid are largely a preference of the hearing aid fitter and not the patient. As mentioned earlier, the ability to fine-tune (or program via computer) the hearing aid allows for less up-front measurements and demands more time in the verification process. It is hard to imagine why a hearing aid dispenser would prefer the inaccurate adjustments of a screwdriver when lower-end programmable hearing aids are no more expensive than conventional technology, yet allow the dispenser the convenience and flexibility of computer programming. For those unable to secure a computer, a variety of programmable technology comes with dedicated programming devices as well.

As indicated in Table 11.3, some decisions soon should be removed from the chart because empiric evidence has provided enough information to determine that these circuitry options do not need to be made on an individual basis. The use of Class D or B receivers are known to produce superior sound quality to that of a Class A receiver (Johnson and Killion, 1994; Palmer et al., 1995), and compression output limiting produces far superior sound quality than analog peak clipping (Hawkins and Naidoo, 1993). If manufacturers are not able to make these circuit choices for all their products, then it is up to hearing aid fitters to ensure that they are not fitting inferior circuitry that will result in poor sound quality.

COUPLING TO OTHER DEVICES

At a minimum, the hearing aid fitter must consider the individual's ability to use the telephone while wearing binaural hearing aids. Many individuals with moderate hearing loss have been using a telephone amplifier successfully before obtaining hearing aids, have been relying on a family member to pass along telephone communication, or have been doing the best they can with the telephone. The hearing aid fitting is an opportunity to improve telephone communication. The hearing aid user should not have to remove his or her hearing aids to use the telephone. With the BTE style, a telecoil (special circuitry that picks up the electromagnetic signal from most telephones) should be included, and the patient must be instructed to switch to the "telephone" setting when using the telephone. The patient should try various orientations of the telephone by the BTE case to get the best signal. The user should not hold the telephone receiver up against the ear, which is now occluded with an earmold. For the ITE and ITC user, the hearing aid fitter should request that a telecoil switch is added to the face plate (Compton, 1994). This should be added to the side used for telephone communication (usually the left ear if the individual is right-handed). The fitter should ask for vertical placement of the telecoil with a preamplifier, if there is room, to get the best response. In many ITCs, the hearing aid will be too small to incorporate telecoil circuitry. This makes this style much less appealing when a telecoil can be obtained in a full ITE. With CICs (deeply inserted), a telecoil would not fit and/or be available to the user in the form of a switch so deeply located in the ear canal. Because of the deep insertion of the CIC, a telecoil is not needed for telephone communication. The other styles require special circuitry because the hearing aid would squeal (feedback) if the user brought the telephone up against the hearing aid microphone. With the CIC, the microphone is far enough away that feedback is avoided. Therefore, the telephone can be amplified by the standard CIC microphone without the need for any special circuitry.

Although the above description portrays the CIC as having a distinct telephone advantage, the lack of telecoil circuitry may limit the user's ability to use various other assistive devices (personal communication systems, large-area systems in theaters). If the user is going to access a variety of assistive technology, telecoils on both hearing aids will be preferable even though only one is needed for the telephone. The HDAN assessment (Fig. 11.6) is the most important component of the evaluation in terms of determining what type of coupling should be included on the hearing aid to access a variety of assistive technologies that will be needed by the listener. If it is determined that the individual will need an FM system (remote microphone and transmitter that send the signal via FM radio waves to a receiver that is then coupler to the listener's ear) to communicate in a very noisy, reverberant lecture hall, then the hearing aid must have the ability to pick up the signal. This may be in the form of a telecoil (the FM receiver would output to a neckloop that produces electromagnetic signal just like a telephone), DAI (a cord leads from the FM receiver to the battery area of a BTE hearing aid, and a "boot" is slipped over the bottom of the hearing aid to make the electrical connection), or a built-in FM receiver (the BTE contains the FM receiver within its casing, making a receiver pack and any cord unnecessary). For the CIC user, assistive technology would have to be coupled via earphones plugged into the receiver. In essence, this would make the least noticeable technology (deeply inserted CICs) the most noticeable (wearing headphones in a public meeting). All these choices and configurations must be considered based on the patient's daily communication demands and preferences. New methods for coupling are being worked on every day, and the reader should review the chapter on assistive technology to get the latest information regarding hearing aid coupling options.

SUMMARY OF UP-FRONT DECISIONS

Table 11.4 provides a summary of the pros and cons associated with the various hearing

Table 11.4
Pros and cons of hearing aid styles, features, and technologies

Pros/cons	Behind-the-ear	In-the-ear	In-the-canal	Completely-in-the-Canal	CROS Family
Based on style alone	Discrete depending on hair style; No cerumen problems; Excellent venting (open ear) options; Good coupling options for telephone and other assistive devices; May be uncomfortable with glasses	Hearing aid fills the ear; Few cerumen problems; Good venting options; Fair coupling options for telephone and other assistive devices	Visible but smaller than ITE; Some cerumen problems; Poor venting options; Poor or no coupling options for telephone and other devices; Good dexterity required for insertion of aid and battery	Not visible; Cerumen problems; No venting options—ear plugged; Can use with telephone as is; No coupling options to other devices; Excellent dexterity required for insertion of aid and battery; Uses more batteries than other styles	Special system allowing for pick-up of the signal from the "dead" ear and transfer to the "better" ear
Conventional	No fine adjustments; New hearing aid needed if hearing changes; Limited, but good circuit choices; Outdated technology in both fitting schemes and signal processing; Life of hearing aid is 3–5 years	No fine adjustments; New hearing aid needed if hearing changes; Limited, but good circuit choices; Outdated technology in both fitting schemes and signal processing; Life of hearing aid is 3–5 years	No fine adjustments; New hearing aid needed if hearing changes; Limited, but good circuit choices; Outdated technology in both fitting schemes and signal processing; Life of hearing aid is 3–5 years	No fine adjustments; New hearing aid needed if hearing changes; Limited, but good circuit choices; Outdated technology in both fitting schemes and signal processing; Life of hearing aid is 3–5 years	No fine adjustments; New hearing aid needed if hearing changes; Wireless; Outdated technology in both fitting schemes and signal processing; Life of hearing aid is 3–5 years
Technology with directional microphone	Better listening in noise; Cannot switch to omnidirectional	Better listening in noise; Cannot switch to omnidirectional	Not available	Not available	Not available
Programmable	Flexible, good fine tuning ability; Variety of excellent circuit choices within one device; Changes in response can be made based on user's experience	Flexible, good fine tuning ability; Variety of excellent circuit choices within one device; Changes in response can be made based on user's experience	Flexible, good fine tuning ability; Variety of excellent circuit choices within one device; Changes in response can be made based on user's experience	Flexible, good fine tuning ability; Variety of excellent circuit choices within one device; Changes in response can be made based on user's experience	Flexible, good fine tuning ability; Wire connecting the hearings

	Life of hearing aid is 3–5 years One step away from state-of-the-art	Life of hearing aid is 3–5 years One step away from state-of-the-art	Life of hearing aid is 3–5 years One step away from state-of-the-art	Life of hearing aid is 3–5 years One step away from state-of-the-art	Excellent sound quality Complete fine tuning Wire connecting the hearing aids
With directional microphone	Better listening in noise Can switch to omnidirectional	Better listening in noise Can switch to omnidirectional	Better listening in noise Can switch to omnidirectional	Not available	Not available
Multiple memory	Ability to use different hearing aid responses in different situations May require remote control	Ability to use different hearing aid responses in different situations May require remote control	Ability to use different hearing aid responses in different situations May require remote control	Ability to use different hearing aid responses in different situations Requires remote control	
Remote Control	Discrete switching of hearing aid functions depending on technology	Discrete switching of hearing aid functions depending on technology	Discrete switching of hearing aid functions depending on technology	Must use remote for any type of function switching	
Digital	Excellent sound quality Complete fine tuning ability Ability to implement new fitting strategies within device Extended life of the hearing aid to 8 years State-of-the-art	Excellent sound quality Complete fine tuning ability Ability to implement new fitting strategies within device Extended life of the hearing aid to 8 years State-of-the-art	Excellent sound quality Complete fine tuning ability Ability to implement new fitting strategies within device Extended life of the hearing aid to 8 years State-of-the-art	Excellent sound quality Complete fine tuning ability Ability to implement new fitting strategies within device Extended life of the hearing aid to 8 years State-of-the-art	
With directional microphone	Better listening in noise Can switch to omnidirectional	Better listening in noise Can switch to omnidirectional	Not available	Not available	
Multiple memory	Ability to use different hearing aid responses in different situations May require remote control	Ability to use different hearing aid responses in different situations May require remote control	Ability to use different hearing aid responses in different situations May require remote control	Ability to use different hearing aid responses in different situations Requires remote control	
Remote control	Discrete switching of hearing aid functions depending on technology	Discrete switching of hearing aid functions depending on technology	Discrete switching of hearing aid functions depending on technology	Must use remote for any type of function switching	

aid styles, features, and technology. The final goal is to take the patient data and find the appropriate combination of hearing aid technology (a specific section of Table 11.4).

Selecting and Ordering the Hearing Aid

Much of the time and effort that once was expended during the hearing aid fitting now must be redirected to the ordering process (Mueller, 1989, 1992). Once the myriad of up-front decisions are made, it is time to select the frequency/gain response and output limit of the hearing aid. In other words, how much gain should the hearing aid produce based on the input level and the frequency range of the input, and at what intensity level should the hearing aid stop amplifying sound altogether?

Audiologists and manufacturers talk about hearing aids with reference to sound pressure level (dB SPL) measurements made in a standard coupler (hard-walled cavity that is meant to mimic an adult, male ear). Any data collected from the patient must either use this same reference or must be converted (as is the case when thresholds are collected with supraural earphones in dB HL).

The individual who will be fitting hearing aids wants to have a clear understanding of the compromises made when using average conversion data versus individual measurements, especially when working with pediatric ears that are very different from the "average ears" used to create the conversions. Generally, if time is spent on individual measures at this stage, less time should be required in verification procedures. Presumably, the inclusion of individual measures will ensure a more ideal fitting without a large amount of manipulation of the recommended hearing aid response. Conversely, the use of average data (thereby saving time at this stage) will result in more time dedicated to the verification process. Presumably, any patient differing significantly from average will require hearing aid parameter manipulation to achieve the appropriate hearing aid response. For these pa-

tients, the original fitting (based on average data) may have gotten the clinician into the range of response, but fine-tuning will be necessary. For the individual who is "average," time has been saved in both the selection stage and the verification stage. It is not clear how common or rare these "average" individuals are, so it is hard to advise the clinician as to where it is best to spend time and energy. It is clear that when conventional (limited ability to fine-tune) hearing instruments are fit, time is probably well spent in individual measures that will modify the recommended 2-cm^3 coupler targets before ordering. The reality in verification is that only limited parameters of this type of hearing aid can be modified so as little error in response as possible is desired. With digitally programmable hearing aids (hearing aids modified via computer or dedicated programming instruments), there is more room for modification based on verification results.

A variety of prescriptive methods are available to the clinician to make decisions regarding the gain/frequency response of the hearing aid. The amount of individual data necessary for a particular fitting method to produce coupler and real ear targets for the purposes of ordering and verifying the response of a hearing aid varies greatly. The type of target generated (coupler, real ear aided response, real ear insertion gain) varies among prescriptive methods. The resulting prescription given an identical hearing loss entered into a variety of prescriptive formulae also will vary widely (Meskan, 1997; Ricketts, 1997). In addition, many manufacturers now either use a device-independent prescriptive method (not linked to a particular hearing aid) as part of their fitting algorithm or use a proprietary fitting algorithm (a fitting method developed specifically by and for a manufacturer that presumably makes full use of the special circuitry in the hearing aid). When defaulting to a manufacturer's fitting algorithm, the clinician should be confident in the premise behind the fitting scheme and have a plan for verification of the method. The decision of which fitting formula to use will depend on the clinician's experience, the patient's hearing loss, and the goals of the hearing aid fitting. As stated earlier, it is most important that the original goals of the fitting dictate the fitting method chosen and the subsequent verification and validation procedures.

Users of a formal prescriptive method ascribe to the belief that the frequency responses that will maximize speech understanding, provide comfort, and/or return a normal loudness perception can be predicted from the unaided auditory measures (e.g., pure-tone thresholds, loudness growth functions). The use of formalized prescriptive methods has increased significantly in recent years. At least four factors have contributed to this increase: (1) the awareness of the unreliability of comparative aided speech audiometry, (2) the greater availability and promotion of prescriptive fitting approaches, (3) the increase in custom hearing aid fitting (this type of fitting does not lend itself to the comparative approach, as it is unreasonable to order multiple custom instruments for every patient), and (4) the development of computerized probe-microphone measures, which have facilitated the real-ear verification of hearing aid performance. The Prescription of Gain/Output (POGO) (McCandless and Lyregaard, 1983), National Acoustical Laboratories Revised (NAL-R) (Byrne and Dillon, 1986), Desired Sensation Level (DSL[i/o]) (Seewald, 1992; Cornelisse et al., 1995), FIG6 (Gitles and Niquette, 1995), and Visual Input Output Loudness Algorithm (VIOLA) (Valente and Van Vliet, 1997) are either popular or gaining popularity. Individuals pursuing what was described in this chapter as two-dimensional hearing aid fittings (gain varying as a function of frequency) will rely on POGO, NAL, and/or DSL (linear mode). Individuals interested in three-dimensional hearing aid fittings (gain varying automatically as a function of input level and frequency) and fittings that attempt to normalize loudness perception will rely on DSL[i/o] (variable compression mode), FIG6, and/or VIOLA. Individuals interested in three-dimensional hearing aid fittings and fittings that attempt to equalize loudness

perception will depend on DSL[i/o] (linear compression mode). Lindley and Palmer (1997) provide a comparison of data needed and target results provided for each of the three-dimensional hearing aid fitting prescriptions.

Figure 11.11 provides a printout from the DSL[i/o] prescriptive formula for the right ear of an example patient. Identifying information including date of birth, which is used to access appropriate average data (UCL, RECD, etc.) as a function of age, is provided at the top. The Assessment Data section provides the thresholds and any other individually measured data. In this case, RECD has been measured. The hearing aid recommendation as calculated by this particular prescriptive method is then provided. It is this information, along with all the features (e.g., telecoil, style) that have been chosen, that is forwarded to the manufacturer. At the bottom of the figure, coupler verification data are provided. These data are used for presetting the hearing aid before fitting the hearing aid on the patient. When the hearing aid arrives from the manufacturer, it has either been preset by the manufacturer (conventional hearing aids) or is programmed by the audiologist (programmable hearing aids) to approximate the targets presented in the Hearing Aid Recommendation section (Fig. 11.12).

The hearing aid is then placed in a coupler, a variety of signal inputs are presented, and the resulting output is recorded. Figure 11.8 provides a picture of an open test box with an ITE hearing aid connected to an HA-1 coupler. A microphone is inserted into the bottom of the coupler and the signal is presented in the test box (lid closed during testing). The coupler mimics the canal portion of the ear between the end of the hearing aid (or earmold with a BTE hearing aid) and the eardrum. The response of the hearing aid is measured and displayed in either output or gain (output minus input) on the screen to the left of the figure. The verification data presented at the bottom of Figure 11.12 are compared with the output measures that are obtained. Figure 11.13 provides a compari-

```
The Desired Sensation Level Method
DSL v4.0 for Windows
Hearing Health Care Research Unit
University of Western Ontario
Canada
```

Patient Information

Patient ID :	Street :
Name : Patient, Joseph	City :
Birth Date : 21-Aug-1919	State/Prov. :
Professional :	Country :
Today's Date : 25-Jan-1999, 12:05:11	Phone :

ASSESSMENT DATA (dB HL)

LEFT EAR

	.25	**.50**	**.75**	**1.0**	**1.5**	**2.0**	**3.0**	**4.0**	**6.0**
Threshold	35	40	45	45	45	50	55	55	60
Upper Limit									
Exponent									
RECD	2	6	5	4	4	3	3	9	1
REUR									
REDD									

HEARING AID RECOMMENDATION

LEFT EAR
Selection Method : DSL [i/o]

HEARING AID		*OTHER*	*OTHER*
Style : ITE		Transducer : ER3	Speech : Cox/Moore
Make :		HL to SPL : Predicted	Compr. Thresh : 40
Model :		HA Style : ITE	Loudness : Predicted
Serial # :		Circuit : WDRC (fixed CR)	
		RE to 2cc : Predicted	Max. Out : Predicted

	.25	**.50**	**.75**	**1.0**	**1.5**	**2.0**	**3.0**	**4.0**	**6.0**
SSPL-90	95	103	104	103	102	106	105	101	98
Full-On Gain (Reserve 0 dB)	11	14	16	15	15	22	23	19	17
User Gain (Input 65 dB)	11	14	16	15	15	22	23	19	17
Comp. Ratio	1.8	1.7	1.8	1.8	1.8	2.0	2.2	2.3	2.7

VERIFICATION DATA

LEFT EAR
Hi-Level (Coupler Output)

	.25	**.50**	**.75**	**1.0**	**1.5**	**2.0**	**3.0**	**4.0**	**6.0**
Target 90 dB	90	94	95	94	94	99	99	95	92
Measured 90 dB									

Mid-Level (Coupler Output)

	.25	**.50**	**.75**	**1.0**	**1.5**	**2.0**	**3.0**	**4.0**	**6.0**
Target 80 dB	85	88	89	88	89	94	94	91	88
Measured									
Target 65 dB	76	79	81	80	80	87	88	84	82
Measured									
Target 50 dB	68	71	73	72	72	79	81	77	77
Measured									

Low-Level

	.25	**.50**	**.75**	**1.0**	**1.5**	**2.0**	**3.0**	**4.0**	**6.0**
Aided SF 0°	12	14	15	16	16	19	22	21	21
Measured									

Comments:

Signature: _____   Date: _____

Figure 11.12. Assessment data, hearing aid gain/frequency response recommendation, and coupler targets as a function of input levels are displayed on the DSL(i/o) printout.

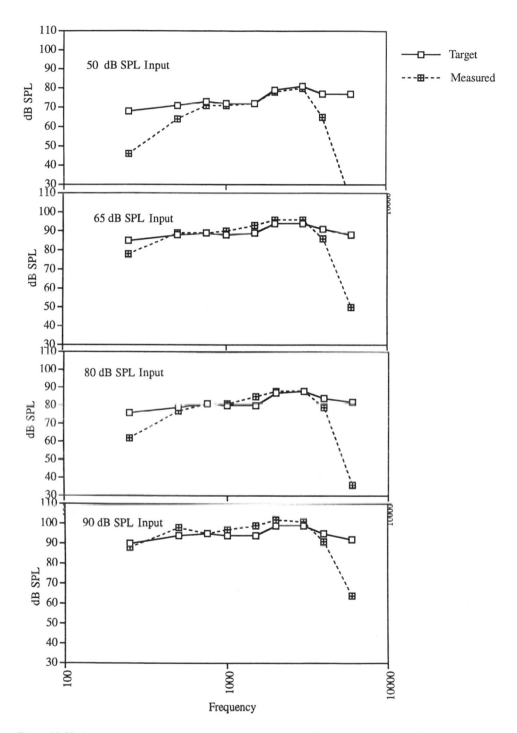

Figure 11.13. Actual measurements in a coupler compared with coupler targets for four input levels.

son of the coupler target data from Figure 11.12 and the measured hearing aid response for this particular patient. The target and measured responses are in good agreement, with the possible exception of the low-frequency response for quiet and moderate input levels and the very-high-frequency response. The clinician may accept this response or may further modify the hearing aid parameters to try to match the targets more closely. The high-frequency response rolls off at the limits of the hearing aid's frequency bandwidth of response. Clinicians do not have time to replot target and measured data onto graphs for comparison, so the DSL[i/o] prescriptive program allows entry of the measured values (see the bottom of Fig. 11.12) and then plots the comparison. In addition, many hearing aid test instruments include popular prescriptive formulae (e.g., NAL-R, DSL, FIG6) and plot the various target curves with the measured responses.

At this point, the hearing aid has been preset and verified in a coupler. If the clinician is using a manufacturer's algorithm, the only verification data available may be related to the response in the real ear. In this case, presetting may only involve entering audiometric data. The hearing aid is programmed via the proprietary algorithm, and then all verification is done in the real ear. This, of course, implies a programmable (flexible) hearing aid that the clinician knows how to manipulate based on various real ear measurement results and patient perceptions.

Verification

In the previous section, we discussed many factors that must be considered during the selection phase of the hearing aid fitting protocol. If these selection decisions are made carefully, one can be relatively certain that when the hearing aids are fitted to the patient, the performance will be at or near the desired level. It is common, however, that to meet desired goals, small adjustments to the hearing aids must be made; this procedure is referred to as the hearing aid fitting.

The adjustments that are made at the time of the fitting are not arbitrary, but rather relate to the gold standard developed by the audiologist. For example, prescriptive fitting approaches often are used to select the electroacoustic characteristics of the hearing aids for a given patient. In this case, the gold standard is the frequency-specific gain and output called for by the selected prescriptive method, and at the time of the fitting the real-ear gain and/or output of the instruments would be measured. Some audiologists might choose not to use prescriptive fitting approaches, but rather to use a gold standard such as loudness restoration or improvement in speech intelligibility. When this is the case, it is necessary to include loudness scaling or speech measures as part of the fitting procedure, and the results of this testing would dictate whether adjustments to the hearing aids are required.

The process of measuring and optimizing the hearing aid fitting is referred to as verification. Regardless of the gold standard that is used, the purpose of the corresponding measurements is to verify that the hearing aids are performing as desired. Later in this chapter, the final component of the hearing aid fitting protocol—validation—will be discussed (that is, the benefit and satisfaction provided by the hearing aids). Often, the distinction between verification and validation is blurred, and sometimes the terms are used interchangeably. Here is an example that might help illustrate the difference. It is Sunday afternoon, and you have decided to make a batch of chocolate chip cookies just like your mom used to make. You use your mom's recipe and carefully measure the butter, flour, sugar, salt, baking soda, and vanilla; you assure that the oven is at 375° and that the dough bakes for precisely 10 minutes. This is all a verification of your mom's recipe. The validation of the recipe occurs when you take the first bite.

As mentioned, verification is related to our fitting goals. Raymond Carhart, the father of audiology, was one of the first to advocate extensive behavioral testing to verify that hearing aid performance was appropriate. Dr. Carhart is known for a classic 1946 publication in which he reported on a residential 12-week hearing aid selection-verification-validation program for hearing-impaired soldiers who were returning from World War II. More relevant to this chapter, however, are the fitting goals that Dr. Carhart presented in 1975:

- To restore to the user an adequate sensitivity for the levels of speech and of other environmental sounds he or she finds too faint to hear unaided.
- To restore, retain, or make acquirable the clarity (intelligibility and recognizability) of speech and other special sounds occurring in ordinary, relatively quiet environments.
- To achieve the same potential insofar as possible when these same sounds occur in noisier environments.
- To keep the higher intensity sounds that reach the hearing aid from being amplified to intolerable levels.

Although hearing aid technology has changed dramatically since 1975, these fitting goals remain the cornerstone of hearing aid fittings today.

VERIFICATION IN THE REAL EAR

Verification of hearing aid performance can range from hours of intensive speech intelligibility testing to speech quality ratings to something as simple as probe-microphone assessment—a procedure that requires no response from the patient. As mentioned earlier, the verification procedure(s) that is used should relate to the method used to select the hearing aids and the audiologist's viewpoint concerning what constitutes a good fitting. In general, verification procedures fall into one of four categories: speech measures of intelligibility, subjective ratings of intelligibility and/or quality, loudness scaling using speech or narrow-band stimuli, and real-ear gain or output measures using probe-microphone equipment or functional gain procedures.

MEASURES OF SPEECH INTELLIGIBILITY

People are fitted with hearing aids because of difficulty understanding speech. It seems reasonable, therefore, that speech testing would be the primary hearing aid verification procedure. Unfortunately, the practical application of this logic is not that simple. Although strong on face validity, speech testing has some inherent weaknesses regarding validity and reliability when the protocol is reduced to the time constraints of a clinical evaluation. These concerns prompted Walden et al. (1983) to examine five basic assumptions of using speech testing for hearing aid verification:

- There are significant differences among hearing aids in terms of how they enable the user to understand everyday speech.
- These differences change from one user to the next, that is, there is an interaction between people and hearing aids.
- These differences can be demonstrated reliably by word intelligibility scores.
- Relative aided performance is stable over time.
- Relative performance in the clinical evaluation predicts relative performance in daily living.

The research of Walden et al. (1983) revealed that many of these assumptions are not met in the typical hearing aid evaluation procedure. Despite these findings, speech testing remains a popular component of the verification process. There are three possible outcomes using speech audiometry which would prompt the audiologist to conclude that the hearing aid fitting is successful:

1. The patient's aided performance is equal to that of persons with normal hearing. Limitation: difficult to achieve with most patients, especially for listening-in-noise speech tasks.
2. The patient's aided performance is maximized. Limitation: difficult to determine unless testing is conducted with many hearing aid settings and/or the audiologist knows the patient's potential maximum performance.

3. Aided results are significantly better than unaided results. Limitation: the audiologist must know what constitutes a significant improvement and recognize that significant may not be maximum.

As can be seen from the above examples, verifying the fitting using speech material can be a challenging experience. If time permits, speech testing should be conducted for listening in quiet and in noise as well as for different presentation levels (e.g., soft, average, and loud speech). As with all speech testing, it is critical to use recorded material—all commonly used tests are available on compact disc.

For testing in noise, the HINT (Soli and Nilsson, 1994), the SIN test (Killion, 1997), or the Speech Perception In Noise (SPIN) test (Kalikow et al., 1979) are all reasonable choices. All these tests use sentence material, standardized with recorded background noise. Both the HINT and the SPIN test have critical difference and normative data that can be used to describe a patient's performance.

SUBJECTIVE JUDGMENTS OF INTELLIGIBILITY AND QUALITY

In the preceding section, the actual measurement of speech intelligibility was discussed. It is possible, of course, to use the patient's judgments of intelligibility instead. Likewise, the patient's judgments of the quality of speech, music, or environmental sounds can be used.

If one has observed or conducted a hearing aid evaluation, one knows that informal subjective judgments are commonly elicited: "Well, Mr. Jones, how does everything sound?" "Let's go out in the waiting room and see how everything sounds." "Why don't you walk outside and see how everything sounds?" It is the old "How does that sound?" test. Done in this informal manner, the responses from the patient probably are worthless (unless there really is a serious problem with the hearing aids), but there is hope.

The key to using patient judgments for either intelligibility or quality ratings is to

use a structured approach—an approach in which the results can be compared scientifically to persons with normal hearing or to other samples of persons with hearing impairment. There are four psychophysical methods for using speech material (or other sound samples) with hearing aid users to provide useful absolute or relative estimates of hearing aid performance (Fabry and Schum, 1994).

- Magnitude estimation—the patient assigns a given value to a speech stimulus that reflects the subjective level (based on intelligibility, quality, etc.).
- Magnitude production—the patient is given a number and instructed to adjust a given parameter (e.g., intensity, SNR) until that number is reached.
- Category scaling—the patient is given a bounded scale (e.g., 0 to 10, 0 to 100) and asked to make a judgment of a speech passage (based on intelligibility, quality, etc.).
- Paired comparisons—two different hearing aids (or different settings of the same hearing aid) are compared directly. The patient must choose one or the other based on some qualitative dimension.

The category scaling technique is used quite frequently in research and easily could be adapted for clinical use. Patients are asked to judge speech and music for such qualities as softness, brightness, clarity, fullness, nearness, loudness, spaciousness, and total impression. Shown in Figure 11.14 is the rating sheet that is used for the clarity rating. The sheet is modified for each one of the other dimensions measured.

At first glance, the reader might think that the goal is always to achieve a score of 10. For the clarity rating in Figure 11.14 this would be true, but consider the rating for softness. A 1 rating would be very harsh, and a 10 rating would be very soft. In this case, the desired rating might be in the 4 to 6 range. This is why it is important to compare the patient's results to those of persons with normal hearing listening to the same material. Depending on the material, per-

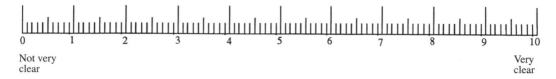

Not very
clear

Very
clear

Figure 11.14. Rating scale for clarity.

Quality of Speech

Distinct	_____	Blurred
Mild/Calm	_____	Sharp
Airy/Open	_____	Shut Up/Closed
Bright		Dull
Quiet	_____	Noisy/Hissing
Clear	_____	Hazy
Near	_____	Far
Full	_____	Thin

Figure 11.15. Bipolar terms that can be used to rate hearing aid processed speech quality. (From Hawkins D. Reflections on Amplification: Validation of Performance. J Acad Rehab Audiol, 1985; 18.)

sons with normal hearing often give clarity ratings well below a 10.

A different type of scaling procedure is to use rating scales that are referred to as semantic differential or bipolar. Figure 11.15 shows an example of this. These scales often are constructed so that there will be five or seven points between the two terms; again, for some of these pairs, the target answer might be at the midway point.

Probably the most extensive work with hearing aids and category scaling has been done by Robyn Cox and colleagues using a procedure called the Speech Intelligibility Rating (SIR) test (McDaniel and Cox, 1992). Several others have used the passages of the SIR in their research.

A procedure other than categoric scaling which commonly is used by audiologists is paired-comparison testing (i.e., while the patient is wearing the hearing aid, two different hearing aid settings are rapidly switched back and forth). During the procedure, the patient is continuously listening to a speech passage. The patient decides which setting provides the best quality or intelligibility, depending on the assigned task. In past years, it was not possible to implement this paired-comparison procedure in clinical settings, because there was no way to change quickly from one hearing aid setting to another. Due to humans' limited auditory memory for such a task, the change must be made in a second or two to obtain reliable judgments. With today's programmable hearing aids, however, it is very easy to conduct paired-comparison testing. With a simple mouse click, one can rapidly go from one setting to another. Kuk and Pape (1992) have listed several potential advantages of the paired-comparison technique:

- Greater sensitivity than speech recognition tasks.
- Good reliability (when compared with other speech tasks).
- Valid verification of the hearing aid fitting.
- Ability to judge several attributes of speech.
- Effectively use a variety of listening conditions.
- Effectively evaluate a wide range of hearing aid parameters.
- Reduced testing time.
- Auditory memory has little effect.
- Task is easy for a wide range of patients.

Whereas paired-comparison testing can be used for judgments of both intelligibility and quality, it is common to find that the setting that provides the best intelligibility will not be the same as the one that provides the best sound quality. This takes us back to the fitting goals and the gold standard of the dispensing audiologist.

These subjective tasks assume a patient-driven fitting protocol. In other words, the hearing aid response is modified based on patient perception/preference. Considering that the adult patient most likely has a long-standing, gradually developing hearing loss, his or her initial preference for sound may not guarantee audibility across the frequency range. A compromise between an audiologist-driven fitting protocol (making a wide range of input levels and frequencies audible) and a patient-driven fitting protocol is most likely the fitting protocol that will lead to successful communication.

VERIFICATION OF LOUDNESS RESTORATION

Verification techniques for speech intelligibility and quality have been outlined. It could be that one of the audiologist's primary fitting goals is loudness restoration—not only for speech, but for environmental sounds (discussed in the selection section). If this is the case, then it is appropriate that aided loudness testing would be part of the overall verification procedure. For the most part, loudness verification can be accomplished using probe-microphone measures (discussed in the next section), but there are three good reasons why behavioral aided loudness testing might be necessary: (1) approximately one-third of audiologists fitting hearing aids do not have access to probe-microphone measurement equipment, (2) probe-microphone testing does not take into account individual variances of loudness summation for speech, and (3) probe-microphone testing does not take into account individual variances of binaural summation.

Aided loudness verification can be conducted for narrow-band signals or for speech, for binaural listening, or for each ear separately. To some point, the extent of testing depends on the importance that the audiologist places on the procedure and how much time he or she is willing to spend.

At the minimum, assuming that probe-microphone measurements already have been conducted, it is reasonable to conduct loudness judgments for speech material. We recommend using meaningful sentences, presented at least at three different input levels. Complete scaling takes a little longer but may provide more reliable findings. The procedures are similar to those that were used in the hearing aid selection phase, except now the signal is presented through a loudspeaker rather than earphones. This means that if we only want to test one ear, we must assure that the non-test ear is not participating.

Figure 11.16 is an example of a patient fitted with WDRC CIC hearing aids. Shown are both the patient's unaided and aided ratings for speech. Our goal was to place the patient's aided judgments within the range of persons with normal hearing; as can be seen, we were quite successful (maybe just a little too much gain for the high-level speech signals). If our fitting goal was loudness restoration, these findings would verify that we had achieved our goal.

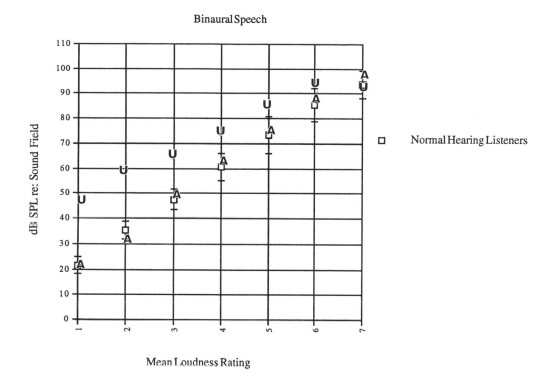

Figure 11.16. Normal-hearing listeners' judgments of loudness for binaural speech. Square symbols represent the mean with standard deviation bars, "A" represents aided results, and "U" represents the unaided results. Normal loudness perception has been returned to this patient through the use of amplification.

MEASUREMENT OF REAL-EAR GAIN AND OUTPUT

As discussed in the selection section, it is common to use a prescriptive fitting approach to obtain desired gain and output across frequencies for a variety of inputs. There are two methods to assess real-ear gain: functional gain and probe-microphone measurements.

Functional gain

When functional gain is conducted, the patient is seated in an audiometric test room and his or her audiometric thresholds are first measured for the unaided condition (it is critical to mask the non-test ear). The hearing aid is then placed on the ear, the gain is adjusted for an average speech signal, and aided thresholds are obtained. The difference between the aided and unaided thresholds is termed functional gain.

When compared with probe-microphone testing, there are many limitations of functional gain. Most notably, gain values are only observed for a single input, and no information is available regarding the actual output of the hearing aid at the patient's eardrum. With today's hearing aids, which continually vary the output of the hearing aid as a function of input, it is important to know how the hearing aid reacts to inputs that vary throughout the intensity range. Additionally, functional gain provides a poor representation of the complete frequency response, and because of head movement and other variables, the results are not very reliable. Nevertheless, if probe-microphone equipment is not available, functional gain testing might be the best method to verify prescriptive targets.

Probe-microphone measurements

In some ways, probe-microphone measurements are similar to functional gain—that is, unaided and aided ear canal SPL measurements can be compared to determine insertion gain, which will be the same value as functional gain. This gain determination, termed real-ear insertion gain (REIG), however, is only one of many useful measurements that can be obtained using this measurement technique. Measurements via probe-microphone can produce results in terms of gain (output minus input) or overall output (absolute measure of SPL in the ear canal). Clinicians often have a preference for evaluating a hearing aid response in terms of either gain or output.

To conduct probe-microphone measurements, a small silicone tube (Fig. 11.9) is placed down the ear canal so that the tip of the tube rests approximately 5 mm from the patent's tympanic membrane. A signal (e.g., speech-shaped noise) is presented from a loudspeaker located approximately 1 meter from the patient's ear. A regulating microphone, located near the ear, maintains the calibration of the speaker output. Ear canal SPL measurements then can be taken for the open ear or when a hearing aid is in place. These various measurements all have names (and acronyms) and are described in ANSI Standard S3.46. We have summarized the various procedures in Table 11.5. There also are three commonly used procedures that are not part of the ANSI standard, and they are included in the bottom portion of the table.

As we mentioned earlier, a fundamental calculation conducted with probe-microphone equipment is the REIG. To make this calculation, one must first measure the real-ear unaided gain (REUG), then put in a hearing aid, and measure the real-ear aided gain (REAG). The difference between the two is the REIG (REAG minus the REUG equals the REIG).

Rather than use a relative measure such as gain, probe-microphone measurements can provide absolute measurements of hearing aid output in the user's ear canal. In this way, the audibility of signals at a variety of inputs can be evaluated. Figure 11.17 shows the real-ear aided response (REAR, an output measure) for an individual wearing a hearing aid. This graph is generated by the DSL[i/o] hearing aid fitting program and provides the target output curves for three inputs (50, 65, and 90 dB SPL) and the subsequent measured responses. In addition, the graph plots the thresholds and UCLs of the patient in SPL so the output measures can be evaluated in terms of audibility (REAR curves must be above threshold symbols) and comfort (REAR curves must be below the discomfort curve).

Figure 11.17 provides the "SPLogram" (threshold and UCL) along with DSL[i/o] generated targets. The SPLogram alone can be used to evaluate hearing aids fit with any fitting scheme because a common goal is to make sounds audible and comfortable. The DSL[i/o] program provides an excellent mechanism for entering and plotting the probe-microphone results, but even more convenient are probe-microphone systems that automatically generate the SPLogram (and DSL[i/o] targets) and overlay the probe-microphone REAR results.

The numerous probe-microphone tests that can be conducted to verify the hearing aid fitting are well beyond the scope of this chapter (see Mueller et al. [1992] for a complete review). We do want to highlight one additional measurement, however, which is invaluable in the hearing aid selection and verification process: the real-ear coupler difference, or the RECD. If we know the difference between the output of a hearing aid in the patient's ear and in a 2-cm³ coupler (which is an easy measurement to make, even with children), then we can preset the hearing aid in the 2-cm³ coupler to match the desired output in the real ear. This presetting can facilitate the verification process, as we know that we are close to the desired levels. This is especially useful when working with a patient who will not tolerate probe-microphone measures.

In general, probe-microphone measurements are the standard for hearing aid verification. Although other verification procedures can substitute for some of the probe-microphone findings, knowing the actual SPL at the ear drum is the most efficient method to assure that prescriptive targets have been obtained and/or audibility at

Table 11.5
Definitions of probe-microphone clinical procedures

Terms from ANSI Standard S3.46
  Real-ear unaided response (REUR)
    SPL as a function of frequency, at a specified measurement point in the ear canal, for a
      specified soundfield, with the ear canal unoccluded
  Real-ear unaided gain (REUG)
    Difference in decibels between the SPL as a function of frequency, at a specified measurement
      point in the ear canal and the SPL at the field reference point, for a specified soundfield, with
      the ear canal unoccluded
  Real-ear occluded response (REOR)
    SPL as a function of frequency, at a specified measurement point in the ear canal, for a
      specified soundfield, with the hearing aid (and its acoustic coupling) in place and turned off.
  Real-ear occluded gain (REOG)
    Difference in decibels, as a function of frequency, between the SPL at a specified measurement
      point in the ear canal and the SPL at the field reference point, for a specified soundfield, with
      the hearing aid (and its acoustic coupling) in place and turned off
  Real-ear aided response (REAR)
    SPL as a function of frequency, at a specified measurement point in the ear canal for a
      specified soundfield, with the hearing aid (and its acoustic coupling) in place and turned on
  Real-ear aided gain (REAG)
    Difference in decibels, as a function of frequency, between the SPL at a specified measurement
      point in the ear canal and the SPL at the field reference point, for a specified soundfield, with
      the hearing aid (and its acoustic coupling) in place and turned on
  Real-ear insertion gain (REIG)
    Difference in decibels, as a function of frequency, between the REAG and the REUG, taken
      with the same measurement point and the same soundfield conditions
Additional probe-microphone terminology
  Real-ear saturation response (RESR)
    SPL as a function of frequency, at a specified measurement point in the ear canal for a
      specified soundfield, with the hearing aid (and its acoustic coupling) in place and turned on,
      with the VC adjusted to full-on or just-below-feedback; the input signal is sufficiently
      intense as to operate the hearing aid at its maximum output level
  Real-ear coupler difference (RECD)
    Difference in decibels, as a function of frequency, between the output of the hearing aid in the
      real ear and in a 2-cm^3 coupler, taken with the same input signal and hearing aid VC setting
  Real-ear dial difference (REDD)
    Difference in decibels, as a function of frequency, between the output from an earphone in the
      real ear and the audiometer dial setting

VC, volume control.

a variety of input levels has been achieved. Probe-microphone measures also allow the audiologist to verify that the hearing aid produces a smooth response (no peaks) across frequency. Peaks are known to affect sound quality and feedback.

OTHER VERIFICATION CONSIDERATIONS

In addition to assessing that speech understanding has been maximized, that sound quality is good, that prescriptive targets have been attained, and that loudness has been normalized, there are some other verification topics that also must be considered. On the surface, these issues may not appear to have a direct effect on the overall goal of improving speech understanding, but in reality they do. If a significant problem is present with any one of these issues, it is probable that the patient will not use his or her hearing aids; this maladaptive strategy, of course, has a very profound effect on speech understanding.

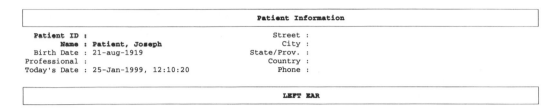

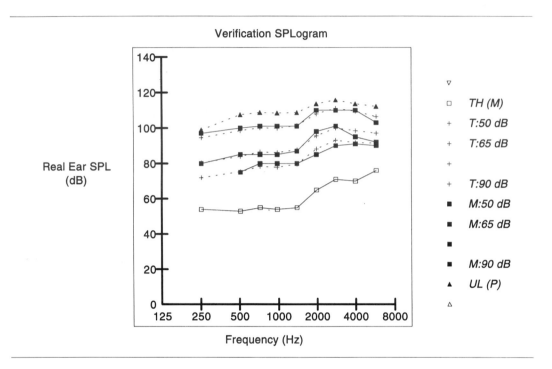

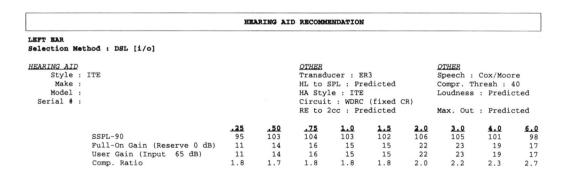

Figure 11.17. SPLogram generated by the DSL(i/o) fitting program. The patient's thresholds and UCLs in dB SPL are displayed, and REARs as a function of input level are displayed against target responses.

Acoustic feedback

Feedback problems will force the patient to use less gain, which will reduce audibility for soft sounds. At the time of the fitting, it is important to assure that no feedback problem exists. The patient should be seated in a quiet room (most hearing aids have maximum gain when the input to the microphone is low) and encouraged to make exaggerated chewing motions to assure that the fitting is not prone to feedback.

Occlusion effect

A hearing aid with minimal venting can cause the hearing aid occlusion effect—an enhancement of low-frequency bone-conducted energy. This enhancement can be as much as 20 dB or more for some patients and will often result in the patient complaint of "my voice sounds like I'm talking in a barrel." This is so bothersome to some patients that they simply stop using their hearing aids. Treatment for this problem is lengthening the ear canal portion of the hearing aids (which helps prevent the cartilaginous portion of the ear canal from vibrating) or increasing the venting of the hearing aid (which helps leak out the bone-conducted energy).

Comfortable fit

The hearing aid should feel comfortable to the patient. In some cases, particularly when deep ear canal fittings are used, shell modification may be necessary. There is some adjustment for the patient, so many times comfort issues are addressed after the patient has had the opportunity to use the hearing aids for a few days.

Cosmetic appeal

Many patients will not wear hearing aids that they believe are unsightly, that is, too big. Although in most cases patients see a sample on the day of the order for the style that they receiving, the actual hearing aid made for their ear might be larger than anticipated (or it just does not look as good as they thought it should when it is set in the ear). It is important to determine that patients are satisfied with the appearance of the hearing aids before they leave the office.

Orientation and Counseling

Palmer and Mormer (1997) provide a systematic program for hearing instrument orientation and adjustment. As indicated above, the dispensing appointment begins by checking the physical and electroacoustic fit of the instruments. This is done before beginning the orientation session. Palmer and Mormer break down the orientation session into two components, including instrument operation and instrument use. The instrument orientation begins with all the visible landmarks on the hearing aids. These might include the battery door, volume control, on/off switch, telephone switch, multiple memory selection button, and remote control. The focus should be on operation (literally manipulating switches and knowing where they are) as opposed to use of the operations. More complex operations (multiple memories and even telephone switches for some users) may be introduced at the follow-up appointment; the focus should be on basic operations for the first week or two. Before the end of the orientation session, the patient (and/or caregiver in some cases) should demonstrate competency in insertion and removal of the batteries and the hearing instruments. Depending on the amount of hearing loss, an assistive listening device may be used during this portion of the orientation, because the individual is not yet wearing the hearing aids.

The next step in orientation is instrument use. The patient should be wearing the hearing aids for this step. Conversation is conducted with the patient and any family members in attendance regarding the altered perception of one's own voice when first using hearing aids. Conversation is continued as the individual experiences the sound quality and loudness of the hearing aids in a fairly quiet environment. Patients may be introduced to listening with competing background noise through the use of a multi-speaker babble tape or performance in noise may be used as part of the verification procedure. The patient should be given ample opportunity to ask questions throughout the orientation session.

The clinician may want to use some sort of wearing schedule (see Palmer and Mormer, 1997) that gradually increases the amount of time a hearing aid is worn for new users. This may help the patient adjust to a foreign body in their ear canal and to the new perception of sound. The goal is to create full-time users who can fully adapt to using hearing aids. Most clinicians find that individuals who wear hearing aids full-time report the most success. A part-time user seems to be introducing new sound perception to his or her brain every time he or she uses the hearing aids. This is especially true if the individual only puts in the hearing aids in very demanding communication situations.

In addition to some sort of wearing schedule, the clinician may want to provide a method by which the patient can record success, problems, and comments about the first few weeks of hearing aid use. This may be used for the purpose of comparing hearing aid memories, hearing aid configurations (monaural, binaural, etc.), and/or coupling options (telecoil, DAI). An individualized worksheet can be created (see Palmer and Mormer, 1997) or a journal could be provided. Some manufacturers provide a journal with specific questions and then provide suggestions regarding response modification based on the patient's answers to the questions. Most manufacturers provide guidance regarding modifications based on specific patient comments. The worksheet or journal aids in collecting the patient's reactions over a week or two rather than asking them to recall their perceptions at the time of the follow-up appointment.

Follow-up and Validation

Patients generally are seen within 2 or 3 weeks of the hearing aid fitting to answer outstanding questions, review the use-journal, and make any necessary physical and/or electroacoustic modifications. In short, the practitioner would like to validate the hearing aid fitting. Additional assistive listening devices and audiologic rehabilitation may be recommended, warranty and insurance programs may be explained, and telephone and special feature use may be reviewed at this time. Palmer and Mormer (1997) provide a sample checklist for the 2-week follow-up appointment. Any posttesting that was planned in the original evaluation should be conducted after the treatment is completed. In other words, if modifica-

tions to the hearing aid response are made or the patient requires reinstruction in the use of some technology (telephone use, multiple-memories, etc.), then posttest measures should be postponed until these items have been completed satisfactorily.

As discussed earlier in this chapter, validation sounds similar to verification (and it is), but when one is concerned with the fitting of hearing aids, there are some distinct differences. Whereas there are some other types of validation measures, in general, when we refer to validation of the hearing aid fitting, we mean outcome measures. Outcome measures, for the most part, consist of subjective ratings by the patient after hearing aid use. These ratings can be obtained through anecdotal comments, informal or formal interviews, or most reliably through a self-assessment inventory. Any measure chosen for this purpose should be related to the original goals of the hearing aid fitting.

For the practicing clinician, outcome measures of hearing aid performance can be very useful in assessing treatment efficacy. For hearing aid fittings, treatment efficacy is tied to three different aspects of the selection and fitting process (Weinstein, 1996):

- Treatment effectiveness: do hearing aids improve speech intelligibility in quiet and for listening in background noise as well as restore normal loudness perceptions?
- Treatment efficiency: are certain hearing aids, or hearing aid settings/adjustments, better than others for improving speech understanding?
- Treatment effects: does the use of hearing aids improve the patient's social or emotional well-being or his or her overall quality of life?

All three of these points must be considered when treatment efficacy is evaluated. As will be discussed shortly, it is unlikely that a single outcome measure will address all the components of efficacy, and different assessment scales will be necessary. The main purpose of validation measures is to use this information for clinical decisions regarding patient care. In some cases, there also might be administrative reasons for maintaining and evaluating this information. The following are six reasons why audiologists currently use outcome measures.

- Comparison of different fitting methods. As stated in the selection section of this chapter, there are several different ways to select hearing aids and hearing aid performance. Outcome measures can help determine if differences exist among these procedures and what procedures are cost-effective.
- Comparison of different technology. Today's hearing aid technology comes with a large range of features and price tags. Manufacturers, audiologists, and consumers all need assistance sorting out what is truly the best and what products have the best value.
- Counseling. Validation measures can assist the audiologist in identifying specific areas in which counseling is needed. In addition, the results of these assessment scales can be used to show the patient how they compare with other hearing aid users or persons with normal hearing.
- Documentation for consumers. As the price of hearing aids becomes higher, consumers are becoming more sophisticated shoppers. Outcome measures from current hearing aid users can show a potential user of hearing aids the degree of success that can be expected.
- Comparison of audiologists or dispensing sites. Multiple dispensing offices under one management structure are very common today. Outcome measures are a method of quality control for the organization as a whole as well as for individual offices and dispensing audiologists.
- Documentation for third-party payers. Although we may think we know the truth, third-party payers want to see some type of documentation that binaural is better than monaural, that multichannel is better than single-channel, and that digital is better than analog.

Some of the assessment scales that can be used for validation of the fitting are mentioned in other chapters of this text and can be found in the Appendix; therefore, the discussion here will be brief. As mentioned in the verification section, there are different fitting goals; for this reason, our validation measures also will focus on different areas. We will address four of these fitting goals in this section:

- Improve speech understanding (in quiet and in noise).
- Achieve loudness restoration for speech and environmental sounds.
- Reduce social and emotional handicap from hearing loss.
- Obtain patient satisfaction for a variety of listening situations/meet patient expectations.

IMPROVE SPEECH UNDERSTANDING (IN QUIET AND IN NOISE)

A scale that is commonly used to assess benefit for listening in quiet and in background noise is the APHAB (Cox and Alexander, 1995). The test is easy to administer and score and can be downloaded from the Web site of Robyn Cox, the developer of the test (www.ausp.memphis.edu/harl). The APHAB is designed to measure disability (the patient first answers the questions with unaided hearing) and subsequent benefit from amplification. Twenty-four questions are divided into four subscales: listening in quiet, in noise, in reverberation, and aversiveness for sounds (how much the patient is bothered by loud sounds—one should not expect this to improve with amplification, but it should not become worse either). Aided results can be scored in terms of benefit for different listening conditions (compared with unaided score) compared to (1) the patient's old hearing aids, (2) aided results for typical hearing aid users, or (3) norms for normal-hearing individuals.

LOUDNESS RESTORATION FOR SPEECH AND ENVIRONMENTAL SOUNDS

If the audiologist's fitting goal is loudness normalization, then it is reasonable to include this as part of the validation procedure. A self-assessment inventory that can be used for this is the Profile of Aided Loudness (PAL) (Mueller and Palmer, 1998; Palmer, Mueller, Moriarty, 1999). The PAL is a 12-item scale designed to determine if loudness restoration has been accomplished for different signal levels. Patients rate their loudness judgments for various real-world sounds (of varying levels of loudness) based on their actual listening experiences. In addition, they rate their satisfaction for the loudness levels provided by the hearing aids. The results are compared with the loudness ratings given for the same sounds by a large group of normal-hearing individuals. The PAL inventory and scoring sheet are provided in Attachment 17 at the end of this book.

REDUCE SOCIAL AND EMOTIONAL HANDICAP FROM HEARING LOSS

A self-assessment scale that is useful for assessing handicap is the Hearing Handicap Inventory for the Elderly (HHIE) (Ventry and Weinstein, 1982), and its cousin, the Hearing Handicap Inventory for Adults (HHIA), which is designed for people younger than 65 years of age (see the chapter on self-assessment for a complete description of these outcome measures). The HHIE and the HHIA are designed to assess the social and emotional handicap that results from hearing loss and the reduction of this handicap that is obtained through the use of hearing aids. One should remember that the APHAB assesses disability; this is why it is advantageous to use both scales. A shortened version (ten questions) of the HHIE (the HHIE-S) is most commonly used in clinical settings.

OBTAIN PATIENT SATISFACTION FOR A VARIETY OF LISTENING SITUATIONS

For the past 10 to 15 years, Sergei Kochkin and the people at Knowles Electronics (Itasca, IL) have been conducting patient satisfaction surveys for all types of hearing aids. To the best of the authors' knowledge, the "n" is now around 20,000 and no doubt growing each month. This large database provides an excellent source for comparison when data are collected for a single patient or clinic. There are several categories of the Kochkin satisfaction ratings, but in general, patients rate their satisfaction for a variety of hearing aid features and listening conditions on a five-point scale ranging from very dissatisfied to very satisfied. An example of the most commonly used subscale is shown in Figure 11.18.

We recently used the Kochkin scale in a study of WDRC multichannel CIC hearing aids (Palmer et al., 1997). In this instance, we were interested in observing how this new product compared with the norms that Kochkin had developed for this type of technology.

Shown in Figure 11.19 are the results of our 50 subjects (half new users, half experienced users) compared to "average" satisfaction. The scale could be used in a similar way to compare the performance of any technology or the performance of a given clinic or dispensing site.

If the Patient Expectation Worksheet (Fig. 11.7) was used in the hearing aid selection process, it can be used as a follow-up measure to document how well patient expectations were met. The patient records "HA" in the box that matches function with the hearing aids. Ideally, the "HA" meets or exceeds the "E" mark (original expectation of treatment). If patient expectations have been met, the hearing aid fitting can be considered a success. If expectations have not been met, alternative technology, configurations, etc. may need to be attempted.

We used this patient expectation evaluation with the same 50 individuals mentioned above. Figure 11.20 illustrates that the majority of expectations for new and previous users were met. A loudness restoration approach was used when fitting these hearing aids. Again, this type of data can be used with individual patients or as a way to track overall clinic or dispensing site performance.

Conclusions

Hearing aid fitting is an ongoing process. The patient may produce new, more demanding expectations as he or she realizes

Situation	Very Satisfied	Satisfied	Neutral	Dissatisfied	Very Dissatisfied
One-to-One	_____	_____	_____	_____	_____
Watch TV	_____	_____	_____	_____	_____
Small Group	_____	_____	_____	_____	_____
Worship	_____	_____	_____	_____	_____
Telephone	_____	_____	_____	_____	_____
In Car	_____	_____	_____	_____	_____
Outdoors	_____	_____	_____	_____	_____
Restaurant	_____	_____	_____	_____	_____
Large Group	_____	_____	_____	_____	_____
Concert/Movie	_____	_____	_____	_____	_____

Figure 11.18. Rating scale and categories from the MarkeTrak survey (Kochkin, 1995).

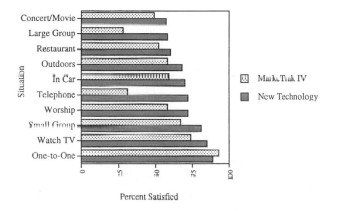

Figure 11.19. Satisfaction results from a group (n = 50) of individuals trying new technology compared with average satisfaction as reported by Kochkin (1995).

communication success, and technology may change and better meet the needs of particular patients. Any of these circumstances require that the patient has access to a knowledgeable hearing aid fitter, and that the hearing aid fitter has an easy communication system with patients to update them regarding advances in technology. Hearing aid fitting should be considered part of an overall aural rehabilitation program. Some patients may access more components of the program than others, but the hearing aid

treatment should be viewed in this larger context. Many patients require more than the fitting and follow-up session to become good users of their hearing aid technology. Further, the individual involved in comprehensive audiologic rehabilitation must understand the original goals of the hearing aid fitting and the audibility and speech understanding that the device provides.

The original goals of both the hearing aid dispenser and the patient should dictate the entire hearing aid fitting process (required

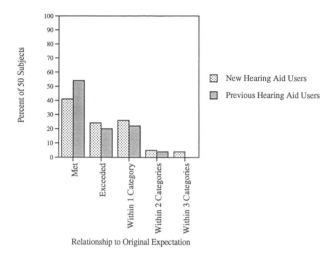

Figure 11.20. Percent of individuals whose expectations were met or exceeded as a result of amplification use.

measurements, up-front decisions, hearing aid response selection, verification, and validation). Goals should be chosen in light of patient needs and abilities, emerging empiric evidence related to the impaired auditory system, and available hearing aid technology. Through the careful selection of the hearing aid candidate, evaluation of the candidate's needs and abilities, consideration of the hearing aids' special features and electroacoustic properties, and use of a reliable verification and validation procedure, we can provide hearing aid fittings that not only will satisfy individuals with hearing impairment but also will maximize their speech understanding ability. The profession of audiology has recently been offered guidelines regarding the hearing aid evaluation and selection process (ASHA Ad Hoc Committee on Hearing Aid Selection and Fitting, 1998); the material offered in this chapter largely follows these guidelines.

The Future

Mead Killion once said that the question is not, "What can a hearing aid do?" but "What should a hearing aid do?" (Killion, 1979) More than a decade later, manufacturers, scientists, and clinicians are starting to understand the important difference between these questions. We are now seeing technology developed specifically in response to new information that is being revealed about the impaired auditory system as opposed to simply applying the latest thing that a hearing aid "can do" and seeing if it helps the impaired auditory system. We see clinical test development that will be appropriate for defining parameters of an individual auditory system, therefore suggesting specific technological solutions. Digital signal processing has just come to ear-level worn hearing aids in the past few years. This technology will greatly affect researchers' abilities to manipulate various parameters and it is hoped that it will provide the clinician with insight into how various parameters should be manipulated based on individual patient data. One exciting aspect of digital technology is the ability to download completely new fitting algorithms that may be found to be superior to a previous version to an existing patient's hearing aid. Microphone development is well underway, and we are sure to see exciting advances in this area in the next few years. The fitter of hearing aid technology must spend a great deal of his or her professional time simply keeping up with information related to the impaired auditory system, testing techniques, and advances in hearing aid technology. Continuing education is now the cornerstone of successful hearing aid dispensing.

REFERENCES

Agnew J. Acoustic advantages of deep canal hearing aid fittings. Hear Instr 1994;45:22–25.

ASHA Ad Hoc Committee on Hearing Aid Selection and Fitting. Guidelines for hearing aid fitting for adults. Am J Audiol 1998;7:5–13.

Bentler R, Pavlovic C. Transfer functions and correction factors used in hearing aid evaluation and research. Ear Hear 1989;10:58–63.

Byrne D, Dillon H. The national acoustics laboratories' (NAL) new procedure for selecting the gain and frequency response of a hearing aid. Ear Hear 1986;7:257–265.

Carhart R. Introduction. In: Pollack M, ed. Amplification for the hearing impaired. New York: Grune and Stratton 1975:xxix–xxxvi.

Compton C. Providing effective telecoil performance with in-the-ear hearing instruments. Hear J 1994;47(4):23–33.

Cornelisse LE, Seewald RC, Jamieson DG. The input/output formula: a theoretical approach to the fitting of personal amplification devices. J Acoust Soc Am 1995;97:1854–1864.

Cox R. Memorandum: administration of the contour test. www.ausp.memphis.edu/harl. 1994.

Cox R, Alexander G. The Abbreviated Profile of Hearing Aid Benefit. Ear Hear 1995;16:176–183.

Davis-Penn W, Ross M. Pediatric experiences with frequency transposing. Hear Instr 1993;44:26–32.

Dillon H. Compression? Yes, but for low or high frequencies, for low or high intensities, and with what response times? [Tutorial]. Ear Hear 1996;17:287–307.

Dillon H, James A, Ginis J. Client Oriented Scale of Improvement (COSI) and its relationship to several other measures of benefit and satisfaction provided by hearing aids. J Acad Audiol 1997;8:27–43.

Fabry D, Schum D. The role of subjective measurement techniques in hearing aid fittings. In: Valente M, ed. Strategies for selecting and verifying hearing aid fittings. New York: Thieme, 1994:136–155.

Feigin J, Kopun J, Stelmachowicz P, et al. Probe-tube microphone measures of ear-canal sound pressure levels in infants and children. Ear Hear 1989;10:254–258.

Gitles T, Niquette P. FIG6 in ten. Hear Rev 1995;2:28–30.

Hawkins D. Selection of SSPL90 from binaural hearing aids fittings. Hear J 1986;39:7–10.

Hawkins D, Naidoo S. Comparison of sound quality with asymmetrical peak clipping and output limiting compression. Am J Audiol 1993;4:221–228.

Hawkins D, Yacullo W. Signal-to-noise ratio advantage of binaural hearing aids and directional microphones under different levels of reverberation. J Speech Hear Disord 1984;49:278–286.

Hawkins D, Cooper W, Thompson D. Comparisons among SPLs in real ears, 2cm³ and 6cm³ couplers. J Am Acad Audiol 1990;1:154–161.

Humes L. Understanding the speech-understanding problems of the hearing impaired system. J Am Acad Audiol 1991;2:59–69.

Johnson W, Killion M. Amplification: is class D better than class B? Am J Audiol 1994;3:11–13.

Kalikow D, Stevens K, Elliot L. Development of a test of speech intelligibility in noise using sentence materials with controlled word predictability. J Acoust Soc Am 1979;61:1337–1351.

Killion, M. Design and evaluation of high fidelity hearing aids. Ph.D. thesis, Northwestern University. Ann Arbor, MI, University Microfilms, 1979.

Killion M. Talking hair cells: what they have to say about hearing aids. In: Berlin C, ed. Hair cells and hearing aids. San Diego: Singular, 1995.

Killion M. The SIN report: circuits haven't solved the hearing-in-noise problem. Hear J 1997;50:28–32.

Killion M, Wilber L, Gudmundsen G. Zwislocki was right . . . a potential solution to the "hollow voice" problem. Hear Instr 1988;39:32–37.

Kochkin S. Customer satisfaction and benefit with CIC hearing instruments. Hear Rev 1995;2:16–26.

Kuk F. Theoretical and practical considerations in compression hearing aids. Trends in amplification. New York: Woodland, 1996.

Kuk F, Pape N. The reliability of a modified simplex procedure in hearing aid frequency response selection. J Speech Lang Hear Res 1992;35:418–429.

Lewis D, Stelmachowicz P. Real ear to 6 cm³ coupler differences in young children. J Speech Hear Res 1993;36:204–209.

Lindley G, Palmer C. Fitting wide dynamic range compression hearing aids: DSL [i/o], the IHAFF protocol, and FIG6. Am J Audiol 1997;6:19–28.

McCandless G, Lyregaard P. Prescription of gain and output (POGO) for hearing aids. Hear Instr 1983;3:16–21.

McCarthy P, Montgomery A, Mueller HG. Decision making in rehabilitative audiology. J Am Acad Audiol 1990;1:23–30.

McDaniel D, Cox R. Evaluation of the speech intelligibility rating (SIR) test for hearing aid comparisons. J Speech Hear Res 1992;35:686–693.

Meskan M. Understanding differences between non-linear fitting approaches. Hear Rev 1997;4:64–72.

Microsonic. Custom ear mold manual. 6th ed. Ambridge, PA: Microsonic, 1998.

Moore B. Perceptual consequences of cochlear hearing loss and their implications for the design of hearing aids. Ear Hear 1996;17:133–161.

Mueller HG. Individualizing the ordering of custom hearing instruments. Hear Instr 1989;40:18–22.

Mueller HG. Individualizing the ordering of custom hearing aids. In: Mueller H, Hawkins D, Northern J, eds. Probe microphone measurements. San Diego: Singular, 1992.

Mueller H. A practical guide to today's bonanza of underused high-tech hearing products. Hear J 1993;46:13–27.

Mueller HG, Bender D. Reasons for obtaining hearing aids: do they relate to subsequent benefit? [Abstract]. Corti's Organ 1988;11.

Mueller H, Bentler R. Measurements of TD: how loud is allowed? Hear J 1994;47:42–44.

Mueller HG, Budinger A. Selection of hearing aid style. Rep Hear Instr Technol 1990;2:5–10.

Mueller HG, Hawkins D. Considerations in hearing aid selection. In: Sandlin R, ed. Handbook of hearing aid amplification, II: clinical considerations and fitting practices. San Diego: College Hill, 1990:31–60.

Mueller HG, Palmer C. The profile of aided loudness: a new "PAL" for '98. Hear J 1998;51:10–19.

Mueller HG, Bryant M, Brown W, et al. Hearing aid selection for high-frequency hearing loss. In: Studebaker G, Bess F, Beck L, eds. The Vanderbilt hearing-aid report II. Parkton, MD: York, 1991:35–51.

Mueller HG, Hawkins D, Northern J. Probe microphone measurements: hearing aid selection and assessment. San Diego: Singular, 1992.

Olsen W, Hawkins D, Van Tasell D. Representations of the long-term spectra of speech. Ear Hear 1987;8:1003–1085.

Palmer C. Curriculum for graduate courses in amplification. Trends Ampl 1998;3:6–43.

Palmer C, Mormer E. A systematic program for hearing aid orientation and adjustment. Hear Rev High Perf Hear Solutions Suppl 1997;1:45–52.

Palmer C, Killion M, Wilber L, et al. Comparison of two hearing aid receiver-amplifier combinations using sound quality judgments. Ear Hear 1995;16:587–598.

Palmer C, Adams S, Durrant J, et al. Managing hearing loss in a patient with Alzheimer disease. J Am Acad Audiol 1998;9:275–284.

Palmer C, Adams S, Bourgeois M, et al. Reduction in caregiver identified problem behaviors in patients with Alzheimer disease post hearing aid fitting. J Speech Hear Res 1999;42:312–328.

Palmer C, Mueller HG, Moriarty, M. Profile of aided loudness: A validation procedure. Hear J 1999;52(6):34–40.

Palmer C, Valente M, Powers T, Mueller G, Nascone M, Potts L (1997). The impact of restoring normal loudness growth on speech understanding as a function of signal-to-noise ratio and input level. 2nd Annual Hearing Aid Research and Development Conference sponsored by the National Institutes of Health and the Veterans Administration, Bethesda, MD.

Pascoe DP. Clinical measurements of the auditory dynamic range and their relation to formulas for hearing aid gain. In: Jensen JH, ed. Hearing aid fitting: theoretical and practical views. Copenhagen: GNDanavox, Inc., 1988:129–151.

Pearsons K, Bennett R, Fidell S. Speech levels in various noise environments. Project report on contract 68 01–2466. Washington, DC: Office of Health and Ecological Effects, U.S. Environmental Protection Agency, 1977.

Pollack M. Special applications of amplification. In: Pollack M, ed. Amplification for the hearing-impaired. New York: Grune & Stratton, 1975.

Ricketts T. Clinical use of loudness growth procedures. Hear J 1997;50:10–20.

Seewald R. The desired sensation level method for fitting children: version 3.0. Hear J 1992;45:36–41.

Silman S, Gelfand SA, Silverman CA. Late-onset auditory deprivation: effects of monaural versus binaural hearing aids. J Acoust Soc Am 1984;76:1357–1362.

Silverman CA, Emmer MB. Auditory deprivation and recovery in adults with asymmetric sensorineural hearing impairment. J Am Acad Audiol 1993;4(5):338–346.

Silverman CA, Silman S. Apparent auditory deprivation from monaural amplification and recovery with binaural amplification: two case studies. J Am Acad Audiol 1990;1:175–180.

Skinner M. Hearing aid evaluation. Englewood Cliffs, NJ: Prentice-Hall, 1988.

Soli S, Nilsson M. Assessment of communication handicap with the HINT. Hear Instr 1994;12:15–16.

Sullivan R. Transcranial ITE CROS. Hear Instr 1988;39:11–13.

Studebaker G, Hochberg I, eds. Acoustical factors affecting hearing aid performance. 2nd ed. Boston: Allyn and Bacon, 1993.

Sweetow R. Some frequently overlooked earmold problems and solutions. Hear Instr 1992;43:19.

Thornton A, Raffin M. Speech discrimination scores modeled as a binomial variable. J Speech Hear Res 1978;21:507–518.

Tyler R. Measuring hearing loss in the future. Br J Audiol 1979;2(Suppl):29–40.

Valente M. Binaural amplification: part I. Audiol J Contin Educ 1982a;7:7–9.

Valente M. Binaural amplification: part II. Audiol J Contin Educ 1982b;7:7–11.

Valente M. Strategies for selecting and verifying hearing aid fittings. New York: Thieme, 1996.

Valente M. Strategies for selecting and verifying hearing aid fittings. New York: Thieme, 1994.

Valente M. The bright promise of microphone technology. Hear J 1998;51:10–19.

Valente M. Treatment strategies for audiology. New York: Thieme (in press).

Valente M, Van Vliet D. The Independent Hearing Aid Fitting Forum (IHAFF) protocol. Trends Ampl 1997;2:6–35.

Valente M, Fabry D, Potts L. Recognition of speech in noise with hearing aids using dual microphones. J Am Acad Audiol 1995a;6:440–449.

Valente M, Valente M, Goebel J. Wireless CROS versus transcranial CROS for unilateral hearing loss. Am J Audiol 1995b;4, 52–59.

Valente M, Potts L, Valente M. Differences and intersubject variability of loudness discomfort levels measured in sound pressure level and hearing level for TDH-50P and ER-3A earphones. J Am Acad Audiol 1997;8:59–67.

Velmans M, Marcuson M. The acceptability of spectrum-preserving and spectrum-destroying transposition to severely hearing-impaired listeners. Br J Audiol 1983;17:17–26.

Ventry I, Weinstein B. The Hearing Handicap Inventory for the Elderly: a new tool. Ear Hear 1982;3:128–134.

Villchur E. Comments on 'the negative effect of amplitude compression in multichannel hearing aids in the light of the modulation-transfer function.' J Acoust Soc Am 1988;86:425–427.

Walden B, Schwartz D, Williams D, et al. Test of the assumptions underlying comparative hearing aid evaluations. J Speech Hear Dis 1983;48:264–273.

Weinstein B. Treatment efficacy: hearing aids and the management of hearing loss in adults. J Speech Lang Hear Res 1996;39(Suppl):37–45.

Westone. The Whole Westone Catalog. Colorado Springs: Westone Laboratories, 1996.

Yund EW, Buckles KM. Enhanced speech perception at low signal-to-noise ratios with multichannel compression hearing aids. J Acoust Soc Am 1995;97:1224–1240.

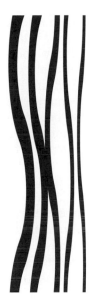

The Hearing-Impaired Adult: Management of Communication Deficits and Tinnitus

Allen A. Montgomery, Ph.D., and K. Todd Houston, Ph.D.

There is a proverbial ancient Chinese curse, "May you live in interesting times." As the new millennium begins, it certainly appears that aural rehabilitation for the adult, in particular, and audiology and speech pathology, in general, are experiencing interesting times!

Exciting Developments

There are exciting developments such as widespread cochlear implants for children, universal newborn screening, truly digital hearing aids, and 500-MHz personal computers with CD-ROM drives fast enough to provide full-screen auditory-visual (A-V) testing and training materials. Also, the advent of true "videophone" A-V speech transmission through fiber-optic telephone lines will make long-distance communication for the hearing-impaired individual much easier. Furthermore, educational audiology and education in general stand to benefit from the available technology and the increasing awareness of the large benefits from improving the classroom signal-to-noise ratio (S/N). Finally, although still problematic, it is likely that near-real-time recognition of speech by computers will become available. This would mean that teachers and presenters at meetings could have their speech displayed on monitors in text form for hearing-impaired persons to read. Obviously hard copies could also be made, which would be especially helpful for literate students in high school or college. These technical breakthroughs are truly exciting and certainly will appear in the next decade.

Continuing Struggles

There are also continuing professional struggles that threaten to derail the efforts of rehabilitative audiologists and speech pathologists to promote and provide services to adults with impaired hearing. There is still much work necessary to establish the AuD degree (and to make sure that aural rehabilitation for the adult is included in the curriculum). The primary battle, however, is to secure reliable third-party support for professional services. Indeed, those of us who believe that it is important to counsel, encourage, and educate our hearing aid clients to achieve their maximum communication potential are increasingly frustrated by the lack of federal, state, and professional support for those activities. Speech pathology is especially hard hit at the moment because of the monetary cap on rehabilitation reimbursement, but adult aural rehabilitative services are not recognized as reimbursable in many states. Audiologists in the authors' home state of South Carolina are currently seeking more comprehensive support for habilitative and rehabilitative services at the state level.

Why is this necessary? Is it because of the old "hearing loss is invisible" problem? The belief that fitting the hearing aid is enough? The lack of dramatic evidence that aural rehabilitation is efficacious—worth the time and effort? The lack of knowledge and skill on the part of the professional? The belief by the client (and sometimes by the professional) that nothing can be done beyond providing amplification?

The answer undoubtedly involves many of these factors, all of which stem from our profession's inability/reluctance to generate and distribute information about adult rehabilitative services. The most important factor, however, can be stated in simple bottom-line terms: it simply is not profitable for audiologists and other providers of hearing aids to spend time in postfitting aural rehabilitation for the adult client. Even the sale of assistive listening devices (ALDs), which can often provide large and immediate gains in communicative effectiveness, are usually not promoted by hearing health professionals for economic reasons: they are expensive to store and demonstrate, and their profit margin is low. Finally, this cost-cutting mindset has also influenced the Veteran's Administration (VA) hospital system and the active-duty military installations that historically were the origin of intensive adult aural rehabilitation.

On the other hand, university-sponsored and community-sponsored clinics are often able to explore extended counseling and training in communication strategies with their clientele (aided by the availability of low-cost student trainees and volunteer workers). Working with adult clients in these settings can be one of the most enjoyable professional experiences available to audiolo-

gists and speech pathologists. Unfortunately, however, the number of clients served in this more comprehensive manner is tiny compared with the huge population of adults receiving hearing aid fittings annually in the United States at for-profit clinics and private practices. Because of this, we have been promoting brief adult aural rehabilitation as a practical way to reach the largest number of clients without placing unrealistic expectations on the hearing health professional.

This chapter presents some background information and reviews techniques used in longer-term approaches to aural rehabilitation, including A-V integration (rather than "single-sense" training). However, the primary intent is to draw attention to the potential benefits of brief aural rehabilitation for the adult client. Finally, some options are presented for audiologists who might wish to expand their rehabilitative services to include the "other" major auditory problem exhibited by the population with sensorineural hearing loss: tinnitus.

Nature of Aural Rehabilitation (Audiologic Rehabilitation)

Traditionally, aural rehabilitation arose in medical settings such as rehabilitation hospitals following World War II. It continues today in rehabilitation centers, in VA medical centers, in community and university clinics, and increasingly in private audiologic practices in which some enterprising audiologists are conducting hearing aid orientations, comprehensive follow-ups, and group meetings of hearing aid users (see Chapter 3 for more information on aural rehabilitation and private practice).

From its early beginnings in the speechreading classes promoted at the turn of the century, aural rehabilitation has always reflected the culture and conditions under which it is practiced. At no time in its 90-year history has this been more true than today. This chapter considers aural rehabilitation in the context of the new millennium and offers not only a description of the many facets of a successful aural rehabilitation program, but also a projection of the changes and challenges that clinicians will face in the 21st century. It is alternately an exciting and a frightening prospect to consider the practice of aural rehabilitation at this time.

Three major developments are likely to have a heavy impact on the conduct of adult aural rehabilitation in the 2000s. These are the social-economic-demographic trends so evident in our society. The social component refers to the rapid development of a multicultural society in which non-White minority members and women will soon be the majority workers and Black, Hispanic, and Asian populations will have established roles. Minority groups almost invariably have a higher prevalence of handicapping conditions, and the need for adult aural rehabilitation services is undoubtedly large and growing. Some minority-oriented programs have emerged, such as the Spanish language HOLA program of Serrano-Navaro et al. (1991). However, the economic legacy of the 1990s is the increasing restriction of funding for rehabilitative services. Finally, the demographic forces produced by the aging population—36 million persons older than age 65 by 2000 (Herer, 1989)—has put a tremendous strain on all rehabilitative services, including aural rehabilitation.

In direct contrast to the education of deaf children, adult aural rehabilitation has suffered from almost a lack of controversy, direction, "schools," and "methods." In the present health care situation, when we (as a society) are forced to choose among care for the elderly, transplants, prolonged neonatal care, drug rehabilitation, and other expensive procedures, we (as audiologists) will be forced to develop brief, effective, accountable, billable activities if aural rehabilitation is to be conducted anywhere outside of subsidized clinics on a widespread basis. In some ways this pressure to produce efficient therapeutic techniques and ways to measure progress (or lack of deterioration) is good. It forces us to examine our clinical procedures critically and develop not only improved rehabilitative methods, but also more sensitive and specific diagnostic and prognostic tests. These new procedures will draw heavily on high technology but also on rehabilitative psychology and cognitive science. On the other hand, it is probably true that such time-honored traditions as the specific speechreading group and isolated auditory training will give way to counseling, assertive situation control, spouse training, audiovisual instruction, and briefer approaches in general.

The authors believe that aural rehabilitation is at a crossroads that could lead either to growth and new directions, such as those seen after World War II, or to a diminution and trivializing effect wherein aural rehabilitation is considered only in the aftermath of hearing aid fitting and available only to financially secure retirees. The growth will come from the high-tech revolution and the elevation of rehabilitation in general accompanying the resolution of the health care crisis. The stagnation will occur if demographics and economic conditions interact in ways that produce financial disincentives for prolonged treatment of any sort. In the long run, however, it is hard to believe that the tremendous general need for rehabilitative services associated with an increasingly older population will not spin off benefits to aural rehabilitation. These benefits, presumably in the form of public awareness, third-party payments, and rehabilitative teams and centers, would be available to us only if we are prepared with (1) accurate, quantitative assessment procedures; (2) efficient treatment methods; and (3) a supply of well-trained personnel (Montgomery, 1994a).

OVERALL GOAL OF ADULT AURAL REHABILITATION

The general overall goal of aural rehabilitation is to increase the probability that successful communication will occur between a hearing-impaired person and his or her verbal environment. This is stated in probabilistic terms because conditions and circumstances change so much from moment to moment and day to day that there is no guarantee that a client will be successful in a given situation, despite the best amplification, speechreading, and assertive listening skills. We strive to increase the odds that communication will take place without difficulty. We seek better communication on the average throughout the client's life. This definition acknowledges that there are many aspects of the situation that are out of anyone's control, that have a statistical rather than a definite predictable basis. Approached in this way, the successes and failures that the hearing-impaired person experiences are viewed realistically. The hearing-impaired person cannot understand everything, but on the average he or she can increase the percentage of "hits" while reducing the frustration and isolation previously experienced.

This overall goal translates into addressing several factors that are emphasized or deemphasized, depending on the client's particular needs, strengths, and weaknesses. Major activities that contribute to increasing the likelihood of communication include the following:

1. Reducing negative emotional reactions such as anger, frustration, fear, and withdrawal related to communication difficulties.
2. Making cognitive processes and attitudes toward hearing impairment more realistic.
3. Increasing knowledge of the context of the communication, including the language/dialect used, current news, the talkers, the topic, the history of the participants, and so on.
4. Maximizing auditory input through professionally fitted hearing aids and through ALDs for specific problems/situations.
5. Improving the listening and viewing (i.e., speechreading) conditions by increasing the auditory and visual S/N through assertive and educational behavior.
6. Optimizing audiovisual input through speechreading and improved viewing habits combined with the amplified auditory signal.
7. Minimizing communication breakdown through preventive action and, when breakdown occurs, using effective repair strategies.

These factors can be viewed in terms of the time frame in which they operate: 1 and 2 (emotion and cognition) are long-term, slowly responding changes that continue through life; 3 and 4 (contextual knowledge and amplification) occur before and while rehabilitation is conducted; 5 (assertive listening) should happen before or immediately on entering a difficult situation; 6 (audiovisual integration) occurs during the situation; and 7 (conversation repair) comes into play only after something is missed or misunderstood. This chapter concentrates on factors 3 through 7 because they are amenable to change.

The successful aural rehabilitation client accomplishes several things. He or she works on long-term goals of emotional and cognitive health, obtains hearing aids and ALDs, works actively to prevent difficult situations before they occur/recur, reacts promptly to improve the overall S/N ratio when entering difficult situations, makes optimal use of audiovisual input during a difficult situation, and repairs misunderstandings immediately after they have occurred. Thus, there is always something that the hearing-impaired person can do when anticipating, encountering, or repairing communication difficulties. This knowledge and the skills that accompany it provide the hearing-impaired client with the confidence and ability to succeed or improve in almost any communication situation.

HEARING LOSS AS A SOURCE OF AMBIGUITY

All seven factors mentioned above increase the likelihood of communication directly or indirectly by reducing the number of alternatives that must be considered in resolving an ambiguous message. If successfully resolved, the message is said to be disambiguated.

The way in which the seven factors come into play can be illustrated by an example. Consider the sentence that occurred in a conversation while two men were watching television: "I_in__e mi_ have _ good year i_ hi_ ba_or_ _om_ _ough." Factors 1 and 2 prevent the listener from trying to figure out what was said: "If I miss it the first time, I never get it" (cognitive discord). If he is wearing a hearing aid, the "s" (z sound) in "his" and "_omes" will become audible as will the unstressed "a" (factor 4). Also, if he can integrate lipreading with the amplified auditory signal (factor 6), he will get the "th" in "thin_" and "through". The sentence now looks like this: "I thin_ _e mi_ have a good year if his ba__or_ _omes through." Of course, if he had been assertive and asked that the volume on the television be turned down (very easy with the remote) during a commercial, he would have heard enough to understand it correctly (factor 5). As it is, he must depend on his knowledge of the context (they are discussing the basketball coach of the local team—factor 3) to supply the key phrase "back court" (speechreading had already ruled out backboard as an option) and decide on "I think he might have a good year if his back court comes through."

The point is that the hearing-impaired person must call on several sources of information and assistance in the search for understanding. If all else had failed, he could have repaired the breakdown by asking a specific question (not just "What?") such as, "If his what comes through?" (factor 7), which reduces the possibilities very quickly to the correct one. Obviously, all seven factors must be addressed in the rehabilitation of hearing-impaired adults, with different emphasis on each factor depending on the client's needs.

MODELS OF AGING

Given the fact that hearing deteriorates over time, even in the absence of active pathology (unless you consider aging itself to be pathologic!), it is not surprising that many adult aural rehabilitation clients are middle-aged or older. It is therefore important that our approach to adult aural rehabilitation consider the aging process and models of aging. Until recently, aging was almost uniformly considered to be characterized by a gradual constant decline in physical,

sensory, and mental capabilities starting as early as age 40. Many studies show exactly such a trend, based on groups of people at each age tested on various characteristics (such as strength, alpha rhythm, memory, and reaction time). This is a decidedly negative model. It implies that one can expect aural rehabilitation clients to degenerate steadily on all fronts despite our efforts. One is fighting a brief holding action at best. This is especially discouraging because sometimes the degenerative physical and mental problems are more serious impediments to rehabilitation than the hearing loss itself.

Recently, however, a much more positive and perhaps more representative model has appeared. It is called the terminal drop model (Smith, 1989). Essentially, it says that many people retain performance levels near those of their middle age long into their 70s and 80s or older. At some point, they then experience a terminal drop—a more rapid decline in capability, often leading to death. In other words, they are relatively healthy until they "drop." Smith believes that the gradual decline data show a misleadingly steep straight-line decline. The steepness in this view is due to the likelihood that the sample of people at each age group included a mix of healthy people and those already in their terminal drop stage. The decline is due primarily to simply having more subjects who have "dropped" in each successive age group. The implications of this are quite profound, suggesting that many people will lead long, healthy lives until late in life. Individuals will experience only minor loss of function until some major catastrophe hits, such as dementing disease, stroke, cancer, broken hip, or heart attack. We have all known people who fit the terminal drop model.

At this point the critical reader will ask, "If the terminal drop model holds so well, why are there so many people who gradually lose their hearing over time?" The answer seems to be that the terminal drop model best describes physical and mental capabilities but not sensory capacity, especially hearing, which does seem to share the gradual loss predicted by the steady decline model. Thus, in a sense, we can have the best of both models in a particular client's sensory loss; clinicians can relieve the consequences to a considerable extent, and the client's capable mind and body can allow the client not only to succeed in rehabilitation but to enjoy the benefits.

Along these lines, it is also encouraging to note that some forms of senility and loss of mobility, which would seem to be the terminal drop itself, are actually reversible in the elderly with a modest, steady program of physical exercise.

The Process of Communication

Verbal communication is an interactive process in which two or more talker-listeners exchange information using a common language and a shared set of rules concerning the manner in which the exchange is conducted. (Note that we do not designate a distinct talker and listener because talking and listening occur simultaneously and roles change very rapidly.). The process includes, among other components, a message to be conveyed, a purpose and intent to convey it, and a medium through which the message is transmitted. The form of the message is spoken sentences and sentence fragments accompanied by verbal and nonverbal pragmatic mechanisms that follow the rules of exchange and streamline the interactive aspects of the communication process. These mechanisms include pauses filled with "uh" or "um" to signal the talker's intent to continue talking, facial expressions indicating understanding or disagreement with the message, and ways to repair the conversation when a misunderstanding or communication breakdown has occurred. The message is thus conveyed between talker-listeners through two channels: the auditory channel, which receives the speech and audible markers, and the visual channel, which receives the dynamic image of the talker's lips (i.e., speechreading) and the visible pragmatic markers, such as facial expression and the information as to who (among three or more participants) is speaking.

UNIMPAIRED COMMUNICATION IS NOT ERROR-FREE!

It is often naively assumed that the process of verbal communication proceeds smoothly in the absence of sensory impairment, but that is far from the truth! A typical communication exchange among two or three people is a constant stream of interruptions, rephrasings, two (or more) people talking at once, corrections, topic shifts, and unclear references to people and things not present. The messages are constantly being checked or verified with facial expressions and phrases such as, "Right?" It is a useful and eye-opening experience for students to transcribe a typical audio recording of a conversation among three people. This exercise illustrates several points. (1) It is sometimes difficult to tell who is speaking without the visual information. (2) Similarly, the visible pragmatic markers are lost, especially head nodding and facial expressions that signal the talker to proceed or back up. (3) If it is a monophonic recording, it is hard to separate the speech from the background noise because the important binaural advantage in separating signal from noise spatially is lost. (4) Much of the speech is in the form of sentence fragments and rephrasings, many of which are redundant. (5) The transcript contains only the words spoken and fails to convey the emotions, spirit, and even the meanings of the conversation itself. That is, a conversation is much more than the words spoken. (6) The talkers share a common knowledge base, whereas the transcribers have no way of knowing such contextual references as to whom "you" or "they" refer or what "my problem" is. (7) Further, if the recording is "impaired" at all (noisy or low fidelity), some of the words are transcribed incorrectly. Errors occur involving speech sounds that are acoustically similar (like "b" or "v"), low intensity ("f," "th," or unstressed "uh"), or have high-frequency energy ("s," "t," "k"). Many of these errors were not made by the actual conversants because they had better acoustic conditions and also could speechread the talker, thereby eliminating the b/v and f/th errors, for example. The transcribers, of course, had the further disadvantage that they could not interact with the talkers and request clarification or repetition; they could not repair the conversation.

IMPLICATIONS FOR AURAL REHABILITATION

From this exercise we can draw several conclusions and glean several implications for aural rehabilitation in cases in which one of the talker-listener's auditory channels is impaired. First, the visual channel is very important—it provides speechreading, contextual clues, pragmatic markers, facial expressions, and eye-gaze direction. The hearing-impaired client must learn to use vision to the greatest extent possible. Therefore, we would expect telephone conversations during which visual cues are absent to be especially difficult for some clients. The availability of a visible image of the talker's face in synch with the audio signal would be of great benefit to the hearing-impaired telephone user.

Maryland is conducting a trial of exactly such an A-V teleconferencing system in its video relay interpreting system for the deaf (*NAD Broadcaster,* 1999). Here, the deaf communicator signs from a remote site to an interpreter at a central location. The interpreter then speaks the message to a hearing recipient through a traditional telephone. The recipient's response is then signed to the deaf individual through the A-V system and a conversation ensues. One can easily envision a conversation directly between two hearing-impaired people each with an A-V telephone with speechreading rather than sign as the visible signal!

Second, the loss of binaural or "stereo" listening has a serious effect on listening in noise. Clients must be fit with two hearing aids if possible (Chapter 11 has more on the advantages of binaural hearing aids).

Third, the communication process involves, indeed is dependent on, interaction among the participants. The aural rehabilitation client must acquire considerable skill in directing—even manipulating—the conversation and in repairing it when it breaks down. The transcribers in the previous example could not ask for a clarification of an indistinct passage, whereas the client can. Furthermore, much of the transcription difficulty in the previous example arose from background noise, which would also severely limit the ability of the client to understand speech. However, if the client has learned assertive listening skills, he or she can act to reduce or eliminate the noise ("Can we move out of the hallway? I'm having trouble hearing you," or "I'm going to turn the radio down for a minute while we are talking"). Assertive noise control can provide as much benefit to an impaired adult as hearing aids and speechreading combined. The successfully rehabilitated adult interacts in an effective, focused way to improve the chances for clear communication. On the other hand, if the aural rehabilitation client is so frustrated or discouraged by the difficulty in hearing that he or she withdraws (physically or mentally) from the conversation or acts inappropriately, then all possibility of constructive interaction, assertive intervention, or repair is lost. In some clients, emotional reactions, fears, and attitudes are the primary obstacles to rehabilitation and must be addressed.

Fourth, much of the meaning is conveyed with tone of voice, manner and rate of speaking, and facial expression. These characteristics are usually available to the hearing-impaired adult and can be used to great advantage.

Fifth, knowledge of the topic and the background and attitude of the talker is a great help in filling in words and phrases that a client might miss. The more the hearing-impaired individual knows about current events, sports, local news, agendas of meetings, and the topic of conversation, the better off he or she is.

A more complete view of the verbal communication environment for the typical hearing-impaired adult thus involves at least six elements: a talker-listener with normal hearing, a message, two-way auditory and visual channels with varying amounts of noise or competing messages, a talker-listener with acquired sensorineural hearing loss, a common language and pragmatic system, and a shared intent to communicate.

Nature of Hearing Loss

For prognostic purposes, hearing loss should be broken down further into three components whose relative rehabilitative impact varies considerably among individuals: hearing threshold, loss of frequency selectivity, and effects of noise.

HEARING THRESHOLD

The first component defines the presence of hearing loss and is shown in the audiogram as the sensitivity curve, that is, the threshold of audibility across frequency. Obviously, a person who cannot hear the high-frequency energy in speech will have reduced speech recognition ability. If a hearing aid is used, the reduction is to the extent that the aid fails to restore normal thresholds in the sound field. There is also some modest effect of distorted loudness relationships among acoustic speech cues due to recruitment. On the whole, it is approximately as if the speech had been filtered (usually low-pass filtered) by the hearing loss. When the filtering is counteracted by frequency-selective amplification, speech recognition is restored to near-normal levels. When the filtering effects of the audiometric threshold are the only pathology, the audiogram is an excellent prognostic factor.

Unfortunately, the two following components prevent many hearing-impaired adults from receiving anywhere near the maximum amount of benefit from amplification. For example, a recent aural rehabilitation client in our adult group had a relatively flat bilateral loss averaging approximately 75 dB HL, yet we could find no level or type of amplification that would produce monosyllabic speech recognition performance above 35% correct. The increased availability of amplified speech energy in his region of audibility was not sufficient to make speech intelligible. Obviously, other distortions are present in his auditory system beyond any threshold filtering that might be present.

LOSS OF FREQUENCY SELECTIVITY

The second component involves the loss of frequency selectivity and can be thought of

as internal distortion of the signal. Here, the client has less than normal ability to discriminate between similar speech sounds, such as "s" and "sh" or "t" and "k," even though the sounds are audible and presented at a comfortable loudness level. The loss of frequency selectivity was clearly demonstrated by Walden et al. (1981b), who experimentally removed the effects of filtering and found that perhaps one-third of patients still had significant loss of speech recognition in addition to that attributable to filtering. The second component probably involves a loss of temporal resolution as well, where the rapid changes in the speech waveform may be distorted or go undetected by the impaired auditory system (Humes, 1982). The loss of spectral and temporal resolving power as a form of internal distortion is present under quiet, ideal amplification conditions and probably is due to cochlear pathology in most cases. More information on this phenomenon can be found in Pickles (1988, chap. 10) and Sachs et al. (1988). Clients who have significant amounts of internal distortion are not likely to receive great benefit from hearing aids and will need aural rehabilitation to reach their full communication potential.

EFFECTS OF NOISE

The third component reflects the difficulty experienced by many hearing-impaired adults (and surprisingly by some people with normal thresholds as well) in separating speech from background noise. This component is often characterized as the S/N problem because the client's speech recognition ability is affected much more seriously by moderate levels of noise than is a normal-hearing individual. Whether the S/N component is truly independent of the loss of frequency resolution ability is debatable. The S/N difficulty may simply reflect the ear's broadened internal tuning curves' inability to reject the noise. However, the well-documented existence of clients whose speech recognition ability in quiet is near normal but deteriorates badly in noise argues strongly for the presence of a specific

S/N component to the individual's hearing loss. Further, many clients report difficulty only in noisy conditions and—for rehabilitation purposes—are most effectively treated as a distinct category of clients with an emphasis on assertive listening, binaural amplification, and speechreading. The prognosis for a pure S/N client depends largely on his or her ability to use these three remedial techniques. Plomp quantifies some aspects of this question in two helpful articles (1978, 1986).

The Practice of Adult Aural Rehabilitation

In the practice of aural rehabilitation for the adult, a hearing-impaired individual seeks help from a specialized professional for the communication breakdowns and emotional reactions caused by a loss of normal hearing function. Typical clients range in age from 20 to 70 years (older clients are discussed in Chapter 13) and have acquired their sensorineural hearing losses over a period of years. Losses may range from mild to severe. Many individuals wear hearing aids and may have been fitted just before enrolling in rehabilitation. This section focuses primarily on the rehabilitation of these representative clients.

THE ADULT AURAL REHABILITATION GROUP

This section describes the aural rehabilitation group as an important, almost essential, part of comprehensive adult rehabilitation. The information is based largely on groups that were formed at the University of South Carolina, although many clinics conduct their own version of the adult aural rehabilitation group (see Binnie and Hession [1990] for a good description of a similar group).

GROUP STRUCTURE

The ideal group involves four or five couples or families with one or both spouses having hearing loss. (One group had a grandmother with a hearing loss, her daughter, and her teenage grandson.) The clinician acts as group leader and facilitator, with two graduate students participating and eventually leading the group as part of their training. The aural rehabilitation group meetings are designed to include several types of experiences. First, the members share feelings, experiences, successes, and failures related to coping with their hearing loss and their spouse's hearing loss. Members actively help each other to identify and solve specific communication problems. Second, some structured therapeutic activities are conducted, such as speechreading, assertive listening practice and role-playing, learning to speak clearly to the hearing-impaired spouse, conversation repair, and situation analysis. Third, the group format allows the administration and discussion of self-administered inventories such as the Communication Profile for the Hearing Impaired (CPHI) (see Chapter 18 for information on other helpful instruments). Finally, each class has some time devoted to didactic information on various topics such as care of hearing aids, ALDs, and other consumer-related issues (Appendices 12.1 and 12.2).

FOUR ESSENTIAL COMPONENTS OF GROUP REHABILITATION

Throughout a series of six classes, it is stressed that there are four essential components to the members' rehabilitation. These primary components of efficient aural rehabilitation are:

1. Effective amplification. This includes properly fitted hearing aids and appropriate ALDs, with orientation and follow-up.
2. A-V integration. Here, the use of speechreading in combination with available auditory information through a variety of exercises is stressed. A handout (available in Appendix 12.3) is discussed and practiced.
3. Assertive listening. Assertive listening is also called situation control or assertiveness for the hearing impaired. It involves the use of assertive control of the com-

munication environment and interactive communication strategies.

4. Consumer awareness. Here, the client is guided through the acquisition of knowledge about hearing loss and the acceptance of responsibility for his or her rehabilitation and growth.

BENEFITS OF GROUP EXPERIENCE

The group situation allows several beneficial things to be experienced by the participating group members:

1. It produces the rapid gains in speechreading and A-V speech recognition that occur in the initial three or four sessions of practice (see "Can Speechreading Be Taught?", below, for a list of reasons why this improvement occurs).
2. It allows group members (hearing-impaired and spouses) to benefit from the group experience. These benefits include (a) sharing feelings of frustration, anger, disappointment, and so on; (b) receiving support and encouragement; (c) gaining perspective on one's situation ("My loss isn't as serious as I thought it was," or "I'm glad I don't have that spouse's problem"); and (d) being exposed to healthy, even inspirational, role models in the group who demonstrate strong, positive approaches to assertive listening and problem-solving in general.
3. It provides an emotionally safe situation in which people can admit their hearing losses and practice communication strategies and assertive behaviors before attempting them in the outside world. Admitting the presence of the hearing loss, we believe, is the single most effective preventive strategy for use in the real world.
4. It provides ongoing contact with an audiologist during the initial hearing aid adjustment period. Anecdotal evidence suggests that one primary reason people reject hearing aids is the cumulative effect of several small malfunctions and irritations coupled with unmet (and per-

haps unrealistic) expectations for hearing aid benefit. Both of these reasons are addressed effectively in the weekly group meetings.

A list of these benefits phrased as goals is used as a handout and discussion guide for the group and is available in Appendix 12.2.

In summary, it is clear that the group experience involves a great deal more than speechreading practice, although some of the members refer to it as their speechreading class. Finally, the authors are convinced that group participation is the most effective form of insurance that a new hearing aid user will continue to use the aid after it is purchased (Montgomery, 1991). It is unfortunate to limit contact with the client after hearing aid fitting and to thus cease rehabilitation with only the first of the four essential components completed.

CONVERSATION REPAIR

The topic of conversation repair has been mentioned previously. It represents an important skill that many hearing-impaired adults seem to lack and is an ideal activity for the aural rehabilitation group as well as for individual therapy. Conversation repair is a modern term for the interactive process that, ideally, follows a conversation breakdown of the type commonly experienced by hearing-impaired individuals. Several interesting studies and reviews have recently appeared that attest to the growing interest in this topic (Tye-Murray, 1994; Caissie and Gibson, 1997; Tye-Murray and Witt, 1997). Gagne and Wyllie (1989) showed that in speechreading, receiving a paraphrase or synonym after an error was more helpful than a repetition. In a similar study, Tye-Murray et al. (1990) indicated that each of five different strategies improved performance but that no one strategy was superior. Asking for a simple repetition, however, remains a popular strategy (Tye-Murray, 1991), although it is not necessarily effective. This is not surprising because as long ago as 1951, Miller et al. showed that simply repeating the controlled presentation of words that had been misunderstood in a list increased overall intelligibility by only a few percentage points. There must be some additional information to supplement the incomplete impression of the word created by the hearing loss. A pure repetition adds nothing to assist the client in the laboratory. However, repetition helps to the extent it does in real life because it buys the client time to think about the context and come up with a better guess, and because the talker often produces the repetition more slowly and loudly in isolation. That is, the repeated word or phrase is said in a different, more intelligible manner (see Picheny et al. [1985] for the substantial benefits of "clear" speech).

One of the most effective ways for the impaired listener to take advantage of the improved repetition of isolated words is to ask as specific a question as possible, rather than just saying, "What?" This latter approach elicits the whole sentence rather than only the single word, which may be all that was missed. Better would be, "You're going *where* on vacation?" than simply "Huh?" Better still, the impaired listener can verify a hunch, "Did you say *George* was there or *Joe*?" These skills can be practiced very effectively in the aural rehabilitation group by having the leader distort a word or phrase in a sentence, and the group members try to come up with the shortest, most specific question possible to elicit only the distorted part. This strategy does much to streamline the dialogue between normal-hearing and hearing-impaired persons. Other strategies such as asking for a synonym or a paraphrase produce much less predictable behavior from the talker and are not generally advisable. Actually, if the talker were willing to paraphrase for a hearing-impaired listener, he or she might be willing to speak in a controlled, clear manner that would eliminate much of the need for repair (Picheny et al., 1985)! (The reader is referred to Erber [1988, chap. 5] for information on training the talker.) Again, conversation repair, like all other interpersonal rehabilitative techniques, works best if the hearing person knows the listener has a hearing loss.

SIMPLE SOLUTIONS

The clinician's role in the group and in individual therapy and counseling is much like a detective, seeking to discover those elements that contribute to the client's communication difficulty. In many cases, ALD consideration and information revealed in the group and in individual/family counseling will indicate specific problems that can be reduced or eliminated with the clinician's knowledge and attention. Sometimes the client's life can be significantly improved (and the spouse's life as well) with simple changes in behavior or through an inexpensive ALD. For example, many couples, in which one or both members is hearing impaired, have fallen into an angry, confrontational reaction style when communication breakdown occurs. Because this may happen several times a day, major improvements in the quality of life can be achieved if better reactions to frustration can be found. It may be as simple as establishing rules for handling the common problem when one person is in another room and the other person calls to him or her: the "I can't hear you when I'm in the kitchen" problem. (The two-room situation is almost always doomed to failure because of (1) lack of speechreading, (2) weak or distorted acoustic signal, (3) interfering noise and resulting poor S/N, (4) poor room acoustics, and (5) lack of a common context or topic.) In the group, we lead the couples to analyze these (and other) reasons for difficulty and help them to come up with an agreed-on set of rules to handle the "kitchen" problem. A typical set might be as follows. Step 1—establish the communication channel: "Can you hear me, Mary?" If yes, proceed with the room-to-room communication; if no, say "I can't hear you, Fred." Step 2—the initiator of the conversation must move to the room where the recipient is, if necessary. We have found that if the group members come up with the rules themselves, with our guidance, they are much more likely to adopt them than if the group leader simply tells them how to handle the situation. Obviously, it is necessary for both spouses to be involved in the process of setting the rules or it does not become "their" solution.

Another example comes out of considering ALDs. A frequent problem involves setting the loudness on the TV audio signal when hearing-impaired and non–hearing-impaired adults watch TV. "Grandma wants the volume up so loud it drives me out of the room!" This is again an important problem because it occurs daily, and it is easily solved with the appropriate ALD. Grandma must be involved in the decision, however, and must help arrive at the solution or she will reject a heavy-handed imposition of the "newfangled headset" (Palmer, 1992).

These examples illustrate several principles: (1) it is most effective to attack the problems that occur often; (2) many communication problems are solved with changes in behavior or attitude, and this is best accomplished in the adult group with the spouses present; and (3) a surprising number of communication difficulties can be resolved quickly and easily once the situation has been analyzed and dialogue between the participants has been opened.

A CASE STUDY

The principles and practices discussed above are probably best illustrated in a case study of a typical adult hearing-impaired client.

During a problem-sharing session in the adult group, Mr. Jones, a 57-year-old man with a moderate high-frequency hearing loss, indicated that he had a recurring, frustrating situation that he was sure had no solution but he would share it anyway. The problem involved a group of six to eight businessmen who met once every 3 or 4 weeks as a dinner club for social conversation at a local restaurant. Mr. Jones reported having considerable difficulty hearing and following the various conversations. The men were all longtime friends, and some were in their 70s. After some questioning, the aural rehabilitation group came up with the following suggestions: (1) start eating earlier or later to avoid the most crowded time in the restaurant; (2) have all the men

learn sign language; (3) encourage Mr. Jones to improve his speechreading skills; (4) get the men to agree to give a verbal signal when a new person starts talking such as "Well . . . "; (5) purchase a personal FM system so that Mr. Jones can pass the microphone around as needed; (6) have Mr. Jones bring up the topic of his hearing loss for discussion among the men; (7) teach the men to announce changes of topics as they occur; (8) have the club ask for a better table (round, not long and rectangular, and away from the kitchen door); and (9) get the men to decide on the likely topics for the evening beforehand.

Obviously, many of the suggestions are impractical (the men are not going to become proficient in sign language), but all suggestions were written on the blackboard for the aural rehabilitation group to consider. The group encouraged Mr. Jones to at least bring up the topic with the men in the dining club and to analyze exactly which factors seem to cause the most difficulty. Mr. Jones reported 2 weeks later that he had brought up the fact of his hearing loss with the men and found, to his surprise, that two other members were also experiencing some difficulty. The club decided to start 30 minutes earlier and requested a better table, which the restaurant owner was happy to provide for his long-term customers. Mr. Jones also seated himself in a better position to speechread and hear the one man he had the most difficulty understanding. Most importantly, Mr. Jones felt much freer than before to ask for clarification, now that the club members knew he had a hearing loss. Finally, by the time of the next club meeting, Mr. Jones had improved his viewing and attending strategies considerably and was able to accommodate more audiovisual integration than previously. He reported having an enjoyable, relaxing experience for the first time, and the aural rehabilitation group applauded him.

Mr. Jones's success illustrates several things: the power of peer pressure in the group to change behavior; the value of assertive listening, starting with admitting that the hearing loss exists; the generally accommodating nature of talkers once they are aware of the listener's difficulty; and the value of analyzing the situation to determine the specific factors that are interfering with communication.

Individual Aural Rehabilitation

Traditionally, aural rehabilitation has focused on lipreading (or speechreading, a more comprehensive term), auditory training, and hearing aid orientation. Much of the therapeutic activity was conducted in individual training sessions, which sometimes extended over weeks or months.

Although the long-term individual-session paradigm may not be cost-effective in the future, many of the techniques can be adapted to a short-term or self-administered therapy format. In this section, unisensory speechreading and auditory training are considered, and circumstances when uni-sensory training may be helpful are discussed. A variety of other clinical activities are then considered briefly and placed in a framework where the client may work to make maximum achievement either individually or in a group setting.

Individual aural rehabilitation takes place under several circumstances. First, much of a rehability nature occurs naturally between audiologist and hearing aid client during the selection and follow-up stages, especially if a formal hearing aid orientation is included. The orientation typically includes information on how the aid works and how to troubleshoot and maintain it. Much time is spent encouraging the client to have realistically low expectations for performance in real-world conditions, and the client may be exposed to noise or taken outside to the street. Also, speechreading and the existence of self-help groups like Self-Help for the Hard-of-Hearing (SHHH) may be mentioned. Second, a client may be scheduled for one-on-one therapy sessions at a university clinic or rehabilitation facility to allow more intensive or long-term exposure to auditory or visual stimuli or for counseling on personal adjustment problems. Finally, a variety of audiovisual materials, such as videocassettes or disks, are available from libraries or other agencies for self-paced practice in speechreading at home or in the clinic (Tye-Murray, 1992).

SPEECHREADING

There is no doubt that speechreading is of vital importance to almost every hearing-impaired person. The crucial questions, however, are whether speechreading can be taught and what is the best way to do it.

Can speechreading be taught?

Several studies indicate that speechreading can be improved with individual, concentrated training (Walden et al., 1977, 1981a), and that most of the improvement comes during the first few hours of therapy. On the other hand, there is a general feeling that adults with acquired hearing losses do not show much improvement beyond some predetermined individual limit (DeFilippo, 1990). These seemingly contradictory observations can be easily reconciled, however.

It seems likely that there are indeed limits to the sensory process—at least in the visual system, although their nature is not clear (Shepherd et al., 1977; Samar and Sims, 1983)—and thus a limit to performance (Gagne, 1994). The gains in speechreading performance with short-term training, then, come from learning to attend and watch effectively, from a willingness to guess (Van Tassel and Hawkins, 1981; Lyxel and Ronnberg, 1987), from increased confidence, and probably from learning the test procedures. If this explanation is correct, it has clinical implications. It means that the improvement is based on important skills (apart from learning the test procedures) that provide more and better visual speech input and a higher probability that the correct word will be included in the ambiguous set of alternatives. These skills could well translate into better speechreading in the real world, and they should be the focus of speechreading instruction. For prognostic purposes, a client with poor viewing habits and restricted guessing should be able to improve considerably in speechreading performance, whereas a person who attends well and guesses well probably has low potential for further progress. A good review of speechreading and whether it can be taught can be found in Arnold (1997).

Speechreading is in no way a substitute for audition. Unfortunately, it is impossible to speechread a conversation without some sound included. This is because many of the phonemes (speech sounds) have little or no visible manifestation. They simply do not appear in the anterior part of the talker's mouth. It is sometimes said that another reason speechreading is so difficult is that the phonemes appear so rapidly that the eye cannot follow the movements. This explanation is incorrect. It is a very "eye-opening" experience to watch a videotape of conversational speech in slow motion and count the number of actual visible movements. As few as one or two per second may be seen for some talkers. The problem is that there are too few visible aspects of speech, not too many! Another difficulty, of course, is that many of the movements look alike. Thus the "s" in "I knew Sue" looks very similar to the "sh" in "a new shoe." The rounded vowel context obscures any natural differences that might exist between "s" and "sh." It is often pointed out that phonemes like "p," "b," and "m" look alike and thus constitute a single visible element, a viseme. This concept unfortunately is confined to sounds occurring in isolation or with open vowels, like "ba," and does not relate well to sounds in more complex contexts like the "s"/"sh" example above (Montgomery et al., 1987). The viseme concept is of limited value in clinical practice in which the emphasis is properly on words and sentences. (Incidentally, the ideal clinical material, in our experience, is the prepositional phrase. A list of prepositional phrases can be generated over the years and is good for several graded speechreading lessons.) Good references for further reading are Massaro (1987, 1998), Montgomery and Demorest (1988), and Campbell et al. (1998).

Analytic and synthetic approaches

The use of simple materials like isolated sounds, consonant-vowel (CV) syllables ("da" or "sa," and so on), or single words may be necessary for some speech-readers who need to gain experience with short-duration clear stimuli. The goal is to move to longer, more realistic stimuli as the client's skill and attention span permit. This approach is called the analytic method because the speech is analyzed into its component parts. This method has been used frequently because it is simple and highly structured. The alternative is the synthetic method, which uses phrases, sentences, and real-life situations as therapeutic material to encourage the client to bring together (synthesize) speech elements into larger units of meaning. Jeffers and Barley (1971) have produced speechreading materials and teaching methods of both types. Many people now believe that speechreading is best taught with some voice added so that the difficulty of the task can be controlled. That is, the client's performance level can be varied from near zero (no voice) to good understanding (strong voice) to suit the client's needs for success and challenge (DeFilippo, 1990).

AUDITORY TRAINING

Much of what has been presented above on speechreading has a direct analogue in auditory training. Analytic approaches are often used to help the client make finer auditory discriminations such as comparing "ba" with "va" (without speechreading, of course) or "sa" and "fa." More severely impaired individuals may benefit from even grosser distinctions, including presence or absence of sound, long or short words, and one or two syllables. Sometimes noise is added to make the task more difficult or more realistic.

It is our experience that the more severely impaired clients benefit from pure auditory training, especially when experiencing amplification for the first time, but that listening in noise is rarely indicated. The trend seems to be toward providing combined

A-V training rather than either sensory channel in isolation. The reader is referred to Garstecki (1981) and Houston and Montgomery (1997) for descriptions of practical ways to perform A-V integration, and to Gagne (1994) for a discussion of clinical issues in A-V speech perception.

Brief Adult Aural Rehabilitation

In the preceding section, a framework for conducting extended versions of both group and individual aural rehabilitation was presented. This represents an almost ideal situation in which professional time and client motivation are abundant. Unfortunately, this is rare in the typical audiologist's practice. Instead, time constraints and reimbursement issues dictate that very little effort is devoted to rehabilitation beyond providing amplification and some orientation to hearing aid care. Thus, there is a gap in the level of professional involvement between extensive and minimal contact with the client after hearing aid fitting.

Brief aural rehabilitation is designed to fill this gap by giving audiologists and speech pathologists the tools—goals, topics, and techniques— to provide a brief exposure of the essentials of aural rehabilitation to the client. Brief aural rehabilitation is based on the belief that adult hearing-aid wearers can benefit from adopting simple strategies that allow them to interact effectively in their day-to-day listening/communicating experiences. Such strategies represent changes in behavior that, with practice, become habitual approaches and reactions to difficult communication situations. It is important to focus on those behaviors that can be changed and adopted and not spend time on long-standing cognitive deficits or attitudes. This issue was addressed above, when a distinction was made between emotional and cognitive characteristics of the client (difficult to change) and speechreading practices and conversational behavior (easier to change).

This version of brief aural rehabilitation, then, is designed to introduce the client to five important aspects of aural rehabilitation in approximately 1 hour. The activities selected are speechreading, adopting clarification strategies, admitting the hearing loss, controlling the conversational situation, and acquiring consumer education. This program has been described in more detail (see Montgomery, 1994b), and a description of the five activities has been reprinted in Appendix 12.4 under the acronym WATCH.

Summary—Aural Rehabilitation

This section presented a variety of clinical aspects of the practice of aural rehabilitation. It can be seen that the goal of aural rehabilitation for the adult is ambitious— to increase the likelihood, the level, of successful communication over the client's lifetime. This is accomplished through giving him or her the skills and the hardware to understand and control the process of communication. All elements of verbal communication are shown to be in the client's domain of influence—the talker, the message, the auditory and visual channels, and the impaired listener himself, whose emotional reactions, cognitive processes, and interactive strategies are tailored to prevent, minimize, and repair communication breakdown.

Because of its potential to help individuals and society, aural rehabilitation offers an excellent opportunity for audiologists and speech pathologists who choose to practice this exciting specialty. Some excellent texts are available for further reading (Erber, 1988, 1998; Schow and Nerbonne, 1995; Hull, 1997; Tye-Murray, 1998; Wayner and Abrahamson, 1998).

Tinnitus

This section considers tinnitus, which audiologists might call the "other" major auditory problem. It is difficult to test and rehabilitate, but it is hoped that this discussion will encourage audiologists to explore it further.

Tinnitus is the sensation of sound in the absence of actual external physical sound. The perception of sound may come from one of two general sources. First, it may be objective tinnitus, which is the result of the presence of physical sound arising internally. Sources for this include blood rush-ing in constricted carotid arteries, low-pitch rumbling from continual contraction of the middle ear muscles, and clicks for the release of air through the eustachian tubes. Objective tinnitus is uncommon in the audiology practice and is appropriately referred for medical or surgical treatment. Our focus is subjective, idiopathic tinnitus, which is the sensation of sound in the absence of physical sound and is of unknown origin. It arises spontaneously, either from peripheral or central sources, and accompanies sensorineural hearing loss. It may take many forms, from broad-band or narrow-band noise to pure-tones and tone complexes with a predominant pitch (Penner, 1995). It is by far the most common form of tinnitus and is responsible for the high incidence of tinnitus. In the United States, it is estimated that 36 million adults have tinnitus, with 7.2 million of them showing a severe, disabling form (Shulman, 1991, Chapter 11). This section provides some introductory information about this interesting and frustrating disor-der and encourages audiologists to consider seeking further knowledge and including treatment in their practices at one of three levels of involvement.

RATIONALE

Why have we included tinnitus in a chapter on adult aural rehabilitation? There are several reasons:

1. It is a common, frequently serious, disorder of the auditory system.
2. Audiologists are often the health care professionals who see it first.
3. Often, no other hearing health professional will even consider tinnitus beyond counseling the client to "learn to live with it."
4. Rehabilitative audiologists may wish to perform tinnitus rehabilitation at varying levels of involvement.
5. At the very least, audiologists should actively be on the lookout for tinnitus in their practices and (1) be informed about making appropriate referrals and (2)

consider tinnitus-masking (which hearing aids often produce) as a factor in their hearing aid evaluation (HAE) protocol and fitting decisions.
6. There are some recent improvements in tinnitus rehabilitation that offer guarded optimism, and audiologists are remiss if they do not inform the serious tinnitus sufferer about them.

This section begins by illustrating some of the strange and seemingly inexplicable characteristics of tinnitus with a personal narrative and discussion of the type of tinnitus likely to be seen by the audiologist. Diagnosis and treatment are then considered, with a focus on some of the newer, more successful approaches to treatment. Following that, several levels of involvement in tinnitus treatment that audiologists might wish to consider are discussed. Finally, some of the excellent sources of information on tinnitus that have recently appeared are mentioned.

PERSONAL NARRATIVE

A personal narrative by one of the authors (A. Montgomery) illustrates some of the unusual characteristics of tinnitus:

I am sitting in a chair in my quiet living room listening to my tinnitus. It is a semi-pure tone with a frequency of approximately 5700 Hz in my right ear. It is matched in loudness to a tone in the left ear with a sensation level (SL) of about 5–6 dB. It is relatively constant over a period of hours although it is more noticeable during stress or fatigue. Its frequency is located on the audiogram approximately half way down my mild/moderate high frequency hearing loss in the right ear. I can easily mask it with an external tone at 10 dB SL at 4000 Hz. But I can also mask it with a 500-Hz tone at 10 dB SL! In fact, it is masked by almost any frequency or noise at a very low sensation level in the right ear. It is even masked by moderate level sounds in the left ear. The masking effect remains for a few seconds after the masker is turned off; that is, it exhibits residual inhibition.

In this mild form, it causes no distress but conveniently exhibits many of the characteristics of more severe tinnitus: it is subjective and idiopathic, arising spontaneously from no external cause; it shows strange, noncochlear masking patterns; it is associated with sensorineural hearing loss; and it varies somewhat with stress and fatigue. Tinnitus is said to be "paradoxically" loud— in this case it certainly seems louder than the 5 dB SL would suggest. (A study of moderate to severe tinnitus showed, amazingly, that 88% of patients matched their tinnitus to SLs of 11 dB or less [Vernon, 1998].)

DIAGNOSIS AND TREATMENT

It seems clear that there is no one simple treatment for tinnitus, partly because there is not a single entity with a single etiology. Instead, there are many types of tinnitus— Shulman (1991) lists 11 types—and diagnosis and treatment are complicated. We believe that one reason for the complications and frustrations is that in many cases the tinnitus does not arise solely from the cochlea. By default it arises centrally in many cases, in our opinion, although the processes are unknown (see Miyamoto et al. [1997] for more evidence of central involvement).

IS TINNITUS PERIPHERAL OR CENTRAL?

There are several reasons why we think that much of the tinnitus seen by audiologists is central in origin:

1. The masking is seen at many frequencies and sometimes even contralaterally. That is, the masking often exhibits a completely noncochlear pattern, much more like the patterns associated with central masking (Feldmann, 1971, 1981).
2. Completely severing the VIIIth nerve does not stop tinnitus in 50% of cases and may make it worse (House and Brackman, 1981).
3. Profoundly deaf people frequently have tinnitus.
4. Central-acting antidepressants and psychotropic drugs sometimes relieve tinnitus.
5. Receiving a cochlear implant (bypassing and/or destroying the cochlea) does not

necessarily stop tinnitus. The percentage of people who do benefit is similar to the number of people whose tinnitus is reduced by using a hearing aid (Ito and Sakakihara, 1998).

The picture is not as clear as it might seem, however, because several forms of tinnitus are at least initially peripheral in origin: spontaneous otoacoustic emissions, tinnitus associated with Ménière's syndrome, tinnitus cased by aspirin and noise exposure, etc.. Many people believe that peripheral (cochlear) tinnitus becomes central over time, so a mixed etiology—peripheral and central—is probably closer to the truth (see Shulman [1991] for a detailed description of possible etiologies).

As might be expected, a subjective symptom that varies greatly across people and whose origin is unknown is very difficult to treat. A variety of medical and surgical treatments (including cutting the auditory nerve!) have been tried. The results are complicated and confusing at best, but no one treatment seems to be successful (a review of current treatment approaches is found in Vernon [1998]).

The one approach that seems to offer relief to most patients, at least in the mild and moderate category, is to supply external masking either in the form of a tinnitus masker or, more frequently, through wearing a hearing aid. Many clients report that their tinnitus is reduced or absent when they are wearing their hearing aids. For example, Surr et al. (1985) found that of 200 new hearing aid users, 62% reported tinnitus; of these, 50% found that the aids produced partial or total relief from tinnitus. Thus, the audiologist is in a position to supply significant benefit to tinnitus sufferers. Indeed, substantial relief from tinnitus should be one criterion for hearing aid fitting, especially in the case of milder, "borderline" hearing losses.

COGNITIVE THERAPY

In many clients, tinnitus is made worse by the client's reaction (overreaction) to it.

The reactions take the form of a cognitive interpretation and an emotional reaction ("I'm going crazy," "I have a brain tumor," "I'll be stuck with this all my life," "It's making me lose my hearing," etc.), which understandably triggers greater distress and frustrations. This may account for some of the paradoxic loudness of tinnitus. Consider an analogy. You are lying in bed alone and about to go to sleep. You hear a creak in the floor in the hallway caused by the house cooling down at night. Do you rationally think, "Oh, that's the house cooling down?" No, you react, "Oh no, what was that?!" When the second creak comes, your heart starts pounding. Your interpretation is cognitive, "There's a stranger in the hallway with a gun. I'll be killed!" The sensation level of the creak might have been 8 dB, but your cognitive reaction to it makes it loud emotionally. So it may be with tinnitus in some cases. Hence, there is the possibility that some simple information and reassurance could help the client to eliminate the cognitive/emotional aspects of the problem. In more serious cases, cognitive therapy may help. A good example is the use of cognitive therapy by Hallam (1994) to reduce the distress caused by reactions to tinnitus (see Wayner [1998] for more information).

TINNITUS LOG

One of the simplest pieces of advice that a hearing-health professional can give to a client with tinnitus is to start a daily tinnitus log. The client is to rate his or her tinnitus three times a day (morning, after work, bedtime). The ratings are to include mood, level of stress felt, tinnitus loudness, and tinnitus annoyance as well as comments on changes in the pitch or nature of the tinnitus if these occur. The ratings each should be based on a three- to five-point scale that can be numbers or adjectives (for example, soft/unnoticeable, moderate, or loud, for the loudness scale, or 1 = unnoticeable, 5 = distressingly loud). The client is to make the ratings every day at the time indicated. The times are selected so that the log can be kept at home. It is especially important to make the stress level ratings and the mood ratings, because stress and depression are frequently associated with making tinnitus worse. After 3 to 4 weeks, the log can be discussed with the client and any patterns noted. Then, if the client is interested, some brief "experiments with an N of one" can be performed. The purpose is to see whether specific dietary or lifestyle factors are involved in exacerbating tinnitus. The possible culprits include caffeine, alcohol, chocolate, and perhaps smoking (Shulman, 1991). The client selects one of these to eliminate from his or her diet (caffeine should be phased out slowly to avoid caffeine-withdrawal headaches), and any effects on tinnitus are noted over a 3-week period. Then another dietary factor can be eliminated (only one at a time), etc. Frankly, this elimination process does not usually result in any startling insights or cures. Nevertheless, in some cases, dietary factors do contribute to tinnitus and can be eliminated. More important, usually, is the knowledge gained about stress and mood, and appropriate referrals can be made. In any event, the log offers an easy way to monitor the tinnitus over time and may result in meaningful clinical information. A more complete description of this can be found in Vernon (1998).

Another encouraging approach related to masking has been developed by Jastreboff and Hazell (1998). In this approach, the tinnitus patient is habituated to (becomes more tolerant/less aware of) the tinnitus through carefully controlled levels of sound that partially mask the tinnitus.

AUDIOLOGIST'S ROLE IN TREATING TINNITUS

It is clear that tinnitus is a common and distressing auditory disorder often associated with sensorineural hearing loss. Audiologists are a natural professional contact for persons with tinnitus. What role, then, should the audiologist play with the client who reports tinnitus? Several roles are possible, depending on the audiologist's equipment, confidence, knowledge, and type of practice.

Level 1: General practice (diagnostic audiology and hearing aid dispensing)

Services: Inquires about tinnitus; encourages American Tinnitus Association membership, makes referrals

Level 2: General practice (same as level 1)

Services: Level 1 services plus offers brief counseling and suggests the personal tinnitus log book; accepts some ongoing responsibility for the client

Level 3: Specialized tinnitus practice within general practice with equipment to perform tinnitus description (loudness and pitch-matching and masking evaluation) as well as auditory brainstem response audiometry

Services: Performs tinnitus description; accepts primary or secondary responsibility for client; has well-established local or regional two-way referral channels to otologists, psychiatrist/psychologists who treat tinnitus patients. Vernon (1987) describes in detail the assessment of the client's tinnitus and also includes a thorough questionnaire.

Several excellent texts and other resources have appeared in the past few years that serve as an introduction and resource for understanding tinnitus. In increasingly technical level they are: Vernon, 1998; Hallam, 1994; Bentler and Tyler, 1987; Doyle et al., 1987; Stephens et al., 1986; Hazell, 1987; Kitahara, 1988; Vernon and Moller, 1994; Shulman, 1991. The American Tinnitus Association (PO Box 5, Portland, OR 97207) is the national consumer organization for tinnitus sufferers (analogous to SHHH for hearing-impaired adults) and produces a good journal. In addition, a good professional journal, *The International Tinnitus Journal,* is available. You can visit the journal's website at www.tinnitus.com.

Summary—Tinnitus

In this final section, a brief introduction to the fascinating topic of tinnitus was provided. It is a complex and little understood phenomenon but one that is extremely common in clinical audiology. It is hoped that clinical audiologists will (1) be interested in acquiring more knowledge about tinnitus, (2) incorporate concerted inquiries and questionnaires about it in their routine clinical protocol, and (3) consider higher levels of involvement in tinnitus treatment in their practices.

Acknowledgments

This chapter is dedicated to the memory of Carl Binnie, an excellent rehabilitative audiologist, influential clinician, and exceptionally nice guy.

REFERENCES

Arnold P. The structure and optimization of speechreading. J Deaf Stud Deaf Educ 1977;2:200–211.

Bentler RA, Tyler RS. Tinnitus management. ASHA 1987; 20:27–32.

Binnie CA, Hession CM. A four-week communication training program. ADA Feedback 1990;Winter:37–41.

Caissie R, Gibson CL. The effectiveness of repair strategies used by people with hearing losses and their conversational partners. Volta Rev 1997;99:203–218.

Campbell R, Dodd BJ, Burnham D. Hearing by eye: the psychology of speechreading and auditory-visual speech. Bristol, PA: Taylor & Francis, 1998.

Doyle PJ, Pijl S, Doyle I, et al. Management of tinnitus: a practical approach. J Otolaryngol 1987;16:127–132.

DeFilippo CL. Speechreading training: believe it or not! ASHA 1990;32:46–48.

Erber N. Communication therapy for adults with sensory loss. San Diego: Singular, 1998.

Erber NP. Communication therapy for hearing-impaired adults. Abbotsford, Victoria, Australia: Clavis Press, 1988.

Feldmann H. Homolateral and contralateral masking of tinnitus by noise-bands and by pure tones. Audiology 1971; 10:138–144.

Feldmann H. Homolateral and contralateral masking of tinnitus. In: Shuman A, ed. Proceedings of the First International Tinnitus Seminar. J Laryngol Otolaryngol 1981;4 (Suppl):60–70.

Gagne JP. Visual and audiovisual speech perception training: basic and applied research. In: Gagne JP, Tye-Murray N, eds. Research in audiological rehabilitation: current trends and future directions. J Acad Rehabil Audiol 1994;27(Monogr):317–336.

Gagne JP, Wyllie KA. Relative effectiveness of three repair strategies on the visual-identification of misperceived words. Ear Hear 1989;10:368–374.

Garstecki DC. Audio-visual training paradigm for hearing impaired adults. J Acad Rehabil Audiol 1981;14:223–228.

Hallam RS. Living with tinnitus: dealing with the ringing in your ears. San Francisco: Thorsons, 1994.

Hazell JWP. Tinnitus. New York: Churchill Livingstone, 1987.

Herer GR. Inventing our future. ASHA 1989;31:35–37.

House JW, Brackman DE. Tinnitus: surgical management.

In: Tinnitus. CIBA Foundation symposium 85. London: Pittman Medical, 1981:204–216.

Houston KT, Montgomery AA. Auditory-visual integration: a practical approach. Semin Hear 1997;18:141–151.

Ito J, Sakakihara J. Suppression of tinnitus by cochlear implant. In: Vernon J, ed. Tinnitus: treatment and relief. Needham Heights, MA: Allyn and Bacon, 1998.

Jastreboff PJ, Hazell JWP. Treatment of tinnitus based on a neurophysiological model. In: Vernon J, ed. Tinnitus: treatment and relief. Needham Heights, MA: Allyn and Bacon, 1998.

Jeffers J, Barley M. Speechreading (lipreading). Springfield, IL: C.C. Thomas, 1971.

Kitahara M, ed. Tinnitus: pathophysiology and management. Tokyo: Igaku-Shoin, 1988.

Lyxell B, Ronnberg J. Guessing and speechreading. Br J Audiol 1987;21:13–20.

Massaro D. Perceiving talking faces. Cambridge: MIT Press, 1998.

Massaro DW. Speech perception by ear and eye—a paradigm for psychological inquiry. Hillsdale, NJ: Lawrence Erlbaum, 1987.

Miller GA, Heise GA, Lichten W. The intelligibility of speech as a function of the contrast of the test materials. J Exp Psychol 1951;41:329–375.

Miyamoto R, Wynne MK, McKnight C, et al. Electrical suppression of tinnitus via cochlear implants. Int Tinnitus J 1997;3:35–38.

Montgomery AA. Aural rehabilitation: review and preview. In: Studebaker G, Bess F, Beck L, eds. The Vanderbilt hearing aid report II. Parkton, MD: York, 1991.

Montgomery AA. Treatment efficacy in adult audiological rehabilitation. J Acad Rehabil Audiol Monogr Suppl 1994a;27:317–336.

Montgomery AA. WATCH: a practical approach to brief auditory rehabilitation. Hear J 1994b;47:10,53–55.

Montgomery AA, Demorest M. Issues and developments in the evaluation of speechreading. In: Sims D, DeFilippo C, eds. New dimensions in speechreading. Volta Rev Monogr 1988;90:193–214.

Montgomery AA, Walden BE, Prosek RA. Effects of consonantal context on vowel speechreading. J Speech Hear Res 1987;30:50–59.

NAD is test site for video relay interpreting. NAD Broadcaster 1999;Feb;21.

Palmer CV. Assistive devices in the audiology practice. Am J Audiol 1992;1:37–57.

Penner MJ. Tinnitus synthesis: fluctuant and stable matches to the pitch of tinnitus. Int Tinnitus J 1995;1:79–84.

Picheny MA, Durlach NI, Braida LD. Speaking clearly for the hard-of-hearing: intelligibility differences between clear and conversational speech. J Speech Hear Res 1985;28:96–103.

Pickles JO. An introduction to the physiology of hearing. 2nd ed. London: Academic Press, 1988.

Plomp R. Auditory handicap of hearing impairment and the limited benefit of hearing aids. J Acoust Soc Am 1978;63:533–549.

Plomp R. A signal-to-noise ratio model for the speech reception threshold of the hearing impaired. J Speech Hear Res 1986;29:146–154.

Sachs MB, Winslow RL, Blackburn CC. Representation of speech in the auditory periphery. In: Edelman G, Gall E, Cowan M, eds. Auditory function: neurobiological bases of hearing. New York: John Wiley & Sons, 1988.

Samar V, Sims D. Visual evoked-response correlates of speechreading performance in normal hearing adults: a replication and factor analytic extension. J Speech Hear Res 1983;26:2–9.

Schow RL, Nerbonne MA. Introduction to audiologic rehabilitation. 3rd ed. Needham Heights, MA: Allyn & Bacon, 1995.

Serrano-Navaro M, Arana M, Cram JE. HOLA: a new trend in aural rehabilitation. Paper presented at the Academy of Rehabilitative Audiology, Summer Institute, Breckenridge, Colorado, June 1991.

Shepherd D, DeLavergne R, Frueh F, et al. Visual-neural correlate of speechreading ability in normal-hearing adults. J Speech Hear Res 1977;20:752–765.

Shulman A, ed. Tinnitus: diagnosis/treatment. Philadelphia: Lea & Febiger, 1991.

Smith MC. Neurophysiology of aging. Semin Neurol 1989;9:64–77.

Stephens SD, Hallam RS, Jakes SC. Tinnitus: a management model. Clin Otolaryngol 1986;11:227–238.

Surr RK, Montgomery AA, Mueller HG. Effect of amplification on tinnitus among new hearing aid users. Ear Hear 1985;6:71–75.

Tye-Murray N. Repair strategy usage by hearing-impaired adults and changes following communication therapy. J Speech Hear Res 1991;34:921–928.

Tye-Murray N. Laser videodisc technology in the aural rehabilitation setting: good news for people with severe and profound impairments. Am J Audiol 1992;1:33–36.

Tye-Murray N. Communication breakdown in conversations: adult-initiated repair strategies. In: Tye-Murray N, ed. Let's converse: a "how-to" guide to develop and expand conversational skills of children and teenagers who are hearing impaired. Washington, DC: Alexander Graham Bell Association for the Deaf, 1994:85–121.

Tye-Murray N. Foundations of aural rehabilitation: children, adults, and their family members. San Diego: Singular, 1998.

Tye-Murray N, Witt S. Communication strategies training. Semin Hear 1997;18:153–165.

Tye-Murray N, Purdy S, Woodworth G, et al. The effect of repair strategies on the visual identification of sentences. J Speech Hear Disord 1990;55:621–627.

Van Tassel DJ, Hawkins DB. Effects of guessing strategy on speechreading test scores. Am Ann Deaf 1981;126:840–844.

Vernon JA. Assessment of the tinnitus patient. In: Hazell JWP, ed. Tinnitus. New York: Churchill Livingstone, 1987.

Vernon JA, ed. Tinnitus: treatment and relief. Needham Heights, MA: Allyn and Bacon, 1998.

Vernon JA, Moller A, eds. Mechanisms of tinnitus. Needham Heights, MA: Allyn and Bacon, 1994.

Walden BE, Prosek RA, Montgomery AA, et al. Effects of training on the visual recognition of consonants. J Speech Hear Res 1977;20:130–145.

Walden BE, Erdman SA, Montgomery AA, et al. Some effects of training on speech recognition by hearing-impaired adults. J Speech Hear Res 1981a;24:207–216.

Walden BE, Schwartz DM, Montgomery AA, et al. A comparison of the effects of hearing impairment and acoustic filtering. J Speech Hear Res 1981b;24:32–43.

Wayner DS. Cognitive therapy and tinnitus: an intensive weekend workshop. In: Vernon J, ed. Tinnitus: treatment and relief. Needham Heights, MA: Allyn and Bacon, 1998.

Wayner D, Abrahamson J. Learning to hear again: an audiologic rehabilitation curriculum guide. Austin, TX: Hear Again, 1998.

APPENDIX 12.1   *Adult Aural Rehabilitation Group Outline*[a]

Session one

1. Introductions, orientation
2. Discussion of what to expect from the group, what situations are difficult; development of list of individual problem areas
3. Presentation of information on hearing and causes of hearing loss

HANDOUTS: Notebooks, diagrams of the ear, list of purposes of the group
OUTSIDE WORK: Begin list of difficult situations

Session two

1. Discussion of difficult situations, introduction of Communication Profile for the Hearing Impaired (CPHI)
2. Presentation of information on the audiogram
3. Performance of brief speechreading test, discussion of speechreading

OUTSIDE WORK: Start on CPHI, speechreading assignment

Session three

1. Discussion of CPHI, discussion of speechreading assignment
2. Demonstration, pep talk on maximizing the chances for speechreading
3. Presentation of information on hearing aids

OUTSIDE WORK: Assertive speechreading assignment

Session four

1. CPHI inventory due
2. Discussion of speechreading assignment, situation analysis
3. Videotape demonstration
4. More information on hearing aids

OUTSIDE WORK: Analyze two situations that you encounter in everyday living

Session five

1. Conversation repair, demonstration and practice
2. Discussion of CPHI inventory results, individual counseling
3. Presentation of information and demonstration of assistive listening devices

HANDOUT: List of assistive listening devices and addresses of suppliers
SUGGESTION: Attend a concert at the Koger Center; use their excellent infrared listening system

Session six

1. Review of specific strategies for difficult listening situations
2. speechreading practice, situation management
3. Course evaluation: "Y'all tell us what you think"
4. Wrap-up

---

[a]Outline handed out to members of adult aural rehabilitation group. This group meets for 2 hours each week for 6 weeks.

APPENDIX 12.2 *Specific Goals and Purposes for the Class*[b]

---

1. To get together and share and discuss problems with other hearing-impaired individuals and couples.
2. To provide a place to practice new communication skills before trying them in the "real world."
3. To gain information and understanding about hearing loss and to have the opportunity to ask questions about your specific situation.
4. To provide a place where you do not have to hide your hearing loss.
5. To give you the opportunity to analyze and practice the art of conversation and conversation "repair."
6. To provide a chance for your spouse/friend/caregiver to gain understanding of your hearing difficulties and learn how to communicate more effectively with you (and you with them).
7. To gain knowledge about new technology in hearing aids and assistive listening devices.

---

[b]Handout for members of adult aural rehabilitation group.

APPENDIX 12.3 *Ways to Maximize Your Chances of Speechreading in Combination With Your Hearing Aid*[c]

---

1. Indicate to the talker in some way that you are hearing impaired.
2. Adjust the communication situation so that noise sources are nearer the talker than to you (all's fair in speechreading). Reduce noise as much as possible.
3. Look around and become familiar with the situation so that you will know what the talkers are referring to.
4. Watch the talker's lips, not his or her eyes. Look around only during pauses (there are plenty of them) and changes of talkers. You can see facial expressions and eye movements without leaving the lips.
5. Adjust the situation so that the light is on the talker's face and not yours. Avoid glare and backlighting that obscure the talker's face or cause you to squint or strain to see.
6. Arrive early for situations that are more formal or structured, such as meetings, religious services, classes, or any place where people will be seated, so that you can stake out the best spot. Do not be afraid to move if you made a mistake or if the structure of the group changes. If there is one primary talker, sit so that you can see him or her without strain. Talk to the organizers beforehand about seating, amplifiers, and so on.
7. Learn to relax, even in tough listening situations. Avoid tension—keep your shoulders down, do not wrinkle your forehead, and so on (one version of this list said, "Work hard at relaxing"; that is not what we mean!).
8. Concentrate on phrases and ideas rather than trying to pick out single words.
9. Make an effort to stay current on recent events, news, sports, and so on. The more you know about likely topics of conversation, the better off you are.
10. Interact with the talker or group to clarify or verify the message when you miss something.
11. Do not wait until you are lost and three sentences behind.

---

[c]Handout for members of adult aural rehabilitation group.

APPENDIX *A Guide to Brief Aural Rehabilitation:*
12.4 *The WATCH Procedure*[d]

W—Watch the Talker's Mouth, Not His Eyes
This serves to introduce the best known, but sometimes least well practiced, of all aural rehabilitation skills—lipreading. Tell your patient that he or she must watch the talker's lips at all times during communication, taking only brief glances around to find the topic of conversation, if necessary. Notice that the emphasis is on the talker's lips. The patient is not to maintain eye contact with the talker.

This usually takes some practice. After introducing the topic, ask your patient to watch your lips (not eyes) as you talk. At some point, get up and walk around the room while talking to see if the patient's eyes follow your movements. If the patient's eyesight appears to be poor, a referral to a vision care specialist may be in order.

Suggest that your patient practice lipreading at home, for example, by turning down (but not off) the volume on the televised evening news and concentrating on the talker's lips for 30 seconds at a stretch. Spend at least 10 minutes on this important topic, being sure to make to patient practice lipreading as well as hearing you talk about its value. Lipreading is the best "noise fighter" available to the patient. Good lipreading skills can increase a person's speech comprehension as much as a 10-dB to 12-dB improvement in the signal-to-noise ratio. That's more than any other technique, except turning off the noise (see below).

A—Ask Specific Questions
Here I suggest to patients that the best way to get clarification of something they missed the first time is to ask as specific a question as possible, instead of saying "Huh?" or "What?" or simply pretending to understand. Here's an example. Suppose a patient heard the sentence, "My wife and I are planning on going to visit my aunt in XXX this fall." With XXX representing the word that he missed. The best response is to ask, "Where does she live?" rather than "What?" which makes the talker repeat the whole sentence and quickly becomes irritating.

Motivated patients usually acquire this skill easily, but some find it hard to abandon the "Huh?" habit. Again, some practice in your office will be helpful in instilling this strategy. You can speak in a low voice if necessary, or even slur or omit an important word on purpose to force the patient to ask you a specific question.

T—Talk About Your Hearing Loss
This brings up the first sensitive topic. In this section of brief aural rehabilitation, we ask the patient to recognize the necessity of frequently mentioning ("admitting") his hearing loss. The purchase of new hearing aids provides an excellent opportunity for a patient to start talking about the hearing loss with friends and family. However, you may find this topic difficult to discuss if you have just sold the patient the smallest available ITC aid, which is designed to be as inconspicuous as possible! Because of this inherent conflict, let me explain why it is so important that the person with impaired hearing be able to mention it to his or her communication partners.

This primary source of a communication breakdown for many hearing aid users is the presence of noise in the listening situation. Lipreading can improve the situation, but it is tiring and not always satisfactory. In general, noise remains a source of difficulty for the vast majority of people with sensorineural hearing loss.

Other sources of difficulty include the inability to see the talker clearly, lack of knowledge about the topic of conversation, competing messages (another form of noise, really), and talkers who speak softly or indistinctly.

No technology can compensate for noise and the other sources of communication breakdown. Therefore, to achieve our goal of increasing the probability of communication, the patient must actively influence the listening situation.

For example, an older man frequently visits his son's family, but has a great deal of difficulty in the family room where they typically congregate. The TV is on, the lighting is poor, several people are talking at once, and the room is very reverberant. Now, no hearing aid can possibly overcome all these problems. That means the older man must actively change the situation. He may say, "You know, I have a hearing loss and the TV makes it hard for me to understand. Can we turn it down a bit?" or "Son, my new hearing aid is picking up all these people. Could we go into the sitting room so we could talk?" or "It helps me if I can read your lips, so I'm going to turn on this light so I can see your face."

This kind of tactful manipulation of the situation can produce more benefit than any amount of noise-reduction circuitry! But these requests all have one thing in common: They require the hearing-impaired person to mention his hearing loss. These strategies are discussed further below, but the point is that before the patient can use any such strategy, he or she must be willing to admit the existence of the hearing loss. The older man's requests make sense only if the other people know the reason for them.

So, how do you convince your patient to admit rather than hide his hearing loss? One approach is simply to present some examples like the one above and illustrate how much improvement can be achieved in such a little time. You might ask patients for some specific situations in which they have difficulty hearing and then explain how admitting the loss could open the door to resolving some of the difficulty. This is a perfect lead-in to our next topic: situation control.

C—Change the Situation

This topic was already introduced in the preceding section. If a patient is willing to admit hearing loss, then the door is open for resolving, or at least reducing, the communication breakdowns that occur in everyday life. Essentially, patients must learn to analyze the communication situations they are in and identify the elements or factors that are causing the difficulty. Often the problem is the result of some type of auditory or visual interference.

You can continue the previous discussion of your patients' specific difficult listening situations and help them understand exactly where the difficulty is coming from and how to address it. This discussion is not as difficult as it sounds. Simply listen to your patients and help them decide why they are having trouble in restaurants (or wherever they encounter difficult listening situations) and how to improve the situation. In a restaurant, the patient could ask the waiter to stand so the patient can see his face.

The hard part is convincing the patient to try some of these "assertive" tactics. At this point, just let your patients know that they can accomplish a lot with some analysis and tactful action, and then turn them loose! But don't turn them loose before you mention the final topic: healthcare knowledge.

H—Healthcare Knowledge

Many older people have been raised to think that the responsibility for their health care lies with the healthcare professional, rather than in themselves. My parents were like that. If the doctor told them to do something, they did it, without question. Today's consumer movement represents the antithesis of this attitude. The emphasis these days is on becoming an informed consumer, whether it be in health care, legal matters, financial planning, whatever.

The final segment of your 1-hour aural rehabilitation session should be devoted to letting your patient know where information on hearing health and technology is available. First of all, patients should feel free to come to you if they have questions of any sort about hearing aids, assistive listening devices, or rehabilitation. Furthermore, they can be encouraged to subscribe to magazines such as *Hearing Health,* which contain a wealth of consumer information on issues and technical advances.

Finally, there is no excuse for not mentioning Self Help for Hard of Hearing People (SHHH), a national consumer group with local chapters throughout the country. SHHH chapters usually meet monthly to discuss common problems and to advocate for the rights of hearing-impaired people. These meetings offer support, information, and encouragement—exactly what your patient will need in the coming months to get the most from his or her new hearing aids!

[d]Reprinted with permission from Montgomery AA. WATCH: a practical approach to brief auditory rehabilitation. Hear J 1994b;47:10,53–55.

Rehabilitative Needs of the Aging Population

Patricia A. McCarthy, Ph.D., and Julie Vesper Sapp, Ph.D.

With the advent of the new millennium, audiologists will finally get the answer to the question that has been the subject of speculation for years: how will the Baby Boom generation respond to the aging process? Through every stage of development, the Baby Boom generation has thrown out the rules of past generations and created its own. The sheer size if not the strength of this demographic group has influenced social policy, politics, education, advertising, marketing, and health care in the United States. Therefore, it is probable that as Baby Boomers become Senior Boomers (Peyser, 1999), the way they respond to hearing loss and audiologic rehabilitation will be different from what has been seen with previous generations.

If history can predict the future, then it is a safe bet to assume that aging Baby Boomers will make their needs known and will demand the best. Throughout their lives, Baby Boomers have witnessed the evolution of technology in communication, entertainment, and health care. Digital cellular phones, pagers, faxes, E-mail, and the Internet have replaced rotary dial telephones. Black and white televisions have become relics replaced by the requisite VCR and wide-screen color televisions. Childhood illnesses like polio are a thing of the past, whereas cures for cancer, spinal cord injuries, and other debilitating diseases are being found each day. Each new technolog-

ical achievement has been embraced by this generation and ultimately accepted as commonplace. Thus, this generation expects results and assumes that technology will be available for their needs. It is probable, therefore, that this generation will welcome technology and expect professional support and services that will improve their communication status. It is not likely that the typical Baby Boomer will be passive about his or her hearing loss and rehabilitation.

The next decades will be particularly challenging for audiologists as the aging population per se becomes a "mixed bag." In 1997, persons older than 65 years numbered more than 34 million or 12.7% of the population; by 2010 that number will grow to 40 million. Between 2010 and 2030, it is projected that there will 70 million Americans older than 65 years of age as the Baby Boom generation reaches 65 years (Profile of Older Americans, 1998). With increasing life spans and better health in general, the aging population is likely to be made up of Baby Boomers and their parents! Consequently, in addition to meeting the new demands of the large Baby Boom generation, audiologists will continue to serve the needs of an aging population that is living longer and growing more numerous.

In the new millennium, relegating all individuals older than 65 years of age to a stereotypical age group will be folly. Can we make generalizations about a demographic group when the age range is 65 to 90+ years? As people live longer, we no longer can assume that the geriatric population is homogenous. For this reason, audiologists in the 21st century will need to recognize that the aging population is the most heterogeneous of any age group given differences in biologic, social, cognitive, and psychologic changes related to age.

Knowledge and respect will be the tools that best will serve the audiologist in meeting the needs of this diverse aging population. Knowledge includes not only facility with amplification and audiologic practices, but also a working understanding of the variant manifestations of the aging process and its effects on communication and ultimately rehabilitation. Respect enhances knowledge. Being knowledgeable of the aging process and its ramifications while at the same time respecting the unique communication needs of the individual will be requirements for effectively serving this population.

This chapter views aging as a process that must be considered in audiologic rehabilitation. Audiologists must know more than just the senescent changes in the auditory system. Therefore, reviews of aging in sensory and psychological processes as well as other issues that affect the rehabilitation process are discussed. Successful rehabilitation strategies are also reviewed.

Theories of Aging and Longevity

Since Ponce de Leon searched for the fountain of youth, the quest for longevity has thrived in our culture. Indeed, with the 20th century came a significant increase in life span. In 1900, the average American could expect to live to the ripe old age of 47 years; in the 1990s, average life expectancy increased to approximately 76 years (Kluger, 1996). Given improvements in diet, health care, and sanitation as well as the discovery of antibiotics, there is optimism that life expectancy will continue to increase.

Despite increases in longevity, there is an overriding assumption that the human body has a maximum life span. Gerontologists believe that although there is some predetermined maximum, there are a number of reasons why most people do not reach this maximum. Schneider (1987) suggests theories of aging range from simple wear and tear to more sophisticated error catastrophe theories. Although a number of theories have been proposed, they generally fall into two categories: programmed theories suggest that aging follows a biologic timetable, and error theories emphasize the role of the environment (NIH, 1998).

There are three major programmed theories. The programmed senescence theory suggests that aging results from a sequential switching "on and off" of certain genes. The endocrine theory states that hormones control biologic clocks that pace aging. The immunological theory suggests that there is a programmed decline in the immune system leading to increased vulnerability, aging, and ultimately death (NIH, 1998).

There are at least six error or damage theories. The wear and tear theory simply states that the body's cells and tissues wear out; the somatic mutation theory points to an accumulation of genetic mutations with increasing age which cause cellular deterioration and malfunction. The cross-linking theory suggests an accumulation of cross-linked proteins damages cells and tissues, thereby slowing bodily processes. The free radical theory pinpoints an accumulation of oxygen radicals as responsible for malfunction of the organs. The error catastrophe theory suggests that damage due to mechanisms that synthesize proteins results in faulty proteins that accumulate and cause catastrophic damage to cells, tissues, and organs. Finally, the rate of living theory simply states the greater an organism's rate of oxygen basal metabolism, the shorter the life span (NIH, 1998).

Are any of these the sole theory responsible for aging? Probably not. It is likely that aging is due to a variety of causes, likely a combination of several of the proposed theories. It is well accepted that we cannot live forever, but improvements in nutrition and health care bode well for increasing life spans in the 21st century. Optimistic demographers predict children born in the United States today can realistically look forward to living to be 100 years old (Kluger, 1996). Scientists are hopeful that with increased knowledge of the causes of aging will come increased quality of life during the aging years. Therein lies the challenge for audiologists. As life spans increase and the aging population burgeons, the demand for effective hearing health care will grow commensurately.

Diversity in the Aging Population

In 1997, approximately 15% of the U.S. population older than 65 years were minorities, with African Americans representing about 8%, persons of Hispanic origin representing about 5%, and Asians or Pacific Islanders representing 2% of the older population (Profile of Older Americans, 1998). In the next millennium, these numbers are expected to grow dramatically. Between 1990 and 1995, the Hispanic population grew 20%, the Asian population grew 23%, and the African American population increased by 8% (Metlife, 1996). It has been projected that by the middle of the 21st century, the minority population will outnumber the non-Hispanic white population (Metlife, 1996).

During the 1980s, Hispanics constituted the fastest growing ethnic segment of the population, with a growth rate 5.5 times greater than that of the general population (Teveris, 1997). Hispanics are expected to outnumber African Americans in the United States within the next 15 years (Metlife, 1996). Therefore, Hispanics have drawn the attention of large companies, such as AT&T, Chevrolet, and Kraft, who have developed successful business in the Hispanic community (Teveris, 1997). American businesses are learning quickly that dealing effectively with a variety of cultures will improve their business success.

The growing racial and ethnic diversity in the U.S. population poses challenges for audiologists. The population increases in minority ethnic groups in the 1980s and 1990s will increase the percentage of minority ag-

ing individuals in need of hearing care in the 21st century. Just as big businesses have done, audiologists must prepare for these changes in their caseloads and consider the cultural implications if they are to be successful.

Myths and Stereotypes of Aging

Perhaps the most daunting task facing the Baby Boom generation as it ages is overcoming the negative images associated with aging. The negative myths and stereotypes surrounding the aging American are pervasive, insidious, and can lead to oversimplification and faulty generalizations. Society tells aging individuals to remain young in mind, body, and spirit while at the same time sending the subliminal message that aging is negative. Television commercials, print advertisements, and situation comedies reinforce the beauty and wonder of youth while often offering a feeble, pitiful image of aging.

In fact, these myths and stereotypes are so deeply entrenched in our society that even aging persons themselves often buy into them. The cosmetic industry is a billion-dollar business built in large part on its claims to reduce the signs if not the effects of aging. Conversely, any product, device, or outward sign associated with aging is to be avoided to escape the image of being "old." Even the American Association of Retired Persons (AARP), truly a powerful voice of the aging population, has allowed these stereotypes to pervade its institutional policy-making. Until 1991, advertisements for hearing aids were not allowed in its publication, *Modern Maturity,* because they were viewed as negative, overt signs of aging.

To date, society in large part has shaped it services to the aging population based on negative stereotypes (Palmore, 1990). Clearly, society's attitudes toward audiologic services often are based on negative stereotypes. The reasoning is simple: hearing aids are associated with aging. Aging is viewed by society as a negative. Therefore, hearing aids are viewed negatively by society. Admitting to a hearing loss is admitting to aging. It is no wonder that young and middle-aged adults eschew hearing aids because they are associated with aging. Older individuals trying to avoid looking "old" do the same. Unfortunately, the logic of "avoiding hearing loss avoids aging" may prevent older hearing-impaired adults from taking advantage of audiologic rehabilitation.

Negative attitudes toward hearing aids and audiologic rehabilitation probably will change only when attitudes toward aging in general change. However, if audiologists allow themselves to make decisions based on these faulty assumptions, opportunities will be lost and inadequate or even inappropriate rehabilitative planning may result. The economic, social, cultural, and ethical costs of these negative stereotypes are apparent. Enlightened attitudes toward aging will benefit not only the hearing-impaired individual but also society at large.

Normal Aging Processes

SENSORY PROCESSES
WITH AGING CHANGES

The auditory system

Whereas traditional thinking regarding presbycusis has focused on the inner ear, aging is accompanied by changes in structure and function throughout the auditory system (Table 13.1). Although no hearing loss results, even the outer ear exhibits age-related structural changes. Loss of elasticity of skin and cartilage often results in enlargement of the auricle, or even the collapse of the external ear canal during placement of supra-aural headphones. Ear canal collapse may result in artifactual conductive hearing loss. Solutions to this problem include the use of insert earphones or sound field audiometry. More troublesome is the impact the loss of elasticity can have on the proper fit of in-the-ear hearing aids or earmolds. The architecture of the auricle and ear canal can distort the ear impression. If the end result is a poor fitting earmold or custom hearing aid, feedback may and most likely will occur. This ultimately may lead to rejection of amplification if modifications are not made.

Histologic studies of the middle ear suggest reduced elasticity of middle ear joints (Harty, 1953) and atrophy of middle ear muscles (Schuknecht, 1955). Arthritic ossicular joints may be seen with advancing age, although without apparent conductive hearing loss (Ethol and Belal, 1974). The effects of aging on the immittance characteristics of the middle ear system, however, are not clear. Results of investigations that have addressed this question have produced divergent results. Some have suggested age-related increases in impedance, others have reported age-related reductions in impedance, and still others have found no age-related changes in impedance (Thompson et al., 1979).

Structural degeneration within the cochlea and stria vascularis occurs with advancing age (Schuknecht, 1974; Willott, 1991). The classic histologic studies of Schuknecht (1955) described atrophic changes involving the membranous labyrinth, including afferent and efferent fibers along the Organ of Corti, spreading from the base to the apex of the cochlea. The slow progression of this process is consistent with the gradual high-frequency hearing loss seen in presbycusis patients. Traveling wave delay within the cochlea, as measured indirectly from distortion products otoacoustic emissions, appears to increase with advancing age (Ramotowski and Kimberley, 1998).

Willott (1996) suggests that age-related hearing loss ultimately results from changes in brain activity. He identifies two contributing factors, which he terms the central effects of biologic aging (CEBA) and the central effects of peripheral pathology (CEPP). The CEBA are the result of direct age-related changes to the central system, such as reduction in synapses or loss of neurons. The CEPP, on the other hand, are central changes caused by loss of peripheral function. In C57 mice, for example, loss of cochlear response in high-frequency regions results in the corresponding high-frequency regions of the inferior colliculus and auditory cortex becoming more responsive to low-frequency stimuli (Willott, 1984). These central changes, originally caused by peripheral pathology in mice, result in further changes

Table 13.1
Sensory changes with aging

Visual	Auditory	Body Sensations
Structural	**Structural**	**Structural**
Depigmentation and atrophy of iris	Loss of elasticity in cartilaginous portion of outer ear	Loss of elasticity in skin and muscles
Yellowing of sclera	Reduced elasticity and atrophy of middle ear muscles	Decreased collagen in connective tissue
Decreased size of pupil	Arthritic middle ear joints	
		Functional
Functional	Atrophy and degeneration of hair cells in basal coil of cochlea	Decreased sensitivity to touch
Decreased acuity	Alteration of motion mechanics of cochlea	Lessened sensitivity to pain
Decreased accommodation	Loss of auditory neurons	Slower healing of wounds due to loss of collagen
Decreased darkness adaptation		
Increased sensitivity to glare	**Functional**	
Decreased ability to discriminate colors	Bilaterally symmetric high-frequency sensorineural hearing loss	
	Inordinate reduction in speech recognition	

in the perception of the sound that continue to be audible (Willott et al., 1994).

Hearing sensitivity

Changes in audition accompany the structural and physiologic changes in the auditory system. Presbycusis, or age-related hearing loss, is typically bilateral, sloping, and sensorineural (Willott, 1996). Both longitudinal and cross-sectional studies have demonstrated that the degree of hearing loss progresses with advancing age (Milne, 1977; Gates et al., 1990; Pearson et al., 1995; Morrell et al., 1996). In other words, individuals in their 80s experience more hearing loss than individuals in their 60s. Studies focusing on gender-based differences have found that men exhibit an earlier onset and more rapid progression of hearing loss than women (Pearson et al., 1995; Morrell et al., 1996). Although older women demonstrate better hearing sensitivity in the high frequencies than older men do, older men demonstrate better hearing sensitivity in the low frequencies than older women do. Despite these trends, individual variability in hear-

ing thresholds is very great. As a result, age alone is a poor predictor of hearing levels.

Both intrinsic and extrinsic factors contribute to the development and progression of hearing loss with advancing age. Mitochondrial DNA deletions have been studied and may show some promise in identifying risk for presbycusis (Bai et al., 1997). Vascular insufficiencies developed throughout a lifetime can contribute to hearing loss. In addition, the longer one lives, the more likely one has been treated with ototoxic medications or experienced excessive noise exposure. Interactions exist between intrinsic and extrinsic variables, and these interactions may be complex. For example, at 70 years of age, men with a history of noise exposure exhibit greater loss of hearing sensitivity than their peers with no history of noise exposure (Rosenhall et al., 1990). The shift in hearing thresholds due to aging accelerates with advancing age, whereas the shift in thresholds due to noise exposure decelerates with advancing age (Dobie, 1994). In fact, by the age of 79, no differences are seen between men with and without a history of noise exposure (Rosenhall et al., 1990).

Despite the risk among older adults, hearing loss in this population is underdiagnosed (Trumble and Piterman, 1992). This highlights the need for appropriate screening programs and for the need to reach out and educate primary care providers and the public at large. Hearing screening programs for the elderly are discussed later in this chapter.

Speech understanding

The loss of ability to understand speech easily is the common complaint of the older person seeking audiologic services. Audibility of speech sounds, as measured by pure-tone thresholds, is the largest contributor to speech understanding problems among older hearing-impaired listeners (Humes et al., 1994; Humes, 1996). Schum et al. (1991) have demonstrated that in quiet, word recognition scores for groups of elderly listeners can be predicted from pure-tone thresholds using an articulation index. Hearing loss accounts for more of the variance in speech understanding seen for women than for men (Dubno et al., 1997). These group findings, however, cannot account for those individuals who do not conform to group averages. Bess and Townsend (1977) found that for older individuals with hearing thresholds worse than 60 dB HL, word recognition scores were worse than for younger listeners with similar thresholds.

The difficulties elderly listeners experience understanding speech in degraded listening conditions are not so easily explained based on audibility alone. In listening situations that have been made more difficult by the presence of background noise or reverberation, peripheral hearing loss accounts for most of the variability in speech understanding measures (Humes, 1996; Humes et al., 1994); however, numerous studies have reported a further decline in speech understanding ability in the presence of competing noise for elderly listeners compared with younger listeners. Schum et al. (1991) found that in the presence of competing babble, the articulation index overestimated word recognition for elderly participants.

The scores for older listeners were, on average, 25% worse than the prediction from the articulation index, based on hearing thresholds and the masking effects of the babble. Consequently, audibility of speech sounds could not be identified as the sole contributor to the decline in speech understanding. Similarly, Wiley et al. (1998) found that a single-talker competing message yielded lower speech understanding scores with advancing age. Although hearing loss was again identified as the factor accounting for the most variation in word recognition scores, age and gender differences were significant even when adjustments were made for hearing levels.

Background noise is not the sole degraded speech condition affecting the elderly listener. Bergman et al. (1976) found that older listeners performed less well than younger listeners when the rate of the speaker increased, when the speech signal was filtered, or in a reverberant listening environment. Nabelek and Robinson (1982) found that across reverberation times, older listeners were affected more adversely than were younger listeners. Most listening in the real world occurs under less than optimal listening conditions. As a result, these findings are important in understanding the communication problems of the elderly hearing-impaired patient.

Controversy surrounds the identification of the cause or causes of the speech understanding decrements that exceed what can be accounted for based on simple audibility. Peripheral distortions, central auditory processing problems, cognitive changes, and attention declines have all been proposed as potential contributors. Willott (1991) suggests that an interactive model including peripheral, central, and cognitive-linguistic factors is most appropriate. As he points out, if the peripheral system is impaired, additional stress is placed on central and cognitive functions, and if cognitive function is impaired, the ability to process sounds is affected. The specific interactions among all the factors are not yet clear.

Rehabilitative intervention with the elderly hearing-impaired patient can address the effects of peripheral hearing loss on the audibility of speech sounds through appropriate amplification. Additional adverse effects caused by the presence of background noise and other degraded listening situations can be addressed through counseling regarding environmental management techniques and through the use of assistive listening technologies.

Central auditory processing

Animal models have identified age-related changes in central auditory structure, function, and neurochemistry (Caspary et al., 1995; Willott, 1996). In elderly humans, changes in the function of auditory structures within the central nervous system, termed central auditory processing disorder (CAPD), are frequently held to be a significant contributing factor to the speech understanding problems of elderly listeners (Marshall, 1981; Humes and Christopherson, 1991). Tests for central auditory dysfunction include dichotic listening tasks, degraded speech tasks, and comparisons of Phonetically Balanced-Max (PB-Max) to Synthetic Sentence Index-Max (SSI-Max). Assessment issues, however, are complicated by the effects of peripheral hearing loss that can affect test results (Marshall, 1981).

Estimates of the prevalence of CAPD among the elderly vary depending on how the sample was selected, what measures were utilized, and what criteria were used to identify CAPD. Among the elderly population, estimates have ranged from as low as 22.6% for persons aged 65 years and older (Cooper and Gates, 1991) to as high as 70% for persons older than 60 years of age (Stach et al., 1990). In both these studies, however, the prevalence of CAPD increased within the elderly population as age increased. Stach et al. (1990) reported prevalence of 95% among persons older than 80 years from a clinical population and 72% for persons older than 80 years from a nonclinical population.

CAPD is a factor that can affect the rehabilitative process. Jerger et al. (1990) found that elderly persons with CAPD reported more hearing handicap on the Hearing Handicap Inventory for the Elderly (HHIE) than elderly persons without CAPD independent of hearing loss. Handicap was even reported within the CAPD group for those individuals who did not experience peripheral hearing loss. These results suggest that the presence of a CAPD can be communicatively handicapping for the elderly in and of itself and can compound the handicapping effects of peripheral hearing loss.

The benefits of amplification for elderly individuals with hearing loss continue to be a debatable issue. When peripheral hearing loss is present, the likelihood of benefit from amplification appeared to be the same for elderly patients with CAPD as for those without CAPD in a study reported by Kricos et al. (1987). In that study, the CAPD group and non-CAPD group produced similar average scores and a similar range of scores on the Hearing Aid Performance Inventory (HAPI). Both groups reported the greatest benefit from amplification in quiet, and the least benefit in noisy environments. Schum (1992) used the HAPI and found that elderly hearing aid users perceived less benefit than the generally younger subjects from the original HAPI normative study (Walden et al., 1984). Chmiel and Jerger (1996) found that the presence of CAPD in elderly persons attenuated the quality of life improvements gained with amplification that prevents them from realizing the full benefits of hearing aids. Using the HHIE to measure reduction in handicap as an outcome of hearing aid use, they found elderly persons with central deficits showed significantly less reduction in hearing handicap than those without CAPD. The reader is referred to Chapter 18 for further discussion of hearing aid benefit in the aging population.

Although the amount of self-perceived benefit from amplification in the elderly population with CAPD cannot be predicted on the basis of these studies, it is clear that some older hearing aid users may experience less benefit than younger hearing aid users. These results, however, should not discourage audiologists from continuing to pursue amplification for the aging hearing-impaired individual. Assistive technology (as discussed in Chapter 16) continues to be a viable alternative to the personal hearing aid for many aging individuals with CAPD. The limited benefit of hearing aids in noisy environments may be discouraging. However, newer technologies and continued research discussed in Chapters 11 and 16 allow for optimism in providing beneficial amplification even for elderly individuals with CAPD.

Vision

By the age of 50 or 55 years, almost everyone needs corrective lenses of some type, with reading glasses being the most common (Timiras, 1972). The decrease in visual acuity after age 40 is a well-accepted aging phenomenon commonly referred to as presbyopia. In fact, after age 60, normal vision even with corrective lenses is rare. Dramatic changes in visual acuity occur with age. However, acuity is not the only aspect of vision that changes with age. Like the ear, almost every structure experiences age-related changes. Huyck and Hoyer (1982) suggest that the effects of aging on vision include reduced visual acuity, reduced accommodation, reduced darkness adaptation, and changes in color vision. As a result, many of these structural changes effect functional changes that have implications for rehabilitation of the hearing-impaired geriatric individual. In the following discussion, a brief review of the anatomy of the eye is provided to facilitate understanding of these structural/functional changes.

The iris, which is situated between the cornea and the lens, is responsible for controlling the amount of light that enters the eye. The lens controls the quality of light by changing its shape, while the size of the pupil (controlled by the iris) dictates the amount of light that will be focused on the retina. The rods and cones of the retina encode the spatial, spectral, and temporal aspects of the visual stimulus. This information is then transmitted from the retina over the optic nerves through the lateral geniculate nuclei to the visual cortex where integration occurs.

Depigmentation and atrophy of the iris, together with a decrease in pupil diameter,

contribute to the diminished amount of light that enters the aging eye. Reduction in pupil size with advancing age, called senile meiosis, is a documented change, although why the pupil shrinks with age is unknown (Sekuler, 1982). It has been estimated that the eye of the average 60-year-old allows only about one-third as much light to enter the eye as that of the average 20-year-old (Atchely, 1988). Consequently, older individuals may need three to four times brighter illumination than their younger counterparts. The retina itself is relatively free of age-related changes (Leopold, 1965).

Yellowing of the lens with age results in a decreased ability to discriminate colors. This yellowing causes the lens to filter out violets, blues, and greens, whereas reds, yellows, and oranges are easier to see (Corso, 1971). Visual adaptation to darkness also changes with age. Botwinick (1978) has suggested that older people adapt as fast as the young, but their adaptation is not nearly as good. A reduced ability of the eye to discriminate detail, called accommodation, has been reported to decrease with age (Bruckner, 1967). Furthermore, the ability to visualize distant objects has been reported to decline in the fifth and sixth decades (Riffle, 1979). Finally, sensitivity to glare reportedly increases with age (Wolf, 1960).

Clearly, these structural and functional changes can undermine the success of rehabilitation of the older hearing-impaired individual. Therefore, these changes should be considered in any rehabilitative planning. Most older individuals will need glasses in addition to large-print reading materials. This includes information given by the audiologist regarding hearing aids and communication strategies. Attention also should be given to levels of illumination in therapy rooms, audiometric test suites, waiting rooms, and offices. Levels of illumination need to be significantly higher for the aged individual to receive the same visual effect as a younger person.

Color discrimination should be taken into account when dealing with the older population. When possible, use of red or orange print for signs and therapy materials will facilitate visualization. Decreases in accommodation with age present a particularly difficult problem during the hearing aid orientation. The older patient's ability to distinguish the external components of the hearing aid may be limited severely. (This represents a challenge for some younger eyes as well!) Some audiologists have enhanced the visualization of these hearing aid components by highlighting them with a red marking pen or nail polish. This technique capitalizes on the older person's ability to see the color red easily. Increased glare sensitivity can also interfere with battery insertion in a hearing aid because the plus sign indicating the correct insertion side may be difficult to see. With some patients, the use of tactile cues to differentiate the positive side of the battery from the negative side may work. For others, marking the "upside" with red, orange, or yellow may be helpful.

Many of the methods, procedures, and strategies used with younger adults in the rehabilitative process are undermined by the visual changes that occur with aging. Therefore, knowledge of these changes in visual structures and functions with age allows audiologists to be creative in rehabilitation planning. The suggestions offered above are but a few of the practical suggestions that can enhance the success of rehabilitation of the older hearing-impaired adult.

Visual perception of speech

Traditional approaches in rehabilitative audiology have included speechreading (lipreading) training (see Chapter 12). The use of visual speech cues can improve perception of the spoken message when hearing loss and/or adverse listening conditions impede understanding, but the effects of aging on the speechreading process must be considered when this approach is used with an older person.

Performance decrements on speechreading tasks have been observed for older subjects when compared with younger subjects across a range of materials including visemes, consonant-vowel monosyllables, and sentences (Farrimond, 1959; Ewertsen and Nielsen, 1971; Pelson and Prather,

1974; Shoop and Binnie, 1979; Kricos and Lesner, 1995). Farrimond (1959), for example, found that for men, speechreading ability declined in each decade after the age of 30. The speechreading performance of older persons is improved, however, when guessing is encouraged (Farrimond, 1989).

The interaction of sensorineural hearing loss with speechreading performance is not as clear. Pelson and Prather (1974) found significantly higher speechreading scores for sentences with older subjects with sensorineural hearing loss than for older subjects with normal hearing. Sapp (Sapp JV. The effects of age, acquired hearing loss, and irrelevant auditory stimuli on the visual perception of speech. Unpublished doctoral dissertation, The University of Georgia, 1997), on the other hand, found significantly higher scores for older participants with normal hearing than for their presbycusis counterparts on the Lipreading Discrimination Test (LDT), a test of viseme discrimination within a sentence context.

Thorn and Thorn (1989) have suggested that age of onset of hearing loss is related to speechreading performance of older adults. Elderly speech-readers with onset of hearing loss in childhood performed better on the speechreading of sentences than elderly subjects who acquired hearing loss during adulthood.

When speech stimuli are presented in the presence of background noise, supplementary speechreading cues improve understanding (O'Neill, 1954). As the signal-to-noise ratio becomes less favorable, reliance on supplementary visual cues increases (Sumby and Pollack, 1954; O'Neill, 1954; Erber, 1969). Older persons also benefit from speechreading cues in a noisy environment, but age-related decrements in the audiovisual speech understanding are still evident (Ewertsen and Nielsen, 1971).

Sapp (Sapp JV. The effects of age, acquired hearing loss, and irrelevant auditory stimuli on the visual perception of speech. Unpublished doctoral dissertation, The University of Georgia, 1997) investigated the effects of irrelevant auditory stimuli on speechreading performance. LDT scores of younger participants (aged 20 to 28 years) with normal hearing, older participants (aged 65 to 75 years) with normal hearing, and older participants (aged 65 to 75 years) with acquired bilateral sensorineural hearing loss were obtained in three conditions: quiet, white noise, and a single talker discourse. No significant differences across conditions were found for the younger subjects. Both groups of older subjects demonstrated a performance decrement in the single talker discourse compared with the quiet condition. Additionally, the older participants with hearing loss were more adversely affected by the competing story than the older participants with normal hearing.

Age-related differences are apparent for visual and audiovisual speech perception. It is important to recall that despite those differences, speechreading cues aid the older person in difficult listening environments. Counseling and training that encourage attention to speechreading cues, and particularly those that facilitate guessing, continue to be appropriate rehabilitative options for the older person with hearing impairment.

Body sensations and wound healing

Evidence suggests that there are age-related changes in the skin senses including touch, pressure, and pain on the skin (Huyck and Hoyer, 1982). Touch and pain, two of the so-called "body sensations" (Atchely, 1988), undergo aging changes that can have an effect on the success of audiologic rehabilitation. The sense of touch starts to become somewhat dulled after about 45 to 50 years of age. In a study by Axelrod and Cohen (1961), sensitivity to light touch on the palm and thumb was significantly less in older subjects (63 to 78 years) than in younger subjects (20 to 36 years). Concomitantly, sensitivity to pain appears to decrease with aging. Although these changes may appear to have little relationship to impaired hearing, they have implications for successful rehabilitation of the older hearng-impaired individual.

Decreased manual touch sensitivity may have a significant effect on the older individual's ability to manipulate a hearing aid. Hearing aid controls are so small that only minimal movement is needed to effect large changes in the hearing aid response. Thus, the older person with decreased touch sensitivity may not be able to make the fine adjustments necessary to set the hearing aid at the most comfortable loudness level. Ultimately, this can lead to rejection of the hearing aid. Hearing aid manufacturers have responded to this situation by adding optional features such as enlarged and stacked volume control wheels, finger grips, removable handles, and screw-set volume control wheels. Fortunately, the evolving popularity of programmable and digital hearing aids negates the necessity for a volume control wheel, thereby eliminating the task of setting the aid to the most comfortable loudness. These features, coupled with the relative ease of inserting a custom in-the-ear hearing aid, should overcome the problem of decreased touch sensitivity in older patients.

Changes in pain sensitivity with age are difficult to quantify because pain is more than a sensory phenomenon. Cognitive and emotional factors as well as individual personality and cultural factors can influence responses to pain (Huyck and Hoyer, 1982). Although it is difficult to generalize about pain sensitivity with age, the clinical impression of gerontologists is that a decrease in pain sensitivity occurs with aging.

There is evidence to suggest that wound healing is delayed in the aging (Kligman et al., 1985). Collagen, a compound tissue found throughout the body, is thought to be involved in healing. Because collagen decreases with age, the loss of collagen may contribute to wounds healing more slowly in the aging (Kimmel, 1974). Although wound repair times are more variable in the elderly, older persons lag behind younger individuals in every stage of repair (Grove, 1982).

Decreased pain sensitivity and slower healing times can have an impact on the hearing aid fitting process and audiologic rehabilitation. If decreased pain sensitivity does occur, then there is an increased likelihood of an older individual ignoring a pathologic condition caused by an improperly fitted earmold or in-the-ear hearing aid.

It is not uncommon to find this auricular irritation among geriatric hearing aid wearers, because elasticity changes in the cartilage of the outer ear may preclude a proper fit of the aid or earmold. If the older patient ignores the condition, it can become chronic, which may preclude wearing the hearing aid until the irritation has healed. Consequently, the older patient may be prevented from wearing his or her hearing aid for a long period as the result of a slow healing process. This situation occurred with a 79-year-old severely hearing-impaired man seen by one of the authors. Unfortunately, the healing process was so slow that this man was without one of his in-the-ear hearing aids for 6 weeks.

The situation described above can be avoided by performing a careful inspection of the initial fit of the aid or earmold and by conducting frequent checks for auricular irritation during the first several weeks of hearing aid wear and on a regular basis thereafter. This type of knowledge incorporated into the audiologic rehabilitation process improves the quality of services provided to the aging population.

CHANGES IN PSYCHOLOGICAL PROCESSES WITH AGING

Selective attention and memory

In the rehabilitative process, the patient must attend to the task at hand and must learn and recall relevant information. Both selective attention and memory, however, exhibit specific age-related decrements that can affect the success of aural rehabilitation.

The term selective attention refers to the ability to ignore irrelevant stimuli while focusing on relevant stimuli. The need for a human ability for selective attention has been attributed to the limited processing capacity of the human brain (Kausler, 1991; Neumann, 1996). Older adults are believed to be more distracted by the irrelevant stimuli (Rabbit, 1965; Kausler, 1991). There appears to be a breakdown in the ability to inhibit processing of the irrelevant stimuli (McDowd and Filion, 1982; Hasher et al., 1991). In visual, auditory, and tactile modal-

ities, older subjects are less successful in performing selective attention tasks, as measured by increases in the number of response errors and increases in the time required to complete a task (Basowitz and Korchin, 1957; Rabbit, 1965; Barr and Giambra, 1990; Kausler, 1991; Madden, 1992). Unlike younger subjects, older subjects perform significantly worse on the LDT in the presence of a linguistic auditory distracter than they do in quiet (Sapp JV. The effects of age, acquired hearing loss, and irrelevant auditory stimuli on the visual perception of speech. Unpublished doctoral dissertation, The University of Georgia, 1997).

Working memory is a limited capacity system that involves the simultaneous storing of recent information and processing of additional information (Hultsch and Dixon, 1990). Due to the breakdown in the ability to use inhibitory attentional mechanisms, older adults can experience difficulty excluding extraneous information from working memory and focusing their attention on the storing and processing of the desired information (Hasher and Zacks, 1988). Additionally, interference from extraneous distracters appears to have a greater effect on elders' ability to retrieve information which has already been stored (Gerard et al., 1991)." Increasing the time allowed to provide a response can improve the performance of older participants (Canestri, 1963).

An important distinction within memory processes is that of automatic versus effortful encoding (Kausler, 1990). Automaticity refers to the encoding of information without the conscious attempt to encode it. In other words, it refers to the way in which individuals "pick up" information without concentrating on attempting to remember it. Effortful encoding, conversely, requires attention and concentration. Automatic processes in auditory memory appear to be little affected by advancing age, whereas effortful processes in auditory memory, requiring attention, decline with age (Amenedo and Diaz, 1998).

Another distinction in the study of memory and aging involves implicit versus explicit memory (Hultsch and Dixon, 1990).

Implicit memory refers to the effect of prior exposure on later performance of a task that does not involve the conscious attempt to recall. Explicit memory involves the conscious attempt to remember. Age-related declines are seen in explicit memory, but little age-related change is seen in implicit memory.

These deficits in attention and memory can affect the audiologic rehabilitation process but do not imply that older individuals cannot participate successfully. Distractions in the environment should be kept to a minimum. Information should be clear and concise. The time allowed for the older patient to process and recall information may need to be increased. These are small accommodations to improve the outcome of the rehabilitation for the older hearing-impaired individual.

Slowing and cautiousness

Slowness of behavior is often observed among older people. Simple reaction time, meaning the simple response to the onset of a stimulus, becomes longer as we age. Older individuals are particularly slow to respond if the stimulus is unexpected (Botwinick and Brinley, 1962). Additionally, the more complex and demanding the task, the slower the response. Reaction time can improve, however, with practice (Botwinick and Thompson, 1967). Rabbit (1996) has reviewed findings across a wide range of functions and has concluded that all mental processes slow with advancing age. As with most age-related changes, of course, individual variability is high, making age alone a poor predictor of the time required for any given task.

An issue related to slowness of response behavior is cautiousness. Although cautiousness among older people is highly task-dependent, on some tasks elderly people are more willing to sacrifice speed for the sake of accuracy (Botwinick, 1984). Among elderly adults, the level of cautiousness on the Stroop Color-Word Interference Test increases with age, and more cautious elderly participants make fewer errors than their less cautious peers (Rush et al., 1987). Cau-

tiousness may also be seen as a failure to respond at all rather than risk making a mistake. This failure to respond is termed the omission error. Rees and Botwinick (1971) have suggested that this tendency among older listeners to make omission errors occurs during pure-tone threshold testing. Elderly listeners do not, however, appear to use more cautious response criteria (Gordon-Salant, 1986) or provide more omission errors during suprathreshold word recognition testing (Sapp and McCarthy, 1993). Further study on omission errors in word recognition testing is needed to determine whether older hearing-impaired subjects perform similarly.

Cautiousness and the slowness of response can affect the elderly patient's progress in the audiologic rehabilitation process. This once again highlights the importance of allowing sufficient time for the older person to master a skill or task, such as hearing aid insertion or manipulation. This may require more patience on the part of the audiologist, but greater rehabilitative success gained by the elderly patient is ample reward.

Motivation

Implicit in the audiologic rehabilitation of individuals of any age is the factor of motivation. Elias and Elias (1977) suggest that the age differences in a variety of human activities may be related to motivation rather than intellectual or physiologic competence.

Included in the definition of motivation are the factors of drive and incentive. Theorists suggest behavior is pushed through the action of motivating drives and pulled through the perception of a goal or valuable object (Bolles, 1967). Drive then appears to be internally generated as from a biologic or psychological need. Incentives are provided externally by the reinforcement of achieving a goal or an object.

Motivation for successful audiologic rehabilitation can be viewed from both a push and pull perspective. Whereas the hearing-impaired individual provides the push or drive, the audiologist can provide the pull or incentive. With hearing loss, a biologic need for better communication is produced.

Theoretically, increased hearing deprivation should result in increased drive to improve communication. In practice, however, this is not always the case. Older hearing-impaired individuals often appear to lack the push or drive necessary for improved communication. To compensate for the lack of drive, the audiologist can provide the pull or incentive. The incentive can be the goal of successful use of amplification, improved use of visual cues, or development of better listening skills and communication.

The audiologist has the responsibility to ensure that the goals for the hearing-impaired individual truly are viewed as valuable to the individual. For this reason, goals for audiologic rehabilitation should be established mutually with the hearing-impaired individual. If input is not obtained from the older client, the value of the goals may be insufficient to provide the incentive and motivation necessary to achieve them. Unfortunately, the input of the client is often not considered in treatment planning. Perhaps this is why so many older clients appear to be lacking motivation.

The audiologist can help increase the older person's motivational level by ensuring that the end goal of treatment is of value to the individual. The use of the Client-Oriented Scale of Improvement (COSI) (Dillon et al., 1997) is an excellent example of tool that incorporates the patient's goals into the audiologic rehabilitation plan. While completing the COSI with the older hearing-impaired individual, it should be apparent that there is sufficient motivation and incentive to ensure success with amplification. Further, completing the COSI allows the audiologist to monitor whether the individual's goals and expectations are realistic and achievable. The COSI is discussed at length in Chapters 11 and 18.

HEALTH CARE ISSUES IN AGING

Physical health of the elderly

Sociologists believe that health is of major importance to aging individuals because it determines their ability to perform those tasks that enable them to participate in family, community, jobs, and leisure activities (Shanas and Maddox, 1976). Participation in audiologic rehabilitation may be included in that statement as well. Consequently, health may be a major determinant of the geriatric individual's ability and or willingness to participate in his or her own hearing rehabilitation. Indeed, our experience has shown this to be true.

In a hearing screening program conducted in a geriatric rehabilitation facility, McCarthy et al. (1995) found a high rate of denial of hearing loss. The protocol included a pure-tone screen and the screening form of the HHIE. Results showed that although 72% of patients failed the pure-tone screening, only 25% had a failing score on the HHIE-S. In essence, a majority of subjects failed the pure-tone screening, suggesting the presence of at least mild hearing loss. However, only a minority of subjects self-reported hearing handicap. The authors concluded that the high prevalence of denial of hearing loss in this population might have been related to the patient's general health status. In fact, these patients were hospitalized for one or more conditions other than hearing loss. As such, their psychic and emotional energy may have been focused on rehabilitation of those conditions, so they were not ready to admit to another possible health problem. Given that health is a major issue in this population and may negatively affect the audiologic rehabilitation process, a discussion of the general health status of the elderly follows.

Unfortunately, there is a strong association between advancing chronologic age and an increased incidence of disease and disability. However, on the average, older people are afflicted with acute disease comparatively less often than younger people. In fact, Ries (1979) reported an average of 1.1 acute conditions per year in the population aged 65 years and older, which represents the lowest occurrence across age groups. However, when this older group experiences an acute condition, they experience more days of restricted activity than do younger individuals. From these data it appears that there is no reason to suspect a higher rate of absenteeism among geriatric patients in an audiology practice. However, when absenteeism is due to an acute illness in the elderly, it may be more long-term than expected.

The incidence of chronic conditions increases with age, and it is estimated that only a small percentage of persons older than 65 years have no chronic conditions. In a 1995 study, more than one-third of older persons reported that they were limited by chronic conditions (Profile of Older Americans, 1998). Hearing impairments were found to be the third most frequently occurring chronic condition in the elderly, exceeded only by hypertension and heart disease (Profile of Older Americans, 1998).

Atchley (1988), however, cautions that a chronic condition is seldom disabling. Therefore, any generalizations about the frequency of occurrence of a chronic condition or the percentage of the geriatric population with chronic conditions must be interpreted in that light. Atchley reports that the number of older individuals with no limitations on activity has increased substantially in recent years. As the "Senior Boom" is included in those studies, the number of older individuals with no chronic conditions is certain to increase dramatically.

Although health is not a seriously limiting factor for most older hearing-impaired patients, general health status should be considered when developing a rehabilitative plan. Rehabilitative goals should be made with respect to the individual's general health status.

Relationship of health to audiologic rehabilitation

The goal of virtually every older person with a disabling condition is restoration of his or her independence and autonomy (Williams, 1989). Concomitantly, a major goal of medical practice is to assist elderly patients in achieving independence (Cluff, 1981). However, a prerequisite to independence and autonomy for the elderly appears to be maintenance of good general health. Whereas such disabilities as cardiac problems and arthritis present known, quantifiable limitations on one's functioning, less is known about the influence of hearing impairment on overall health status and functioning. Nonetheless, given the ubiquitous presence of hearing impairment among the elderly, this is clearly an issue of interest to all health care professionals working with this population.

Studies of the impact of hearing impairment on the overall health status of the elderly have garnered conflicting results. Herbst and Humphrey (1980) found that hearing loss in the elderly was associated with poor health, increased depressive symptoms, as well as a reduction in mobility, activities, interpersonal relations, and enjoyment of life. Yet, Salomon (1986) found no direct relationship between hearing level in the elderly and life satisfaction, self-perception, and general activity level. Neither of these studies, however, adjusted for confounding variables (Bess et al., 1989).

Given these conflicting results, Bess et al. (1989) conducted a study to clarify whether hearing loss imposes adverse functional and psychosocial consequences on elderly patients. The impact of hearing impairment was analyzed on 153 patients older than 65 years of age. Pure-tone audiometry was conducted to determine hearing levels, and functional health status was assessed using the Sickness Impact Profile (SIP). The SIP, a 136-item standardized questionnaire that assesses physical and psychosocial function, has 12 subscales: ambulation, mobility, body care, movement, social interaction, communication, alertness, sleep/rest, eating, work, home management, and recreation/pastimes. Three main scales are formed by combining subscales: physical (ambulation, mobility, body care, movement), psychosocial (social interaction, communication, alertness), and overall (combining all 12 subscales). The higher the SIP score, the higher the level of functional impairment (Bess et al., 1989).

Results of this study demonstrate that poor hearing was associated with higher SIP scores and increased overall dysfunction. Furthermore, progressive hearing impairment in elderly patients was associated with progressive physical and psychosocial dysfunction. The authors conclude that hearing loss appears to be an important determinant of function in elderly persons.

If hearing impairment is such a strong determinant of physical and psychosocial function, then all health care professionals working with aging individuals should have a vested interest in the audiologic assessment of their older patients. This can happen only if audiologists educate other health care professionals about the incidence of hearing impairment and the possible deleterious effects of hearing loss on overall daily functioning. Clearly, the impact of ignoring a hearing impairment in an elderly person may extend beyond the simple inability to hear. Indeed, the neglected hearing loss may contribute to a diminished overall quality of life for the elderly person.

Use of medication by the elderly

Polypharmacy, the concurrent use of several drugs, is common in the aging population (American Nurses Association, 1997). Patients older than 65 years use an average of 2 to 6 prescribed medications and 1 to 3.4 nonprescription medications (Stewart and Cooper, 1994). Unfortunately, polypharmacy often includes the inappropriate use of multiple and interacting drugs that can cause sensory and cognitive side effects. Montamat and Cusack (1992) found that 12% of older patients being evaluated for dementia were actually suffering from adverse drug reactions. Further, 10% of elderly people admitted to the hospital are there because of adverse drug reactions, with one-fifth of those admissions due to over-the-counter medications (Montamat and Cusack, 1992).

Given the incidence of chronic diseases and disorders, it is not surprising that use of medication by the elderly is higher than among younger patients (Vestal, 1984). As the geriatric population grows, so will the expenditures for drugs and medications. In 1976, the elderly population spent approximately 25% of the national total for drugs and drug sundries; it has been estimated that by the year 2030, expenditures for drugs by the elderly in the United States will reach 30

to 40% of the national total (Vestal, 1978). Furthermore, multiple drug use by elderly individuals is the rule rather than the exception. Consequently, the potential for medication errors among the elderly is great. Complicating the situation is the fact that older adults are prone to increased drug sensitivity (Schumacher, 1980; Braithwaite, 1982). These factors contribute to the higher incidence of adverse drug reactions in the elderly than in the young (Vestal, 1978).

Polypharmacy including the misuse of medications, adverse drug reactions, and aging changes related to drug sensitivity all can have negative effects on the elderly person both physiologically and behaviorally. Table 13.2 displays many of the commonly observed side effects associated with several classes of drugs. Although these side effects can occur with any age group, the elderly may be particularly at risk.

Patients whose medication errors are chronic are considered to be noncompliant (Cooper, 1994). Noncompliance with drug therapy has been the subject of several investigations. In a review of more than 50 studies, Blackwell (1972) found that complete failure to take medication occurred in 25 to 50% of all outpatients. A study by Parkin et al. (1976) found that a lack of understanding of the drug regimen was the greatest problem in medication compliance. Schwartz et al. (1962) found that error-prone patients were likely to make multiple mistakes more than single mistakes. The most frequent mistake was omission of medication, followed by lack of knowledge about the medications, use of medications not prescribed by the physician, and errors of dosage, timing, or sequence. Medication errors can be made by professionals and patients (Cooper, 1993).

In addition to misuse, older patients have a higher incidence of adverse effects due to medication errors (Cooper, 1994). Chronic health problems combined with a decline in physiologic functioning of the elderly may predispose elderly adults to adverse drug reactions (Cherry and Morton, 1989). Physiologic changes with aging can have dramatic effects on the absorption and distribution of

Table 13.2
Possible adverse effects of prescription drugs

Drug Class	Adverse Effects

Antihypertensives
    Reserpine
    Methyldopa
    Propranolol
    Clonidine
    Hydralazine
	Sedation, fatigue, depression, constipation, confusion, weakness

Analgesics
    Narcotics
        Morphine
        Codeine
        Meperidine
        Pentazocine
        Propoxyphene
	Sedation, hallucinations, confusion, withdrawal, constipation

Nonnarcotic Indomethacin	Headache, dizziness, confusion, depression

Antiparkinsonian
    L-Dopa
    Carbidopa
    Bromocriptine
    Trihexyphenidyl
	Confusion, hallucinations, depression

Antihistamines
    Diphenylpyraline
    Hydroxyzine
	Sedation, anxiety, confusion

Antimicrobials
    Gentamicin
    Isoniazid
	Psychosis, depression, agitation, hallucination, memory disturbance

Cardiovascular
    Digitalis
    Lidocaine
    Atropine
	Fatigue, psychosis, irritability, confusion

Hypoglycemics
    Insulin
    Sulfonylureas
	Anxiety, irritability, confusion, lethargy

Laxatives	Habituation, withdrawal, irritability, insomnia, confusion

Reprinted with permission from Ouslander JG, Jarvick LF, Small GW. Illness and psychopathology in the elderly. Psychiatr Clin North Am 1982;5:155.

drugs in the body. Dosages of medications often have to be adjusted up or down to achieve desirable levels in the body. Less of a drug may be needed to achieve the same effect as with a younger person (National Council on the Aging, 1997).

Another issue in medication compliance is the complexity of the language used in the directions found on the labels of the bottles and containers. Tymchuk (1990) investigated the readability of over-the-counter medications using a standard readability formula. His results showed that elderly persons using some common over-the-counter medications would have to have a reading ability anywhere between grade 6 and college level to comprehend the information. Previous studies in medical decision-making found that the average reading comprehension levels of competent elderly people were between fourth and fifth grade (Tymchuk et al., 1986, 1988). In addition, Tymchuk (1990) reported that the obtained grade levels found on the labels actually masked the complexity of some of the medical, technical, and scientific language used. Therefore, only a very well informed layperson, pharmacist, or physician would understand most of the language. Tymchuk suggests that lack of understanding may contribute to of misuse of medication among the elderly.

Polypharmacy can severely compromise communication if the elderly patient is experiencing any of the adverse effects shown in Table 13.2. Given the prevalence of polypharmacy, audiologists must be cognizant of it effects. Elderly patients experiencing any of these adverse effects may have difficulty participating in their own rehabilitation. Unfortunately, audiologists may be tempted to consider such behaviors as confusion, irritability, memory loss, or depression as normal albeit negative aspects of aging. As a consequence, the elderly person's rehabilitation potential may appear limited, and recommendations for amplification and communication therapy may not be made. Thus, the elderly person in this situation may experience "double jeopardy." Not only has this older person experienced serious side effects from prescribed medication, but he or she may have appropriate rehabilitative recommendations withheld by the audiologist.

The problems of polypharmacy in the aging population underscore the importance of a comprehensive case history complete with information about the patient's medication regimen. Audiologists working with elderly patients must be aware of the potentially serious side effects that older patients may experience from medications. They must be knowledgeable about the medications that their patients are taking and look for signs of these behavioral side effects that may occur during the rehabilitation process. Although attributing irritability and confusion to aging may be the easy answer, it may lead to inappropriate rehabilitative decision-making by the audiologist.

Health care providers' relationships with the elderly

The continuing growth of the geriatric population suggests a great need for health care providers who are knowledgeable about care of the elderly. It has been estimated that even with minimum use, more than 24,000 primary care physicians knowledgeable about geriatric medicine will be needed by the year 2010, when there will be as many as 35 million people in the United States 65 years of age and older (Belgrave et al., 1982). This projection implies more than the demand for a large number of physicians; it suggests that these physicians must be knowledgeable of and sensitive to the special medical needs of the geriatric population. Furthermore, the importance of physicians' attitudes toward the elderly is underscored by the critical role physicians play in the lives of older persons. Indeed, the elderly use about three times more of the health care resources than the rest of the population (U.S. Department of Health and Human Services, 1983). Older people accounted for 40% of all hospital stays in 1995 and had over twice as many contacts with physicians as people younger than 65 years (Profile of Older Americans, 1998).

Health care professionals have responded to the rapidly growing older population by attempting to change health care delivery systems. One innovative program designed to address the health care needs of the aging is the Geriatric Interdisciplinary Team Training Program (GITT) at the Rush-Presbyterian-St. Luke's Medical Center, Chicago, IL. This program was underwritten by The John A. Hartford Foundation as a grant to prepare health care practitioners for geriatric health care. The program curriculum offers clinical experiences in a variety of health care settings and emphasizes the value of interdisciplinary teams in serving the geriatric population. Trainees and practitioners from medicine, nursing, social work, occupational therapy, clinical nutrition, speech-language pathology, and audiology as well as a number of other disciplines participate. Whereas traditional models of health care delivery have centered on the physician as the "captain of the ship," this model emphasizes that every member of the team brings unique knowledge, experience, and skills. The point of the interdisciplinary geriatric team is to tap into the talents of each team member in providing high-quality care to older patients. The focus on the patient as a whole person, with decisions made by a team, is thought to be the model of the future in geriatric medicine. Given the incidence of hearing loss in this population, the role of the audiologist on an interdisciplinary team is essential.

An interdisciplinary approach to training health care professionals represents the most hopeful approach for the future of geriatric health care. This approach will provide reciprocal benefits to both participating professionals and geriatric patients. To that end, all allied health care professionals need to be resolute in (1) eliminating stereotypes about the elderly as patients, (2) improving the educational preparation of health care professionals by expanding curricula to include interdisciplinary training in geriatric health care, and (3) improving the quality of health care service delivery to the burgeoning geriatric population.

Successful Rehabilitation Strategies

SCREENING

Hearing screening programs traditionally have targeted two groups: the pediatric and the geriatric populations. Chapter 4 discusses the national effort to initiate a universal hearing screening for newborns. Although hearing loss among the aging population is much more prevalent than in newborns, no systematic, large-scale hearing loss identification program exists for the aging. The U.S. Preventive Services Task Force (1989) has recommended that aging persons be screened for hearing impairment, as have the American Academy of Audiology (1991) and the American Speech-Language-Hearing Association (1989).

Currently, older persons with hearing loss enter the hearing health care system in a number of ways, ranging from physician referral to self-referral. Audiologists, primary care physicians, nurses, public and community health services, and nursing home professionals are among those interested in identification of hearing loss in this population. Unfortunately, however, no

standard hearing screening protocol or referral criteria have been adopted widely by those involved in making referrals or conducting hearing screenings. Although some primary care physicians may conduct formal hearing screenings, many rely only on the complaints of the patient. Given Weinstein's (1994) contention that older adults may minimize the functional effects of their hearing impairment, this latter method for screening may largely be ineffective.

Hearing screenings have evolved as a viable method for identifying older individuals with hearing loss. The goal of any screening program is to reach as large a proportion of the target population as possible (American Academy of Audiology, 1991). Hearing screenings are conducted in a variety of settings including health fairs, physicians' offices, nursing facilities, community health programs, and homes. However, the methods used to screen for hearing impairment and the criteria for referral to audiology are variable. Consequently, a variety of hearing screening protocols have evolved with varying degrees of success. A discussion of various screenings methods follows.

Traditionally, hearing screenings have consisted of pass/fail pure-tone audiometric tasks. A criterion level is determined, and the patient who responds at this level passes; the patient who does not respond fails and is referred for further testing. For the screening to be effective, the criterion level must be chosen so that those who pass are not experiencing communication problems due to hearing loss. Those who fail, on the other hand, should be those who will benefit from follow-up testing and rehabilitative services.

Pure-tone screenings can be done using a calibrated audiometer in a sound-treated room or using a portable audiometer or a hand-held audiometer in a quiet environment. The Audioscope, an otoscope with a built-in audiometer, delivers pure tones at 500 Hz, 1000 Hz, 2000 Hz, and 4000 Hz at one of three intensity levels. Overall accuracy for the Audioscope has been reported to be between 75 and 80% (Bienvenue et al., 1985; Frank and Peterson, 1987).

The selection of an effective criterion level for use with the elderly imposes an interesting dilemma. Unlike young children, all of whom have intense communicative demands placed on them by the need for language acquisition and successful education, hearing handicap for the elderly is not easily predictable from pure-tone thresholds alone. An older individual may be working or retired, may be socially active, and may live with family, in a retirement community, in a nursing home, or alone. These lifestyle factors will affect the degree of hearing loss that the individual will be able to cope with before the loss affects the ability to communicate successfully. In reviewing literature related to the issue of selecting a criterion level, Schow (1991) suggests that a 40-dB HL screening level at 1000 and 2000 Hz may be appropriate for elderly persons living in an institutional setting.

Lowering the criterion level to 25 dB HL, as is commonly used when younger adults are screened, causes concern for overreferrals. A single criterion level for pure-tone screening cannot take into account the variability within the elderly population, which has an impact on determining the communicative needs of the elderly individual.

An alternative or adjunct to pure-tone screening with the elderly is the screening self-assessment inventory. These screening scales are designed to separate those who perceive themselves as having communication problems resulting from their hearing loss from those who do not. The Hearing Handicap Inventory for the Elderly Screening Version (HHIE-S) (Ventry and Weinstein, 1982, 1983; see Attachments 22 and 23) and the Self-Assessment of Communication (SAC) (see Attachment 1) (Schow and Nerbonne, 1977) were suggested in proposed ASHA Guidelines (1996) as examples of tools for screening hearing handicap in the elderly population. The ASHA Guidelines state that the choice of the instrument to be used should be based on the population to be screened. However, the SAC purportedly can be used with individuals from 20 to 80 years of age, whereas the HHIE-S was standardized on individuals

age 65 years or older. Consequently, a choice between the HHIE-S and SAC must be made when screening the elderly population. Lee and McCarthy (1991) investigated whether differences exist between these two inventories in their ability to screen hearing handicap in individuals age 65 years or older. Results of this study showed no significant differences between the HHIE-S and the SAC. Schow et al. (1990) compared these two inventories using large groups of young and elderly adults. Test predictive measures such as sensitivity, specificity, positive predictive value (PPV), and negative predictive value (NPV) were examined when pure-tone findings were used as a criterion measure. Results of this study suggested that the overall efficiency of the SAC was slightly higher than that of the HHIE-S. However, Schow et al. (1990) concluded that the SAC and the HHIE-S perform very similarly, even though the SAC was standardized on a broad age range and the HHIE-S was standardized on the elderly. Furthermore, Frank et al. (1989) reported a high correlation (0.918) between the HHIE-S and the SAC.

Although there are no significant differences between these two inventories in screening hearing handicap, qualitative differences may exist. For example, the response format of the HHIE-S may be more suitable for the elderly population. The yes/no/sometimes format of the HHIE-S may be easier and less-time consuming than the five-point multiple-choice format of the SAC for some older individuals. This may be particularly true if the inventory is administered face-to-face rather than as a paper-and-pencil screening tool.

Lichtenstein et al. (1988) evaluated the utility of the HHIE-S as a tool for screening hearing loss. They compared HHIE-S results from 178 elderly subjects with audiometric results obtained during the same visit. The diagnostic performance of the HHIE-S was compared against five different definitions of hearing loss. They found that the HHIE-S is a valid, robust screening tool for identifying hearing-impaired elderly irrespective of the audiometric definition used.

Sangster et al. (1991) screened the hearing of ambulatory patients older than 65 years who were patients in a family practice. They compared the effectiveness of the HHIE-S versus a Welch-Allyn Audioscope. They found both screening tests to be important in detection of hearing impairment. A subset of subjects had been previous hearing aid users. These subjects were referred to an audiology clinic and agreed to have their hearing aids analyzed. Of the 11 subjects wearing hearing aids, 10 were found to either require a new device or a significant modification to their existing hearing aids.

Jupiter (1989) used both a pure-tone task and a self-assessment scale (HHIE-S) in a screening protocol. She found that based on the HHIE-S, 36.2% of the elderly screened fell into referral priority categories, whereas 66% failed a pure-tone screening. When comparing a group screened using both the pure-tone task and HHIE-S to a group screened using only a pure-tone task, equal percentages were referred for follow-up. Of those referred for follow-up from either group, most who chose to proceed (approximately 30% of those who failed) went to physicians for follow-up. Few of these were seen for further testing or obtained a hearing aid. Use of other rehabilitative services was not surveyed. These findings suggest the need for greater education for older patients failing a hearing screening. Patients should be informed of audiologic services and the potential benefits of amplification. Clearly, a hearing screening program for the elderly can be considered successful only if it ultimately leads to appropriate rehabilitation.

Typically, the hearing of elderly patients in long-term care facilities is screened by nursing personnel as part of admissions or in-take physical examinations. Assessment of auditory function, however, is often limited to a single question during the patient interview (Newman, 1990). Unfortunately, nonaudiologists in health care often fail to recognize hearing loss as a problem that needs assessment and rehabilitation in aging people (Salomon, 1986). Given this scenario, Newman (1990) looked at the feasibility of nurses administering a hearing screening test. A screening tool, the Hearing Assessment Test (HAT), was developed to be administered by nurses to elderly patients at bedside. The HAT consisted of four sections: self-assessment items, a word discrimination task, a sound identification test, and an observation checklist. Although the HAT is in need of further validity and reliability testing, results of this study suggest this it is a potentially useful tool for nurses to use in identify elderly patients with hearing impairment. Tolson (1997) suggests that nurses can make a measurable contribution to identification of hearing impairment through the implementation of relatively simple, low-cost procedures. Of course, identification of hearing loss through any screening program must be followed by appropriate audiologic referral, diagnostic, and rehabilitative processes.

The case for development of a systematic audiometric screening of all nursing home residents was made by Voeks et al. (1990) in their study of hearing assessment practices in nursing homes. To determine whether audiometric screenings duplicated the observations of other medical personnel, audiometric results for each resident were compared with the nursing and physician assessments. Nurses' observations of hearing status were either "good" or "impaired," and physicians' observations were either "within normal limits" or "impaired." Results indicated that 16% of nursing home residents with significant hearing loss (PTA > 40 dB HL) were not identified using either the nursing or physician assessments. Furthermore, 76% of patients admitted to nursing homes were at risk or significantly hearing impaired, and 60% complained of hearing difficulties during daily activities. The authors concluded that because standard practice fails to identify many individuals in need of hearing health care, a systematic audiometric screening program should be instituted. Moreover, the authors contend that when more than three-fourths of the individuals in an institution share the same disability, institutional policy should be directed toward accommodating the disability in question.

Jupiter and DiStasio (1998) used the HHIE-S as a substitute for pure-tone screening to initiate hearing health care with the homebound elderly population. They found that pure-tone sensitivity correlated most highly with the situational subscale of the HHIE-S. Given that this population of aging individuals is typically underserved by audiologists, the authors conclude that the HHIE-S is a reasonable approach to identifying those in need of further audiologic services.

The ideal screening protocol appears to be the use of both a pure-tone screen and a hearing handicap scale. Because there often is a disparity between hearing impairment and hearing handicap, combining the two techniques may increase the overall accuracy of the screening program (Lichtenstein et al., 1988). Finally, the ultimate goal of any screening program should not be forgotten. Individuals identified through screening programs should be referred to an audiologist for a thorough audiologic evaluation and audiologic rehabilitation (American Academy of Audiology, 1991). Identification of hearing loss in the aging population is only the first step.

USE OF HEARING HANDICAP INVENTORIES WITH ELDERLY LISTENERS

The use of inventories to assess the subjective aspects of hearing loss has become a well-accepted methodology in the past decade. In fact, self-report inventories and scales have become the tool of choice in measuring handicap, hearing aid benefit, satisfaction, and outcome in general. A plethora of self-report tools have merged with various formats, purposes, target populations, and psychometric properties. The reader is referred to Chapter 18 for an excellent discussion of these instruments in outcome measurement.

The handicapping effects of hearing impairment extend not only to the person with hearing loss, but also to his or her communication partners. As such, the perceptions of family members and significant others are important to the success of the audiologic

rehabilitation process. Attempts to quantify the perceptions of family members and significant others have typically shown a disparity in the degree of handicap reported (Schow and Nerbonne, 1977; McCarthy and Alpiner, 1983; Newman and Weinstein, 1986). In fact, Chmiel and Jerger (1993) found that older hearing-impaired persons tended to rate themselves as less handicapped than did their significant others. These results underscore the importance of inclusion of family members and/or significant others in the rehabilitation process. A better understanding of the extent of the communication problems of the individual can lead to more effective intervention, thus ensuring more success in rehabilitation.

Evaluating the effects of hearing loss on communicative and psychosocial function is imperative before planning and conducting a rehabilitative program. This is no less true for older listeners than for younger listeners, but the instrument selected should be appropriate for the individual being served. Hearing handicap scales have been specifically designed for use with elderly patients, and others have been developed through modification of existing questionnaires. In general, inventories for the elderly tend to use fewer items, most notably omitting vocational questions. Fewer response choices are used for each item to simplify administration. Face-to-face presentation is often recommended rather than the more traditional paper-and-pencil format (Weinstein et al., 1986). A review of these scales highlights the unique qualities of each of these instruments for the elderly (see Chapter 18 for further discussion of these tools as outcome measures).

One of the first scales designed specifically for the older population was the Denver Scale of Communication Function for Senior Citizens Living in Retirement Centers (Attachment 18). J.M. Zarnoch and J.G. Alpiner (The Denver scale of communication function for senior citizens living in retirement centers. Unpublished study, 1977) modified the original Denver Scale of Communication Function for use with older individuals. It was designed for presentation through an individual interview, because self-scoring scales often are not feasible with older persons. This scale consists of seven major questions covering the topics of family, emotions, other persons, general communication, self-concept, group situations, and rehabilitation. These are scored by a plus (yes) or minus (no). Under each main question are a "probe effect" and an "exploration effect." The probe effect attempts to specify the problem areas related to the general question. The exploration effect determines how applicable the general question is to the individual. This aspect of the scale helps to eliminate questions that are irrelevant to the individual and consequently unnecessary in establishing goals for aural rehabilitation. A scoring form is included to help in interpretation of the responses. This scale does not provide norms or group comparisons. Rather, it allows the individual to provide his or her communication performance before and after any rehabilitative procedures.

Kaplan et al. (1978) also modified the Denver Scale of Communication Function (DSCF) for use with older individuals. To make the DSCF more usable for older people living in retirement settings or with their families, several basic modifications were made. First, the interview technique was adopted. Second, the seven-point scale was reduced to five points with each point defined for the patient. Third, all items concerned with vocation were eliminated, because most older persons are not employed. Fourth, the "family" category was changed to "peer and family attitudes," because many older people do not live with their families. Fifth, the "self" and "socialization" categories were combined into one category aimed at probing degrees and feelings of participation in social activities. Finally, a new category, "specific difficult listening situations," was added. Although the DSCF-Modified (Attachment 19) was found to be reliable when using group data, individual test-retest reliability was variable. Therefore, the authors caution against using the scale as a premanagement or postmanagement evaluation tool.

The unique problems of the elderly living in nursing homes are the focus of the Nursing Home Hearing Handicap Index (NHHI) developed by Schow and Nerbonne (1977) (Attachment 20). The 20-item scale is divided into two sections titled "self" and "staff." The premise of the NHHI is that input from both of these sources is superior to either one alone. Both sections can be administered as a paper-and-pencil test. A five-point rating scale for each item is used. In evaluating the scale, the authors found that the staff members' ratings of hearing handicap correlated much better with the pure-tone average than did the residents' self-perception scores. They concluded that staff members were probably more objective observers of residents' hearing difficulties. However, that there was a discrepancy between the ratings may be of rehabilitative value. Therefore, this scale may provide information for treatment planning that includes nursing home staff in-service education.

Alpiner and Baker (1981) developed the Communications Assessment Procedure for Seniors (CAPS) (Attachment 21). It attempts to evaluate communication status in terms of both attitudes and specific communication situations. CAPS enables the clinician to evaluate subjectively how a person living in an extended care facility reacts to his or her hearing loss. Questions are included for five communication areas: general communication, group situations, other persons, self-concept, and family. A final section is included to determine if an individual is interested in and could benefit from remediation. CAPS is also an interview-type scale and is interpreted subjectively.

One of the best-designed and most widely researched assessment instruments is the HHIE by Ventry and Weinstein (1982) (Attachment 22). This scale was developed to assess the social and emotional effects of hearing impairment in the noninstitutionalized older person. The HHIE is composed of an emotional and a social/situational subscale. It was standardized on 100 noninstitutionalized individuals older than 65 years of age. It was found to be highly reliable and contains a high degree of content validity.

Scoring involves "yes" (4 points), "sometimes" (2 points), and "no" or "not applicable" (0 points). The total score can range from 0 to 100, wherein the higher the score, the greater the self-assessed hearing handicap. This scale can be administered in either a face-to-face or a paper-and-pencil format (Newman and Weinstein, 1989). The HHIE-S is the screening version of the scale and consists of five emotional items and five social/situational items (Attachment 23). Statistical analysis suggests this short form is of comparable reliability and validity to the long form.

One of the most exciting uses for the HHIE and HHIE-S is in the area of assessing hearing aid benefit. Weinstein et al. (1986) determined that the 95% confidence interval for change on the HHIE is 18%. In a pre/postintervention comparison, a change of 18% can therefore be considered significant clinically. In group studies, Newman and Weinstein (1988) and Malinoff and Weinstein (1989) assessed hearing handicap among elderly clients before hearing aid fitting and again after hearing aid fitting. Newman and Weinstein found that after 1 year of hearing aid use, the perception of hearing handicap as measured by the HHIE was significantly reduced. Malinoff and Weinstein assessed benefit following 3 weeks, 3 months, and 1 year of hearing aid use. They found that after 3 weeks of hearing aid use, a sharp reduction in hearing handicap occurred. Perception of handicap increased between 3 weeks and 3 months but still represented a significant improvement over the pre-fit scores. The perception of handicap remained stable between 3 months and 1 year. These findings suggest that the typical return visit by the new hearing aid user after 2 to 3 weeks of hearing aid use may not be sufficient to monitor the elderly client's long-term adjustment to and success with amplification. Additional follow-up at longer intervals may allow the audiologist to provide the elderly client with further rehabilitation once the perceived benefit from the hearing aid has stabilized. Further discussion of hearing aid benefit with the aging population is presented in Chapter 18.

The HHIE-S, being a shorter scale, requires less time for the audiologist to administer and for the elderly patient to complete. To determine whether the HHIE-S also could be used to assess hearing aid benefit, Newman et al. (1991) administered this scale to new hearing aid users before hearing aid fitting and 3 weeks after hearing aid fitting. They established a 95% confidence interval of 9.3 points on the HHIE-S as indicating true change from the pre-fit to post-fit scores. They found significant reductions in perceived handicap on both the emotional and social/situational subscales of the HHIE-S after 3 weeks of hearing aid use.

These studies suggest that self-assessment inventories are viable tools to be used to measure hearing aid outcome. Because providing amplification is the cornerstone of effective audiologic rehabilitation, it is important that success with hearing aids be measured and documented (McCarthy, 1990). Therefore, use of self-assessment inventories in measuring hearing aid benefit is recommended for use with the geriatric population.

HEARING AIDS

Technology versus use

As discussed in Chapter 11, advances in hearing aid technology and hearing aid fitting practices have revolutionized our ability to select amplification for hearing-impaired patients. Despite these advances, however, hearing aids continue to be underused by the hearing-impaired elderly population. Various studies generally report that less than one-fourth of older potential candidates for amplification actually have hearing aids (Ward et al., 1993; Popelka et al., 1998).

Fino et al. (1992) looked at audiometric data, hearing aid status, and follow-up from 178 elderly individuals who had been screened in primary care facilities. Eighty-three of these individuals (47%) were considered candidates for amplification. Of the 83 hearing aid candidates, 58 simply opted not to obtain amplification. Of the remaining 25 elderly hearing-impaired patients, 14 already owned a hearing aid, and only 1 purchased a hearing aid as a result of audiologic recommendations. In all, 67% of the elderly hearing-impaired patients who were considered candidates for amplification chose not to obtain a hearing aid. Commonly reported reasons for elderly individuals choosing not to obtain a hearing aid include concerns regarding cost, amplification of background noise, fear of drawing attention to a hearing handicap, deceptive dealer practices, and where to obtain a hearing aid (Franks and Beckman, 1985; Fino et al., 1992).

The negative stigma associated with hearing aid use, labeled the "hearing aid effect," has been reported in several studies (Blood et al., 1977; Johnson et al., 1982). In their study of the hearing aid effect in older women, Doggett et al. (1998) found that older women perceived their aided peers significantly more negatively than their unaided peers when rating measures of confidence, intelligence, and friendliness. As the 20th century closes, it is frustrating that although amplification technology has made tremendous strides, social attitudes toward hearing aid use are changing very slowly.

Amplification and quality of life

The data on hearing aid use and satisfaction raise important issues for the rehabilitative audiologist who works with the geriatric population. How can we predict which elderly patients will use hearing aids and which will not? How can we improve the rate of success and the level of satisfaction for elderly hearing aid users? How can older persons with hearing loss be convinced of the auditory and quality-of-life benefits that often accompany amplification?

If hearing impairment can indeed contribute to a reduction in quality of life as discussed earlier in this chapter, then it could be hypothesized that amplification and audiologic rehabilitation should help restore quality of life diminished by hearing impairment. Bridges and Bentler (1998) investigated this notion in their study of the relationship between successful hearing aid use and a sense of "well-being" in older subjects

as measured by the Geriatric Depression Scale and the Satisfaction with Life Scale. Results suggested that subjects who reported no hearing loss indicated significantly less depression than those older subjects with hearing loss. Older subjects who had not been successful hearing aid users showed significantly higher depression than the successful hearing aid users. Most importantly, successful hearing aid users reported higher ratings of life satisfaction than the unsuccessful users. These results underscore the contribution of hearing aids to improving the general well-being of the older person with hearing loss. Thus, the authors believe that hearing aids should be viewed as a necessary part of good health care rather than as an elective.

In a large-scale study of older male veterans, Mulrow et al. (1990) studied the impact of hearing aids on quality of life. Subjects were assigned to either a hearing aid fitting group or a waiting list group. Each subject was given the HHIE, the Quantified Denver Scale of Communication Function, the Short Portable Mental Status Questionnaire, the Geriatric Depression Scale, and the Self-Evaluation of Life Function. Subjects who were fitted with hearing aids showed significant improvements on the HHIE and the Quantified Denver Scale compared with subjects without amplification. Mulrow et al. concluded that hearing aids are effective in reversing social, emotional, and communication dysfunction that accompany hearing impairment.

Chmiel and Jerger (1996) investigated the extent to which the presence of CAPD limited hearing aid benefit in older hearing-impaired persons. The HHIE was used to measure a reduction in hearing handicap as a result of hearing aid use. Older subjects without central auditory disorders obtained a significant improvement in HHIE scores after 6 weeks of hearing aid use. In subjects who had not performed well with a dichotic listening task (Dichotic Sentence Identification Test), average HHIE scores did not change significantly after hearing aid use. The authors suggest that these results affirm the value of amplification as having a positive value in reducing hearing handicap. However, as discussed earlier in this chapter, the negative impact of central auditory disorder may undermine the value of amplification.

For the elderly individual with a mild to moderate hearing loss, the level of perceived hearing handicap is a factor in determining candidacy, once again highlighting the usefulness of hearing handicap scales with the elderly population. In looking at elderly individuals after they had obtained amplification, Nabelek et al. (1991) identified three groups: full-time hearing aid users, part-time hearing aid users, and nonusers. They compared them with each other and with an elderly normal hearing group and a young normal hearing group. Unaided, under headphones, the subjects listened to a story and were asked to set the highest intensity of various background noises that they could "put up with." The full-time users tolerated a lower signal-to-noise ratio with music as the background noise than any other group. With speech-spectrum noise, the full-time users tolerated more noise than the part-time users and nonusers. Overall, the full-time hearing aid users were more tolerant of relatively high noise levels. Because these measures were made after hearing aid fitting, the predictive ability of these measures cannot be addressed. Additionally, the HHIE was given to the hearing-impaired subjects. No significant differences on hearing handicap were found among the full-time, part-time, and nonusers as measured by the HHIE. Comparing perceptions of hearing handicap without amplification and with amplification using the HHIE, only the full-time users demonstrated a significant reduction of handicap with the hearing aid. These data suggest that there may be a relationship between the ability to tolerate background noise and hearing aid benefit.

Although not all older patients may experience a dramatic improvement in quality of life as a result of amplification, data from these studies suggest that for many older people improved communication translates into improved quality of life. Further research is needed to establish the relationship

between the psychosocial consequences of hearing impairment and the effects of rehabilitative intervention (see Chapter 18 for a comprehensive discussion of outcome measures and audiologic rehabilitation).

Hearing aid counseling and follow-up

Ultimately, orientation and counseling are the keys to successful hearing aid use by the older individual. Without adequate orientation and follow-up, a hearing aid is much more likely to be rejected. As with all hearing aid counseling, time must be spent discussing hearing aid parts and function; rehearsing hearing aid insertion and removal, battery changing procedures, and manipulation of the controls; and emphasizing realistic expectations for the benefits and limitations of the hearing aid. The client who expects more than the hearing aid alone can achieve will be a dissatisfied hearing aid owner. Additional counseling regarding adjustment to amplification should be stressed. The counseling should be tailored to the unique listening needs, skills, and strategies of the individual.

The greatest difference in counseling and follow-up between older and younger hearing aid purchasers is in the time that will need to be allotted to the task. Smedley and Schow (1990) recommend a minimum of three follow-up visits within the first month after fitting an elderly patient with a hearing aid. This schedule will allow the audiologist to repeat vital information and will allow the new hearing aid owner to rehearse hearing aid care skills with needed supervision and reinforcement. The goal for the elderly hearing-impaired user is to master the skills necessary to use the hearing aid and to develop a thorough understanding of how to use the aid and what to expect from it. Almost all elderly individuals will be able to learn to use a hearing aid independently, but many will require a longer time to master the necessary skills and information.

In cases in which hearing aid use will require assistance, a significant other must also be trained. The individual chosen must be someone who is regularly available to assist the patient. This may be the spouse or other family member. In a nursing home, these tasks will fall within the duties of staff members. Because of high turnover rates in institutional settings and reassignments within a nursing home, frequent, periodic in-services may be necessary to ensure that the hearing-impaired patient will be able to use his or her hearing aid consistently. The need for these follow-up services within the nursing home is clear. Thibodeau and Schmitt (1988) found that 72% of hearing aids in a sample of nursing homes and retirement centers were malfunctioning, with dead/weak batteries and clogged vents and sound openings composing the majority of the problems. Clearly, the importance of in-service education of nursing home personnel cannot be overemphasized.

GROUP THERAPY

Although group therapy is not a new concept in audiology, audiologists are increasingly finding it an effective strategy for working with older hearing-impaired individuals after they have been fit with amplification. Many audiologists are offering group sessions that focus not only on rehabilitation, but also on hearing health education for both the hearing aid user and his or her family. Group sessions serve the purpose of offering rehabilitation strategies for effective communication, providing information about hearing loss and hearing aids, and offering a "support group" atmosphere with older hearing-impaired peers.

Kricos (1997) views organized group sessions as an opportunity for "a collaborative problem-solving orientation to working with the hearing-impaired elderly." In particular, she reports that group sessions can be an effective means for the audiologist to work with new hearing aid users and their families to identify problems and find solutions. She feels the peer support and inclusion of family/significant others are the advantages of this approach to audiologic rehabilitation.

Further support for the effectiveness of group therapy is provided in Northern's study of the effect of audiologic rehabilita-

tion after hearing aid fittings (Northern and Beyer, 1999). In a large-scale study of new hearing aid wearers, Northern compared the return rate of new users who had completed a series of group rehabilitation sessions with the return rate of new users who did not attend these sessions. Of the 7187 new hearing aids users in this study, 4107 chose not to attend a postfitting audiologic rehabilitation class, and 3080 attended at least one of three classes offered. The hearing aid return rate for those who attended follow-up rehabilitation sessions was only 3%; the rate for new users who did not attend these sessions was 9%. Further, national data suggest that return rates for hearing aids may be as high 12 to 24%. These data underscore the importance of audiologic rehabilitation following the hearing aid fitting. Furthermore, these results serve to remind us that the hearing aid fitting is only the first step in the rehabilitation process.

TREATMENT EFFICACY

In Chapter 18, Weinstein presents a comprehensive review of outcome methodology and research in rehabilitative audiology. To a large extent, much of the outcome research has focused on hearing aids and follow-up rehabilitation programs. Traditional audiologic treatment strategies have not been the focus of most outcome research studies. A well-done study by Kricos and Holmes (1996), however, specifically focused on the efficacy of such traditional methods as analytic auditory training and active listening training with older hearing-impaired adults. They were not able to document the efficacy of analytic auditory training for older adults with hearing handicap but did find the use of an active listening approach was effective for improving audiovisual speech recognition in noise. This study represents a well-designed, initial effort to determine the efficacy of the rehabilitation methods espoused since the beginning of the 20th century. In the 21st century, more studies examining the efficacy of our methods will be necessary and possibly mandated. The reader is referred to Chapter 18 for further discussion on this topic.

Innovative Service Delivery

TELEHEALTH

Given the technology explosion and the dramatically changing state of health care policy in the United States, it is not surprising that traditional service delivery is giving way to innovative delivery models. Cost, access, and distance have triggered an increase in alternative sites for delivering services to the elderly (Weinstein and Clark, 1989). Consequently, health care services not previously available in rural, remote areas are becoming increasingly available through telecommunications technology. Service delivery in the home has also become a viable option.

Advances in telecommunications have allowed the concept of telemedicine to evolve into a fast-growing reality. As more and more health care providers participate in this type of health care, the term telemedicine has been broadened to "telehealth." Any doubts about the future of telehealth were erased with passage of the 1997 Comprehensive Telehealth Act. The federal law funds Medicare reimbursement for professional teleconsultants to beneficiaries living in rural areas with shortages of health professionals (Goldberg, 1997).

The possibilities for engaging in telehealth by audiologists and speech-language pathologists are vast. Although the opportunities for consultation and direct patient care will depend on the technology available, the impetus to acquire the technology will be great. Reducing travel costs and making health care accessible and affordable will be behind this growing delivery model. Given the active participation of the federal government to date, it is probable that third-party reimbursers will follow suit in reimbursing for these services. Goldberg (1997) suggests that modification of digital hearing aids over the telephone represents an area of telehealth that may become commonplace with audiologists in the future. The possibilities seem endless: post-hearing aid rehabilitation sessions, reprogramming of hearing aids, and patient education appear to be possible aspects of telehealth

for hearing-impaired individuals in underserved, remote areas.

HOME HEALTH CARE

Another delivery model not typically considered by audiologists is home health care. Speech-language pathologists have developed a successful delivery model for the provision of in-home services to patients with neurogenic speech and language disorders due to strokes and traumatic brain injury. In fact, the American Speech-Language-Hearing Association Task Force on Home Care (1986) characterized home health care as the most dynamic segment in health care in the 1980s. They provided four reasons for the growth of home care. First, it is a response to the rapidly expanding elderly population. Second, there is pressure on hospitals to decrease costs by reducing length of stay and limiting the number of beds. Third, there is a strong consumer need or preference for receiving services within the home. Fourth, government agencies and private businesses are stressing cost-containment in health care. This task force stressed that given the unique characteristics of the home, speech-language pathologists and audiologists need to work with the family and other professionals to ensure continuity of patient care. Indeed, Selker (1987) states that home care requires adaptation of treatment regimens and training of caregivers/family members to ensure proper care.

Although home health care in general is not new, its growth in the past 10 years has been phenomenal. Waldo et al. (1985) estimate that the average annual growth rate of the home care industry in recent years has been 20 to 25%. For example, in 1961 there were only 208 agencies in the United States providing home care; in 1990, there were an estimated 12,000 to 14,000 providers (Applebaum and Phillips, 1990).

Unfortunately, as the home health care trend continues to grow and become more profitable for health care providers, audiologists are somewhat hesitant to engage in this model because of the past. The specter of the door-to-door hearing aid salesperson of 40 years ago colors our perception of home health care. Whether it was deserved or not, hearing aid dealers who went door to door often developed unscrupulous reputations. Therefore, audiologists may think there is a negative stigma associated with the provision of audiologic services in the home. In the new millennium, hearing home health care may represent an excellent alternative for many hearing-impaired older individuals, especially those with mobility problems. The accuracy of diagnostic and hearing aid evaluations performed in the home may be questionable. However, given insert earphones and portable equipment, some of these obstacles can be eliminated (Kirkwood, 1995). Further, hearing aid fittings and orientations as well as audiologic rehabilitation could be conducted ideally in the patient's home. Indeed, the face validity of these procedures might increase greatly if rehabilitative decisions and planning were done in the patient's own communication environment. As the home health care industry grows, audiologists must overcome resistance to offering services in the patient's home and develop appropriate models for effective delivery of a full range of audiologic rehabilitation services in that environment.

COMPUTERS AND THE INTERNET

In Chapter 17, computer applications to rehabilitative audiology are discussed in-depth. In the elderly, however, some questions about "computer phobia" and access to technology linger. Can older individuals who are experiencing so many aging changes use a computer to assist in their own rehabilitation? As Baby Boomers become Senior Boomers, can audiologists afford not to use computers and cyber resources? What role will computers and the Internet play in audiologic rehabilitation in the future?

Hurvitz and Goldojarb (1988) attempted to answer the first question by comparing two methods of providing audiologic re-

habilitation to elderly residents of a Veterans Administration nursing home. Subjects were assigned to one of three groups. The first group received a six-lesson audiologic rehabilitation program presented on an Apple IIC computer with a color display monitor. Lessons were designed to be user-friendly, and only a few keystrokes were required. Topics included mechanisms of the ear, audiograms, management of hearing problems, speechreading, hearing aids, and communication skills training. Group two also had a six-lesson program covering the same material, but it was led by an instructor. A third group served as a control group and received no therapy. The effectiveness of the methods was measured by administering a 25-question pre/post-test to each subject. Questions required remembering specific information and giving problem-solving answers to situational questions. Results showed that both the first and second groups achieved significantly higher performance after instruction than did the third group. No significant difference was found between the first and second groups' performances.

The authors of this study concluded that each method of offering audiologic rehabilitation was valuable and offered unique advantages. Whereas the class offered greater opportunity for support and socialization, the computer-assisted method allowed each subject to proceed through the material at his or her own pace. In addition, an audiologist was not required to be present while subjects were working on the computer.

Perhaps an even more important finding of this study relates to the fact that elderly nursing home residents were successful with user-friendly software. Moreover, they were able to learn via this method. These encouraging results suggest that audiologists should not make presumptions about their older patients' facility with technology.

Answers to the second and third questions posed above are already being answered. The number of computer and Internet users continues to increase. The availability of information about hearing loss, hearing aids, and audiologic rehabilitation currently available on the Internet is already limitless. In a search of available audiologic rehabilitation resources on the Internet, Wojcik (1999) found a wealth of information available to the hearing-impaired consumer using a simple key word approach. Using such key words as hearing loss, hard of hearing, hearing aids, and hearing impaired, Wojcik was able to find Websites that provided information spanning such topics as anatomy of the ear, how to read your hearing test, everything you want to know about hearing aids, and support groups for people with hearing impairment. Wojcik suggests two approaches to online rehabilitative audiology. With a clinician-structured approach, the audiologist compiles an individualized database for the patient, considering the sophistication and needs of the user. Instructions and a sample printout of a Webpage are provided. The database can be tailored to include Websites with such diverse topics as travel tips for persons with hearing impairment or using cellular telephones with hearing aids. With the client-structured approach, the patient is provided with a comprehensive database from which he or she can choose appropriate Websites of interest. This approach may be most appropriate for the individual with some computer and Internet experience.

In the recent experience of the authors, once seniors are exposed to computers and the Internet, they embrace the technology with enthusiasm. We have observed seniors who are fascinated with the Internet and use it for information retrieval and pleasure. An increasing number of our patients bring us information about hearing and hearing aids that they found on the Web! It could be argued that access is limited only to those seniors with the income to afford computers. This increasingly is not the case. More and more libraries are on-line and make Internet access available to all library patrons. Even "cyber coffee shops" offer the chance for seniors to surf the net. Audiologists will be remiss in not using computers and the Internet as resources in rehabilitation planning in the near future. Audiologists should be prepared to direct their aging patients to Websites that will provide patient education and information.

Summary

The underlying premise of this chapter has been that hearing health care delivery can be improved if the effects of aging are known, understood, respected, and incorporated into the rehabilitation process. As the aging population continues to expand in the 21st century, indeed as we all become part of it, quality services that meet the unique needs of the elderly will be demanded. Survival of audiology as a profession may, in large part, be dependent on how we respond to meeting the rehabilitative needs of the growing elderly hearing-impaired population in the 21st century.

REFERENCES

Alpiner JG, Baker B. Communication assessment procedures in the aural rehabilitation process. Semin Speech Lang Hear 1981;2:189–204.

Amenedo E, Diaz F. Automatic and effortful process in auditory memory reflected by even-related potentials: age-related findings. Electroencephalogr Clin Neurophysiol 1998;108:361–369.

American Academy of Audiology. Position statement: aged persons with hearing impairment. Audiol Today 1991;6:3.

American Nurses Association. Position statements: polypharmacy and the older adult. http://www.ana.org, 1997.

American Speech-Language-Hearing Association. Guidelines for audiologic screening, 1996.

American Speech-Language-Hearing Association. The delivery of speech-language and audiology services in home care. ASHA 1986;28:49–52.

American Speech-Language-Hearing Association. Guidelines on audiology service delivery in nursing homes. 1997.

Applebaum R, Phillips P. Assuring the quality of in-home care: the "other" challenge for long-term care. Gerontologist 1990;30:444–450.

Atchley R. Social forces and aging. Belmont CA: Wadsworth, 1988.

Axelrod S, Cohen LD. Senescence and embedded-figure performance in vision and touch. Percept Psychophysiol 1961;12:283–288.

Bai U, Seidman M, Hinojosa R, et al. Mitochondrial DNA deletions associated with aging and possibly presbycusis: a human temporal bone study. Am J Otol 1997;18:449–453.

Barr RA, Giambra LM. Age-related decrement in selective attention. Psychol Aging 1990;5:597–599.

Basowitz H, Korchin SJ. Age differences in the perception of closure. J Abnorm Soc Psychol 1957;54:93–97.

Belgrave L, Lavin B, Breslau N, et al. Stereotyping of the aged by medical students. Gerontol Geriatr Educ 1982;3:37–44.

Bergman M, Blumenfeld V, Cascardo D, et al. Age-related decrement in hearing for speech: sampling and longitudinal studies. J Gerontol 1976;31:533–538.

Bess F, Townsend T. Word discrimination for listeners with flat sensorineural hearing losses. J Speech Hear Disord 1977;42:232–237.

Bess F, Lichtenstein J, Logan S, et al. Hearing impairment as a determinant of function in the elderly. J Am Geriatr Soc 1989;37:123–128.

Bienvenue GR, Michael PL, Chaffinch JC, et al. The audioscope: a clinical tool for otoscopic and audiometric examination. Ear Hear 1985;6:251–254.

Blackwell B. The drug defaulter. Clin Pharmacol Ther 1972;13:841.

Blood G, Blood I, Danhauer J. The hearing aid "effect." Hear Instr 1977;28:12.

Bolles RC. Theory of motivation. New York: Harper & Row, 1967.

Botwinick J. Aging and behavior. New York: Springer, 1978.

Botwinick J. Aging and behavior: a comprehensive integration of research findings. 3rd ed. New York: Springer, 1984.

Botwinick J, Brinley J. Aspects of RT set during brief intervals in relation to age, sex and set. J Gerontol 1962;17:295–301.

Botwinick J, Thompson J. Practice of speeded response in relation to age, sex, and set. J Gerontol 1967;22:72–76.

Braithwaite R. The pharmacokinetics of psychotropic drugs in the elderly. In: Wheatly D, ed. Psychopharmacology of old age. New York: Oxford University Press, 1982.

Bridges JA, Bentler RA. Relating hearing aid use to well-being among older adults. Hearing J 1998; 51:39–44.

Bruckner R. Longitudinal research on the eye. Gerontol Clin 1967;9:87–95.

Canestri R. Paced and self-paced learning in young and elderly adults. J Gerontol 1963;18:165–168.

Caspary DM, Milbrandt JC, Helfert RH. Central auditory aging: GABA changes in the inferior colliculus. Exp Gerontol 1995;30:349–360.

Cherry K, Morton M. Drug sensitivity in older adults: the role of physiologic and pharmacokinetic factors. Int J Aging Hum Dev 1989;28:159–174.

Chmiel R, Jerger J. Some factors affecting assessment of hearing handicap in the elderly. J Am Audiol 1993;4:249–257.

Chmiel R, Jerger J. Hearing aid use, central auditory disorder and hearing handicap in elderly persons. J Am Acad Audiol 1996;7:190–202.

Cluff L. Chronic disease, function and quality care. J Gerontol 1981;34:299.

Cooper JW. Community and nursing home drug monitoring guidelines—1993. Watkinsville, GA: Consultant Press, 1993.

Cooper JW. Drug related problems in the elderly patient. http://www.scn.org/hsw-cgi/m2n.pl/fp/senior/Info.files/caregiving/drugs, 1994.

Cooper JC, Gates GA. Hearing in the elderly: the Framington cohort, 1983–1985: Part II. Prevalence of central auditory processing disorder. Ear Hear 1991;12:304–311.

Corso JF. Sensory processes and age effects in normal adults. J Gerontol 1971;260:90–105.

Craik FIM. Age difference in human memory. In: Birren JE, Schaie KW, eds. Handbook of the psychology of aging. New York: Van Nostrand Reinhold, 1977.

Dillon H, James A, Ginis J. Client oriented scale of improvement (COSI) and its relationship to several other

measures of benefit and satisfaction provided by hearing aids. J Am Acad Audiol 1997;8:27–43.

Dobie RA. Separating noise-induced from age-related hearing loss. West J Med 1994;160:564–565.

Doggett S, Stein R, Gans D. Hearing aid effect in older females. J Am Acad Audiol 1998;9:361–366.

Dubno JR, Lee F, Matthews LJ, et al. Age-related and gender-related changes in monaural speech recognition. J Speech Lang Hear Res 1997;40:444–452.

Elias MF, Elias PL. Motivation and activity. In: Birren J, Schaie K, eds. Handbook of the psychology of aging. New York: Van Nostrand Reinhold, 1977.

Erber NP. Interaction of audition and vision in the recognition of oral speech stimuli. J Speech Hear Res 1969;12:423–425.

Ethol B, Belal A. Seniles changes in the middle ear joints. Ann Otology 1974;83:49–54.

Ewertsen HW, Nielsen HB. A comparative analysis of the audiovisual, auditive and visual perception of speech. Acta Otolaryngol 1971;72:201–205.

Farrimond T. Age differences in the ability to use visual cues in auditory communication. Lang Speech 1959;2:179–192.

Farrimond T. Effect of encouragement on performance of young and old subjects on a task involving speech reading. Psychol Rep 1989;65:1247–1250.

Fino MS, Bess FH, Lichtenstein JJ, et al. Factors differentiating elderly hearing aid wearers and non-wearers. Hear Instr 1992;43:6–10.

Frank T, Bennett S, Blood L. Relations between hearing handicap and impairment. Paper presented to the annual convention of the American Speech-Language-Hearing Association, St. Louis, 1989.

Frank T, Peterson DR. Accuracy of a 40dBHL Audioscope and audiometer screening for adults. Ear Hear 1987,8. 180–183.

Franks J, Beckman N. Rejection of hearing aids: attitudes of a geriatric sample. Ear Hear 1985;6:161–166.

Gates G, Cooper J, Kannell W, et al. Hearing in the elderly: the Framingham cohort 1983–1985. Ear Hear 1990;11:247–256.

Gerard L, Zacks R, Hasher L, et al. Age deficits in retrieval: the fan effect. J Gerontol 1991;46:131–136.

Goldberg G. Up with telehealth. ASHA 1997;39:26–31.

Gordon-Salant S. Effects of aging on response criteria in speech-recognition tasks. J Speech Hear Res 1986;29:155–162.

Grove GL. Age-related differences in healing of superficial skin wounds in humans. Arch Dermatol Res 1982,272:381–385.

Harty M. Elastic tissue in the middle ear cavity. J Laryngol Otol 1953;67:723–729.

Hasher L, Zacks R. Working memory, comprehension, and aging: a review and new view. In: Bower GH, ed. The psychology of learning and motivation. New York: Academic Press, 1988;22.

Hasher L, Stoltzfus E, Zacks R, et al. Age and inhibition. J Exp Psychol Learn Mem Cogn 1991;17:163–169.

Hultsch D, Dixon R. Learning and memory in aging. In: Birren JE, Schaie KW, eds. Handbook of the psychology of aging. San Diego: Academic Press, 1990.

Humes L. Speech understanding in the elderly. J Am Acad Audiol 1996;7:161–167.

Humes L, Christopherson L. Speech identification difficulties of hearing-impaired elderly persons: the contributions of auditory processing deficits. Speech Hear Res 1991;34:686–693.

Humes LE, Watson BU, Christensen LA, et al. Factors associated with individual differences in clinical measures of speech recognition among the elderly. J Speech Hear Res 1994;37:465–474.

Hurvitz H, Goldojarb M. Comparison of two aural rehabilitation methods in a nursing home. Paper presented to the annual convention of the American Speech-Language-Hearing Association, Boston. Massachusetts, 1988.

Huyck M, Hoyer W. Adult development and aging. Belmont, CA: Wadsworth, 1982.

Jerger J, Jerger S, Mauldin L. Studies in impedance audiometry: 1. normal and sensorineural ears. Arch Otolaryngol 1972;96:513–523.

Jerger J, Oliver T, Pirozzolo F. Impact of central auditory processing disorder and cognitive deficit on the self-assessment of hearing handicap in the elderly. J Am Acad Audiol 1990;1:75–80.

Johnson C, Danhauer J, Edwards R. The "hearing aid effect" in geriatrics—fact or fiction? Hear Instr 1982;33:24–36.

Jupiter T. A community hearing screening program for the elderly. Hear J 1989;42:14–17.

Jupiter T, Distasio D. An evaluation of the HHIE-S as a screening tool for the elderly homebound population. J Acad Rehabil Audiol 1998;31:11–21.

Kaplan H, Feely J, Brown J. A modified Denver scale: test retest reliability. J Acad Rehabil Audiol 1978;11:15–32.

Kausler DH. Automaticity of encoding and episodic memory processes. In: Lovelace EA, ed. Aging and cognition: mental processes, self-awareness and interventions. North Holland: Elsevier Science, 1990.

Kausler DH. Experimental psychology, cognition, and human aging. 2nd ed. New York: Springer-Verlag, 1991.

Kimmel DC. Adulthood and aging. New York: John Wiley & Sons, 1974.

Kirkwood D. Is home hearing care an idea whose time has come again? Hear J 1995;48:13–24.

Kligman AM, Grove GL, Balin AK. Aging of the human skin. In: Finch CE, Schneider EL, eds. Handbook of the biology of aging. New York: Van Nostrand Reinhold, 1985.

Kluger J. Can we stay young? Time 1996;November:90–98.

Kricos P. Audiologic rehabilitation for the elderly. Hear J 1997;50:10–11.

Kricos PB, Holmes AE. Efficacy of audiologic rehabilitation for older adults. J Am Acad Audiol 1996;7:219–229.

Kricos PB, Lesner SA. Age effects of the perception of visemes. Poster session presented at the annual convention of the American Academy of Audiology, Dallas, Texas, 1995.

Kricos PB, Lesner SA, Sandridge SA, et al. Perceived benefits of amplification as a function of central auditory status in the elderly. Ear Hear 1987;8:337–342.

Lee J, McCarthy P. A comparison of self-reported handicap in two hearing handicap inventories. Paper presented to the annual convention of the American Speech-Language-Hearing Association, Atlanta, Georgia, 1991.

Leopold L. The eye. In: Freeman JT, ed. Clinical features of the older patient. Springfield, IL: Charles C. Thomas, 1965.

Lichtenstein M, Bess F, Logan S. Diagnostic performance of the HHIE-S against differing definitions of hearing loss. Ear Hear 1988;9:208–211.

Madden DJ. Selective attention and visual search: revision of an allocation model and application to age differences. J Exp Psychol Hum Percept Perform 1992;10:821–836.

Malinoff RL, Weinstein BE. Changes in self assessment of hearing handicap over the first year of hearing aid use by older adults. J Acad Rehabil Audiol 1989a;22: 54–60.

Marshall L. Auditory processing in aging listeners. J Speech Hear Disord 1981;46:226–240.

McCarthy P. Self-assessment inventories as quality assurance tools. Rocky Mount J Commun Disord 1990;6: 17–21.

McCarthy P, Pass C, Klodd D. Denial of hearing loss in the aging population: rehabilitative implications. Poster session presented to the American Academy of Audiology, Dallas, Texas, 1995.

McCarthy PA, Alpiner JG. An assessment scale of hearing handicap for use in family counseling. J Acad Rehab Audiol 1983;16:256–270.

McDowd J, Filion D. Aging selective attention, and inhibitory processes. A psychophysiological approach. Psychol Aging 1992;7:65–71.

Metlife statistical bulletin recap: the changing U.S. population. http//:www.metlife.com/, 1996.

Milne JS. A longitudinal study of hearing loss in older people. Br J Audiol 1977;11:7–14.

Montamat SC, Cusak B. Overcoming problems with polypharmacy and drug misuse in the elderly. Clin Geriatr Med 1992;8:143–158.

Morrell CH, Gordon-Salant S, Pearson JD, et al. Age- and gender-specific reference ranges for hearing level and longitudinal changes in hearing level. J Acoust Soc Am 1996;100:1949–1967.

Mulrow C, Aguilar C, Endicott J, et al. Quality of life changes and hearing impairment. Ann Int Med 1990;113: 188–194.

Nabelek AK, Robinson PK. Monaural and binaural speech perception in reverberation for listeners of various ages. J Acoust Soc Am 1982;71:1242–1248.

Nabelek AK, Tucker FM, Letowski TR. Toleration of background noises: relationship with patterns of hearing aid use by elderly persons. J Speech Hear Res 1991;34: 679–685.

National Council on the Aging. Polypharmacy. http://www.ncoa.org/caregiving/polypharm.htm, 1997.

National Institutes of Health. In search of the secrets of aging. http://www.nih.gov/health/chip/nia/aging/quest.html, 1998.

Neumann O. Theories of attention. In: Newmann O, Saunders AF, eds. Handbook of perception and action. London: Academic Press, 1996.

Newman C, Weinstein B. Judgements of perceived hearing handicap by hearing-impaired elderly men and their spouses. J Acad Rehabil Audiol 1986;19:109–115.

Newman CW, Weinstein BE. The hearing handicap inventory for the elderly as a measure of hearing aid benefit. Ear Hear 1988;9:81–85.

Newman CW, Weinstein BE. Test-retest reliability of the hearing handicap inventory for the elderly using two administration approaches. Ear Hear 1989;10:190–191.

Newman CW, Jacobson GP, Hug GA, et al. Practical method of quantifying hearing aid benefit in older adults. J Am Acad Audiol 1991;2:70–75.

Newman D. Assessment of hearing loss in elderly people: the feasibility of a nurse administered screening test. J Adv Nurs 1990;15:400–409.

Northern J, Beyer C. Reducing hearing aid returns through patient education. Audiol Today 1999;11:10–11.

O'Neill JJ. Contributions of the visual components of oral symbols to speech comprehension. J Speech Hear Disord 1954;19:429–439.

Ouslander JG, Jarvick LF, Small GW. Illness and psychopathology in the elderly. Psychiatr Clin North Am 1982;5:155.

Palmore EP. Ageism: negative and positive. New York: Springer, 1990.

Parkin D, Henney C, Quirk J, et al. Deviation from prescribed drug treatment after discharge from hospital. Br Med J 1976;2:686–688.

Pearson JD, Morrell CH, Gordon-Salant S, et al. Gender differences in longitudinal study of age-associated hearing loss. J Acoust Soc Am 1995;97:1196–1205.

Pelson RO, Prather WF. Effects of visual message-related cues, age, and hearing impairment on speech reading performance. J Speech Hear Res 1974;17:518–525.

Peyser M. Home of the gray. Newsweek 1999;March:50–53.

Popelka M, Cruikshanks K, Wiley T, et al. Low prevalence of hearing aid use among older adults with hearing loss: the epidemiology of hearing loss study. J Am Geriatric Soc 1998;46:1075–1078.

Profile of Older Americans: 1998. Administration on Aging. National Aging Information Center Database. http://www.ageinfo.org, 1998.

Rabbit P An age-decrement in the ability to ignore irrelevant information. J Gerontol 1965;20:233–238.

Rabbit P. Speech processing and aging. In: Woods RT, ed. Handbook of the clinical psychology of aging. New York: John Wiley & Sons, 1996.

Ramotowski D, Kimberley B. Age and the human cochlear traveling wave delay. Ear Hear 1998;19:111–119.

Rees JN, Botwinick J. Detection and decision factors in auditory behavior of the elderly. J Gerontol 1971;26:133–136.

Ries PW. Acute conditions: incidence and associated disability, U.S., 1977–1878. Vital and health statistics, series 10, no. 132. Washington, DC: U.S. Government Printing Office, 1979.

Riffle KL. Physiological changes in aging and nursing assessment. In: Reinhardt AJ, Guinn MD, eds. Current practice in gerontological nursing, St. Louis: CV Mosby, 1979.

Rosenhall U, Pedersen J, Russell JE. Cautiousness and visual selective attention performance among older adults. Ear Hear 1990;11:257–263.

Rush MC, Panek PE, Russell JE. Cautiousness and visual selective attention performance among older adults. J Genet Psychol 1987;148:225–235.

Salomon G., Hearing problems in the elderly. Special supplement series, 3. Danish Medical Bulletin I 1986.

Sangster JF, Gerace TM, Seewald RC. Hearing loss in elderly patients in a family practice. Can Med Assoc J 1991;144:982–984.

Sapp JV, McCarthy PA. A comparison of young and elderly listeners on omission rates in word recognition testing. J Am Acad Audiol 1993;3:308–314.

Schnedier E. Theories of aging. a perspective. In: Butler RN, Schnedier EL, Sprott RL, et al., eds. Modern biological theories of aging. New York: Raven Press Books, 1987.

Schow RL. Consideration in selecting and validating an adult/elderly hearing screening protocol. Ear Hear 1991; 12:337–347.

Schow R, Nerbonne MA. Assessment of hearing handicap by nursing home residents and staff. J Acad Rehabil Audiol 1977;10:10–12.

Schow R, Smedley T, Longhurst T. Self-assessment and impairment in adult/elderly screening: recent data and new perspectives. Ear Hear 1990;11(Suppl):17–27.

Schuknecht H. Pathology of the ear. Cambridge: Harvard University Press, 1974.

Schuknecht H. Presbycusis. Laryngoscope 1955;65:419–420.

Schum DJ. Responses of elderly hearing aid users on the Hearing Aid Performance Inventory. J Am Acad Audiol 1992;3:308–314.

Schum DJ, Matthes LJ, Lee FS. Actual and predicted word-recognition performance of elderly hearing-impaired listeners. J Speech Hear Res 1991;34:636–642.

Schumacher G. Using pharmacokinetics in drug therapy. VII. Pharmacokinetics factors influencing drug therapy in the aged. Am J Hosp Pharmacol 1980;33:559–562.

Schwartz D, Wang M, Feitz L, Goss M. Medication errors made by the elderly chronically ill patients. Am J Public Health 1962;52:2018–2029.

Sekular R. Vision as a source of simple and reliable markers for aging. In: Reft ME, Schneider EL, eds. Biological markers of aging. NIH publication no. 82–2221. Washington, DC: U.S. Department of Health and Human Services, 1982.

Selker L. Special issue: An aging society. Implications for health care needs impacts on allied health practice and education. J Allied Health 1987;16.

Shanas E, Maddox GL. Aging, health and organization of health resources. In: Binstock R, Shanas E, eds. Handbook of aging and the social sciences. New York: Van Nostrand Reinhold, 1976.

Shoop CD, Binnie CA. The effects of age upon the visual perception of speech. Scand Audiol 1979;8:3–8.

Smedley TC, Schow RL. Frustrations with hearing aid use: candid observations from the elderly. Hear J 1990,41, 21–27.

Stach BA, Spretnjak ML, Jerger J. The prevalence of central presbycusis in a clinical population. J Am Acad Audiol 1990;1:109–115.

Stewart RB, Cooper JW. Polypharmacy in the aged: practical solutions. Drug Aging 1994,4.449–461.

Sumby WH, Pollack I. Visual contributions to speech intelligibility in noise. J Acoust Soc Am 1954;26:212–215.

Teveris E. Hispanic consumers in the U.S.: a $220 billion high growth market. Business Intelligence Program. http://future.sri.com/, 1997.

Thibodeau LM, Schmitt J. A report on condition of hearing aids in nursing homes and retirement centers. J Am Acad Audiol 1988;21:99–112.

Thompson DJ, Sills JA, Recke KS. Acoustic admittance and the aging ear. J Speech Hear Res 1979;22:29–36.

Thorn F, Thorn S. Speech reading with reduced vision: a problem of aging. J Optic Soc Am 1989;6:491–499.

Timiras P. Developmental physiology and aging. New York: Macmillan, 1972.

Tolson D. Age-related hearing loss: a case for nursing intervention. J Adv Nurs 1997;26:1150–1157.

Trumble SC, Piterman L. Hearing loss in the elderly: a survey in general practice. Med J Aust 1992;157: 400–404.

Tymchuk A, Ouslander L, Rader N. Informing the elderly: a comparison of four methods. J Am Geriatr Soc 1986;34: 818–822.

Tymchuk A, Ouslander L, Rahbar B, et al. Medical making among elderly people in long term care. Gerontologist 1988;28(Suppl):59–63.

Tymchuk AJ. What information is actually found on the labels of commonly used children's over-the-counter drugs. J Assoc for the Care of Children's Health 1990;19: 174–184.

U.S. Department of Health and Human Services. Health, United States 1983. Washington, DC: U.S. Government Printing Office, 1983.

U.S. Preventive Services Task Force. Screening for hearing impairment. In: Guide to clinical preventative services: an assessment of the effectiveness of interventions. Baltimore: Williams & Wilkins, 1989.

Ventry L, Weinstein B. The hearing handicap inventory for the elderly: a new tool. Ear Hear 1982;3:128–134.

Ventry L, Weinstein B. Identification of elderly people with hearing problems. ASHA 1983;25:37–42.

Vestal R. Drug use in the elderly: a review of problems and special considerations. Drugs 1978;16:358–382.

Vestal R. Geriatric clinical pharmacology: an overview. In: Vestal R, ed. Drug treatment in the elderly. Sydney, Australia: ADIS Health Science Press, 1984.

Voeks S, Gallagher C, Langer E, et al. Hearing loss in the nursing home. J Am Gerontol Soc 1990;38:141–145.

Walden BE, Demorest ME, Hepler EL. Self report approach to assessing benefit derived from amplification. J Speech Hear Res 1984;27:49–56.

Waldo D, Levit K, Lazenby H. National health care. Health Care Financ Rev 1985;80:1–21.

Ward J, Lord S, Williams P, et al. Hearing impairment and hearing aid use in women over 65 years of age. Med J Aust 1993;159:382–384.

Weinstein B. Age-related hearing loss: how to screen for it, and when to intervene. Geriatrics 1994;49:40–45.

Weinstein B, Clark L. An aging society. ASHA 1989;4:67–69.

Weinstein B, Spritzer J, Ventry I. Test-retest reliability of the hearing handicap for the elderly. Ear Hear 1986;7:295–299.

Wiley TL, Cruickshanks KJ, Nondahl DM, et al. Aging and word recognition in competing message. Am Acad Audiol 1998;9:191–198.

Williams TF. Teamwork for the problems of aging. ASHA 1989;31:77–78.

Willott JD. Aging and the auditory system: physiology and psychophysics. San Diego: Singular, 1991.

Willott JF. Anatomic and physiologic aging: A behavioral neuroscience perspective. J Am Acad Audiol 1996;7:141–151.

Willott JF. Changes in frequency representation in the auditory system of mice with age-related hearing impairment. Brain Res 1984;309:159–162.

Willott JF, Carlson S, Chen H. Prepulse inhibition of the startle response in mice: relationship to hearing loss and auditory system plasticity. Behav Neurosci 1994;108:703–713.

Wojcik C. Rehabilitative audiology on the Internet. Presented to the Illinois Speech-Language-Hearing Association, Chicago, Illinois, 1999.

Wolf E. Glare and age. Arch Ophthamol 1960;64:514–520.

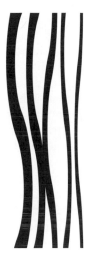

Counseling Adults With Hearing Impairment

Sue Ann Erdman, M.A.

Counseling is the process within which clinicians facilitate clients' adjustment. The ultimate goal of rehabilitative audiology is to facilitate adjustment to the auditory and nonauditory consequences of hearing impairment. The focus of rehabilitative audiology is on the individual who has a hearing impairment and on what it means to live with a hearing impairment. Successful rehabilitation is the product of the following:

1. Establishing the therapeutic conditions that facilitate change.
2. Actively engaging patients in the rehabilitation process.
3. Identifying pertinent communication and concomitant adjustment problems.
4. Conducting appropriate intervention procedures.
5. Ensuring adherence to and benefit from treatment regimens.

In each area, the pivotal ingredient is effective counseling. Not only is it an important clinical skill, counseling is the essence of successful rehabilitation.

Although the emphasis in this chapter is on adults with postlingually acquired hearing loss and their families, the theoretical and practical considerations are applicable with other populations. Individuals who seek audiologic intervention may be referred to as clients or patients. The term used is typically a function of the setting in which services are provided. Individuals seen in hospitals are more frequently referred to as patients, whereas those seen in private practices are referred to as clients. The terms are used interchangeably in this chapter. Counseling is also often referred to as psychotherapy or therapy. A difference in severity is inferred by some. Psychotherapy tends to imply intervention for more serious problems such as personality disorders or other psychopathologies, whereas counseling suggests help in adjusting to specific or situational problems. In fact, the same theories and methods pertain to each; hence, the terms are generally used interchangeably as they are here.

Are Audiologists Counselors?

Scope of practice statements, standards for certification, minimal competencies for the provision of audiologic rehabilitation services, and preferred practice patterns all emphasize the importance of counseling in audiologists' professional roles. It is the audiologist's professional responsibility to counsel individuals with hearing impairment and the members of their families about hearing loss and its subsequent communication and adjustment problems. Although it is an integral part of clinical practice, counseling in audiology is only now beginning to evolve into a well-defined and systematic process. The inclusion of counseling in training influences clinicians' professional identity (i.e., their conceptualization of their responsibilities and role as audiologists). Training in counseling affirms several key principles:

1. Counseling is fundamental to rehabilitation.
2. Audiologists are the professionals responsible for counseling those who seek intervention for hearing problems.
3. Effective counseling enhances treatment outcomes.
4. Effective counseling skills can be learned and developed.

Some audiologists have had qualms about their responsibilities and capabilities as counselors. A program of study in which one obtains the knowledge and skills needed to provide effective counseling replaces such qualms with competence and confidence.

REQUISITE KNOWLEDGE AND SKILLS FOR COUNSELORS

Specifically, what knowledge and skills does one need to provide counseling to individuals who have hearing problems? Critical, of course, is a solid understanding of hearing impairment, audiologic tests, hearing aids, and the full array of hearing assistive technologies. Also vital is insight into the communication and adjustment problems experienced by those who have hearing impairment and by their families. Without this core knowledge base, the audiologist cannot convey expertise in the field, which is critical to establishing credibility. Clinicians must have a thorough understanding of the communication process and the variables that affect it. Clinicians must also have knowledge of counseling theories and methods and the role of process variables. Clinicians must be skilled in applying cognitive and behavioral strategies in counseling due to their particular relevance to adjustment and rehabilitation. They must be knowledgeable in the areas of human development, personality, and psychological adjustment. They must have

expertise in administering and interpreting assessment measures that delimit the nature and extent of clients' disabilities or handicap. Clinicians must have the ability to identify intervention targets, to define rehabilitation goals, and to implement intervention strategies that are appropriate for specific target problems and treatment goals. The ability to monitor progress and to redirect intervention as needed is also essential. Clinicians must have the competencies necessary to assess treatment effectiveness and outcomes through quality assurance procedures, program evaluation, and clinical research and to document, utilize, and disseminate their findings. Clinicians must be able to engage clients in the rehabilitation process. This requires the ability to establish rapport with clients and to win clients' trust. To do so, clinicians must have the interpersonal skills necessary to convey empathy, understanding, and a willingness and ability to help. Indeed, Carl Rogers, throughout his entire professional life, maintained that an attitude of warmth and empathy from the clinician is the most powerful ingredient in the therapeutic process.

COUNSELING IN THE AUDIOLOGIC REHABILITATION PROCESS

Sanders (1975, 1980) first described counseling in audiologic rehabilitation in terms of informational counseling and personal adjustment counseling. This distinction is often still made. Definitions of counseling describe it as a process designed to facilitate resolution of problems by enabling individuals to identify and achieve appropriate solutions for their problems. Patterson (1986) maintains that counseling includes the affective realm (i.e., attitudes, feelings, and emotions), and that when these are not involved, the process does not constitute counseling but rather "teaching, information giving, or an intellectual discussion." Few individuals report an absence of emotional reactions to the problems hearing impairment can pose. Thomas' findings (1984, 1988) indicate that adjustment to hearing loss is a psychological process consisting of numerous affective factors for which counseling is indeed warranted. Further, he places the counseling responsibility on providers of audiologic services, stressing that rehabilitation success is not likely if the social and psychological factors relevant to each individual are not considered. Noble (1996) advocates a psychosocial approach in which the individual's interactional needs and concerns are identified and addressed. Stephens (1996), even more pointedly, asserts that it is the audiologist's role to help clients identify their problems and set realistic expectations. He describes counseling as the key to providing clients with the information needed to identify and understand problems they have experienced.

The distinction between informational and personal adjustment counseling is diluted even further when counseling is specifically viewed as problem-solving. An initial step in problem-solving is problem identification. The ease with which this first step is accomplished depends on the individual's awareness of the problem. Many individuals with hearing impairment, for example, simply are not aware of how much they are missing. Consider the gentleman who sincerely believes that his wife now mumbles, because he can hear her talking but he cannot understand her. He and his wife must be aware of the problem and must understand it before they, as a couple, can accept it and make the accommodations necessary to resolve it.

Acceptance of and adjustment to hearing impairment is facilitated immensely simply by increased understanding of the effects of hearing loss. Many people do not have a clear understanding of the relationship low and high frequencies have with speech loudness and clarity. They equate hearing loss with decreased "volume" or audibility as opposed to a lack of clarity and intelligibility. Understandably, they then find it hard to realize that they have a significant hearing problem. By explaining the varied effects that hearing loss can have on the ability to hear and understand speech, the clinician enables the client to understand a problem. Understanding facilitates acceptance. Acceptance of a problem is a pre-requisite to assuming responsibility for resolving the problem. Problem-solving approaches to counseling are designed to facilitate personal adjustment but rely heavily on the dissemination or sharing of information. This approach consists of systematic resolution of pertinent problems using any and all available resources. The versatility and goal-orientedness of these problem-solving approaches are ideal for rehabilitation counseling. Rather than being a separate entity or distinctly different function, informational counseling in rehabilitative audiology is an essential and integral aspect of the overall process that is intended to facilitate personal adjustment. Categorizing or labeling specific facets of the overall process limits, rather than enhances, awareness of the scope and nature of counseling.

Very different approaches to counseling do exist. Karasu (1986) put the number at approximately 400, and there is every indication from the literature in the helping professions that this number has continued to rise. Clinicians often find that a combination of various aspects of different counseling approaches is useful. This is in contrast to adhering to a specific theory or model regardless of the patient's particular adjustment problems or the counselor's philosophy and skills. Traditionalists and those who strongly adhere to specific counseling models have cautioned against approaches that are atheoretical and unsystematic. Notwithstanding these debates, there is a growing awareness that approaches are converging. Moreover, common features and trends in practice are being identified. These trends have created a foundation on which an integrative approach to counseling can proceed.

The integrative psychotherapy movement has gained considerable momentum in the past several years (Arnkoff and Glass, 1992; Beutler and Consoli, 1992; Norcross and Goldfried, 1992; Thomas et al., 1992; Garfield and Bergin, 1994; Prochaska and DiClemente, 1994; Bongar and Beutler, 1995; Garfield, 1995; Gold, 1996; Ford and Urban, 1998). To appreciate the converging trends and commonalties in counseling, a basic familiarity with existing methodologies and their theoretic underpinnings is needed. The following review is presented to introduce the major counseling approaches in use today, to stimulate interest in counseling theory, and to introduce theories and methods that have particular relevance and potential for facilitating adjustment to hearing impairment.

Counseling: Theories and Methods

How counseling approaches are categorized varies. It can be based on common underlying theories, the school of thought to which its originator subscribed, the type of methodologies used, or the learning modality involved. Because counseling in rehabilitation is approached from a problem-solving perspective, the counseling methods outlined here are generally categorized on the basis of how the adjustment process is primarily facilitated: by modifying behaviors, thoughts, or feelings. Cognitive or rational approaches, for example, focus on thought processes, reasoning, and logic to facilitate adjustment by enabling clients to think differently. Affective or humanistic approaches are aimed at modifying feelings and emotions. Behavioral approaches, in turn, emphasize the body and physical actions as opposed to the mind, intellect, or affective realm. There are, of course, limitations to such categorizations. As discussed below, the lines that divide the categories are, in many cases, fading.

It is generally believed that psychoanalysis is not appropriate for counseling that is specifically rehabilitative in nature. Hence, classical Freudian analysis is not addressed here. Cognitive, behavioral, and affective approaches to counseling do, however, have roots in psychoanalytic theory; some (e.g., Adler's individual psychology) are referred to as "neo-psychoanalytic" therapies. Despite its widespread influence, psychoanalysis is often not a viable or appropriate option for intervention. Among its limitations are cost, length of therapy, and the level of cooperation required from the patient. Psychoanalysis is not usually recommended in re-

habilitation counseling because it is too time-consuming to be applied efficiently and requires education and training atypical of most professionals in rehabilitation settings. Nonetheless, some familiarity with psychoanalytic theory (particularly in terms of personality structure, defense mechanisms, and the unconscious) is relevant in understanding personality and behavior as well as the counseling process in general. Freudian ego defenses, including repression, projection, reaction formation, and regression, are often discussed in relation to adjustment to disability. Research findings in support of Freudian explanations of adjustment to disability are equivocal at best (Cook, 1992; Thomas et al., 1992). The influence of psychoanalytic theory on other therapy approaches has been widespread. Nonetheless, its limitations have resulted in a host of other varied approaches.

COGNITIVE APPROACHES

Cognitive methods in counseling emphasize intellectual or logical means of resolving problems. Cognitions include thoughts, ideas, beliefs, opinions, interpretations, values, and perceptions, which may or may not be conscious. From the cognitive perspective, abnormal behavior and emotional disturbance are caused or mediated by cognition. Cognitions can be modified by active means, such as self-analysis, or by passive means in which the counselor assumes an essentially didactic role. Cognitive therapy assumes that:

1. Cognitions and cognitive functioning have a mediating role.
2. Peoples' responses to events are affected by their cognitive assessment of the events.
3. Cognitive functioning can be monitored and modified.
4. Changes in attitudes, interpretations, and thoughts can promote changes in actions.

Table 14.1 outlines approaches to counseling that are generally viewed as cognitive in nature. The individuals to whom the ap-

Table 14.1
Cognitive approaches to counseling

Approach	Originator	Landmark Publications
Individual psychology	Alfred Adler	Adler (1963)
		Ansbacher and Ansbacher (1964)
Cognitive therapy	Aaron T. Beck	Beck (1976)
		Beck and Emery (1985)
		Beck et al. (1979)
Rational-emotive therapy	Albert Ellis	Ellis (1962)
		Ellis and Grieger (1977)

proaches are attributed and seminal publications are included for those who wish to explore the therapies more fully. Beck's (1976) cognitive therapy and Ellis' (1962) rational-emotive therapy (RET) use active, directive methods to address patients' irrational or dysfunctional assumptions and beliefs. Both therapies are present-oriented and utilize a reality testing approach to problem-solving. In Beck's cognitive therapies and RET, the counselor assumes an accepting yet confrontational role in which persuasion and argument are used to help explore the inappropriateness of clients' perceptions. This confrontational role is somewhat more didactic in RET than in Beck's approach, in which a collaborative relationship between counselor and client is encouraged. In both approaches, the patient is aided in identifying, confronting, and modifying inappropriate underlying assumptions that have triggered emotional distress or behavior problems.

Ellis acknowledges Adler's individual psychology (1963) as a precursor to RET. Both view emotions as a product of thought processes; in as much as people are capable of reason, they can control their feelings by controlling their thoughts. Adler's ideas on self-worth, including the view that inferiority feelings result when differences exist between concepts of ideal self and actual self, are clinically relevant in counseling individuals who have not accepted their disability. Adlerian theory is viewed as a collaborative educational enterprise with specific goals including fostering social interest, changing faulty motivation, reducing feelings of inferiority, overcoming discouragement, rec-

ognizing and using one's resources, encouraging individuals to recognize equality among people, and helping individuals become contributing members of society (Mosak, 1995; Corey, 1996). Adler's individual psychology addresses modifications of motivation through changing goals and concepts. Techniques utilized include paraphrasing, encouraging, confronting, interpreting, developing contracts, and giving assignments. Because of his emphasis on the social nature of human beings, Adler himself was interested in applying his methods to groups of patients. This is discussed in more detail below.

RET is specifically intended to minimize irrational consequences (i.e., emotional disturbances) such as anxiety (self-blame) and hostility (blaming others or circumstances) that result from impossible "shoulds," "oughts," and "musts" that people inflict on themselves. The positive effects of alleviating, if not eliminating, these emotional tolls may include recognition of the rights of others, self-direction, independence and responsibility, flexibility and openness to change, scientific thinking, commitment to something outside oneself, willingness to try things, and self-acceptance (Patterson, 1986). Here too, the emphasis is on modification of cognitive patterns.

The appeal of cognitive approaches is their logical, indeed common sense, approach to what people think, say, and do. This is illustrated in Ellis' A-B-C model of adjustment difficulties. When a highly charged emotional consequence (C) follows a significant activating event (A), A may seem to but actually does not cause C. Emotional consequences, in fact, are caused by the person's belief system (B). Undesirable emotional consequences can be eliminated or alleviated by effectively disputing the irrational beliefs via rational or behavioral challenges. The cognitive skills required in RET might preclude using this approach with some people. Its appropriateness for individuals with low self-esteem or those having difficulties adjusting to specific situations or problems (e.g., a disability) make it useful in rehabilitative counseling. Ellis' theories and methods have not been adequately subjected to rigorous investigations (Dobson and Shaw, 1995; Haaga and Davison, 1995); hence, his impact as a scientist is uncertain. Ellis, himself, has a reputation for being somewhat abrasive and outrageous (Corey, 1996). Nevertheless, among clinicians he is regarded to be the most influential of psychotherapists (Smith, 1982). RET has been well-received by the public as a "self-help" tool (Ellis and Harper, 1975) and, as noted above, RET has been applied to a very wide range of clinical problems. Nonetheless, his RET is used widely and has profoundly influenced the evolution of cognitive therapies

Beck's approach was called "cognitive therapy" long before an entire category of therapies became known as such. Beck (1976) differentiates among three levels of cognition: automatic thoughts, schemata (underlying assumptions), and cognitive distortions. He maintains that emotional distress and other psychological problems can be precipitated by characteristic errors in logic that lead to cognitive distortions such as arbitrary inferences, selective abstraction, overgeneralization, catastrophizing and minimizing, personalization, labeling and mislabeling, and polarized thinking result from errors in reasoning (Beck and Weishaar, 1995). The goal of Beck's cognitive therapy is to identify and eliminate maladaptive ways of thinking and to learn new effective and rational ones. To do so, clients are encouraged to gather and examine evidence that they contend supports their faulty thinking. The clinician examines that evidence together with the client and then helps the client identify disparities, determine the need for change, and initiate a plan of action. The client-clinician relationship in Beck's cognitive therapy is a facilitative and interactive one; the clinician challenges and encourages and frequently gives homework assignments. Although cognitive behavior is particularly renowned for its use in the treatment of depression and anxiety, it has also been used successfully in a wide range of other areas including marital distress, abuse, phobias, panic attacks, substance abuse, chronic pain, eating disorders, suicidal behavior, health-care problems, and posttraumatic stress disorder. Unlike Ellis, Beck is an empiricist. His theories and measures (e.g., Beck Depression Inventory) have been thoroughly investigated; Beck may be the most widely read of the cognitive theorists.

These contributors to cognitive approaches to psychotherapy and counseling—Adler, Beck, and Ellis—departed from their original psychoanalytic orientation with the intention of enhancing the therapeutic process. The constructs of cognitive approaches are more easily explained than those of psychoanalytic or humanistic methods. Cognitive methods are expedient and effective, and although systematic and structured, they are more flexible than many of the behavioral approaches. Additionally, cognitive therapy is typically a short or brief process, which may also contribute to its popularity.

BEHAVIORAL APPROACHES

Behavioral counseling is based on learning theory to an even greater extent than are the cognitive methods. Behavior therapies use learning principles to change inappropriate behaviors and to teach adaptive behaviors. Although approaches differ widely, behavioral counseling is typically described as having roots in experimental and social psychology, and as being analytic and empiric in nature. The focus of intervention is on the observable and measurable. Table 14.2 outlines selected behavioral therapies and the individuals with whom they are generally associated. Familiarity with the work of

Table 14.2
Behavioral approaches to counseling

Approach	Originator	Landmark Publications
Behavior therapy	Joseph Wolpe	Wolpe (1958, 1982)
Social learning methods	Albert Bandura	Bandura (1969, 1977, 1986)
Multimodal therapy	Arnold Lazarus	Lazarus (1976, 1981)
Cognitive behavior modification	Donald Meichenbaum	Meichenbaum (1974, 1977)

Pavlov (1927, 1928) and Skinner (1938, 1953, 1971) is warranted to appreciate behavioral counseling methods. A Russian biologist with interests in nutrition and digestion, Pavlov contributed to the conceptualization of classic conditioning and extinction following his observations of salivation responses in dogs. Skinner's instrumental or operant conditioning, exemplified in experiments with key-pecking pigeons and bar-pressing rats, is fundamental to an understanding of token economics and other behavior modification programs. The work of these renowned behaviorists is basic to introductory psychology courses.

Joseph Wolpe, yet another psychoanalyst, first introduced behavioral concepts into the clinical arena. A South African who became interested in Pavlov's theories, Wolpe developed what is now known as systematic desensitization, originally termed reciprocal inhibition (Wolpe, 1958). This method is used to treat phobias and anxiety by introducing an incompatible response such as relaxation paired with a hierarchy of stimuli that evoke the undesirable emotional response. Wolpe's original model involved having clients imagine feared stimuli progressing through hierarchies from the least to the most anxiety-provoking stimulus conditions. In vivo desensitization, often used to assess the successfulness of intervention, involves exposure to the actual stimulus rather than imagining it. Other behavioral strategies used by Wolpe (1982), which have been used to treat a wide range of problems, include aversion therapy and assertiveness training. The latter has been applied to hearing-impaired populations in a number of settings (Erdman, 1980; DiMichael, 1985). Wolpe has been criti-

cized for not acknowledging the probable impact of cognitive and relational variables inherent in his or any behavioral approach. Indeed, behavior therapy often includes cognitive and affective variables such as correction of misconceptions, teaching, acceptance, expressions of concern and interest, reassurance, suggestions, persuasion, and a desire to help, all of which are known to influence counseling outcome.

During the 1970s, emphasis on the cognitive processes increased among the behavioral approaches. Bandura's social learning theory (1969, 1977), Lazarus' multimodal therapy (1976, 1981), and Meichenbaum's cognitive behavior modification (1974, 1977) were developed in response to limitations inherent in strictly behavioral explanations of emotional disturbances and other aspects of human functioning. Bandura (1986) believes learning is cognitively mediated rather than an automatic association of a stimulus with a response. His theory of social learning includes learning through observation, imitation, and modeling, and acknowledges the role of expectations and environmental considerations in understanding behavior. Social learning models promote performance and observational approaches to learning over verbal (didactic or persuasive) methods. Meichenbaum's (1974, 1977) cognitive behavioral modification approach is based on self-instructional procedures. Clients engage in self-observation to monitor thoughts, feelings, and behaviors. In therapy, internal communication or "self-speech" is modified, thus enabling the person to adapt a flexible rather than fixed set of coping strategies. The versatility of this approach is evidenced by its successful use in hyperactivity, chronic pain, anxiety disorders, depression, obsessive-compulsive disorder, tension headache, irritable bowel syndrome, and sexual disorders (Corey, 1996).

The overlapping of behaviorism with the cognitive perspective is evident in social learning theory, Meichenbaum's methods, Ellis' RET, and Beck's cognitive therapy. Lazarus, a behaviorist, considers his multimodal approach to therapy (1976, 1986, 1992, 1996) to be responsive to the multitude of problems with which patients often present. To address the range of problems adequately, a multimodal assessment is conducted to determine the individual's "BASIC I.D." (behavior, affect, sensation, imagery, cognition, interpersonal relationships, and drugs/biology). The BASIC I.D. is an assessment and intervention model as well as Lazarus' view of personality dimensions. Lazarus (1989) contends that the assessment provides an operational means of determining what works, for whom, and under what conditions. In that respect, the multimodal approach is touted as being flexible and versatile, if not eclectic. Because it is based on observations, testing of hypotheses, and empirically derived data, Lazarus maintains multimodal therapy is a behavioral approach. The original label, "multimodal behavior therapy," has been dropped, however, in favor of the term "technical eclecticism." Lazarus (1986) maintains that the goal of behavior therapy is to develop a stable conceptual framework that allows for:

1. Specification of problems and treatment goals.
2. Specification of treatment strategies to resolve the problem and achieve the goals.
3. Systematic assessment of the successfulness of the intervention.

In many instances, behavioral approaches to counseling have made shorter, cost-effective treatment a possibility. Specific treatment methods spawned by behavioral approaches have been particularly beneficial in clinical settings. Among these are many aspects of behavioral medicine including biofeedback. Behavioral therapy has also led to a resurgence of interest in the use of hypnosis in treatment. Behavioral therapists respond to criticism that they are "social control agents" by pointing out that clients determine their own therapy goals. Although this would not always apply to children, or some mentally retarded and institutionalized individuals, Bohart and Todd (1988) acknowledge the egalitarian nature of behavior therapy and cite evidence that behavior therapists are rated as highly as other therapists in warmth, empathy, and genuineness. As in any counseling relationship, this may be one of the most salient ingredients of the therapeutic process. Some believe behavioral therapy is passé; others believe its potential is only now beginning to be realized. The effect it has had on behavioral medicine is one indication of such potential.

AFFECTIVE APPROACHES

Affective or humanistic approaches to counseling focus on emotion or feelings to facilitate adjustment rather than on behavior or thought processes. An inherent problem in affective approaches is that emotions can only be dealt with indirectly. The premise underlying affective counseling methods is that clients can redirect their lives given an empathic, therapeutic climate conducive to self-exploration. The client is viewed as the agent of change in humanistic counseling models. Examples of the humanistic approaches to counseling are shown in Table 14.3.

Carl Rogers' client-centered therapy, now frequently referred to as person-centered therapy, is based on extensive theories of personality and development (1942, 1951). Rogerian theory is another distinct departure from psychoanalysis; individuals are viewed as innately good, basically realistic or rational, constructive, and growth oriented. Also considered to be a phenomenologic approach (i.e., one which holds that although a real world may exist, its existence is inferred on the basis of perceptions), the intent of person-centered therapy is to change the way the client perceives his or

Table 14.3
Humanistic approaches to counseling

Approach	Originator	Landmark Publications
Person-centered therapy	Carl Rogers	Rogers (1942, 1951, 1961, 1980)
Gestalt therapy	Friedrich Perls	Perls et al. (1951)
		Perls (1969, 1973)
Existential psychotherapy	Rollo May	May (1961, 1977)

her phenomenal field. Rogers' approach differs significantly from cognitive counseling approaches in terms of the counselor's role. The client-centered counselor is characteristically nondirective. This is entirely consistent with the overall goal of enhancing the self-directed growth process, self-actualization. Concepts central to Rogers' client-centered therapy include congruence, unconditional positive regard, and empathy—critical factors in the therapist's role that are essential to the therapeutic process. Self-concept, locus-of-evaluation, and experiencing are concepts that apply to the client. These constructs have been carefully investigated with respect to outcome of the counseling process. Outcome is enhanced when clients receive congruence, unconditional positive regard, and empathy from the counselor as this enables them to become more positive, realistic, self-expressive, self-directed, and open in their experiencing. Rogers' methods have been used with a wide range of patients and in a variety of settings. Because personal attributes rather than extensive training in psychotherapy are considered to be essential counselor ingredients, this approach is within the purview of counselors in rehabilitation settings (Thomas et al., 1992). The impact of Rogers' theories on rehabilitation counseling has been enormous. Rogers' concepts regarding ideal versus real-self discrepancies (i.e., differences in how people view themselves and how they wish to view themselves) are central to understanding why people react differently to physical disabilities; it is not the disability, but the significance one attaches to it that determines acceptance and adjustment. Rehabilitation is impeded when the realities of disability are unacceptably inconsistent, or incongruent,

with ideal-self (Cook, 1992). Self-acceptance (wherein real-self, if not consistent with, is satisfactory or acceptable compared with ideal-self) is instrumental in adjustment to disabilities including hearing impairment. Erdman and Demorest (1986, 1998c) found strong relationships between self-acceptance and overall psychological adjustment to hearing impairment, maladaptive compensatory strategies, and perceptions of others' attitudes and behavior. Among the potential benefits of person-centered therapy are greater self-acceptance and effectiveness in problem-solving, more realistic and objective perceptions, less defensiveness, maturity, a greater capacity for dealing with stress, and a sense of self-control (Rogers, 1986, 1993; Raskin and Rogers, 1989). Corsini (1995) contends that those considering careers in counseling, regardless of their philosophical orientation, would do well to begin with Rogers' *Counseling and Psychotherapy* (1942).

If Rogers' methods are person-centered, then Gestalt therapy (Perls et al., 1951; Perls, 1969, 1973) should be called present-centered. A phenomenologic-existential approach, Gestalt therapy is somewhat similar to person-centered therapy. The goal of this holistic approach is to integrate the individual to the point that he or she is self-directive. The counselor's role and the therapeutic process are, however, distinctly different from person-centered therapy. Gestalt therapy focuses on the here and now to increase the person's ability to remain in contact with the current situation. This includes an awareness of all the elements that configure one's gestalt or whole field. The exercises used in Gestalt therapy—including enactment, exaggeration, and guided fantasy—are experiential and are designed to enhance awareness. Counselors are confrontational, probing, and authoritative to the point of actively frustrating patients so they can find the support and resources they seek within themselves. Extensive training and personal therapy are requirements to be a Gestalt therapist. This, in and of itself, limits its application in rehabilitation settings. The process is neither easy nor pleasant; many who begin treatment reportedly do not continue. Unlike person-centered counseling, Gestalt therapy has not been the subject of systematic investigations. Nonetheless, this approach has also made its contributions. Expressions that have become idiomatic, such as "getting in touch with" and "consciousness-raising," have roots in Gestalt techniques. Experiential exercises used in Gestalt therapy have been adapted for a wide variety of purposes in workshops. The Gestalt focus on nonverbal communication has been influential in many arenas. Although there is some evidence that many previously rigid stances in Gestalt methods are softening, particularly with respect to "frustrating" the patient (Patterson, 1986), Gestalt therapy continues to be controversial. Corey (1995) cites several concerns including the tendency to discount the cognitive aspects of counseling, the potential danger of abusive techniques, and the possibility manipulating the client with some of these techniques. Despite early perceptions that the approach was appropriate for individuals stereotypically viewed as rigid, inhibited, or perfectionistic, Gestalt therapy experienced an almost surprising degree of popularity with the public.

Although Rogers' and Perls' approaches can be considered existential in nature, there are those who espouse a more distinctly existential approach. In the United States the most influential of these has been Rollo May (1961, 1977), whose writings reflect the existential philosophy of Husserl, Kierkegaard, and Nietzsche. May and Yalom (1989) predict existential therapy will be absorbed into other approaches in as much as it deals with presuppositions underlying counseling of any kind. One might say the approach constitutes a philosophy of therapy that understands humans as being. Because existential therapy is meant to transcend the therapy process, there are no specific methods. The significance of its philosophical underpinnings are such, however, that the writings of May are strongly recommended to those who will consider adapting converging trends in counseling to their own practice.

The contributions of humanistic, phenomenologic, and existential counseling are many. The critical nature of counselor characteristics and their importance to the counselor-client relationship are especially noteworthy. Rogers' influence in this domain may well be unsurpassed. Similarly, his theory of self, and the rigorous study to which the concepts embodied in this have been subjected, are now cornerstones in the understanding of personality. Role-playing and the "empty chair" technique have proven to be effective therapy tools that have been adapted from Gestalt therapy by counselors of various orientations.

Toward an Integrative Model of Counseling

As evidenced in the preceding descriptions, there is considerable overlap in counseling approaches. The "eclectic approach" is cited most often as the approach used by clinicians in practice. The second most frequently cited is "cognitive-behavioral." Beck's approach is now designated as cognitive-behavioral, and Lazarus' approach is now formally termed "technical eclecticism" although "multimodal" is still commonly used. In many ways, these approaches both demonstrate some "meeting of the minds" as to the ingredients necessary for therapy to be effective. A variety of factors have given rise to the eclectic, or integrative, movement, not the least of which is the increased awareness of the distinct similarities among the various counseling approaches. Although there are still those who adhere to their own school of thought, increasingly, efforts are being made to build on an apparent convergence of concepts and methods and the discovery of multiple common factors. Cognitive and behavioral approaches have many similarities;

they tend to be present-centered, problem-oriented, systematic, structured, efficient, empiric, and less esoteric than other approaches. Self-acceptance and self-growth are goals common to humanistic, psychoanalytic, and cognitive approaches. Each of these orientations also considers adjustment problems to be the result of rigid, maladaptive, or similarly inadequate, inappropriate perceptions of reality.

Patterson (1986) cites seven implicit commonalties among counseling approaches:

1. An agreement that humans can change or be changed.
2. An agreement that some behaviors are undesirable, inadequate, or harmful or result in dissatisfaction, unhappiness, or limitations that warrant change.
3. An expectation that clients change as a result of their particular techniques and intervention.
4. An agreement that those who seek counseling experience a need for help.
5. An agreement that clients believe change can and will occur.
6. An expectation that clients will be active participants.
7. Interventions characteristically include persuasion, encouragement, advice, support, and instruction.

In addition to the features that these approaches have in common, there are other factors that are pressing the various theories and methods toward integration. Norcross and Newman (1992), for example, note the following:

1. A proliferation of different approaches.
2. The appropriateness of each approach for some but not all clients or problems.
3. Socioeconomic realities of the managed care era and increased demand for accountability.
4. Commonalties in the therapeutic factors that appear to influence outcome the most.
5. The popularity of time-effective, problem-focused therapy.

6. Evidence that therapy works, but a lack of evidence of differences in effectiveness among therapies.
7. Enhanced communication with and increased opportunities to share with colleagues from other schools of thought and to experiment with different therapies.
8. Development of organizations and publications to facilitate the integration of therapies.

The ultimate goal of the integration movement is to enhance treatment. One school of thought, to which the term eclectic best applies, is to expand and enhance the methodologies of therapy techniques that can be used without a significant modification of one's ideology or theoretical orientation. The integration movement is more intent on creating a theoretical model from a merger of what is best in some approaches so as to achieve outcomes superior to that which would be obtained otherwise. Goldfried and Norcross (1995) describe the integration efforts as being characterized by disillusionment with single-school approaches and a corresponding readiness to look at other approaches with different theoretical orientations. The readiness is key; there is a history of rivalry, if not outright animosity, among those who adhered to different theoretical groups. The acrimonious sparring among factions was drawn up short, however, when study after study demonstrated that although counseling was effective, the different approaches were all equally effective (Bugental, 1964; Luborsky et al., 1975; Smith and Glass, 1977; Kazdin and Bass, 1989; Whiston and Sexton, 1993). Fortunately, once it was shown that no one therapy was superior to the others, the period of self-important contentiousness yielded to an era of earnest cooperation.

In 1983, the Society for the Exploration of Psychotherapy Integration (s.e.p.i.) was formed. It is both interdisciplinary and international. Journals have also appeared, such as the *Journal of Integrative and Eclectic Psychotherapy* and *Journal of Psychotherapy Integration.* From these interactions, progress towards integration is proceeding. At this time, there are three primary thrusts: technical eclecticism, theoretical integration, and common factors. Goldfried and Norcross (1995) stress that the three are interrelated rather than distinctly different. Proponents of the movement are hopeful that, over time, integration can occur by merging the basic commonalties as well as the useful differences across the various therapies. This would permit psychotherapy to maximize the common factors associated with successful outcomes while capitalizing on techniques that prove to be effective differentially. Readers who would like to obtain a more in-depth perspective of the integration movement are referred to Beutler and Consoli (1992), Norcross and Goldfried (1992), Garfield and Bergin (1994), Prochaska and DiClemente (1994), and Goldfried (1995).

TRANSTHEORETICAL MODEL

Several outgrowths of the integration movement have emerged. Among these are Lazarus' technical eclecticism (1989a,b), systematic eclectic psychotherapy (s.e.p.) (Beutler, 1979, 1983, 1986; Beutler and Clarkin, 1990; Beutler and Consoli, 1992), constructivist theory (Mahoney, 1991, 1995, 1996; Neimeyer, 1993, 1995; Neimeyer and Mahoney, 1995), and the transtheoretical model (Prochaska, 1979; Prochaska and DiClemente, 1982; Prochaska et al., 1992). Because the transtheoretical model has been applied to enhance adherence to health-related treatment recommendations, it is presented here as an example of one approach that can be applied across different therapies.

The transtheoretical model evolved from an analysis of 24 different psychotherapy theories and empiric and clinical data (Prochaska, 1994). The model is based on three dimensions of change: level of change, stage of change, and process of change. The term "transtheoretical" represents the model's applicability to behavioral change regardless of the theoretical orientation of the clinician or intervention techniques. The model's utility has been established in areas such as cessation and acquisition of behaviors, addictive and nonaddictive behaviors, frequent and infrequent behaviors, and socially acceptable and less socially acceptable behaviors (Prochaska and DiClemente, 1992; Prochaska, 1994; Prochaska et al., 1994). Readiness for change consists of a decision-making process that is driven by shifts in balance between the individual's perceived pros and cons of changing behavior. The point at which readiness for change occurs, referred to as "decisional balance," marks the shift in balance between the negative and positive perceptions. The model's stages of change provide an outline for specific strategies that can be directed at appropriate targets at the appropriate time. For example, cognitive interventions designed to effect change in attitude toward one's behavior are more appropriate during the precontemplation and contemplation stages. Evidence also suggests that information pertaining to negative consequences of the behavior is more effective during precontemplation, whereas during the contemplation stage, the individual becomes more receptive to the potential benefits of behavior change. Independent requests for validating information indicate that the decisional balance is being reached. At this juncture, intervention that encourages and reinforces behavioral change becomes more relevant. Until this shift in balance occurs, however, noncognitive intervention is not likely to be effective.

Eclectic and integrative theorists advocate the use of existing scientific theory and clinical evidence from the range of psychotherapies to guide the integration process. In Ford and Urban's (1998) estimation, the transtheoretical model lacks emphasis in areas other therapy approaches deem important and for which there is considerable empiric data. They cite maladaptive levels and types of emotions as examples. They are of the opinion that the integrative models, in general, reveal infrequent use of available empiric knowledge and theories in the areas of emotion, cognition, perception, and development. Prochaska and Norcross (1994) observe that the insight therapies focus on subjective processes (i.e., those within the individual). From that perspective, change is largely viewed as inner-directed. There are, however, limits imposed by the environment that call for an emphasis on action. According to Prochaska and Norcross, in the integrative model, a synthesis of awareness and action processes promotes inner change while taking limits imposed by the environment into account. Readers who would like a more in-depth look at the transtheoretical model should see Prochaska and DiClemente (1992, 1994) as well as Di Clemente and Prochaska (1998).

INTEGRATING MULTICULTURAL AND SPIRITUAL PERSPECTIVES INTO COUNSELING PRACTICE

A matter of increasing importance for counselors concerns the integration of multicultural and spiritual perspectives into counseling theory and practice. Corey's (1995, 1996) reviews of different approaches to counseling include discussions of the contributions to, and limitations of, each approach in multicultural counseling. Primary issues include cultural differences with respect to verbalizing thoughts and feelings, discussing family matters, perceiving internal versus external control, adhering to cultural values and beliefs, and expecting the clinician rather than the client to propose resolutions. Corey points out that Adler's focus on social interest, family, goal orientation, and striving to belong is consistent with Eastern cultures. Person-centered therapy allows clients to determine what will be dealt with in counseling, values cultural pluralism, and fosters respect for individual differences. Behavior therapy's emphasis on behavior rather than feelings is compatible with many cultures. Tanaka-Matsumi and Higginbotham (1994) also view the focus on the relationship between behavior and environment to be particularly compatible with multicultural counseling. In cognitive-behavior therapy, the focus on teaching and learning circumvents the stigma some cultures associate with mental illness and therapy.

Individuals from cultures that differ from the clinicians may encounter verbal and/or nonverbal obstacles to communicating their thoughts and needs. The combination of these potential liabilities with hearing impairment puts these individuals at even greater risk for communication difficulties. The problem is confounded further for non–English-speaking clients and for clients for whom English is a second language. Clinicians must be sensitive to cultural differences and the ways in which outcomes may be affected by such differences. Moreover, clinicians must be alert to the fact that hearing impairment is likely to be more handicapping to individuals whose language and/or culture differ from the society in which they are living. Multicultural issues related to counseling have received considerable attention in the literature in recent years. For excellent discussions of clinical implications of multicultural differences, readers are also referred to the following: Paunonen et al. (1992); Sue et al. (1992); Atkinkson et al. (1993); Dana (1993); Westbrook et al. (1993); Feist-Price and Ford-Harris (1994); Pedersen (1994); Brodsky and Steinberg (1995); Casas (1995); Kashima et al. (1995); Rhee et al. (1995); Singelis and Brown (1995); Alston et al. (1996); Doyle and Wong (1996); Fowers and Richardson (1996); Gergen et al. (1996); Katigbak et al. (1996); and Mays et al. (1996).

Spiritual and religious orientation, often the source of one's beliefs and values, can be associated with cultural background. It can also, however, reflect a highly personal and individual set of convictions. Including the spiritual component of clients' belief systems in counseling provides insight into the values and beliefs that influence their thinking and behavior. Although religion can be a source of spiritual strength, it can also be the source of guilt, shame, and conflict. Many therapists are advocating the need for a spiritual dimension to counseling theories (Bergin, 1988; Grimm, 1994; Mattson, 1994). Readers who are interested in this dimension of multicultural counseling are also referred to Miller and Martin (1988), Pate and Bondi (1992), Faiver and O'Brien (1993), Mattson (1994), and Pedersen (1994).

Process Variables

What are the best predictors of the eventual outcome of counseling? Regardless of theoretical orientation, it is agreed that client variables, clinician variables, the client-clinician relationship, and intervention techniques are key. There is also a general consensus that counselor variables are the most influential. The questions underlying the integration movement are basically these: "What works?" and "For whom does it work?" Orlinsky and Howard (1986, 1987) identify four variables that can characterize every therapy: the therapeutic contract, the therapeutic interventions, the therapeutic bond, and treatment compliance. Understanding process variables (i.e., the factors that have an effect on outcome) is key to understanding how counseling works. In an extensive literature review, Corsini and Rosenberg (1955) identified nine mechanisms of change in therapy. Corsini (1995) maintains that these are equally applicable despite four decades of intervening innovations in counseling. He describes the mechanisms as cognitive, affective, and behavioral and indicates that these mechanisms of change are apparent in individual as well as group therapy. The cognitive factors include universalization, insight, and modeling. Universalization is the recognition that human suffering is universal; one benefits from realizing that "I'm not alone." Insight relates to the benefits incurred through increased understanding of one's self and others. Modeling facilitates change because people learn and benefit from watching others.

Affective factors that facilitate adjustment include acceptance, altruism, and transference. Acceptance pertains to a sense of belonging and receiving unconditional positive regard from others, notably from the counselor. Change is engendered altruistically by the awareness that one is loved and cared for, and that one loves and cares for others. Transference, a global recognition of the significance attached to the counselor by the client (not limited here to strict psychoanalytic connotations), is another factor to which change is frequently attributed.

The behavioral mechanisms identified as effecting change include reality testing, ventilation, and interaction. Reality testing facilitates change when new behaviors and concepts can be experimented within the safety of the counseling session and are subsequently reinforced or modified as a result of success, feedback, and support. Ventilation refers to benefits derived from the opportunity to express pent-up emotions or previously unvoiced fears and preoccupations. Lastly, interactions with a counselor or group members, in which clients essentially admit to a problem, facilitate adjustment.

CLINICIAN VARIABLES

Psychologists, social workers, and psychiatrists are not the only professionals whose occupations involve counseling. Teachers, nurses, physical therapists, ministers, probation officers, attorneys, and many others have counseling responsibilities. Almost by definition, those in the "helping professions" find that counseling is an integral aspect of their work. Awareness of this reality is evidenced in the literature. Brammer and MacDonald's (1996) *The Helping Relationship* and Egan's (1994) *The Skilled Helper* both stress that individuals who possess the critical characteristics can learn the concepts and skills needed to provide effective counseling. Findings, replicated in varied settings, with varied populations, in varied contexts, and in varied languages, simply and categorically demonstrate that those who communicate warmth, genuineness, and accurate empathy are more effective in interpersonal relationships regardless of their role or the purpose of the interaction (Rogers, 1957, 1980; Truax et al., 1966; Truax and Mitchell, 1971; Gerson, 1996; Lewin, 1996; Fierman, 1997). This may explain why several therapy outcome studies found that paraprofessionals achieved as good or better outcomes than did formally trained professionals (Gomes-Schwartz, 1978; Durlak, 1979; Hattie et al., 1984; Berman and Norton, 1985). Brammer and MacDonald summarize two levels of characteristics that are generally viewed as conducive to effective counseling. The first group of general personal characteristics includes the following:

1. Awareness of self and values.
2. Awareness of cultural experiences.
3. Ability to analyze his or her own feelings.
4. Ability to serve as model and influencer.
5. Altruism.
6. Strong sense of ethics.
7. Responsibility.

More specific counselor qualities that many view as being essential to facilitate growth and adjustment include:

1. Empathy.
2. Warmth and caring.
3. Openness.
4. Positive regard and respect.
5. Concreteness and specificity.
6. Communication competence.
7. Intentionality.

Clearly, many of these characteristics are not things one can study so as to learn how to be an effective counselor. In fact, they are characteristic of one's personality. Not surprisingly, individuals with these characteristics often choose a career in a helping profession. Audiologic rehabilitation certainly falls into that category; it is a career in which the clinician helps others adjust to their hearing impairment. It is quite likely that those who enter this field possess most if not all of the above characteristics.

Some of the skills exemplified by those who are rated highly empathic can be learned. Two methods of pacing (i.e., following the client's expressed thoughts and feelings) that promote empathic understanding are skills in which counselors receive training. Reflection of feeling and restatement of content exemplify the emotional reactivity and accurate perspective-taking facets of empathy essential to the counselor-client relationship as discussed below. Also termed active or reflective listening, these counseling skills can be modeled, practiced

through role-playing, and evaluated by peers or supervisors.

Clinicians must also be aware of non-verbal cues that influence counseling and communication effectiveness. Facial expression, eye contact, gestures, body posture, proximity, speaking rate, and tone of voice influence perceptions of clinician empathy, genuineness, and unconditional positive regard. To provide optimal care, counselors' interpersonal skills must be inextricably interwoven with technical skills. The quality of audiologists' relationships with patients tempers the impersonal isolation of the audiometric test suite, the intimidating effects of electronic and computerized technology, and the apprehension patients' experience when faced with the diagnosis of hearing impairment and the prospect of hearing aid use.

The clinician can control many environmental variables that affect communication with clients. Messages communicated in a quiet, private area such as an office or test suite will be heard more easily and will be taken more seriously than messages delivered in noisy, public areas such as lobbies or waiting areas. Above and beyond the fact that effectiveness is precluded, *in view of patients' absolute right to privacy and confidentiality, counseling—regardless of its purpose or nature—should not be conducted in a public area.*

THE CLIENT-CLINICIAN RELATIONSHIP

The most frequently cited and discussed variables in counseling involve the nature of the counselor-client relationship that, many believe, defines and determines the counseling process (e.g., Rogers, 1957; Squier, 1990; Hall et al., 1993; Bordin, 1994; Gelso and Carter, 1994; Henry and Strupp, 1994; Orlinsky et al., 1994; Orlinsky and Howard, 1995; Lewin, 1996; Fierman, 1997; Patterson and Hidore, 1997; Gelso and Hayes, 1998; and Safran and Muran, 1998). Patterson (1986) claims that those who debate evidence supporting the counseling relationship as the most powerful, effective variable in the counseling process are simply threatened by the implications of this incontrovertible fact. These findings indicate that warmth, empathy, trust, respect, and unconditional positive regard—personal attributes that the effective counselor presents to the client and which, thereby, define the working alliance in counseling—are more salient than any other variables in the treatment process. For those whose theories and methodologies are trivialized by what Patterson feels is perhaps the most well-documented and supported conclusion in the psychology of human behavior, some resistance is largely understandable. Although the evidence does not confirm that these relational conditions are sufficient for therapeutic change, it also does not confirm that they are not. More importantly, there is no evidence of the effectiveness of any other treatment variables in the absence of these relational conditions.

The role of the counseling audiologist should be supportive and facilitative and will, at times, be directive. These requisite elements and the implications for audiologist-patient relationships have been discussed by many practicing audiologists (Erdman et al., 1984; Caccavo and Geist, 1986; Wylde, 1987; Skinner, 1988; Roberts and Bouchard, 1989; Erdman et al., 1994). Nevertheless, the effects of relational variables have not been explored in audiology. Moreover, development of effective interpersonal skills in clinician-client relationships typically receives little attention in audiologists' clinical training. There are notable exceptions. In the graduate program in audiology at the University of Memphis, for example, a course in interpersonal communication precedes more advanced courses in counseling and audiologic rehabilitation. Course content includes literature (e.g., Jourard, 1971, 1974; Adler and Towne, 1990; Verderber and Verderber, 1992; Knapp and Vangelisti, 1995; Johnson, 1997) and exercises related to interpersonal communication effectiveness and the variables that influence interpersonal communication. In view of the importance of counselor self-awareness, emphasis is also placed on self-disclosure and self-actualization. Without such training, clinicians may not recognize

which aspects of their relationships with clients are effective and beneficial or they may simply lack the confidence to foster such relationships (Squier, 1990; Northouse and Northouse, 1992; Dunbar-Jacob, 1993; Egan, 1994; Gordon and Edwards, 1995; Brammer and MacDonald, 1996). Consequently, clients may receive appropriate technical care on a physical level but inadequate psychological care on a personal level. The end result is dissatisfaction with treatment.

Swan and Gatehouse (1990) and Brink et al. (1996) have found that hearing-impaired patients seek audiologic assistance because of the disabilities and handicap they are experiencing. They are managed, however, on the basis of pure-tone thresholds. "Treating the audiogram" is analogous to providing technical care for a physical problem while ignoring the very reasons the individual sought treatment. Clients are much more likely to adhere to, benefit from, and be satisfied with treatment that is relevant to them.

Younger, less experienced practitioners tend to exhibit more empathy than do those who are older and more experienced (Hall and Dornan, 1988). To gain insight into clients' hearing problems and adjustment difficulties, listening attentively is crucial. Listening to clients communicates care and concern, which are critical elements of empathic rapport. Clinicians' time constraints are often viewed as a legitimate excuse for not listening to clients' problems. When feeling rushed, clinicians may seem harried and distracted. This demeanor may be interpreted to be a lack of interest, concern, or understanding. In short, the clinician is perceived as lacking empathy.

Empathy has two characteristic facets or stages that are critical to the counseling process. One is the capacity to respond affectively to another's emotional state. Squier (1990) refers to this aspect of empathy as emotional reactivity. This is different from sympathy, which implies feeling sorry for someone else's problem or situation. The word empathy is derived from the German word *Einfühlung,* which can best be translated as "feeling into." Having empathy means feeling the other's pain. The second aspect of empathy, perspective-taking, involves the ability to take another's point of view. This is a cognitive rather than affective level of relating to the other person. Squier analyzed well-documented findings on relational variables and treatment outcome. On the basis of this analysis, he constructed a model of empathic understanding in practitioner-patient relationships and adherence to treatment regimens. The model indicates that clinicians' cognitive and affective empathy facilitate patients' awareness and understanding of their problems, which in turn facilitates the motivation to resolve them. The increased understanding and motivation enhance clients' confidence that they can cope and adjust. Increased insight into the problems, on the part of clinician and client, also facilitates discussions about how the problems can be managed. When clients sense that clinicians care and understand, a level of trust develops that permits clients to be more relaxed and more optimistic about treatment outcome. It is the interaction between increased knowledge and motivation that promotes adherence to treatment programs. Empathic understanding is particularly critical in cases of chronic, long-term illness and handicapping conditions, because clients will need to adhere to the treatment recommendations on an ongoing basis (Falvo, 1985; Squier, 1990; Sherbourne et al., 1992; Thomas et al., 1992).

CLIENT VARIABLES

Clients' expectations and level of motivation are critical variables in the counseling process. Unrealistic expectations and a lack of motivation immediately indicate a poor prognosis. Not surprisingly, there can be deterrents to the development of a constructive bond between clinicians and clients. Some patients simply elicit more empathy from clinicians than others. Pettegrew and Turkat, 1986 describe three patient types—assertive, ideal, and stoic. Assertive patients see health care providers more frequently, receive more medication, apply for more disability payments, and are perceived by raters to be pushy and contentious if not manipulative. Ideal patients are described as such because they are attentive, are precise in delivering and requesting information, and do not exaggerate their health problems. The stoic topology is characteristically relaxed, exhibits passive communication in the health care relationship, and is viewed as easily controlled. Although therapeutic empathy is primarily generated by the clinician, these types suggest that patients' communication styles may have mitigating effects on this critical variable.

Managing clients who are seemingly uncooperative or otherwise difficult is a challenge best met by striving even more to see things from their perspective. Missed appointments are a frequent problem in clinical settings. Clients often attribute this to forgetfulness. Given that people tend to forget what they do not want to remember, chronic missed appointments should alert clinicians to the possibility of difficulty accepting a diagnosis or a lack of motivation to follow a specific treatment regimen.

Barriers erected by clients are often indicative of efforts to cope with a situation that they perceive (on some level) to be unmanageable or overwhelmingly stressful. Falvo (1985) discusses a multitude of patient reactions that can negatively affect adherence to treatment regimens, including denial, forgetting, detrimental- or over-compensation, retreating or withdrawing, regression, ascribing blame, self-blame, rationalization, hiding feelings, projection, and hyperactivity. Counselors must be alert to these behaviors. Denial of significant communication difficulties and/or related adjustment problems, for instance, should not be taken at face value. Clients may be disinclined to discuss problems due to the implications of the diagnosis or they may try to downplay the significance of the problem by not focusing on the negative. Rather than refute the client's stance, efforts should be made to focus on issues he or she is willing to discuss.

Denial can be adaptive or maladaptive. If negative aspects of a situation are merely downplayed to maintain optimism and adjustment, it may be an adaptive coping mechanism. Denial that precludes addressing issues affecting health, job performance, or interpersonal relationships is maladaptive. Audiologists should anticipate denial of adjustment related problems and minimization of communication difficulties. *Denial should not be interpreted to mean that the individual does not experience these problems.*

Living With Hearing Impairment

AUDITORY AND NONAUDITORY CONSEQUENCES OF HEARING IMPAIRMENT

Counseling in audiologic rehabilitation addresses what it means to live with a hearing impairment and its auditory and nonauditory consequences. The terminology used to describe the consequences of hearing impairment has stimulated considerable debate and confusion over the years. The discussions have focused on the terms "disability" and "handicap" and the need to clarify their definitions so as to facilitate the exchange of clinical and research findings (Erdman, 1993a,b; Erdman et al., 1994; Hyde and Riko, 1994; Giolas, 1990; Schow and Gatehouse, 1990; Noble, 1988; Stephens and Hétu, 1991; Ward, 1983, 1988; Weinstein, 1996). Stephens and Hétu, in particular, have stressed the need for consensus. As a result, there has been a trend toward common usage of the World Health Organization (WHO) (1980) definitions of the four domains of auditory dysfunction: disorder, impairment, disability, and handicap. Disorder refers to the specific diagnosis in anatomic, physiologic, and diagnostic terms (e.g., otosclerosis). Appropriate remedial intervention for a disorder is most likely to entail medical or surgical treatment. Impairment refers to the resulting abnormal function of the auditory system. This may be manifested as reduced hearing sensitivity or discrimination, localization difficulties, or tinnitus. The extent of auditory impairments can be measured. Medical intervention may be indicated; however, remediation could also be rehabilitative in nature (e.g., hearing aids). Disability refers to impairment effects on one's ability to use hearing in everyday activities, be it in speech perception or environmental awareness. Disability may vary as a function of communication need, environmental conditions, and other situational variables. Hearing disabilities are the auditory consequences of the individual's hearing impairment. The negative impact on well-being and quality of life, the nonauditory effects of hearing impairment and hearing disability, constitute handicap. This may include repercussions on interpersonal relationships, on emotional health, and on educational, social, or occupational interactions and aspirations. In short, handicap amounts to the psychosocial consequences of the dysfunction. This interpretation is consonant with the rehabilitation counseling view of handicap as the cumulative negative fallout of psychological and sociologic barriers.

Ironically, just as some degree of uniformity in the terms' usage is being achieved, the WHO has proposed modifications to the classification system. The proposed changes include replacing the term "disability" with "activities limitation," and "handicap" with "participation restrictions." In as much as these changes are still in the proposal stage, use of the original 1980 WHO terms and definitions is continued here.

Disability and handicap are inextricably interwoven. Adjustment is predicated on the person's capacity to cope with a disability. Lazarus and Folkman (1984) define coping as "constantly changing cognitive and behavioral efforts to manage specific external and/or internal demands that are appraised as taxing or exceeding the resources of the person" (p. 141), an appropriate working definition for what is involved in contending with hearing impairment. The ability to cope effectively can be affected by the very psychological and sociologic variables one endeavors to control (Lazarus and Folkman, 1984; Scheier and Carver, 1992; Taylor and Aspinwall, 1996). For example, depression (not an uncommon reaction to long-standing stress, loneliness, or isolation) can result in apathy. Apathy and lethargy inhibit the effort and energy needed to compensate effectively for hearing difficulties and thereby lead to further failure, isolation, and depression. In short, handicap can exacerbate disability, which in turn, further exacerbates handicap.

Dispositional optimism has been linked to effective coping that is characteristically varied and spontaneous (Scheier and Carver, 1985, 1987, 1992; Scheier et al., 1986). Individuals who are optimistic, by definition, have positive outcome expectancies that provide ongoing motivation to continue the coping behavior. Erdman and Demorest (1986, 1994, 1998c) found strong correlations between self-acceptance and acceptance of hearing loss. Optimism, in conjunction with perceived control and sense of security, is associated with how individuals with impaired hearing cope in simulated stressful communication tasks (Scott et al., 1994) as well as with individuals' ratings of their own abilities to cope with hearing difficulties (Andersson et al., 1995). Others have also demonstrated that negative affect portends more frequent and more severe symptom reports (Watson and Clark, 1984, 1992; Watson, 1988; Watson and Pennebaker, 1989). Negative affect is consistently correlated with neuroticism and poor self-esteem. Just as those with positive self-esteem are accepting of themselves and their imperfections and are optimistic about their ability to cope and solve problems, the opposite holds true for those with poor self-esteem. These individuals typically use avoidant coping strategies, have diffuse complaints, and are chronically pessimistic. Schow and Gatehouse (1990) found that neuroticism is predictive of poor adjustment to hearing impairment. How such personality variables affect decision-making, problem-solving, and successful behavioral changes is of vital importance in setting treatment goals and determining the most appropriate intervention techniques. Rehabilitation counseling attempts to prevent or minimize handicap by focusing on the elimination or alleviation of these psychosocial problems so as to facilitate adjustment (Thomas et al., 1992).

COMMUNICATION NEEDS OF ADULTS WITH HEARING IMPAIRMENT

Recent reports confirm what clinicians have suspected for some time: the "Baby Boomer" generation is experiencing hearing impairment at an earlier age than did their parents or grandparents. Age effects are not occurring earlier; the generation of rock bands, boom boxes, Walkmen, snowmobiles, and high-powered appliances and tools has sustained noise-induced hearing impairment. What are the implications of hearing impairment for this generation? Typical Baby Boomers have not reached retirement age and are actively employed. Not surprisingly, employment portends greater communication need and more difficult communication environments (Erdman and Demorest, 1998b). Consequently, hearing impairment can be expected to be more problematic than it would be otherwise. This is particularly worrisome in view of the potential consequences to family harmony, job performance, and career progression. Between the ages of 18 and 65, adults typically experience peak communication demands in relation to education, occupation, marriage, and child-rearing. Hearing impairment can complicate any of these major life endeavors. Ineffective communication may preclude career progression or marital happiness. Stress, withdrawal, or anger related to continued communication difficulties can ruin relationships, result in dismissal from a job, or suppress the motivation necessary to succeed in any aspect of life.

EMPLOYMENT ISSUES

Thomas et al. (1982) found that although hearing impairment may not result in unemployment, it does contribute to work-related problems. Their results suggest that individuals with hearing impairment are often underemployed. The authors were unable to discern whether underemployment was specifically related to hearing difficulties, to performance issues unrelated to hearing, or to discrimination on the basis of hearing impairment. Scherich (1996) reports inadequate knowledge among employers and employees about accommodations that can be made in the workplace to facilitate communication. Although group situations were reportedly the most difficult, it was those types of situations in which accommodations were least often made. Dowler and Walls (1996) conclude that accommodations (whether a product or a procedure) in the workplace are made most successfully when the product or procedure follows from the specific needs posed by the essential job function. Listening demands associated with the average workday result in complaints of fatigue, irritability, and stress from individuals with even mild hearing impairments. Active-duty service members with mild to moderate hearing impairments frequently report feeling stressed, frustrated, incompetent, angry, embarrassed, and discouraged as a result of work-related hearing problems (Erdman et al., 1984).

Hearing conservation efforts in noise-hazardous work environments focus on individuals at risk for noise-induced hearing impairment and those who have already sustained impairment. This complicates workers' ability to hide hearing impairment, a tendency related to the stigma attached to hearing impairment, and to workers' need to protect their self-image (Hétu et al., 1988, 1990; Hétu, 1996). In these studies, individuals working in mines, lumber mills, and wood and metal products factories were preoccupied with the demeaning attitudes and comments of coworkers. Hallberg and Jansson (1996) contend that women who work in noise-hazardous areas may be even more likely than men to give the appearance of normal hearing due to concerns about stigmatization.

Beaudry and Hétu (1990) reviewed the literature related to attitudes of those with normal hearing toward the hearing impaired. Their findings suggest that attitudes toward persons with hearing impairment are generally positive. Kyle et al. (1985) report that manual laborers are less likely to acquire hearing aids than are nonmanual workers. The latter engage in more verbal activities, recognize the effects of hearing impairment more readily, and are more apt to acquire hearing aids. This pattern is evident among military personnel as well; officers are more likely to obtain hearing aids that the military provides gratis than are enlisted personnel.

The gradual onset of hearing impairment and the insidious way in which concomitant communication problems develop cause many individuals to attribute difficulties to something other than hearing ability. By exerting extra effort and energy, these individuals compensate when necessary, believe they are hearing what they need to hear, and are often oblivious to how much they are missing. They are slow to recognize others' reactions to their apparent inattentiveness, forgetfulness, or aloofness. They fail to realize that others may view them as "slow" or uninformed when they do not understand what is said. Such reactions can affect career progression. The reluctance to reveal hearing impairment in the work setting is often associated with worries about career advancement. The consequences of hearing impairment on job performance and career progression have not, as yet, been systematically investigated.

It is easy to take patients' assertion that they have no difficulties at face value. Those individuals who are reluctant to admit to hearing-related problems can be counseled by focusing on the documented hearing impairment and on the prevention of problems hearing impairment might precipitate. Stoic patients who maintain an "everything's just fine" attitude are, in part, why practitioners end up treating the pathology rather than the patient. Conflicting messages between the diagnostic report and the patient's smiling face do not facilitate appropriate treatment. Patients may inadvertently belittle their problems by trying to appear cheerful and nonproblematic so health care providers will like them and, subsequently, take good care of them. Clinicians must focus on covert messages from patients and help them explore the impact hearing impairment has had on job performance, social life, relationships, energy level, and motivation to meet new challenges. Comprehensive self-assessment inventories such as the Communication Profile for the Hearing Impaired (CPHI) (Demorest and Erdman, 1986, 1987) and the Hearing Performance Inventory (HPI) (Giolas et al., 1979) can be administered to determine the extent of communication difficulties experienced in work-related settings and the use of adaptive and/or maladaptive coping strategies. The CPHI's Denial and Problem Awareness scales provide clinicians with additional insight into patients' willingness to acknowledge specific communication difficulties typical of hearing impairment and related adjustment problems. This information is useful in interpreting other scale scores and in recognizing a priori patients' reluctance to admit to hearing problems. This awareness facilitates counselors' perspective-taking and emotional reactivity.

Lalande et al. (1988) emphasize the importance of meeting the unique needs of those with high-frequency sensorineural hearing impairment incurred as a result of occupational noise exposure. Specifically, they recommend the following:

1. Information and counseling to promote understanding of the nature of the problem and greater acceptance and adjustment to the hearing handicap.
2. Development of skills and strategies to reduce communication breakdown.
3. Stress management.

Industrial audiologists are responsible for increasing awareness of the hazards of noise exposure. They also have a role in increasing awareness of the consequences of hearing impairment and subsequent implications for productivity. Individuals who have attended rehabilitation programs after acquiring noise-induced hearing impairment not only become strong proponents of hearing conservation efforts, they also enhance participation in rehabilitation efforts (Lalande et al., 1988). Counseling is a critical element of hearing conservation efforts. The success of hearing conservation programs is directly related to compliance with the recommended use of hearing protection in the workplace and other noise-hazardous areas. Improving adherence to hearing protection guidelines is a critical

aspect of the industrial audiologist's counseling activities.

MARITAL AND FAMILY ISSUES

Until quite recently, the effects of hearing impairment on family life have received little attention in the literature. All family members are affected by one person's hearing impairment. Communication difficulties occur as a direct result of hearing impairment and because of misconceptions about hearing problems. The marital relationship probably represents the most intensely interactive communication dyad in society. The successful growth and development of this relationship depends on the quality of partners' communication with one another. Although couples may be expected to understand each other's weaknesses and limitations, it is also quite likely that they take certain things about one another for granted. When one partner is hearing impaired, the quality of their communication is affected by that impairment as well as by the couple's overall understanding of, and adjustment to, the limitations it imposes. Spouses' perceptions of the handicapping effects of hearing impairment are often inconsistent with those of their hearing-impaired partners (McCarthy and Alpiner, 1983; Newman and Weinstein, 1986; Hétu et al., 1987, 1993; Erdman and Demorest, 1994, 1998c; Erdman et al., 1995); there is a tendency for spouses to underestimate the degree of difficulty their hearing-impaired partners report, although the mean scores for spouses and individuals with hearing impairment are remarkably similar. The correlations between the hearing-impaired individuals and spouses, however, are low, often in the 0.2 to 0.3 range (McCarthy and Alpiner, 1983; Erdman and Demorest, 1994, 1998c). These correlations confirm the disparate views that couples so often have of communication and adjustment difficulties. Spouses also characteristically respond in contradictory ways to their partner's hearing difficulties. They may complain about the extent of the hearing problem and a spouse's refusal or reluctance to do anything about it.

At the same time, they may claim that the spouse:

1. Hears just fine when he or she wants to;
2. Just does not pay attention;
3. Does not care enough to listen; or
4. All of the above.

These same spouses do not repeat or speak up, fail to get the hearing-impaired person's attention before they speak, talk from other rooms, and say "forget it" or "never mind" when the hearing-impaired partner asks them what they said. The hearing-impaired individual's ability to hear well at times can negate the significance of a diagnosed hearing problem. In view of not sharing the same perceptions, it is not surprising that hearing-impaired individuals and their partners fail to resolve their shared communication problems satisfactorily. As Hétu et al. (1987) point out, couples do not spontaneously attempt to find mutually acceptable solutions. Consequently, it is essential that family members be included in at least some phases of the counseling process.

Hallberg and Barrenäs' (1994) recommendation is even stronger. They conclude that spouses should be included in "every audiological rehabilitation programme concerning males with noise induced hearing loss" (p. 260) and that attention should be paid to nonattendees as they might be those most in need of rehabilitation intervention. Four strategies were identified that depict wives' reactions to their husbands' hearing problems. The co-acting spouse participates along with her husband in the rejection or denial of hearing problems. The spouse who exhibits minimizing strategies downplays the hearing difficulties but also admits that the hearing impairment has had an effect on the couple's close relationship. She is likely to do everything possible to avoid conflict. The mediating spouse attempts to control the situation by listening for herself and her partner. She navigates the husband away from difficult situations and advises him what to do and say. The fourth strategy involves a spouse who uses distancing strategies; this results in a marriage that is almost nonexistent. The spouse does not deny her partner's hearing problems and she readily admits that the hearing impairment has affected their relationship. These four types resulted from combinations of two variables: (a) the husband's reluctance to admit to hearing problems and (b) the impact of the hearing impairment on the intimate relationship.

Intimate relationships are vulnerable to the auditory and nonauditory effects of hearing impairment. In counseling individuals who are hearing impaired and their spouses (or other family members), all parties' perceptions must be considered. To do so, self-assessment inventories can be administered to the patient and the significant other. This approach has been advocated by many clinicians. McCarthy and Alpiner (1983) developed a scale specifically for use in family counseling. The disparity in hearing-impaired patients' and their partners' perceptions as assessed by both the CPHI and the McCarthy-Alpiner Scale exemplifies the difficulties couples and families experience in adjusting to hearing impairment. The hearing-impaired person may be more or less aware of hearing difficulties than family members are, differences may exist relative to their perceptions of the nature of the problems, or family members may differ in their views of how to cope with hearing difficulties. Screening instruments including Schow and Nerbonne's (1982) Self-Assessment of Communication and the Hearing Handicap Inventory for the Elderly (Newman and Weinstein, 1986) have also been used to assess discrepancies in couples' perceptions of hearing handicap.

Audiologists' role in counseling couples who are dealing with hearing impairment is a delicate one; both parties live with the effects of the hearing impairment but view the problems from different perspectives. In addition to providing an empathic, supportive atmosphere, clinicians can:

1. Furnish objective information about hearing impairment.
2. Evaluate the disparate views of hearing problems.

3. Identify common ground.
4. Offer potential explanations for the disparities.

Counseling sessions provide neutral time and territory in which alternative solutions can be generated with guidance from an informed mediator who can empathize with each person, and with the couple as a unit, to facilitate adjustment. Scores from self-assessment inventories help identify disparities in couples' perceptions of their communication difficulties. They are also invaluable in describing each party's perception to his or her partner in an objective manner. Once the partners are aware of the differences in their perceptions, they can begin to focus on the problems these differences have caused. For example, a hearing-impaired person who has worked all day in a busy office, straining to listen in meetings, on the telephone, to irate customers, and a demanding boss, arrives home in dire need of time out, during which listening is the last thing he or she wants to do. Meanwhile, spouse and children are anxiously waiting to share news, to ask for help with homework, to discuss family crises, to interact, in short, to be heard. Unfortunately, the family members' need to be heard coincides with the hearing-impaired person's need to "tune out." In as much as not listening to someone communicates a disinterested, uncaring attitude, the family's solidarity can be shaken severely. Family members are insensitive to the fatigue, often specifically related to listening, and unknowingly place unreasonable demands on the hearing-impaired person. The family's failure to recognize and address the necessity for time out results in communication problems far more significant than the degree of hearing impairment. These issues and similar ones are common in families with a hearing-impaired member. Ironically, the milder the impairment, the less likely everyone in the family is to attribute the problems to hearing loss.

Group counseling affords couples an opportunity to learn that other families grapple with the same frustrations and difficulties as a result of hearing impairment. This arrangement facilitates adjustment for individual partners and couples as they discover that other hearing-impaired persons, other spouses, and other couples can identify with the individual and shared problems experienced in a marriage. In a couples' group, clinicians must attend to individual reactions, couples' interactions, and of course interactions among all group members. The therapeutic advantages of shared insights, problem-solving, and commiseration are particularly effective and efficient when counseling groups of couples and outweigh any potential disadvantages posed by the complexities of the groups member composition.

Beyond the Hearing Aid Orientation

Counseling, the facilitative process used to resolve problems experienced secondary to hearing impairment, is the cornerstone of audiologic rehabilitation. The effectiveness of counseling determines the extent to which all other rehabilitative measures—from hearing aid use to speechreading succeed or fail. Counseling enables individuals to cope effectively with the communicative difficulties they have experienced and the extent to which they can resolve subsequent adjustment problems. In essence, counseling effectiveness determines the outcome of one's clinical services.

Audiologists' counseling skills are critical in facilitating acceptance of and adjustment to hearing impairment and hearing aid use. Allaying patients' concerns relative to diagnosis and instilling an optimistic, yet realistic, awareness that the personal experience of hearing disability and handicap can be managed effectively requires empathic understanding.

The course of adjustment to hearing impairment cannot be predicted. It is possible to generalize and describe problems typically experienced by hearing-impaired individuals; however, no one adjustment pattern can be determined from a given audiometric configuration. Individuals with a particular type and/or degree of hearing impairment may tend to report similar communication problems and adjustment difficulties. It is not uncommon for individuals with identical audiograms, however, to experience dissimilar communication difficulties and adjustment patterns.

The unpredictable nature of adjustment to hearing loss is not atypical; there is considerable evidence that adjustment to disability is universally unpredictable. Moreover, there is multidisciplinary evidence that type and degree of disabilities are not associated with type or degree of personality traits (Shontz, 1977; Wright, 1983; Falvo, 1985; Cook, 1992). This applies to hearing impairment as well (Thomas, 1984; Erdman and Demorest, 1998c). These results also reveal that disability affects individual behavior and can have a profound psychosocial impact. Thomas et al. (1992) identify several factors that impinge on adjustment to disability:

1. Negative reactions from others (stigma).
2. Dependency on others.
3. Changes in interpersonal relationships.
4. Isolation or lack of accessibility to the environment.
5. Acceptance of the disability.
6. Low self-esteem or difficulty reintegrating the self-concept.

These variables are all associated with the individual and his or her environment, not with characteristics of the disability per se. Similarly, Knutson and Lansing (1990) found that among those with profound acquired hearing impairment, specific communication strategies and accommodations to hearing impairment contribute to individuals' psychological adjustment as opposed to the hearing impairment.

Notwithstanding this multidisciplinary evidence, many studies have been conducted to examine the relationship between hearing impairment and its resultant communication and adjustment difficulties. Correlations between audiometric variables and self-report measures—obtained to explore the predictive capability of audiometric data or the validity of self-assessment tools—

albeit significant, have typically not been strong (Speaks et al., 1970; Weinstein and Ventry, 1983a,b; Brainerd and Frankel, 1985; Hawes and Niswander, 1985; Rowland et al., 1985; Erdman and Demorest, 1990, 1998b; Kielinen and Nerbonne, 1990). Although one can infer that there is a relationship between hearing loss and its concomitant communication and adjustment problems; the relationship is not one that permits prediction of communication difficulties or adjustment problems for a given individual. Regardless of how much more expedient it might be, degree and nature of handicap cannot be determined from audiometric data alone. Information regarding auditory variables, as Thomas (1988) stresses, does not suffice when it comes to explaining the psychological stress that results from hearing loss.

ASSESSING DISABILITY AND HANDICAP

If hearing impairment is a handicapping condition and audiologists are the appropriate professionals to manage this condition, how is this responsibility to be shouldered? First and foremost, audiologists must view each hearing-impaired patient as a unique individual with idiosyncratic needs. In addition to documenting the degree of hearing impairment, the full effects of that impairment on communication ability and psychosocial functioning must also be ascertained.

Interviews, clinical observations, and formal and informal assessment procedures are indispensable when formulating an initial impression of a client's perception of his or her hearing difficulties. The high incidence of hearing impairment in the general population, coupled with clinicians' daily exposure to those with hearing impairment, must not result in a nonchalant or complacent attitude regarding the implications of the diagnosis for the client. Discounting patients' personal reactions to the diagnosis of hearing impairment by inadvertently implying that hearing loss is just an ordinary, everyday problem is the antithesis of empathic understanding. For the individual, the diagnosis and its implications are intensely personal. Although the person may have been aware of hearing-related difficulties for some time, the formal diagnosis of a clinically significant hearing loss may cause distress. In all probability, the individual would much rather learn there is no problem or that it is an insignificant one. The manner in which the clinician deals with a patient's overt and covert concerns is vitally important in enhancing the likelihood that hearing aid use will be viewed as a positive and plausible option.

Timing is an extremely critical variable at this juncture. Clinicians sometimes forge ahead and schedule another appointment for a hearing aid evaluation without establishing patients' readiness to accept the diagnosis and the responsibility for doing something about it. Readiness is a prerequisite to accepting the option of amplification with enthusiasm, optimism, and motivation. The clinician can alleviate patients' concerns by suggesting that the actual significance of hearing impairment be viewed in terms of the specific communication problems that have arisen and the implications of those problems for patients and their families, coworkers, and friends. This encourages patients to assume an active role in decision-making and problem-solving, and dispels any sense of their not having a choice relative to the treatment options. By actively engaging patients in this process, it is more likely that the decisions made will be acceptable to them.

Self-assessment inventories are invaluable in facilitating the identification of pertinent communication difficulties and the variables that contribute to those problems. The audiogram, as an explanation of hearing impairment, is not particularly meaningful to most clients. Descriptions of the kind of communication difficulties and frustrations they have experienced, as found in various self-assessment inventories, provide meaning and relevance to the diagnosis. Indeed, completion of a self-assessment questionnaire can be beneficial in focusing patients on the extent to which hearing difficulties have actually progressed. It also assists them in verbalizing vague complaints that they have downplayed and tried to ignore to cope with their hearing difficulties. Scores from instruments such as the HPI (Giolas et al., 1979; Lamb et al., 1983), The Denver Scale of Communication Function (Alpiner et al., 1974; Alpiner, 1982), and the CPHI (Demorest and Erdman, 1986, 1987, 1988, 1989a,b) can be used as a baseline to assess the extent and nature of hearing disability and handicap, to outline counseling goals, and to monitor progress. In most instances, patients can complete these questionnaires in approximately 20 minutes with little or no supervision. They may do so in the clinic or at home. Automated scoring procedures typically take less than 2 minutes per patient. With a minimal amount of time and effort, clinicians can obtain a wealth of information relative to an individual's specific communication difficulties, coping behaviors, and adjustment problems. This information is of fundamental importance in facilitating emotional reactivity and perspective-taking, the key ingredients of empathic understanding. A comprehensive assessment of hearing disability and handicap is a prerequisite to treatment of the communicative consequences of hearing impairment and resultant adjustment problems.

Clinicians should select standardized instruments appropriate for their clinical population's characteristics and needs. The clinical use of psychometric instruments carries certain responsibilities. Most importantly, the clinician should have a thorough knowledge of the instrument's content, scope, applications, psychometric properties, and administration and scoring procedures to ensure valid measurement and interpretation (Demorest and Walden, 1984).

Routinely using a particular assessment tool with a particular clinical population is beneficial in a number of ways. In addition to quantifying and documenting the pertinent adjustment difficulties of each client, the cumulative results yield normative data that describe the characteristic needs and problems of one's clientele. These local norms provide a basis for determining appropriate treatment goals and procedures, a reference for interpreting individuals' scores and progress, and a baseline for monitoring program effectiveness.

One concern relative to using specific criteria to designate disability or handicap is the subsequent use of these criteria to determine eligibility for services. This is a legitimate concern. Even those with minimal hearing impairment should be viewed as having a potentially handicapping condition that could manifest itself insidiously, gradually, or suddenly as personal circumstances or environmental conditions change. Patients can experience a sudden significant decrease in hearing ability that may or may not be not evident from the audiologic reassessment. A multitude of factors may precipitate sudden difficulties. Something as innocuous as installing air conditioning can lead to sudden, significant hearing difficulties with a rash of new frustrations and emotional strain for the entire family. Prevention of handicap involves familiarizing clients with the typical auditory and nonauditory effects of hearing impairment, the variables that facilitate or exacerbate adjustment to hearing impairment, and the skills necessary to minimize the difficulties that may develop as communication needs or personal circumstances change. Prevention is a legitimate rehabilitation endeavor.

SERVICE DELIVERY MODELS

Incorporating routine assessment and management of hearing disabilities and handicap into audiologists' practice is limited by the fact that audiology reflects a medical model of service delivery (Illich, 1976) as opposed to a rehabilitation/helping process model (Anderson, 1977). The clinical implications of the differences in these two approaches warrant consideration.

Professionals functioning within a rehabilitation model of treatment react differently to the adjustment problems experienced by a patient secondary to illness or disability than do professionals in a medical model of service delivery. In a rehabilitative model, health care reflects a facilitative, collaborative helping process; patients partici-

pate actively in the identification and resolution of pertinent problems. In the medical model, patients are passive recipients of diagnostic and treatment procedures. The patient may not agree with, understand, or accept the professional's diagnosis (identification of the problem) or regimen (solution to the problem.) Not surprisingly, the traditional medical model can contribute to noncompliance because patients are not participants in the decision-making process relative to their treatment.

The pattern of communication between clinician and client is key. In the traditional medical model, communication is top-down. In the rehabilitation model, communication takes place horizontally. Where the medical model is authoritarian, the rehabilitation model is facilitative and interactive. In one, the clinician does something to a client; in the other, the clinician does something with the client. Research suggests that the more authoritative the professional is, the less compliant the client is likely to be.

Counselor characteristics are the key to engaging patients in the management (i.e., identification and resolution) of their problems which enhances adherence to treatment programs. The essential relational conditions of empathy, warmth, understanding, and respect provide a basis of trust that patients need to accept, assimilate, and act on the information given them. This complex interaction exemplifies the rehabilitation model and helping process. The professional's role in compliance is a critical one (Falvo, 1985; Meichenbaum and Turk, 1987; Squier, 1990; Sherbourne et al., 1992; Al-Darmaki and Kivlighan, 1993; DiMatteo et al., 1993; Dunbar-Jacob, 1993; Charles et al., 1997; DiClemente and Scott, 1997).

Recent focus on the role of behavior in disease emphasizes the importance of compliance in prevention and treatment of health problems. The cost of noncompliance to society is staggering. Consider, for example, the cost to society for hearing aids that are sitting in dresser drawers. This problem exists throughout the health care professions. Particularly for those with chronic disease or disability, failure to adhere to treatment regimens increases the cost of treatment over time enormously.

Engaging clients in the management of their problems not only promotes compliance with treatment recommendations, it also enhances patient satisfaction with services and improves treatment outcomes. Erdman et al. (1994) also encourage a transition to a rehabilitative model of service delivery because this would provide a framework within which audiologists can begin to focus more closely on the communication and adjustment problems that their clients report.

Clients can also be engaged in the treatment process by analyzing the problems they experience. Problem-solving exercises can facilitate the identification and analysis of clients' hearing difficulties and resultant adjustment problems. The exercises shown in Table 14.4 have been used with hearing-impaired clients in a variety of clinical settings. Reviewing assignments with clients engages them in the problem-solving process while enhancing clinicians' awareness of maladaptive coping strategies and adjustment problems.

Identifying and analyzing difficulties experienced secondary to hearing impairment can be therapeutic in and of itself. Rehabilitative counseling, however, must also include mechanisms to ensure resolution of the problems that have been identified. Problem-solving can be designed for use in individual, group, or family counseling.

Integrating Counseling Into Audiologic Services

As in rehabilitation counseling, counseling in rehabilitative audiology can effectively be conducted using an eclectic, problem-solving approach. Intervention is designed to resolve or minimize communication and adjustment problems experienced secondary to hearing loss. Counselors proceed on the assumption that patients' problems, behavior, and adjustment are products of their idiosyncratic psychological make-up, life histories, and environments. This "somatopsychological" perspective, which uses a "person by situation" paradigm to analyze adjustment to disability, stresses the personal meaning of the disability (Cook, 1992). The empathic counselor must determine the personal meaning of disability to facilitate adjustment, or in audiology, what it means to live with hearing impairment.

The importance of viewing rehabilitative needs as a function of the personal needs and psychosocial influences of individuals with hearing impairment has been acknowledged more readily in recent years (Erdman et al., 1994; Noble and Hétu, 1994; Noble, 1996; Stephens, 1996). The philosophical and practical underpinnings of clinical services in audiology, however, have been slow to reflect this. Focus remains primarily on diagnosis of hearing impairment. In light of evidence that patients seek assistance because of the disability and handicap experienced that may not correspond to their hearing impairment (Swan and Gatehouse, 1990), the clinical focus in audiology needs to be expanded.

Evaluations of the disabling and handicapping effects of hearing impairment, when conducted, are often intended to assess hearing aid candidacy. The scope and nature of hearing problems are relevant in as much as they provide a rationale for the clinician to present to the client when recommending amplification. For this purpose, "screening" tools, which can be administered routinely in an expedient fashion, are often employed. Among the instruments that can be used for this purpose are the Hearing Handicap Scale (High et al., 1964), the Hearing Measurement Scale (Noble and Atherley, 1970), the Social Hearing Handicap Index (Ewertsen and Birk-Nielsen, 1973), the Hearing Handicap Inventory for the Elderly (HHIE) (Ventry and Weinstein, 1982; Weinstein and Ventry, 1983a,b; Weinstein et al., 1986; Newman and Weinstein, 1989), and the Hearing Handicap Inventory for Adults (HHIA) (Newman et al., 1990).

Screening instruments are not diagnostic tools. They are specifically designed to answer a particular question that requires a yes-no or pass-fail response. A "fail" on a hearing screening test can confirm the direction

Table 14.4
Problem-solving exercises

Problem identification
1. Describe a situation in which your hearing loss has affected your ability to communicate. Include:
   (a) Environment (immediate surroundings, adjacent areas, ambient noise)
   (b) Communication need (nature of communication, purpose, importance)
   (c) Behavioral reaction (what you do as a result)
   (d) Cognitive reaction (what your immediate thoughts are)
   (e) Affective reaction (how you feel when the problem occurs)
2. Communication is a two-way process. It involves a sender and a receiver. Describe the other person's reaction to your communication difficulty. Include:
   (a) Behavioral reaction 1 (what others do and/or say when this happens)
   (b) Covert reaction (what you suspect they are thinking or feeling)
   (c) Behavioral reaction 2 (what you do or say in response to others' reactions)
   (d) Cognitive reaction (what you think about their reaction)
   (e) Affective reaction (what you feel about their reaction)
Exploring potential solutions
1. Hearing aids will not resolve all of your hearing problems, but there are other possible solutions. Examine potential solutions for the problems you have identified. Describe:
   (a) Environmental changes (how you can modify your environment)
   (b) Behavioral changes (what you can do or say differently)
   (c) Cognitive changes (what you think about these situations)
   (d) Communication changes (other communication means, e.g., face to face, in writing)
   (e) How the above changes will eliminate or minimize your hearing problems.
2. Even people who know you have a hearing problem cannot understand what it is like. As a result, they do not know how to make communicating with you easier. Explain to others:
   (a) Environmental factors that interfere (background noise, distance, no visual cues, etc.)
   (b) Benefits of behavioral strategies (getting your attention, eliminating other noise, etc.)
   (c) Hearing aids are not substitutes for normal hearing
   (d) Hearing loss is fatiguing and frustrating
   (e) Joint ways to resolve communication difficulties for both parties

treatment should take or it can indicate additional evaluation. To assess the actual extent and types of communication and adjustment problems experienced by those with hearing impairment, a more comprehensive assessment is required. Such assessments make it possible to establish treatment goals and to select appropriate intervention procedures. With that information in hand, one can decide when and how to provide the necessary counseling and rehabilitative intervention.

Although the specific problems experienced by hearing-impaired clients vary, the ultimate goals in counseling these patients are similar:

1. Acceptance of and adjustment to hearing impairment.

2. Acceptance of and adjustment to amplification.
3. Effective communication ability.

Audiologists are responsible for ensuring that hearing-impaired clients attain these goals. Empathic understanding in clinician-client relations and a problem-solving approach to facilitating adjustment to hearing impairment constitute an appropriate framework for intervention designed to achieve them.

To achieve the ultimate or long-term goals that define successful rehabilitative intervention in audiology, it is necessary to establish concrete short-term goals. For example, the following goals and strategies might be set:

1. Understanding hearing impairment (explain auditory system and audiogram).
2. Awareness of effects of hearing impairment (explain audibility and clarity of speech in terms of vowel and consonant energy, effects of background noise).
3. Understanding communication variables (explain importance of visual input, audiovisual integration, environmental conditions, listening behavior).
4. Identification of pertinent difficulties (problem-solving exercises and self-assessment inventories completed and discussed).
5. Awareness of adaptive/maladaptive compensatory behaviors and consequences (explore present strategies and alternatives).

The specific techniques used in counseling will necessarily vary by virtue of the patients' orientation, the audiologists' expertise and comfort level with various concepts and methods, the nature of the difficulties identified, the structure of the counseling sessions, and what does or does not seem to be working. A problem-solving framework is flexible and compatible with an assortment of methods (Erdman, 1993) including assertiveness training, stress management, traditional "aural rehabilitation" techniques including speechreading and auditory training, and behavioral training as in communication repair strategies.

Counseling is a necessary and integral aspect of rehabilitation; how (not if) it is provided is dictated by the needs of the patient and the available resources. Successful outcomes result in satisfied clients who return and who refer others. Dissatisfied clients do not refer other patients; they may also influence potential new clients to go elsewhere. Problem-solving approaches to counseling, as described earlier in this chapter, are well-suited to rehabilitation counseling because the emphasis is on systematic resolution of the specific problems with which clients present. Problem-solving approaches have been used in counseling hearing-impaired patients in a variety of settings including teaching hospitals (Alberti et al., 1984), mil-

itary hospitals (Erdman et al., 1984), programs for those with occupational hearing loss (Lalande et al., 1988), elderhostel programs (Kaplan, 1983; Bally and Kaplan, 1988), hospital hearing clinics in Sweden (Eriksson-Mangold et al., 1990), and private practices (Caccavo and Geist, 1986).

GROUP COUNSELING

In many clinical practices, including audiology, economic considerations preclude the provision of extended individual counseling to every patient. Maximum use of available resources is possible with group counseling because more patients receive treatment in less time from fewer counselors. An inherent advantage of individual counseling is the opportunity it provides for an empathic counselor-client relationship in which perspective-taking and emotional reactivity can readily occur. Conducting initial counseling on an individual basis fosters the counselor-client relationship. Individuals who are particularly troubled by their hearing problems may initially be more responsive to the attention received in individual sessions. From the clinician's perspective, it is usually easier to focus on patient's complaints and problem-solving strategies on an individual basis.

In addition to efficiency and the variety of perspectives afforded by group counseling, there are other advantages that are particularly relevant when groups are primarily supportive or therapeutic in nature. Jacobs et al. (1988) describe seven types of groups that are differentiated on the basis of their inherent goals: mutual sharing or support groups, education groups, discussion groups, task groups, growth (encounter) groups, therapy groups, and family groups. Groups are particularly effective because they offer concentrated opportunities for mechanisms of change (Corsini, 1995) to affect the adjustment process. Yalom (1985) characterizes operant variables in group counseling as "curative factors" that apply to most effective group approaches. These factors include altruism, group cohesiveness, universality, sharing information, guidance, catharsis, identification, family and social reenactment, instillation of hope, interpersonal learning, self-understanding, and existential factors.

Rapport tends to develop easily in groups of hearing-impaired patients (Erdman et al., 1994). This promotes interaction, ventilation, and reality testing in a safe, supportive environment. The shared experience of hearing impairment establishes a common ground that promotes universalization, the realization that one is not alone. It also provides opportunities for insight and modeling. Vicarious learning and feedback within groups are especially valuable as members get ideas from one another on how to resolve communication difficulties. Individuals in a group often learn more from each other than they do from the counselor or group leader.

Facilitating group counseling sessions is a demanding process that requires leadership ability and excellent communication skills in addition to the usual attributes of effective counselors. Other highly desirable features include good organization and planning skills, prior experience with groups, an understanding of group dynamics and group process, and insight into the variables that influence groups' therapeutic value.

A number of factors have to be considered when implementing group counseling sessions (Corey, 1995). These include group composition and size, length and time of sessions, physical setting, and options for group leadership. The composition of a group can be determined in a variety of ways. Clinic schedules may dictate the days and times group sessions can be held. Patients may need to meet at times that do not conflict with work or family schedules. Groups can be formed on the basis of patients' clinical needs as determined by evaluations of communicative handicap. Selected groups might focus on work-related hearing difficulties or on consequences of hearing impairment on social life, for example. There is also merit, however, in having groups with members whose problems and coping skills are somewhat divergent. This enhances members' ability to benefit from one another's strengths and facilitates generating alternative solutions to problems. Most groups have fixed membership, with the number of sessions established in advance and the intervention expected to follow a specific course. Ongoing groups, on the other hand, often have open membership wherein individuals periodically join and others depart. A series of group counseling sessions is strongly recommended for new hearing aid users and individuals who have not succeeded in adjusting to amplification in the past.

Any initial trepidations or skepticism members might have before attending group sessions dramatically resolve as members discover mutual problems and concerns. Level of motivation and commitment to the group sessions are extremely important variables. The optimal size of discussion, support, and therapy groups ranges from 5 to 8 members; education groups often range up to 12 members. Group size can impinge negatively on treatment outcome if they are larger than is appropriate for the purpose. The potential for antitherapeutic effects must be considered to ensure that large groups are not formed for the sake of convenience. When groups are too small, it can put too much pressure on individual members to participate and can reduce opportunities for interaction and vicarious learning. Sessions for support and discussion groups ideally range from 1.5 to 3 hours. This permits interactions to be more than superficial and encourages all members to participate. Convenience, privacy, and comfort are important variables to consider for all group meetings; with hearing-impaired clients acoustics, ambient noise levels, and proximity and visibility of other members are also critical considerations.

One disadvantage of group counseling is the counselor's limited ability to be responsive to each member of the group, to interactions between specific members, and to overall group dynamics all at the same time (Corey, 1995). Group counselors must be prepared to deal with members who tend to dominate or monopolize discussions; clients who are withdrawn, negative, or resistant; individuals who rescue or enable others in the group; prolonged silences; hostility within the group; overt and covert reactions; and tangentially related discussions. Effective counselors are able to draw out reticent members and cut off those who ramble, monitor nonverbal reactions by visually scanning the group, maintain a therapeutic atmosphere, establish and shift the focus of discussions, set the tone, energize the group, clarify, summarize, provide information, encourage, support, and actively listen (Jacobs et al., 1988). They are informed, prepared, and flexible. In view of the myriad responsibilities involved, it is useful to have cofacilitators, particularly when a group's needs, size, and composition warrant additional monitoring.

Group counseling is complex; it can be a stimulating and draining experience for counselors. Fortunately, the common focus on hearing difficulties, the structure afforded by the problem-solving process, and prior insight into each group member's specific problems (through intake interviews, individual meetings, self-assessment scores, or problem-solving exercises) provide a solid framework for conducting group counseling sessions. Nonetheless, the complexities of group counseling warrant considerable forethought, planning, and preparation. The proliferation of self-help groups for hearing-impaired persons (Finisdore, 1984) and the reports of hearing-impaired clients who have participated in group counseling are testimony to the efficacy of group dynamics in facilitating adjustment to the consequences of hearing impairment. Increased inclusion of group counseling in audiology practices is warranted given their effectiveness and efficiency.

CONCLUSION

Comprehensive audiologic services imply assessment and treatment of all aspects of auditory dysfunction. Focusing on the hearing impairment to the exclusion of the ensuing communication and adjustment problems has undermined the extent to which audiologic services can be effective and successful. Awareness of these limitations has renewed emphasis on the role counseling plays in facilitating adjustment to hearing impairment.

In summary, counseling, a facilitative problem-solving process, is the essence of successful rehabilitative intervention. Many aspects of affective, cognitive, and behavioral counseling methods have direct applications in audiologic rehabilitation. An empathic counselor-client relationship and cognitive-behavioral, problem-solving approaches are fundamental aspects of rehabilitation counseling that audiologists can use to address the auditory and nonauditory consequences of hearing impairment. The need to address the problems that actually prompt individuals to seek audiologic intervention dictates a refocusing of service delivery in audiology. Specifically, facilitating adjustment to hearing disability and handicap necessitates a model of service delivery that is rehabilitation oriented. Maximizing the benefits of counseling in audiology practices will permit greater emphasis on what it means to live with a hearing impairment and will enable individuals who seek audiologic intervention to communicate and function more effectively in their day-to-day lives.

REFERENCES

Adler A. The practice and theory of individual psychology. Paterson, NJ: Littlefield, Adams, 1963.

Adler RB, Towne N. Looking out/looking in. 7th ed. Fort Worth: Harcourt Brace Javanovich, 1993.

Alberti PW, Pichora-Fuller MK, Riko K. Aural rehabilitation in a teaching hospital: evaluation and results. Ann Otol Rhinol Laryngol 1984;93:589–594.

Al-Darmaki F, Kivlighan D. Congruence in client-counselor expectations for relationship and the working alliance. J Counsel Psychol 1993;40:379–384.

Alpiner JG. Evaluation of communication function. In: Alpiner J, ed. Handbook of Adult Rehabilitative Audiology. Baltimore, MD: Williams & Wilkins, 1982.

Alston RJ, Bell TJ, Feist-Price S. Racial identity and African Americans with disabilities: theoretical and practical considerations. J Rehabil 1996;62:11–15.

Anderson TP. An alternative frame of reference for rehabilitation: the helping process vs. the medical model. In: Marinelli RP, Dell Orto AE, eds. The psychological and social impact of physical disability. New York: Springer, 1977.

Andersson G, Melin L, Scott B, et al. A two-year follow-up examination of a behavioral treatment approach to hearing tactics. Br J Audiol 1995;29:347–354.

Ansbacher HL, Ansbacher R. The individual psychology of Alfred Adler. New York: Harper Torchbooks, 1964.

Arnkoff DB, Glass CR. Cognitive therapy and psychotherapy integration. In: Freedheim DK, ed. History of psychotherapy: a century of change. Washington, DC: American Psychological Association, 1992:657–694.

Atkinkson DR, Morten G, Sue D. W. Counseling ethnic minorities: a cross-cultural perspective. 4th ed. Dubuque, IA: William C. Brown, 1993.

Bally SJ, Kaplan H. The Gallaudet University aural rehabilitation elderhostels. J Acad Rehabil Audiol 1988;21:99–112.

Bandura A. Principles of behavior modification. New York: Holt, Rinehart & Winston, 1969.

Bandura A. Social learning theory. Englewood Cliffs, NJ: Prentice-Hall, 1977.

Bandura A. Social foundations of thought and action: a social cognitive theory. Englewood Cliffs, NJ: Prentice-Hall, 1986.

Beaudry J, Hétu R. Measurement of attitudes of those with unimpaired hearing towards the hearing impaired: a critical examination of the available scales. J Speech Lang Pathol Audiol/ROA 1990;14:23–32.

Beck AT. Cognitive therapy and emotional disorders. New York: International Universities Press, 1976.

Beck AT, Emery G. Anxiety disorders and phobias. New York: Basic Books, 1985.

Beck AT, Weishaar ME. Cognitive therapy. In: Corsini RJ, Wedding D, eds. Current psychotherapies. 5th ed. Itasca, IL: FE Peacock, 1995:285–320.

Beck AT, Rush AJ, Shaw B, et al. Cognitive therapy of depression. New York: Guilford Press, 1979.

Bergin AE. Three contributions of a spiritual perspective to counseling, psychotherapy and behavior change. Counsel Values 1988;33:21–31.

Berman JS, Norton NC. Does professional training make a therapist more effective? Psychol Bull 1985;98:401–407.

Beutler LE. Toward specific psychological therapies for specific conditions. J Consult Clin Psychol 1979;47:882–897.

Beutler LE. Eclectic psychotherapy: a systematic approach. New York: Pergamon Press, 1983.

Beutler LE. Systematic eclectic psychotherapy. In: Norcross JC, ed., Handbook of eclectic psychotherapy. New York: Brunner/Mazel, 1986:94–131.

Beutler LE, Clarkin J. Systematic treatment selection: toward targeted therapeutic interventions. New York: Brunner/Mazel, 1990.

Beutler LE, Consoli AJ. Systematic eclectic psychotherapy. In: Norcross JC, Goldfried MR, eds. Handbook of psychotherapeutic integration. New York: Basic Books, 1992:264–299.

Bohart AC, Todd J. Foundations of clinical and counseling psychology. New York: Harper & Row, 1988.

Bongar B, Beutler LE, eds. Comprehensive textbook of psychotherapy: theory and practice. New York: Oxford University Press, 1995.

Bordin ES. Theory and research on the therapeutic working alliance: new directions. In: Horvath AO, Greensberg LS, eds. The working alliance: theory, research, and practices. New York: Wiley, 1994:13–37.

Brainerd SH, Frankel BG. The relationship between audiometric and self-report measures of hearing handicap. Ear Hear 1985;6:89–92.

Brammer LM, MacDonald G. The helping relationship: process and skills. 6th ed. Englewood Cliffs, NJ: Prentice-Hall, 1996.

Brink RHS van den, Wit HP, Kempen GIJM, et al. Attitude and help-seeking for hearing impairment. Br J Audiol 1996;30:313–324.

Brodsky AM, Steinberg SL. Psychotherapy with women in theory and practice. In: Bongar B, Beutler LE, eds. Comprehensive textbook of psychotherapies: theories and practice. New York: Oxford University Press, 1995:295–310.

Bugental JFT. The person who is the therapist. J Consult Psychol 1964;28:272–277.

Caccavo MT, Geist P. Adjustment strategies for hearing-impaired people. Hear Instr 1986;37:46–52.

Casas JM. Counseling and psychotherapy with racial/ethnic minority groups in theory and practice. In: Bongar B, Beutler LE, eds. Comprehensive textbook of psychotherapies: theories and practice. New York: Oxford University Press, 1995:311–335.

Charles C, Gafni A, Whelen T. Shared decision-making in the medical encounter: what does it mean? (or it takes at least two to tango). Soc Sci Med 1997;44:681–692.

Cook D. Psychosocial impact of disability. In: Parker RM Symanski EM eds. Rehabilitation counseling: basics and beyond. Austin, TX: Pro-Ed, 1992:249–272.

Corey G. Theory and practice of group counseling. 4th ed. Pacific Grove, CA: Brooks/Cole, 1995.

Corey G. Theory and practice of counseling and psychotherapy. 5th ed. Pacific Grove, CA: Brooks/Cole, 1996.

Corsini RJ. Introduction. In: Corsini RJ, Wedding D, eds. Current psychotherapies. 5th ed. Itasca, IL: FE Peacock, 1995.

Corsini RJ, Rosenberg B. Mechanisms of group psychotherapy. J Abnorm Soc Psychol 1955;51:406–411.

Dana RH. Multicultural assessment perspectives for professional psychology. Boston: Allyn & Bacon, 1993.

Demorest ME, Erdman SA. Scale composition and item analysis of the Communication Profile for the Hearing Impaired. J Speech Hear Res 1986;29:515–535.

Demorest ME, Erdman SA. Development of the Communication Profile for the Hearing Impaired. J Speech Hear Disord 1987;52:129–143.

Demorest ME, Erdman SA. Retest stability of the Communication Profile for the Hearing Impaired. Ear Hear 1988; 9:237–242.

Demorest ME, Erdman SA. Relationships among behavioral, environmental, and affective communication variables: a canonical analysis of the CPHI. J Speech Hear Disord 1989a;54:180–188.

Demorest ME, Erdman SA. Factor structure of the Communication Profile for the Hearing Impaired. J Speech Hear Disord 1989b;54:541–549.

Demorest ME, Walden BE. Psychometric principles in the selection, interpretation, and evaluation of communication self-assessment inventories. J Speech Hear Disord 1984;49:226–240.

DiClemente CC, Prochaska JO. Toward a comprehensive, transtheoretical model of change. In: Miller WR, Heather N, eds. Treating addictive behaviors. 2nd ed. New York: Plenum, 1998.

DiClemente CC, Scott CW. Stages of change: interactions with treatment compliance and involvement. In: Onken LS, Blaine JD, Boren JJ, eds. Beyond the therapeutic alliance: keeping the drug-dependent individual in treatment. NIDA research monograph 165. Rockville, MD: National Institute on Drug Abuse, 1997:131–156.

DiMatteo MR, Sherbourne CD, Hays RD, et al. Physicians' characteristics influence patients' adherence to medical treatment: results from the medical outcomes study. Health Psychol 1993;12:93–102.

DiMichael SG. Assertiveness training for persons who are hard of hearing. Rockville, MD: SHHH Publications, 1985.

Dobson KS, Shaw BF. Cognitive therapies in practice. In: Bongar B, Beutler LE, eds. Comprehensive textbook of psychotherapy: theory and practice. New York: Oxford University Press, 1995:159–172.

Dowler DL, Walls RT. Accommodating specific job functions for people with hearing impairments. J Rehabil 1996;62:35–43.

Doyle J, Wong LLN. Mismatch between aspects of hearing impairment and hearing disability/handicap in adult/elderly Cantonese speakers: some hypotheses concerning cultural and linguistic influences. J Am Acad Audiol 1996;7:442–446.

Dunbar-Jacob J. Contributions to patient adherence: is it time to share the blame? Health Psychol 1993;12:91–92.

Durlak JA. Comparative effectiveness of paraprofessional and professional helpers. Psychol Bull 1979;86:80–92.

Egan G. The skilled helper: a systematic approach to effective helping. 5th ed. Pacific Grove, CA: Brooks/Cole, 1994.

Ellis A. Reason and emotion in psychotherapy. New York: Lyle Stuart, 1962.

Ellis A, Grieger R. Handbook of rational-emotive therapy. New York: Springer, 1977.

Ellis RW, Harper RA. A guide to rational living. N. Hollywood, CA: Wilshire Book Company, 1972.

Erdman SA. The use of assertiveness training in adult aural rehabilitation. Audiol Audio J Contin Educ 1980;5.

Erdman SA. Counseling the hearing-impaired adult. In: Alpiner JG, McCarthy PA, eds. Rehabilitative audiology: children and adults. Baltimore: Williams & Wilkins, 1993a:374–413.

Erdman SA. Self-assessment in audiology: the clinical rationale. Semin Hear 1993b;14:303–313.

Erdman SA, Demorest ME. Self-acceptance: correlates in the Communication Profile for the Hearing Impaired [Abstract]. ASHA 1986;28:160.

Erdman SA, Demorest ME. CPHI manual: a guide to clinical use. Baltimore: University of Maryland, Baltimore County, 1994.

Erdman SA, Demorest ME. Adjustment to hearing impairment I: Description of a heterogeneous clinical population. J Speech Lang Hear Res 1998a;41:107–122.

Erdman SA, Demorest ME. Adjustment to hearing impairment II: Audiological and demographic correlates. J Speech Lang Hear Res 1998b;41:123–136.

Erdman SA, Demorest ME. Psychological and marital adjustment among adults with hearing impairment. Presented at the Academy of Rehabilitative Audiology Summer Institute, Fontana, WI, June 1998c.

Erdman SA, Crowley JM, Gillespie GG. Considerations in counseling the hearing impaired. Hear Instr 1984;35:50–58.

Erdman SA, Wark DJ, Montano JJ. Implications of service delivery models in audiology. J Acad Rehabil Audiol 1994;27:45–60.

Erdman SA, Binzer S, Demorest ME, et al. Communication Profile for the Hearing Impaired (CPHI): spousal forms. Presented at the Academy of Rehabilitative Audiology Summer Institute, Howey-in-the-Hills, Florida, June 1995.

Eriksson-Mangold M, Ringdahl A, Björklund A-K, et al. The active fitting (AF) programme of hearing aids: a psychological perspective. Br J Audiol 1990;24:277–285.

Ewertsen HW, Birk-Nielsen H. Social Hearing Handicap Index: social handicap in relation to hearing impairment. Audiology 1973;12:180–187.

Faiver CM, O'Brien EM. Assessment of religious beliefs form. Counsel Values 1993;37:176–178.

Falvo DR. Effective patient education: a guide to increased compliance. Rockville, MD: Aspen Systems, 1985.

Feist-Price S, Ford-Harris D. Rehabilitation counseling: issues specific to providing services to African American clients. J Rehabil 1994;60:13–19.

Fierman LB. The therapist is the therapy: effective psychotherapy. Northvale, NJ: Jason Aronson, 1997;2.

Finisdore M. Self-help in the mainstream. Volta Rev 1984;86:99–107.

Ford DH, Urban HB. Contemporary models of psychotherapy: a comparative analysis. 2nd ed. New York: Wiley, 1998.

Fowers B, Richardson FC. Why is multiculturalism good? Am Psychol 1996;51:609–621.

Garfield SL, Bergin AE, eds. Handbook of psychotherapy and behavior change. 4th ed. New York: Wiley, 1994.

Gelso CJ, Carter JA. Components of the psychotherapy relationship: their interaction and unfolding during treatment. J Counsel Psychol 1994;41:296–306.

Gelso CJ, Hayes JA. The psychotherapy relationship: theory, research, and practice. New York: Wiley, 1998.

Gergen KJ, Gulerce A, Lock A, et al. Psychological science in cultural context. Am Psychol 1996;51:496–503.

Gerson B, ed. The therapist as a person: life crises, life choices, life experiences, and their effects on treatment. Hillsdale, NJ: Analytic Press, 1996.

Giolas TG. "The measurement of hearing handicap" revisited: a 20-year perspective. Ear Hear 1990;11(Suppl):2–5.

Giolas TG, Owens E, Lamb S, et al. Hearing Performance Inventory. J Speech Hear Disord 1979;44:169–195.

Gold JR. Key concepts in psychotherapy integration. New York: Plenum, 1996.

Goldfried MR. From cognitive behavior therapy to psychotherapy integration. New York: Springer, 1995.

Goldfried MR, Norcross JC. Integrative and eclectic therapies in historical perspective. In: Bongar B, Beutler LE, eds. Comprehensive textbook of psychotherapies: theories and practice. New York: Oxford University Press, 1995:254–273.

Gomes-Schwartz B. Effective ingredients in psychotherapy: prediction of outcome from process variables. J Consult Clin Psychol 1978;46:1023–1035.

Grimm W. Therapist spiritual and religious values in psychotherapy. Counsel Values 1994;38:154–164.

Haaga DAF, Davison GC. Disappearing differences do not always reflect healthy integration: an analysis of cognitive therapy and rational-emotive therapy. J Psychother Integr 1991;1:287–303.

Hall JA, Dornan MC. Meta-analysis of satisfaction with medical care: description of research domain and analysis of overall satisfaction levels. Soc Sci Med 1988;27:637–644.

Hall JA, Epstein AM, DeCiantis ML, et al. Physicians' liking for their patients: more evidence for the role of affect in medical care. Health Psychol 1993;12:140–146.

Hallberg LR-M, Barrenäs M L. Group rehabilitation of middle-aged males with noise-induced hearing loss and their spouses: evaluation of short- and long-term effects. Br J Audiol 1994;28:71–79.

Hallberg LR-M, Jansson G. Women with noise-induced hearing loss: an invisible group. Br J Audiol 1996;30:340–345.

Hattie J, Sharpley C, Rogers H. The comparative effectiveness of professional and paraprofessional helpers. Psychol Bull 1984;95:534–541.

Hawes NA, Niswander PS. Comparison of the Revised Hearing Performance Inventory with audiometric measures. Ear Hear 1985;6:93–97.

Henry WP, Strupp HH. The therapeutic alliance as interpersonal process. In: Horvath AO, Greensberg LS, eds. The working alliance: theory, research, and practices. New York: Wiley, 1994:51–84.

Hétu R, Lalonde M, Getty L. Psychosocial disadvantages associated with occupational hearing loss as experienced in the family. Audiology 1987;26:141–152.

Hétu R, Riverin L, Lalande N, et al. Qualitative analysis of the handicap associated with occupational hearing loss. Br J Audiol 1988;22:251–264.

Hétu R, Riverin L, Getty L, et al. The reluctance to acknowledge hearing difficulties among hearing-impaired workers. Br J Audiol 1990;24:265–276.

High WS, Fairbanks G, Glorig A. Scale for self-assessment of hearing handicap. J Speech Hear Disord 1964;29:251–230.

Illich I. Medical nemesis. New York: Pantheon, 1976.

Jacobs EE, Harvill RL, Masson RL. Group counseling: strategies and skills. Pacific Grove, CA: Brooks/Cole, 1988.

Johnson DW. Reaching out: interpersonal effectiveness and self-actualization. Boston: Allyn & Bacon, 1997.

Jourard SM. The transparent self, revised ed. New York: Van Nostrand Reinhold, 1971.

Jourard SM. Healthy personality: an approach from the viewpoint of humanistic psychology. New York: Macmillan, 1974.

Kaplan H. Elderhostel for the hearing impaired. ASHA 1983;25:46–49.

Karasu T. The specificity versus nonspecificity dilemma: toward identifying therapeutic change agents. Am J Psychiatry 1986;143:695–698.

Kashima Y, Yamaguchi S, Kim U, et al. Culture, gender, and self: a perspective from individualism-collectivism research. J Pers Soc Psychol 1995;69:925–937.

Katigbak MS, Church AT, Akamine TX. Cross-cultural generalizability of personality dimensions: relating indigenous and imported dimensions in two cultures. J Pers Soc Psychol 1996;70:99–114.

Kazdin AE, Bass D. Power to detect differences between alternative treatments in comparative psychotherapy outcome research. J Consult Clin Psychol 1989;57:138–147.

Kielinen LL, Nerbonne MA. Further investigation of the relationship between hearing handicap and audiometric measures of hearing impairment. J Acad Rehabil Audiol 1990;23:89–94.

Knapp M, Vangelisti A. Interpersonal communication and interpersonal relationships. Boston: Allyn & Bacon, 1995.

Knutson JF, Lansing CR. The relationship between communication problems and psychological difficulties in persons with profound acquired hearing loss. J Speech Hear Disord 1990;55:656–664.

Kyle JG, Jones LG, Wood PL. Adjustment to acquired hearing loss: a working model. In: Orlans H, ed. Adjustment to adult hearing loss. San Diego: College-Hill, 1985.

Lalande NM, Riverin L, Lambert J. Occupational hearing loss: an aural rehabilitation program for workers and their spouses, characteristics of the program and target group (participants and nonparticipants). Ear Hear 1988;9:248–254.

Lamb SH, Owens E, Schubert ED. The revised form of the Hearing Performance Inventory. Ear Hear 1983;4:152–157.

Lazarus AA. Multimodal behavior therapy. New York: Springer-Verlag, 1976.

Lazarus AA. The practice of multimodal therapy. New York: McGraw-Hill, 1981.

Lazarus AA. Multimodal therapy. In: Norcross JC, ed. Handbook of eclectic psychotherapy. New York: Brunner/Mazel, 1986:65–93.

Lazarus AA. Multimodal therapy. In: Corsini RJ, Wedding D, eds. Current psychotherapies. 4th ed. Itasca, IL: FE Peacock, 1989a.

Lazarus AA. The practice of multimodal therapy. Baltimore: Johns Hopkins University, 1989b.

Lazarus AA. Multimodal therapy: technical eclecticism with minimal integration. In: Norcross JC, Goldfried MR, eds. Handbook of psychotherapy integration. New York: Basic Books, 1992:231–263.

Lazarus AA. The utility and futility of combining treatments in psychotherapy. Clin Psychol Sci Pract 1996;3:59–68.

Lazarus RS, Folkman S. Stress, appraisal, and coping. New York: Springer, 1984.

Lewin RA. Compassion: the core value that animates psychotherapy. Northvale, NJ: Jason Aronson, 1996.

Luborsky L, Singer B, Luborsky L. Comparative studies of psychotherapy. Arch Gen Psychiatry 1975;32:995–1008.

Mahoney MJ. Human change processes: the scientific foundations of psychotherapy. New York: Basic Books, 1990.

Mahoney MJ. Theoretical developments in the cognitive psychotherapies. In: Mahoney MJ, ed. Cognitive and constructive psychotherapies: theory, research, and practice. New York: Springer, 1995:3–19.

Mahoney MJ. Constructivism and the study of complex self-organization. Constr Change 1996;1:3–8.

Mattson DL. Religious counseling: to be used, not feared. Counsel Values 1994;38:187–192.

May R. Existential psychology. New York: Random House, 1961.

May R. The meaning of anxiety, revised ed. New York: Norton, 1977.

May R, Yalom I. Existential psychotherapy. In: Corsini RJ, Wedding D, eds. Current psychotherapies. 4th ed. Itasca, IL: FE Peacock, 1989.

Mays VM, Rubin J, Sabourin M, et al. Moving toward a global psychology: changing theories and practice to meet the needs of a changing world. Am Psychol 1996;51:485–487.

McCarthy PA, Alpiner JG. An assessment scale of hearing handicap for use in family counseling. J Acad Rehabil Audiol 1983;16:256–270.

Meichenbaum D. Cognitive behavior modification. Morristown, NJ: General Learning Press, 1974.

Meichenbaum D. Cognitive behavior modification: an integrative approach. New York: Plenum Press, 1977.

Miller WR, Martin JE, eds. Behavior therapy and religion: integrating spiritual and behavioral approaches to change. Newbury Park, CA: Sage, 1988.

Mosak HH. Adlerian psychotherapy. In: Corsini RJ, Wedding D, eds. Current psychotherapies. 5th ed. Itasca, IL: FE Peacock, 1995.

Neimeyer RA. Constructivist psychotherapy. In: Kuehlwein KT, Rosen H, eds. Cognitive psychotherapies in action. San Francisco: Jossey-Bass, 1993:268–300.

Neimeyer RA. An appraisal of constructivist psychotherapies. In: Mahoney MJ, ed. Cognitive and constructive psychotherapies: theory, research, and practice. New York: Springer, 1995:163–194.

Neimeyer RA, Mahoney MJ, eds. Constructivism in psychotherapy. Washington, DC: American Psychological Association, 1995.

Newman CW, Weinstein BE. Judgments of perceived hearing handicap by hearing impaired elderly men and their spouses. J Acad Rehabil Audiol 1986;19:109–115.

Newman CW, Weinstein BE. Test-retest reliability of the Hearing Handicap Inventory for the Elderly using two administration approaches. Ear Hear 1989;10:190–191.

Newman CW, Weinstein BE, Jacobson GP, et al. The Hearing Handicap Inventory for Adults: psychometric adequacy and audiometric correlates. Ear Hear 1990;11:430–433.

Noble W. What is a psychosocial approach to hearing loss? Scand Audiol 1996;25:6–11.

Noble WG, Atherly GRC. The Hearing Measure Scale: a questionnaire for the assessment of auditory disability. J Aud Res 1970;10:229–250.

Noble W, Hétu R. An ecological approach to disability and handicap in relation to impaired hearing. Audiology 1994;33:117–126.

Norcross JC, Goldfried MR, eds. Handbook of psychotherapy integration. New York: Basic Books, 1992.

Norcross JC, Newman CF. Psychotherapy integration: setting the context. In: Norcross JC, Goldfried MR, eds. Handbook of psychotherapy integration. New York: Basic Books, 1992:3–45.

Northouse PG, Northouse LL. Health communication: strategies for professionals. 2nd ed. Norwalk, CT: Appleton & Lange, 1992.

Orlinsky DE, Howard KI. Unity and diversity among psychotherapies: a comparative perspective. In: Bongar B, Beutler LE, eds. Comprehensive textbook of psychotherapies: theories and practice. New York: Oxford University Press, 1995:3–23.

Orlinsky DE, Grawe K, Parks BK. Process and outcome in psychotherapy—noch einmal. In: Bergin AE, Garfield SL, eds. Handbook of psychotherapy and behavior change. 4th ed. New York: Wiley, 1994:283–329.

Pate RH, Bondi AM. Religious beliefs and practice: an integral aspect of multicultural awareness. Counsel Educ Supervis 1992;32:108–115.

Patterson CH. Theories of counseling and psychotherapy. New York: Harper & Row, 1986.

Patterson CH, Hidore SC. Successful psychotherapy: a caring, loving relationship. Northvale, NJ: Jason Aronson, 1997.

Paunonen SV, Jackson DN, Trzebinski J, et al. Personality structure across cultures: a multimethod evaluation. J Pers Soc Psychol 1992;62:447–456.

Pavlov IP. Conditioned reflexes. London: Oxford University Press, 1927.

Pavlov IP. Lectures on conditioned reflexes. New York: International Publishers, 1928.

Pedersen P. A handbook for developing multicultural awareness. 2nd ed. Alexandria, VA: American Counseling Association, 1994.

Perls FS. Gestalt therapy verbatim. Lafayette, CA: Real People Press, 1969.

Perls FS. The Gestalt approach. Palo Alto: Science and Behavior Books, 1973.

Perls FS, Hefferline R, Goodman P. Gestalt therapy. New York: Julian Press, 1951.

Pettegrew LS, Turkat ID. How patients communicate about their illness. Hum Commun Res 1986;12:376–394.

Prochaska JO. Systems of psychotherapy: a transtheoretical analysis. Homewood, IL: Dorsey Press, 1979.

Prochaska JO. Strong and weak principles for progressing from precontemplation to action on the basis of twelve problem behaviors. Health Psychol 1994;13:47–51.

Prochaska JO, DiClemente CC. Transtheoretical therapy: toward a more integrative model of change. Psychother Theory Res Pract 1982;19:276–288.

Prochaska JO, DiClemente CC. Stages of change in the modification of problem behaviors. In: Hersen M, Eisler RM, Miller PM, eds. Treating addictive behaviors. 2nd ed. New York: Plenum, 1992.

Prochaska JO, DiClemente CC. The transtheoretical approach: crossing traditional boundaries of therapy. Malabar, Florida: Krieger, 1994.

Prochaska JO, DiClemente CC, Norcross JC. In search of how people change: applications to addictive behaviors. Am Psychol 1992;47:1102–1114.

Prochaska JO, Velicer WF, Rossi JS, et al. Stages of change and decisional balance for 12 problem behaviors. Health Psychol 1994;13:39–46.

Raskin NJ, Rogers CR. Person-centered therapy. In: Corsini RJ, Wedding D, eds. Current psychotherapies. 4th ed. Itasca, IL: FE Peacock, 1989.

Rhee E, Uleman JS, Roman RJ. Spontaneous self-descriptions and ethnic identities in individualistic and collectivistic cultures. J Pers Soc Psychol 1995;69:142–152.

Rogers CR. Counseling and psychotherapy. Boston: Houghton Mifflin, 1942.

Rogers CR. Client-centered therapy. Boston: Houghton Mifflin, 1951.

Rogers CR. The necessary and sufficient conditions of therapeutic personality change. J Consult Psychol 1957;21:95–103.

Rogers CR. On becoming a person. Boston: Houghton Mifflin, 1961.

Rogers CR. A way of being. Boston: Houghton Mifflin, 1980.

Rogers CR. Client-centered therapy. In: Kutash IL, Wolf A, eds. Psychotherapist's handbook: therapy and technique in practice. San Francisco: Jossey-Bass, 1986.

Rogers CR. Client-centered therapy. In: Kintash IL, Wolf A, eds. Psychotherapist's casebook. Northvale, NJ: Jason Aronson, 1993:197–208.

Rowland JP, Dirks DD, Dubno JR, et al. Comparison of speech recognition-in-noise and subjective communication assessment. Ear Hear 1985;6:291–296.

Safran JD, Muran JC. The therapeutic alliance in brief psychotherapy: general principles. In: Safran JD, Muran JC, eds.. The therapeutic alliance in brief psychotherapy. Washington, DC: American Psychological Association, 1998:217–229.

Sanders DA. Hearing aid orientation and counseling. In: Pollack MC, ed. Amplification for the hearing impaired. New York: Grune & Stratton, 1975.

Sanders DA. Hearing aid orientation and counseling. In: Pollack MC, ed. Amplification for the hearing impaired. 2nd ed. New York: Grune & Stratton, 1980.

Scheier MF, Carver CS. Optimism, coping, and health: assessment and implications of generalized outcome expectancies. Health Psychol 1985;4:219–247.

Scheier MF, Carver CS. Dispositional optimism and physical well-being: the influence of generalized outcome expectancies on health. J Pers 1987;55:169–210.

Scheier MF, Carver CS. Effects of optimism on psychological and physical well-being: theoretical overview and empirical update. Cogn Ther Res 1992;16:210–228.

Scheier MF, Weintraub JK, Carver CS. Coping with stress: divergent strategies of optimists and pessimists. J Pers Soc Psychol 1986;6:1257–1264.

Scherich DL. Job accommodations in the workplace for persons who are deaf or hard of hearing: current practices and recommendations. J Rehabil 1996;62:27–35.

Schow RL, Gatehouse S. Fundamental issues in self-assessment of hearing. Ear Hear 1990;11(Suppl):6–16.

Schow RL, Nerbonne MA. Communication screening profile: use with elderly clients. Ear Hear 1982;3:135–147.

Scott B, Lindberg P, Melin L, et al. Control and dispositional style among the hearing-impaired in communication situations. Audiology 1994;33:177–184.

Sherbourne C, Hays R, Ordway L, et al. Antecedents of adherence to medical recommendations: Results from the medical outcomes study. J Behav Med 1992;15:447–467.

Shontz FC. Physical disability and personality: theory and recent research. In: Marinelli RP, Dell Orto AE, eds. The psychological and social impact of physical disability. New York: Springer, 1977.

Singelis TM, Brown WJ. Culture, self and collectivist communication: linking culture to individual behavior. Hum Commun Res 1995;21:354–389.

Skinner BF. The behavior of organisms. New York: Appleton-Century, 1938.

Skinner BF. Science and human behavior. New York: Macmillan, 1953.

Skinner BF. Beyond freedom and dignity. New York: Knopf, 1971.

Skinner MW. Hearing aid evaluation. Englewood Cliffs, NJ: Prentice-Hall, 1988.

Smith D. Trends in counseling and psychology. Am Psychol 1982;37:802–809.

Smith ML, Glass GV. Meta-analysis of psychotherapy outcome studies. Am Psychol 1977;32:477–483.

Speaks CS, Jerger J, Trammell J. Measurement of hearing handicap. J Speech Hear Res 1970;13:768–776.

Squier RW. A model of empathic understanding and adherence to treatment regimens in practitioner-patient relationships. Soc Sci Med 1990;30:325–339.

Stephens D. Hearing rehabilitation in a psychosocial framework. Scand Audiol 1996;25(Suppl 43):57–66.

Stephens D, Hétu R. Impairment, disability and handicap in audiology: towards a consensus. Audiology 1991;30:185–200.

Swan IRC, Gatehouse S. Factors influencing consultation for management of hearing disability. Br J Audiol 1990;24:155–160.

Sue DW, Arredondo P, McDavis RJ. Multicultural counseling competencies and standards: a call to the profession. J Counsel Dev 1992;70:477–486.

Taylor SE, Aspinwall LG. Mediating and moderating processes in psychosocial stress: appraisal, coping, resistance, and vulnerability. In: Kaplan HB, ed. Psychosocial stress: perspectives on structure, theory, life-course, and methods. San Diego: Academic Press, 1996:71–110.

Thomas AJ. Acquired hearing loss: psychological and psychosocial implications. London: Academic Press, 1984.

Thomas AJ. Rehabilitation of adults with acquired hearing loss: the psychological dimension. Br J Audiol 1988;22:81–83.

Thomas AJ, Lamont M, Harris M. Problems encountered at work by people with severe acquired hearing loss. Br J Audiol 1982;16:39–43.

Thomas K, Thoreson R, Butler A, et al. Theoretical foundations of rehabilitation counseling. In: Parker RM, Symanski EM, eds. Rehabilitation counseling: basics and beyond. 2nd ed. Austin, TX: Pro-Ed, 1992:207–247.

Truax CB, Mitchell KM. Research on certain therapist skills in relation to process and outcome. In: Bergin AE, Garfield SL, eds. Handbook of psychotherapy and behavior change: an empirical analysis. New York: Wiley, 1971.

Truax CB, Wargo DG, Frank JD, et al. Therapist empathy, genuineness, and warmth and patient therapeutic outcome. J Consult Psychol 1966;30:395–401.

Ventry IM, Weinstein BE. The Hearing Handicap Inventory for the Elderly: a new tool. Ear Hear 1982;3:128–134.

Verderber RF, Verderber KS. Inter-act: using interpersonal communication skills. 6th ed. Belmont, CA: Wadsworth Publishing, 1992.

Ward WD. The American Medical Association/American Academy of Otolaryngology formula for determination of hearing handicap. Audiology 1982;22:313–324.

Ward WD. Correspondence: answer to Noble. Audiology 1988;27:61–64.

Watson D, Clark LA. Negative affectivity: the disposition to experience aversive emotional states. Psychol Bull 1984;96:465–490.

Watson D, Clark LA. Affects separable and inseparable: on the hierarchical arrangement of the negative affects. J Pers Soc Psychol 1992;62:489–505.

Watson D, Pennebaker JW. Health complaints, stress, and distress: exploring the central role of negative affectivity. Psychol Rev 1989;96:234–254.

Weinstein BE, Ventry IM. Audiologic correlates of hearing handicap in the elderly. J Speech Hear Res 1983a;26:148–151.

Weinstein BE, Ventry IM. Audiometric correlates of the Hearing Handicap Inventory for the Elderly. J Speech Hear Disord 1983b;48:379–384.

Weinstein BE, Spitzer JB, Ventry IM. Test-retest reliability of the Hearing Handicap Inventory for the Elderly. Ear Hear 1986;7:295–299.

Westbrook MT, Legge V, Pennay M. Attitudes towards disabilities in a multicultural society. Soc Sci Med 1993;36:615–623.

Whiston SC, Sexton TL. An overview of psychotherapy outcome research: implications for practice. Prof Psychol Res Pract 1993;24:43–51.

WHO. International classification of impairments, disabilities and handicaps: a manual of classification relating to the consequences of disease. Geneva: World Health Organization, 1980.

Wolpe J. Psychotherapy by reciprocal inhibition. Stanford, CA: Stanford University Press, 1958.

Wolpe J. The practice of behavior therapy. 3rd ed. New York: Pergamon Press, 1982.

Wright BE. Physical disability: a psychosocial approach. New York: Harper & Row, 1983.

Wylde MA. Psychological and counseling aspects of the adult remediation process. In: Alpiner JG, McCarthy PA, eds. Rehabilitative audiology: children and adults. Baltimore: Williams & Wilkins, 1987.

Yalom ID. The theory and practice of group psychotherapy. New York: Basic Books, 1985.

TECHNOLOGY IN AUDIOLOGIC REHABILITATION

Cochlear Implants

Anne L. Beiter, M.S., and Judith A. Brimacombe, M.A.

Cochlear implants are biomedical electronic devices that convert sound into electrical current to stimulate remaining auditory nerve elements directly, thereby producing hearing sensations. Research in the area of electrical stimulation of the auditory system has an extensive history (see Simmons, 1966, for a review of early investigations); however, it has been only in the past 25 years that implantable devices have been developed for the purpose of long-term electrical stimulation in humans. During this relatively short period, cochlear implants have evolved from single-channel systems to more complex multichannel devices. A number of authors have summarized these developments (Luxford and Brackmann, 1985; Staller, 1985; Shallop and Mecklenburg, 1987; Mecklenburg and Shallop, 1988; House and Berliner, 1991; Mecklenburg and Lehnhardt, 1991; Tyler and Tye-Murray, 1991).

Today, multichannel cochlear implantation is considered a safe and effective medical treatment for severe to profound bilateral, sensorineural hearing loss in appropriately selected adults and for profound bilateral hearing loss in children. Therefore, cochlear implants are not viewed as experimental; rather, they are regarded as an important component in routine clinical practice for the management of severe to profound hearing loss (National Institutes of Health, 1995). Otologists, audiologists, speech-language pathologists, educators of the hearing-impaired, and other interested professionals are collaborating to provide services that will enable cochlear im-

plant recipients to maximize benefit from their devices.

Currently, there are several different multichannel cochlear implant systems available commercially or under clinical investigation. The systems that have received approval for commercial distribution by the United States Food and Drug Administration (FDA) are the (1) Nucleus 22 and Nucleus 24 Cochlear Implant Systems, manufactured by Cochlear Limited, Sydney, Australia, and (2) the Clarion Multi-Strategy Cochlear Implant System, manufactured by Advanced Bionics Corporation, Sylmar, CA, USA. These are the systems discussed in this chapter. Single-channel cochlear implant systems are no longer used in the United States.[a]

Although the design features of specific devices exhibit some elemental differences (see Tyler and Tye-Murray, 1991), there are general principles that characterize cochlear prostheses. All systems are composed of an implantable, internal component and an externally worn microphone and processor. Acoustic signals picked up by the microphone are electrically transduced and sent via cabling to the processor so that they may be filtered, analyzed, or processed in some manner. The electrical outputs from the processor are delivered to the electrodes im-

---

[a]In November 1984, the FDA approved the 3M/House single-channel device for commercial use in adults. The 3M Company ceased manufacturing of their system in 1987. The AllHear single channel device, also developed by Dr. William House, is not being used in the United States.

planted in the cochlea. The application of electrical current at the electrode site results in direct stimulation of remaining neural elements. The resultant electrical discharge of auditory neurons proceeds up through the central auditory system, reaches the brain, and is interpreted as sound.

Nucleus 22 and Nucleus 24 Cochlear Implant Systems

The Nucleus 22 and Nucleus 24 Cochlear Implant Systems were developed with collaboration between the University of Melbourne, Melbourne Australia, and Cochlear Limited. Historical reviews may be found in Clark et al. (1987a), Patrick and Clark (1991), and Clark (1997). The Nucleus 22 Cochlear Implant System is the most widely used system, with more than 20,000 implant recipients worldwide. The Nucleus 22 System includes the Nucleus 22 cochlear implant, the Spectra body-worn speech proces-

sor, and in the future an ear-level (ESPrit 22) speech processor (Fig. 15.1). The Nucleus 24 Cochlear Implant System is the newest Nucleus system and was approved for use in adults and children by the FDA in June 1998. The Nucleus 24 cochlear implant builds on many of the proven design features of the Nucleus 22 implant, including the same 22-band intracochlear electrode array and the use of robust materials, such as titanium. The system includes the Nucleus 24 cochlear implant as well as the SPrint (body-worn) and ESPrit (ear-level) speech processors (Fig. 15.2).

INTERNAL COMPONENTS

The Nucleus 22 and Nucleus 24 cochlear implants consist of the implantable receiver/stimulator and a banded electrode array. The receiver/stimulator is an electronic device composed of a custom-designed integrated circuit and a small number of passive com-

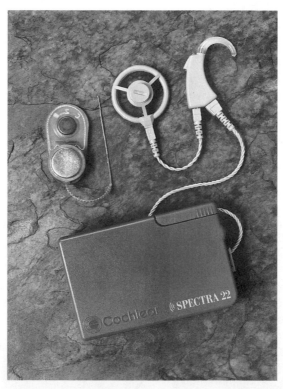

Figure 15.1. The Nucleus 22 System consists of the receiver/stimulator and electrode array, a miniaturized speech processor, and an ear-level microphone and transmitting coil.

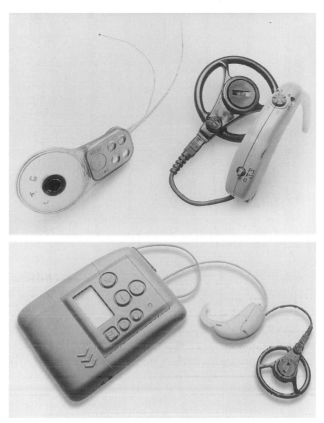

Figure 15.2. The Nucleus 24 System includes the CI24 implant (top) as well as the ESPrit and SPrint speech processors (bottom.)

ponents. The Nucleus 24 implant includes a new custom integrated circuit that allows stimulation of the auditory nerve at rates up to 14,400 Hz. The electronic circuitry of both implants is hermetically sealed within a titanium and ceramic capsule. A platinum receiving coil and rare earth magnet are external to the hermetically sealed capsule and are embedded in biocompatible, medical-grade silicone rubber used to encase the entire package. Connected to the receiver/stimulator by ceramic feedthroughs within the package is the smooth, flexible electrode array. It has 22 evenly spaced platinum electrode bands supported on a silicone rubber carrier. The electrodes vary in a smooth taper from 0.6 to 0.4 mm and are spaced equally along the distal 17 mm of the silicone carrier. A separate, insulated platinum-iridium wire is welded to each of the electrodes, and these wires run through the carrier, connecting each band separately to the receiver/stimula-

tor. On the proximal 8 mm of the silicone carrier are 10 additional nonstimulating platinum bands that provide extra mechanical stiffness to the array to aid in its insertion into scala tympani.

The Nucleus 24 cochlear implant includes two independent extracochlear ground electrodes to provide the capability of monopolar stimulation. The first ground (MP1) is a small ball electrode on a separate lead wire that is placed under the temporalis muscle during surgery. The second ground (MP2) is a plate electrode on the implant body. Each of these extracochlear electrodes may be used independently or linked electrically to form a third grounding option (MP1+2). In monopolar stimulation, the active or stimulating electrode is intracochlear and the ground or reference electrode is outside the cochlea. Both the Nucleus 22 and Nucleus 24 implants provide bipolar and common ground stimulation modes. In bipolar modes, the stimulating and ground electrodes are both within the cochlea.

In comparison to the Nucleus 22 implant, the shape of the Nucleus 24 cochlear implant reduces the overall size of the required surgical bed that must be drilled in the mastoid bone. It has a thin profile and is precurved to conform to the shape of a very young child's head. The cochlear implant is placed under the skin in a surgically created depression in the mastoid bone, and the electrode array can be inserted up to 25 mm into the cochlea. The surgeon places the extracochlear ball electrode under the temporalis muscle. Clark et al. (1987b; 1991a,b; 1997) and Webb et al. (1990) discuss surgical considerations and techniques for the Nucleus 22 and 24 cochlear implants.

The Nucleus 24 cochlear implant incorporates a sophisticated multipurpose telemetry system. Telemetry refers to the method by which the implant receives data from the external system and how it sends back diagnostic information about implant function to the Nucleus 24 Clinical Programming System. The N24 telemetry function provides electrode impedance, voltage compliance, and an innovative neural response telemetry (NRT). The programming audiologist can identify short- or open-circuit electrodes with electrode impedance measurements. These measurements can be obtained during surgery to assure that the device and electrodes are functioning properly. The clinician also makes impedance measurements during device programming. Electrodes that are short circuited or have too high an impedance will be eliminated from psychophysical testing. In addition, during device setting, ongoing voltage compliance measurements alert the clinician if the implant does not have sufficient voltage to deliver the amount of electrical current specified. This information is helpful so that programming parameters may be refined to suit individual needs. The NRT measures physiologic responses generated by the electrical stimulation of neural tissue within the cochlea. It uses the cochlear implant electrodes as both stimulating and recording electrodes, thus eliminating the need for the placement of scalp electrodes or an interface to additional evoked potential equipment. Currently, clinicians are using NRT to gather electrophysiologic data for the purpose of comparing these data with subjects' behavioral responses to electrical stimulation. After sufficient data have been collected from a large group of cochlear implant recipients, guidelines will be developed that may assist in the programming for adults and children.

The Nucleus 24 and the most recent version of the Nucleus 22 implant have a removable magnet and specific design characteristics to allow implant recipients to undergo magnetic resonance imaging (MRI) up to 1.5 Tesla, but not higher. If the implant's magnet is in place, it must be removed surgically under local anesthesia before any MRI studies. The feature of a removable magnet is an important design consideration, because there is a high likelihood that young children receiving implants today will require at least one MRI study during their lifetimes.

EXTERNAL COMPONENTS

The external components of the Nucleus 22 system include an ear-level directional microphone, transmitting coil, cables, and a body-worn speech processor, the Spectra 22. A single rechargeable AA battery powers the system. The transmitting coil is kept against the skin by a rare earth magnet that attracts to the companion magnet in the implant. The speech processor receives the electrical signals sent from the microphone, performs an analog-to-digital (A-D) conversion, then digitally extracts and encodes specific information about the acoustic input signal. The resulting digital code is routed to the transmitting coil and then to the implanted receiver/stimulator via radio frequency (RF) transmission. This system uses the spectral peak (SPEAK) speech-coding strategy.

The Nucleus 24 system has two speech processors. The SPrint is a fully digital body-worn processor that holds up to four independent programs or MAPs. The headset used with the processor includes a directional microphone, cables, and transmitting coil. The advanced circuitry and flexibility of this speech processor make it possible to program the SPrint using different advanced speech coding strategies. Additionally, the processor contains many user-selectable features, such as microphone sensitivity and loudness controls, a noise reduction feature, and programmable alarms and locks. The ESPrit is a cosmetic ear-level speech processor connected by a short cable to the transmitting coil. Two high-power 675-zinc air batteries power the ESPrit. It stores two user-selectable programs, accessible with a small toggle switch on the unit. The programmable rotary control functions independently as either a loudness or microphone sensitivity control. The ESPrit implements the SPEAK strategy. As with the Nucleus 22 speech processor, the SPrint and ESPrit processors send a stream of digital code to a transmitting coil and then across the skin by RF transmission.

In the Nucleus 22 and 24 systems, the cochlear implant receives power and the digital code from the speech processor, decodes the digital pulses, and sends constant current, biphasic electrical pulses to selected electrodes along the implanted array. For a more detailed description of the transmission of the digital signals to the cochlear implant, see Brimacombe and Beiter (1994) and Patrick et al. (1997).

The Clarion Multistrategy Cochlear Implant System

The Clarion Multistrategy Cochlear Implant System, manufactured by Advanced Bionics Corporation, is based on earlier research from the University of California San Francisco cochlear implant project. Additional development assistance came from collaborative efforts from the Neuroscience Program Office of the Research Triangle Institute (RTI) in North Carolina and MiniMed Technologies, Sylmar, CA, USA, a manufacturer of implantable insulin pumps.

INTERNAL COMPONENT

The internal portion of the system, referred to as the implantable cochlear stimulator (ICS), includes a precurved intracochlear electrode array, receiving coil, and the electronics package. The receiving coil and electronics are encased in a hermetically sealed ceramic case. A magnet also is included to allow coupling to the external headpiece. The ICS has an extracochlear ground electrode, which is a platinum band that goes around the implant package. There is a cochlear implant specifically for the right and left ears, because the electrode array's silicone rubber carrier is precurved to fit the shape of the cochlea. Theoretically, this places the array closer to the modiolus once it has been inserted into scala tympani. The electrode array consists of 16 platinum-iridium ball electrode contacts; each contact is 0.3 mm in diameter. The contacts are arranged in eight near-radial pairs with the two contacts of each pair separated by 0.5 mm. The electrode contacts are arranged in this manner to focus the electrical stimulation closer to remaining auditory neural elements. The eight pairs are spaced 2.0 mm apart (Schindler and Kessler, 1989; Kessler and Schindler, 1992, 1994). The Clarion system is an eight-channel device, and the implant can produce stimulation on the eight channels sequentially or simultaneously using either monopolar or bipolar stimulation. In monopolar stimulation, the active or stimulating electrode is intracochlear and the ground or reference electrode is outside the cochlea. Bipolar stimulation refers to passing current between two electrodes where the active and ground electrodes are both inside the cochlea. The first version of the Clarion system (version 1.0) became commercially available for adults in 1996. Shortly thereafter, a slightly smaller implant and processor (version 1.2) was introduced. The FDA approved this version for children in June 1997.

A more recent version of the ICS, the Clarion S-series, incorporates a change to the electrical connection of the electrodes to widen the spacing between the radial bipolar pairs effectively. An electrode from one pair is connected electrically to a contact of an adjacent pair to form what has been called "enhanced bipolar coupling." Enhanced bipolar coupling widens the spacing between the active and ground electrodes of the bipolar pair. The purpose is to stimulate a greater number of neural elements and, it is hoped, to increase the recipient's perceived loudness sensations as the amount of delivered current increases. However, this mode of stimulation reduces the total number of available channels from eight to seven when using bipolar as compared with monopolar stimulation (Advanced Bionics Corporation, 1997b).

All three versions (1.0, 1.2, and the S-series) of the ICS include a telemetry function that sends information back to the external processor regarding ICS status and electrode impedances. The audiologist uses this information when programming the device. Electrodes that are shorted or open circuit cannot be used in the recipient's programs.

The electronics package of the cochlear implant is placed under the skin in a surgically created well in the mastoid and occipital bones. During surgery, the preformed array is straightened mechanically using a special insertion tool. A large cochleostomy into scala tympani is required for use of this tool. Once inserted, the array returns to its original precurved shape. The array can be inserted up to 25 mm into the cochlea. The device is tested intraoperatively to assess the ICS status and measure electrode impedances before and after closure of the surgical wound (Schindler and Kessler, 1989; Lalwani et al., 1998).

EXTERNAL COMPONENTS

The external components of all three versions of the Clarion system include a body-worn speech processor, one-piece headset, cable, and battery pack to power the processor and implant. The headpiece incorporates an omnidirectional microphone and transmitting antenna in one unit. It also houses the companion magnet to keep the headpiece aligned over the cochlear implant. The headpiece connects to the speech processor by a single cable. The microphone picks up sound, and the electrical signal goes through the cable to the speech processor. The processor has an overall bandwidth

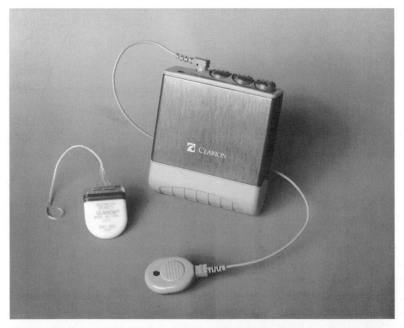

Figure 15.3. The Clarion System consists of the implantable cochlear stimulator, the one-piece headset, and body-worn speech processor.

from 250 to 5500 Hz. It processes the signal through a maximum of eight programmable bandpass filters, digitizes the information, and then sends the information to the transmitting coil where the digital code is sent across the head by RF transmission. The version 1.0 speech processor was larger and held two programs. The 1.2 and S-series processors have been miniaturized and store up to three independent user-selectable programs on the electrical erasable programmable read-only memory (EEPROM) chip in the processor. The processors also feature user-adjustable microphone sensitivity and volume controls. The Clarion S-series is shown in Figure 15.3.

Speech Coding Strategies for the Clarion and Nucleus 22 and 24 Cochlear Implant Systems

In cochlear implant systems, the principal function of the processor is to prepare and code the incoming acoustic information for delivery to the implant. When the signal is speech, the signal processing should deliver electrical stimulation to the auditory system that produces percepts that are speech-like for the cochlear implant recipient. For a review of speech perception related to signal processing, see Millar et al. (1990).

The Nucleus 22 and 24 systems use digital signal processing and incorporate several different speech-coding strategies. These coding strategies represent a set of "rules" that define how the incoming acoustic speech signal will be analyzed and coded by the speech processor. Historically, the Nucleus 22 system used speech-coding strategies that encoded specific speech features that were known empirically to be important for speech recognition. This family of strategies was referred to as speech feature extraction coding strategies. The reader is referred to Beiter and Brimacombe (1993), Brimacombe and Beiter (1994), and Patrick et al. (1997) for a review of these strategies.

Currently, the Nucleus 22 and 24 systems implement the SPEAK speech-coding strategy. In addition, the Nucleus 24 implements various other strategies, including contin-

uous interleaved sampling (CIS) and advanced combination encoder (ACE) strategies. All these strategies stimulate the auditory nerve with short-duration pulses of varying amplitude (i.e., varying amounts of electrical current) to represent the ongoing acoustic signal. The SPEAK strategy is a spectrally based strategy that takes advantage of the place pitch selectivity of the cochlea. It continuously analyzes the incoming acoustic signal (150 to 7.8 kHz) and divides it into 20 bandwidths. During each scan, the energy in each band is measured to determine which bands contain the highest amplitudes or maxima at that point in time. Each electrode along the array (up to 20 of the 22 available) is assigned to a band in accordance with the tonotopic order of the cochlea. The most apical electrode or channel, which will stimulate low-frequency neural elements, is assigned to the lowest frequency bandwidth, and the remaining channels are assigned to progressively higher frequency bands. During each scan cycle, the maxima, or peaks of energy, are determined and presented sequentially to the appropriate electrodes in tonotopic order from high to low frequency. As the spectral characteristics of the input signal vary, different electrodes along the array will be stimulated to represent the ongoing changes in the acoustic input. Depending on the signal level and spectral composition of the input, on average 6 channels (and up to 10) are stimulated for each scan cycle. The SPEAK coding strategy stimulates the cochlea at a modest rate that varies depending on the number of maxima delivered during each scan cycle. The average rate is 250 Hz.

In contrast to SPEAK, CIS strategies (Wilson et al., 1991a,b; 1994) attempt to reproduce the ongoing fine temporal changes in the acoustic waveform, as opposed to changes in the frequency domain. The Nucleus 24 implements a 4-, 6-, 8-, or 12-channel CIS strategy. In CIS strategies, the overall signal bandwidth is divided by the number of electrodes to be used (in this case 4, 6, 8, or 12) to determine the bandwidth for each filter or channel. The clinician selects a subset of the 22 electrodes on the array and assigns one electrode to each filter, following the tonotopic order of the cochlea. During each scan cycle, the output amplitudes from each filter are determined and represented as changes in the amount of electrical current sent to the selected electrodes. In contrast to SPEAK, in which place of stimulation varies along the array, in CIS strategies the same subset of electrodes or channels is always stimulated sequentially during each scan of the filters, regardless of the amount of energy detected in the filter. To represent temporal variations, CIS strategies stimulate the auditory nerve at rates of more than 800 Hz per channel. The maximum stimulation rate available with the Nucleus 24 implant is 14,400 Hz across all channels. To date, results across different cochlear implant devices indicate that SPEAK and CIS speech coding strategies provide equivalent performance on tests of open-set speech recognition, suggesting that the central auditory system can process spectrally or temporally based information.

The Nucleus 24 system implements strategies referred to as advanced combination encoders (ACE). When using ACE, the audiologist manipulates various parameters for coding speech information in an attempt to optimize individual performance. This family of strategies allows the clinician to combine some of the best features of spectrally and temporally based strategies, such as selection of the number of maxima and stimulation sites along the array with overall higher stimulation rates. Clinical research is in progress to compare in a controlled manner individual subject performance across SPEAK, CIS, and ACE speech-coding strategies.

The Clarion system incorporates two basic types of signal processing: compressed analog (CA)—more recently referred to as simultaneous analog stimulation (SAS)—and, nonsimultaneous, pulsatile processing CIS. In SAS, the input signal is divided into seven frequency bands, processed, and then the output of each band is presented simultaneously as a continuous reconstructed analog waveform to the seven electrode

pairs. One filter is assigned to each pair of electrodes along the array, following the normal tonotopic organization of the cochlea. The lowest frequency bandwidth is assigned to the most apically placed electrode pair, and progressively more basally placed electrodes are assigned higher-frequency bandwidths (Schindler and Kessler, 1993; Kessler and Schindler, 1994; Advanced Bionics Corporation, 1997b). The CA or SAS strategy used with the 1.0 and 1.2 implants was successful for only a small proportion of implant recipients, primarily because many recipients did not receive sufficient loudness when stimulated in a bipolar mode (Tyler et al., 1996). Monopolar stimulation is less suited to strategies that use simultaneous stimulation due to the wider spread of current in this mode, which can result in distortions due to overlapping current fields and channel interactions. With the introduction of enhanced bipolar coupling in the S-series implant, a larger proportion of recipients may be fit with the SAS (Battmer, 1997; Osberger and Kessler, 1998). Monopolar stimulation is used in the implementation of the CIS strategy in the Clarion system. Again, the input signal is processed through the eight filters, and the output from each determines the pulse amplitude of the short-duration electrical pulses that are sent sequentially to the eight active electrodes along the array. Assignment of filters to electrodes follows the tonotopic organization of the cochlea. The maximum stimulation rate per channel is 833 Hz, for a total stimulation rate of 6664 Hz.

Programming the Systems for Daily Use

Following cochlear implant surgery, there is a 4- to 6-week recuperative period before the programming of the speech processor. Once the surgical incision has healed and swelling over the area of the receiver/stimulator has reduced, the cochlear implant recipient returns to the clinic for the fitting of the external equipment.

Speech processors are miniature personal

computers. In the Nucleus systems, they contain random access memory (RAM) to store patient-specific programs, or MAPs. In the case of the Clarion systems, the processors use an EPROM to hold and update programs. In both Nucleus and Clarion systems, an IBM PC-compatible computer, a specialized interface unit, and customized software make up the programming system. The clinician uses these to obtain the necessary information to create each individualized MAP and program the speech processor for daily use. Both the Nucleus and Clarion programming systems are very flexible. They allow the clinician to make adjustments easily to the programs as the cochlear implant user becomes a more experienced listener. The RAM or EPROM within the speech processor can be updated almost instantaneously with a new MAP.

Both Nucleus and Clarion systems use customized software to perform specific psychophysical tests; based on the individual's responses, a program or MAP is configured that defines the parameters of electrical stimulation. Specifically, measurements of the amount of current needed to obtain a threshold and a maximum comfortable loudness level for electrical hearing are made for each electrode pair or channel. These values define the electrical dynamic range of hearing for each channel. Dynamic ranges vary within an individual across the electrode array and from patient to patient. Measurements of thresholds and comfortable loudness levels define the endpoints of the loudness growth function. This function defines how the on-going loudness variations in speech and environmental sounds will be mapped onto the individual's electrical dynamic range and, therefore, how important loudness cues will be perceived. Electrical dynamic ranges are narrow, typically on the order of 6 to 25 dB (Simmons, 1966; Shannon, 1983; White et al., 1984), whereas the amplitude variations in speech are on the order of 30 dB.

After dynamic ranges for each stimulating electrode have been established, the software automatically assigns a frequency range or bandwidth to each channel that will be used in the program. This assignment is made in an orderly fashion, with the high frequencies allocated to the more basally placed electrodes and the lower frequencies assigned to the more apically placed electrodes. As discussed in the section on coding strategies, for both the Nucleus and Clarion systems, frequency to channel allocation also is influenced by the number of channels used in the program and the type of speech-coding strategy selected. Stimulation of the electrodes normally results in perceptions that follow the tonotopic organization of the cochlea, wherein the lowest place-pitch percept will be the most apical electrode and the highest place-pitch percept will be the most basal electrode. For the Nucleus devices and the Clarion using the CIS strategy, electrodes are differentially stimulated in rapid succession based on the speech processor's extraction of information from the ongoing acoustic signal and the type of speech-coding strategy selected (i.e., SPEAK, CIS, or ACE for the Nucleus 24 and CIS for Clarion). When the Clarion device is programmed using SAS, the seven electrode pairs are stimulated simultaneously. More information on programming the Nucleus and Clarion speech processors for adults and children can be found in Roberts (1991), Beiter et al. (1991), Staller et al. (1991a), Rance and Dowell (1997), and Shapiro and Waltzman (1998).

Candidate Selection

Initially, cochlear implants were indicated only for those adults and children who demonstrated bilateral, profound, or total sensorineural hearing loss who gained no benefit from well-fit amplification. Individuals diagnosed with profound hearing loss will obtain varying degrees of benefit from traditional amplification (Fujikawa and Owens, 1978, 1979). Although hearing aid benefit can be more difficult to quantify objectively in this population, it is clear that simple audiologic measures of pure-tone sensitivity are insufficient to predict which individuals may benefit from powerful, appropriately fit amplification (Moeller, 1982;

Sims, 1982; Owens et al., 1985a; Owens and Raggio, 1988; Boothroyd, 1989; Geers and Moog, 1989). Thus, careful speech perception testing with appropriately fit hearing aids is a prerequisite to any consideration of cochlear implantation. An additional complicating factor is that, currently, the degree of benefit an individual might expect to receive from a cochlear implant cannot be predicted accurately preoperatively (Gantz et al., 1988; Fritze and Eisenwort, 1989; National Institutes of Health, 1995). Having said this, it should be pointed out that one of the main objectives of the preoperative evaluation is to select those candidates who are most likely to benefit from receiving an implant.

Today, multichannel cochlear implant technology has evolved to include more sophisticated speech-processing strategies that provide improved outcomes of enhanced speech recognition for most individuals with cochlear implants. As researchers have accumulated additional speech perception data and experience with cochlear implant recipients using these more sophisticated technologies, the audiologic criteria for implantation have expanded to include individuals who have more residual hearing and demonstrate some benefit from acoustic amplification. It is expected that the indications for prescribing a cochlear implant for both adults and children will continue to evolve as devices improve and additional experience with implant recipients accumulates.

ADULT PREOPERATIVE SELECTION AND EVALUATION PROCESS

The recommended patient selection criteria vary somewhat across the Clarion and Nucleus devices and in comparison are slightly expanded for the Nucleus 24 system. Thus, to give a broader overall picture, the criteria for the Nucleus 24 cochlear implant are presented in Table 15.1. These criteria are guidelines for the selection of those individuals who are most likely to benefit from cochlear implantation. With respect to adults with severe to profound hearing impairment, the expected benefits of a cochlear implant differ dramatically depending on the age at onset of deafness. Adults with a postlinguistic onset of hearing loss and those individuals who experienced an early onset, progressive hearing impairment and used hearing aids for some period are expected to receive substantial benefit in terms of hearing-only speech understanding. On the other hand, congenitally deafened adults who have never derived benefit from hearing aids and, therefore, experienced long-term sensory deprivation typically receive marginal benefit. Thus, the selection criteria differ considerably for these two populations.

The preoperative evaluation consists of medical/surgical and audiologic assessments as well as evaluations by other professionals, such as a speech-language pathologist, psychologist, or social worker, as needed on a case-by-case basis. Typically, several appointments will be required before a decision regarding candidacy can be

Table 15.1
Preoperative patient selection criteria for postlinguistically deafened adults

Severe to profound sensorineural hearing loss, bilaterally
Postlinguistically deafened
18 years of age or older
Marginal benefit from appropriate amplification (as defined by test scores of 40% correct or less in the best-aided condition on tape-recorded tests of open-set sentence recognition)
Psychologically and motivationally suitable
Medical examination should not reveal the following contraindications:
    Deafness due to lesions of the acoustic nerve or central auditory pathway
    Active middle ear infection or tympanic membrane perforation in the presence of active middle ear disease
    Absence of cochlear development

made. Throughout the evaluation process, the prospective candidate and family receive educational counseling from both the surgeon and audiologist regarding the risks and benefits of the procedure (Pope et al., 1986). It is important that the candidate be familiarized with the external hardware, counseled regarding the need for long-term repair maintenance of the equipment, and told of the remote risk of internal device failure.

It is critical that adequate time be devoted to answering any questions the candidate or family has and to questioning them regarding their expectations for use of the device. A series of expectations questionnaires have been developed for use with adults who are considering a cochlear implant (Cochlear Corporation, 1998a). The intent of these questionnaires is to quantify both the prospective candidate's and the family's expectations of device benefit. If expectations are unrealistically high in regard to what the implant can potentially provide a given individual, a decision regarding candidacy should be delayed until the team completes further counseling to bring expectations into line. In this respect, it is extremely helpful if the prospective implant recipient and members of the family can meet and talk privately with a cochlear implant user and his or her family.

MEDICAL/SURGICAL EVALUATION

During the initial clinical visits, the surgeon obtains a detailed medical history and performs a thorough otologic examination. One of the aims of this evaluation is to determine the etiology of deafness and to establish the age at onset and duration of severe to profound hearing loss. This kind of information is important for the team to take into consideration when counseling the candidate and family preoperatively. Although individual patient variables viewed in isolation have not proven to be good predictors of postoperative performance, certain patient characteristics in combination (e.g., early onset and long duration of deafness) do affect the degree of postoperative benefit. At

the University of Iowa Cochlear Implant Project, Gantz (1992) found that 21% of the variance in postoperative open-set speech perception scores was accounted for by the variable of duration of deafness. In their study, other variables accounted for considerably less variance; however, these researchers identified a number of factors that when taken in combination may allow better prediction of postoperative performance.

During the physical examination, it is important to note any potential complicating factors, such as any previously created surgical defects, congenital anomalies, or other conditions that could require alterations to the surgical plan. In general, preexisting ear conditions should be treated before final determination of candidacy (Gray, 1991). In addition to severe to profound hearing impairment, some candidates may also be blind (Martin et al., 1988), report vestibular problems, experience tinnitus, or have some other medical condition that needs to be taken into consideration during the evaluation. In most cases, a holistic approach is helpful in evaluating the overall risk/benefit for the individual considering implantation. During the workup, the necessary laboratory tests will be completed and the results reviewed. At some point during the evaluation process, a general physical examination also must be performed to establish that the patient is healthy enough to undergo surgery without undue risk.

Careful radiologic assessment of the cochleae is one of the most important components of the medical evaluation. High-resolution computed tomography (CT) scans are essential for studying the structures of the inner ear, specifically the basal turn of the cochlea, and identifying any malformations or disease processes, such as cochlear otosclerosis. The results of imaging will be important from the standpoint of candidate exclusion, ear selection, presurgical counseling, and general surgical planning and management (Balkany et al., 1986; Balkany and Dreisbach, 1987; Pyman et al., 1990). Cochlear agenesis and absence of an auditory nerve are contraindications to cochlear implantation (Jackler et al., 1987b). Other conditions, such as cochlear dysplasia and partial or complete obliteration of the basal turn of the cochlea, are considered relative contraindications. When osteoneogenesis is present, the surgeon can usually drill forward 8 to 10 mm in scala tympani through the new bone or fibrotic tissue and achieve at least a partial insertion of the electrode array (Balkany and Dreisbach, 1987; Balkany et al., 1988). In some instances, surgeons have found an obliterated scala tympani but an open scala vestibuli and have successfully placed the array into that scala (Steenerson et al., 1990).

When physical or radiographic evaluations suggest the presence of a preexisting condition, as noted above, the candidate must be fully informed and agree to proceed in light of the possibility of a less than complete insertion of a multichannel electrode array. After the surgeon has explained the cochlear implant surgical procedure, the candidate should ask any questions he/she has and then read and sign an informed consent document.

The status of the auditory nerve can be evaluated preoperatively using electrical stimulation of the promontory or round window. This procedure involves the transtympanic placement of a needle electrode onto the promontory, or alternatively, placement of a ball electrode into the round window niche. A small amount of electrical current is passed between the stimulating electrode and a surface electrode that is placed on the ipsilateral cheek or earlobe. The patient should report a consistent hearing sensation that is time-locked to the presentation of the stimulus and increases in perceived loudness as the amount of current increases. Individuals who do not exhibit responses to promontory or round window stimulation generally are not considered candidates for cochlear implantation, as a negative result suggests there is an insufficient number of remaining auditory nerve fibers to elicit a hearing percept (Lambert et al., 1987; Cochlear Corporation, 1994; Pyman et al., 1990; Kileny et al., 1991, 1992). Promontory or round window stimulation is not indicated in all cases. For example, if a candidate

demonstrates clear auditory thresholds that are described as hearing rather than tactile, it is not necessary to perform a promontory test. However, whenever there is concern regarding the integrity of the auditory nerve (e.g., auditory adaptation is present or the etiology is temporal bone fracture) or when the patient exhibits a complete total hearing loss in the ear that is being considered for implantation, promontory stimulation should be performed. Promontory testing is essential when the deafness is due to head trauma because it is possible that fracture of the temporal bone could be concomitant with severing of the acoustic nerve (Gray, 1991).

AUDIOLOGIC EVALUATION

Level I: air- and bone-conduction audiometry and immittance testing

The initial audiologic assessment consists of measurements of residual hearing and middle ear function. Residual hearing is assessed using standard techniques for obtaining air- and bone-conducted puretone thresholds bilaterally. Air-conduction thresholds should be determined for the frequencies ranging from 125 to 8000 Hz using a calibrated audiometer that has an output greater than 115 dB at 500 through 4000 Hz. Bone conduction and immittance testing are performed to rule out a significant conductive component to the hearing loss. Stapedial reflex test findings should be consistent with severe to profound sensorineural hearing loss. Most commonly, reflexes will be absent at frequencies greater than 250 Hz bilaterally. If reflexes are obtained at frequencies greater than 250 Hz, auditory brainstem response testing should be performed to rule out a nonorganic component to the hearing loss. Stimuli should consist of both unfiltered clicks and frequency-specific tone pips to ascertain the general configuration of the hearing loss. Otoacoustic emission testing should also be performed. If emissions are present, further evaluation is required to determine potential candidacy (Starr et al., 1996).

Level II: aided audiometric and speech testing

Once a severe to profound or profound bilateral sensorineural hearing loss has been determined, the degree of benefit obtained from amplification should be measured. The audiologist conducts a hearing aid evaluation to establish whether the candidate's hearing aids are appropriate for the degree of hearing loss. If alternative amplification would be more appropriate, a trial period of at least 1 month is recommended. For postlinguistically deafened adults, a trial with a tactile device is not recommended due to the limited benefit derived by current technology (Skinner et al., 1988).

The hearing aid evaluation should consist of standard electroacoustic measurements (e.g., frequency response curve, maximum power output, and harmonic distortion), sound field warble-tone thresholds, insertion gain, and an assessment of speech discrimination ability. For a thorough discussion of hearing aid selection and evaluation, the reader is referred to Pollack (1980), Skinner (1988), and Skinner et al., 1994a.

Sound field testing should be carried out in a monitored environment, using a measuring microphone attached to a sound level meter. Typically, the candidate is seated facing a loudspeaker in a sound-treated room at a distance of 1 meter. The measuring probe microphone should be placed in close proximity to the hearing aid microphone. Warble-tone thresholds are assessed at frequencies ranging from 250 through 4000 Hz. A speech detection threshold is also obtained.

The speech discrimination test battery is generally administered in the best-aided condition, unless there is more residual hearing in an ear, warranting a monaural workup to assess the contribution of each ear to the binaural listening condition. In this situation, a screening test that measures monaural and binaural open-set sentence recognition is recommended before the more complete workup (Shallop, personal communication, Shallop JK, 1994). For those candidates with severe to profound hearing loss, the speech perception battery focuses on open-set, auditory-only, mono-syllabic word and sentence recognition. However, for candidates with very limited aided residual hearing, the audiologist may include some closed-set tests and an assessment of speechreading ability. Recorded materials are recommended over live-voice presentations, so that results can be compared across cochlear implant centers and for a given patient over time.

Historically, a thorough test battery, referred to as the Minimal Auditory Capabilities (MAC) battery, designed by Owens et al. (1985b), has been used with postlinguistically deafened adults. It includes 14 subtests that evaluate the perception of both suprasegmental and segmental aspects of speech, environmental sound recognition, and speechreading enhancement. The battery includes easier closed-set and more difficult open-set measures. Another audiologic battery developed at the University of Iowa incorporates tests from the MAC Battery and other measures devised by Tyler et al. (1983). This battery consists of 15 subtests; again, closed-set and open-set measures are used. Some of the subtests in the Iowa test battery are available on video laser disc (Tyler et al., 1986). Although these test batteries are excellent for research purposes, they may be impractical in a routine clinical setting. For this reason, a shorter version (Cochlear Corporation, 1998a) incorporates portions of the MAC and Iowa batteries. These tests are listed in Table 15.2 and are distributed on compact disc.

Once the medical and audiologic assessments have been completed, the cochlear implant team meets to discuss the candidate's preoperative profile. The medical findings are reviewed, paying close attention to the results of the high-resolution CT scans. The results of the audiologic tests are discussed in relation to the potential for individual postoperative benefit from the cochlear implant. Comparisons are made between the individual's aided performance and the average results obtained from a large pool of multichannel cochlear implant recipients. Particular attention should be paid to the individual's aided open-set word and sentence recognition when materials are

Table 15.2
Recommended audiologic test battery for evaluation of adult candidates

Level I   Air- and bone-conduction audiometry and immittance testing
          Pure-tone thresholds under headphones
          Bone conduction thresholds
          Tympanomety
          Middle ear reflexes
          Otoacoustic emissions
          Auditory brainstem response testing (optional)
Level II Aided audiometric and speech testing
          Initial hearing aid evaluation
          Trial with an appropriate hearing aid (when indicated)
Level III Speech recognition testing
          Closed-set
              Four-choice spondee
              Vowel identification
              Medial consonant identification
          Open-set
              Monosyllabic words (NU 6)
                  Word score
                  Phoneme score
              CID Sentences
              Iowa Sentences without Context
          Speechreading enhancement (recommended only for those individuals who score 0%
              on open-set sentence measures)
              CID Sentences
                  Speechreading only
                  Speechreading with sound

presented at 70 dB sound pressure level (SPL). If the presentation level must be higher than 70 dB SPL for the candidate to understand any speech, this suggests possible implant candidacy.

PEDIATRIC PREOPERATIVE SELECTION AND EVALUATION PROCESS

The clinical evaluation of potential pediatric cochlear implant candidates involves professionals from otolaryngology, audiology, speech-language pathology, psychology, and education. Other disciplines may be added to the team as necessary on a case-by-case basis. The family also plays an integral role on the team. When the candidate is a young child, the parents assume the responsibility of making the decision of whether to pursue cochlear implantation. Ideally, the parents have accepted their child's deafness, have been informed regarding the various treatment options available, and understand the long-term commitment to the child's (re)habilitation and support it fully. When the child is an adolescent or teenager, the team members must carefully examine the child's own feelings, expectations, and desires surrounding implantation. Older children who are going through the evaluation process solely because of parental wishes are not considered good cochlear implant candidates.

Questionnaires have been developed to assess the expectations of the parents and the child, when appropriate. If the parents' expectations for device benefit are unrealistic, additional counseling is needed. One common expectation is that the child will begin to speak intelligibly following device implantation. Although this goal may be realized long-term, it is important to counsel parents that this is a secondary benefit of implantation. Depending on the child, it may take many months or years of strong auditory/oral (re)habilitation before it is achieved. When counseling regarding the long-term commitment to (re)habilitation, an effective strategy is to arrange for the family to meet with another family who has gone through the same decision-making process and has a child with a cochlear implant.

Written material also should be provided to the family. It should include information on the impact of deafness, how a cochlear implant functions, how children are evaluated before implantation, the surgery, the device-fitting process, equipment trouble-shooting suggestions, and the postimplantation (re)habilitation (Cochlear Corporation, 1999a).

The educator plays an important role on the team during the preoperative evaluation as well as during the postoperative habilitation and long-term management of the child. Early in the selection process, the school system and the child's teacher should be informed that the child is being considered for a cochlear implant and be invited to the team meetings. The educator may be unfamiliar with cochlear implants and have somewhat ambivalent feelings in regard to working with a child with an implant. Thus, specific information about the cochlear implant must be provided and any misconceptions resolved. Written materials are available describing how a cochlear implant operates and how to care for it in the classroom (Coch-

lear Corporation, 1999b). Preoperatively, the teacher provides information to the team regarding the child's functional use of amplification, his or her general learning style, the existence of any learning difficulties, and his or her overall communication abilities within the classroom. Before surgery, the child's teacher should introduce the entire class to the concept of what a cochlear implant is and how it works. The fact that surgery is required should be explained as well. This will help the child successfully integrate into the class following the surgery and the initial fitting of the external equipment. During the school day, the classroom teacher will be responsible for verifying that the external equipment is functioning and performing basic trouble-shooting of the equipment.

The recommended selection criteria for children being considered for cochlear implantation are found in Table 15.3. They are fairly general, allowing the pediatric cochlear implant team to evaluate each child within a more individualized context. Recently, candidacy criteria for children have been broadened to include children who are profoundly hearing impaired but demonstrate a small amount of aided open-set, auditory-only word recognition. Initial postoperative results with children fitting this profile suggest that children who have had

---

Table 15.3
Preoperative pediatric patient selection criteria

Profound sensorineural hearing loss, bilaterally

Between the ages of 18 months and 17 years

Patients should demonstrate little or no benefit from hearing aids as defined by obtaining 20% or less on appropriate open-set measures. In younger children, little or no benefit is defined as lack of progress in development of simple auditory skills in conjunction with appropriate amplification and participation in intensive aural habilitation.

Medical examination should not reveal the following contraindications:
  Deafness due to lesions of the acoustic nerve or central auditory pathway
  Active middle ear infection or tympanic membrane perforation in the presence of active middle ear disease
  Absence of cochlear development

Candidates should have received consistent exposure to input from a sensory aid (e.g., hearing aid, vibrotactile device, or cochlear implant). A 3- to 6-month hearing aid trial is required for children without previous aided experience

Candidates should be enrolled in educational settings that emphasize oral/aural training

Families and (if possible) candidates should be psychologically and motivationally suitable

increased auditory experience make earlier gains in speech recognition than those who do not demonstrate benefit from amplification (Zwolan et al., 1997; Beiter et al., 1998). Whether this initial advantage is maintained has not been demonstrated. In addition, the age limit for pediatric implantation for the Nucleus 22 and 24 Systems has been lowered from 2 years to 18 months of age. The decision to lower the age limit was supported by the excellent postoperative benefit obtained by children who received implants at a relatively young age (Waltzman et al., 1992, 1994; Dowell and Cowan, 1997; Staller et al., 1997). In addition, it reflects the importance of early intervention to minimize the effects of sensory deprivation and maximize the potential for development of oral speech and language skills during the early formative period. From a surgical perspective, the cochlea is adult-size at birth and maturation of the skull is sufficient to accommodate the device, even at this young age. However, some alterations to surgical technique are recommended in the pediatric patient (Cochlear Corporation, 1998b). Although implantation before 18 months of age is theoretically possible, it may be difficult to verify profound bilateral deafness or quantify the amount of benefit the child receives from amplification.

The recommendation that the child be enrolled in an educational program that places strong emphasis on the development of auditory/oral communication underscores the fact that such abilities will not develop without the appropriate (re)habilitation. This may suggest modifications to the individualized educational plan. In some cases, it may be necessary to implement changes in the child's educational placement before proceeding with cochlear implantation (Beiter et al., 1991; Boothroyd et al., 1991).

MEDICAL/SURGICAL EVALUATION

The preoperative medical evaluation consists of a comprehensive history, physical examination, all necessary laboratory tests, and high-resolution CT scans as described earlier. The history should include infor-

mation regarding the pregnancy, developmental milestones, any postnatal problems, additional handicaps, and a family history related to hearing loss. During the medical examination, any malformations of the ear should be noted. The incidence of otitis media should also be reviewed (Clark and Pyman, 1997). High-resolution CT scans are essential for the evaluation of any inner ear malformations such as Mondini's dysplasia (Jackler et al., 1987a). The finding of a very narrow internal auditory canal may be a contraindication to cochlear implantation, as it may indicate that only the facial nerve is present (Jackler et al., 1987b). In older children, the viability of the auditory nerve can be assessed behaviorally using the promontory or round window stimulation procedure, described in section "Adult Preoperative Selection and Evaluation Process." Kileny and Kemink (1987), Kileny et al. (1994), and Mason et al. (1997) use electrically elicited brainstem responses to make measures of eighth nerve viability during preoperative or perioperative promontory stimulation testing. Although these procedures are somewhat challenging from a technical point of view, they prove useful in the assessment of very young children when there is concern regarding the status of the auditory nerve.

AUDIOLOGIC EVALUATION

The audiologic evaluation of children for a cochlear implant follows many of the same steps described for adults, with the exception that the test materials for the assessment of benefit from amplification will be different and the evaluation process may take longer. In addition, if the child has never worn appropriate amplification, an extended trial (i.e., 3 to 6 months) is recommended, during which time the child receives consistent auditory habilitation. Ideally, this program stresses the meaningful use of audition and involves the parents to teach them how to provide daily auditory skill development throughout the child's day. For very young children, pretraining may be an important component of the trial period (Beiter et al., 1991; Staller et al., 1991a). During pretraining, basic auditory concepts are taught, leading to the development of conditioned responses to acoustic stimuli. If progress with traditional amplification is noted, the decision regarding implant candidacy may be postponed until a more thorough evaluation of benefit from hearing aids can be completed.

Once a bilateral, profound hearing loss has been determined using standard behavioral audiometry, immittance testing should be performed to identify any conductive component to hearing loss and to confirm the profound nature of deafness through stapedial reflex testing. Electrophysiologic measures may be used to substantiate the diagnosis but should not be used exclusively to determine candidacy. That is, some behavioral audiometric testing must be performed under earphones so that frequency-specific information can be obtained for each ear. Also, tests for otoacoustic emissions should be incorporated into the routine evaluation of these children. If emissions are present in the face of other diagnostic evidence suggesting a severe to profound hearing loss, additional evaluation is required before determining candidacy (Starr et al., 1996; Stein et al., 1996).

The speech perception tests used to evaluate the benefits obtained from traditional amplification will vary depending on the age, cognitive level, and language abilities of the child. A hierarchy of tests is shown in Table 15.4. For the very young child with

Table 15.4
Recommended audiologic test battery for evaluation of pediatric candidates

Level I	Air- and bone-conduction audiometry and immittance testing
	Pure-tone thresholds under headphones
	Tympanomety
	Middle ear reflexes
	Otoacoustic emissions
	Auditory brainstem response testing (optional)
	Hearing aid evaluation
	Hearing aid trial (when indicated)[a]
	Pretraining (when indicated)[b]
Level II	Speech perception Evaluation
	Closed set
	CID Early Speech Perception Battery
	Low Verbal Version (use only with those children who do not have enough language to take the standard version)
	Standard Version
	NU-CHIPS
	Open -set
	GASP Words
	MAC Spondee Recognition
	CID Sentences
	PBK Words
	Lexical Neighborhood Monosyllable Word Test
	Multisyllable Lexical Neighborhood Test
	Measure of Speechreading (with and without sound)
	Craig Lipreading Inventory word subtest
	Visual Enhancement Subtest of the MAC Battery
	Parent inventory
	Meaningful Auditory Integration Scale

[a]If the child has not been fitted with appropriate amplification, a minimum 3- to 6-month trial with hearing aids is recommended under most conditions. An exception would be in the case of a postmeningitic child who is showing evidence on CT scans of ongoing ossification of the cochlea.

[b]Children who demonstrate minimal attending skills or who are not under stimulus/response control should receive pretraining to develop these skills before beginning the speech perception evaluation.

extremely limited receptive vocabulary, the low-verbal version of the CID Early Speech Perception (ESP) Battery (Moog and Geers, 1990) may be the most appropriate measure. In addition, the parents should be interviewed using the Meaningful Auditory Integration Scale (MAIS) (Robbins et al., 1991) or the Infant Toddler version (IT-MAIS). This scale provides information regarding the child's use of hearing during routine daily activities. For children with a richer receptive vocabulary, the standard version of the ESP is used. The battery consists of three closed-set subtests that evaluate the child's ability to use suprasegmental and segmental information. The ESP Battery has several strengths: (1) it incorporates a hierarchy of skill levels, (2) the vocabulary is appropriate for young deaf children, (3) pictures or objects depict the auditory stimuli, and (4) stimuli are recorded but may be presented via live voice if necessary (Staller et al., 1991a). The Northwestern University Children's Perception of Speech (NU-CHIPS) test is a standardized, recorded, closed-set test (Elliott and Katz, 1980) consisting of monosyllabic words. It is appropriate only for children with more extensive vocabularies.

Tests of open-set word or sentence recognition range in difficulty and include the Glendonald Auditory Screening Procedure (GASP) (Erber, 1982), Spondee Recognition subtest from the MAC Battery, CID Sentences, and the phonetically balanced kindergarten list of monosyllabic words (PBKs) (Haskins, 1949) and Lexical Neighborhood Tests (Kirk et al., 1995). The GASP word and sentence subtests are the easiest of the open-set measures, primarily due to the use of simple vocabulary. The remaining tests require that the child possess a more sophisticated lexicon. A measure of speechreading ability may be obtained. This can prove difficult, especially with young children, given their short attention spans and the difficulty of the task. The Craig Lipreading Inventory (Jeffers and Barley, 1977) uses a picture-pointing task and relatively simple vocabulary. Older children with late onset deafness may be tested using adult material such as the Visual Enhancement Subtest of the MAC Battery.

Osberger et al. (1991) have devised other test measures. They include the closed-set Change/No Change test, the Screening Inventory of Perception Skills, the Minimal Pairs test, the Hoosier Auditory Visual Enhancement test, and the modified open-set Common Phrases test. In addition, the closed-set Monosyllable Trochee Spondee (MTS) test (Erber and Alencewicz, 1976), and the Word Intelligibility by Picture Identification (WIPI) (Lerman et al., 1965) have been used to assess suprasegmental and segmental discrimination abilities. It is not recommended that candidates be administered all the measures discussed. Rather, testing should be tailored to each child's age and cognitive and linguistic level.

Auditory Rehabilitation

Following the fitting of the external equipment, the audiologist plans an individualized program of follow-up that includes visits for any necessary reprogramming and auditory training with the device, if needed. For adults with postlinguistic onset of hearing loss, little formal training is typically required. However, most recipients will need counseling regarding use of the device and direct practice for listening in difficult situations. In addition, clinicians can provide advice, support, and some practice on use of the telephone. On the other hand, adults with prelinguistic deafness or long-term sensory deprivation will require more extensive, structured practice to achieve maximum benefit from the cochlear implant. In addition to appointments with the audiologist for reprogramming, it is important for these recipients to receive auditory rehabilitation either through their audiologist or another clinician/therapist. It is important to begin auditory rehabilitation at a level at which the tasks are not too difficult for the individual. In this way, progress can be based on achievements, and discouragement on the patient's part can be minimized. Screening tests can be used to determine the level at which an individual should begin his or her training.

For adults with long-term sensory deprivation, a multisensory approach to rehabilitation is recommended, as individuals will use all cues available to them in their everyday environment. Training often begins in the auditory-visual modality. After success at this level, auditory-only activities may be introduced, if appropriate. Initially, the therapist presents material in a closed-set and will work toward the introduction of contextually based open-set material. Strauss-Schier and Rost (1996) and Fugain et al. (1996) provide excellent suggestions for working with postlinguistically and prelinguistically deafened adults.

For children, the type and frequency of auditory (re)habilitation must be based on the needs of the child. Factors such as age at onset of hearing loss, length of sensory deprivation, and the dependence on spoken language affect the course of training and the rate of progress that can be expected for a given child. Brackett (1991) has divided children into four training categories based on these factors affecting progress. The categories are (1) postlinguistic, short-term deafness, age-appropriate language; (2) congenital or prelinguistic, short-term deafness (2 to 4 years of age), limited to poor language; 3) postlinguistic, long-term deafness (older than 4 years of age), fair to good language; and (4) congenital or prelinguistic, long-term deafness (greater than 4 years old), limited to poor spoken language. Each of these groups will make progress over time but the rates will vary. In general, Brackett recommends a synthetic, integrated approach that incorporates listening into all daily activities.

Lowell and Stoner (1960) have developed specific activities for auditory skill development in children (Erber [1982], Schuyler et al. [1985], Stout and Windle [1986]). More recently, many educators, therapists, and clinicians have published excellent articles and books on the subject of (re)habilitation for children with severe to profound hearing impairments who use hearing aids or cochlear implants. Moog et al. (1994) and McConkey-Robbins (1994) have provided guidelines for developing speech perception skills and general oral communication abilities in children with cochlear implants. Allum (1996) has edited a comprehensive text on rehabilitation for adults and children using cochlear implants. Estabrooks (1994, 1998) has edited two texts that provide useful and important information related to the auditory habilitation of children with severe to profound hearing impairments. Both are good resources for parents and professionals. Nevins et al. (1991) provide information from the educator's perspective as a member of a pediatric cochlear implant program. A complete listing of aural rehabilitation materials for adults and children can be ordered from the American Speech-Language-Hearing Association (1990). Materials are also available through the Alexander Graham Bell Association for the Deaf. Finally, the reader is referred to Chapter 7 for further discussion of rehabilitation strategies for children with significant hearing impairment.

Results

POSTLINGUISTICALLY DEAFENED ADULTS

More than 25,000 adults and children have been implanted with various types of cochlear implants worldwide; more than 22,000 have received the Nucleus 22 or 24 multichannel system. The benefit obtained from cochlear implants has been found to vary depending on the type of device (e.g., single-channel versus multichannel systems) (Gantz et al., 1988; Brimacombe et al., 1989; Mangham and Kuprenas, 1989; Tyler et al., 1989). In fact, single-channel cochlear implants are no longer used in most countries. Benefit also varies across the population of patients, regardless of the specific multichannel device used (Cohen et al., 1985; Gantz et al., 1988; Dorman et al., 1989; Staller et al., 1991a,b; Gantz, 1992; Skinner et al., 1994b; Kessler et al., 1995; Waltzman et al., 1995; Tyler et al., 1996; Lalwani et al., 1998). Factors affecting this interpatient variability may include the age at implantation, the age at onset of profound deafness, the years of sensory deprivation, the degree of auditory nerve survival, and the cognitive processing abilities of the individual.

Despite the interpatient variability observed across devices, the benefits obtained from intracochlear, multichannel implants by postlinguistic, severe to profoundly hearing-impaired adults have increased significantly in the past several years. Improvements in technology—including more powerful integrated circuits, digital signal processing, and sophisticated speech processing strategies—have contributed in large part to improvements in postoperative outcomes (National Institutes of Health, 1995; Patrick, 1998; Rubenstein, 1998). Skinner et al. (1994b) reported statistically significant increases in individual performance on a variety of measures in quiet and noise for 63 adults who participated in a carefully controlled ABAB study comparing the earlier Multipeak (MPEAK) speech feature-extraction strategy with SPEAK using the Nucleus 22 system. The proportion of subjects showing statistically significant improvements with SPEAK varied from 25 to 80%, depending on the difficulty of the measure. The largest increases in performance were seen on more difficult measures, such as open-set sentence tests administered in background noise. Staller et al. (1997) reported on a large series of postlinguistic, severe to profoundly hearing-impaired adults who received the Nucleus 22 cochlear implant and were initially stimulated with SPEAK. Most subjects demonstrated relatively high levels of open-set speech recognition after only a short period of exposure to the coding strategy. After 2 weeks of device use, the mean monosyllabic word score was 19.2% and the mean sentence score was 53.5%. Performance increased with additional experience to 35.6% on monosyllabic words and 74.4% on sentences after 6 months of experience. Thirty-eight percent of the subjects scored greater than 90% and only 1 subject scored less than 10% on sentence recognition.

Tyler et al. (1996) have shown comparable results for 19 postlinguistically deafened adults implanted with the Clarion device after a similar amount of experience (9 months). They reported mean scores of 37.2% for monosyllabic words and 61.5% on sentence recognition. These subjects used version 1.0 of the Clarion system. Recently, Lalwani et al. (1998) reviewed postoperative outcomes for 31 subjects with 6 months of device experience. Open-set mean scores were 32% and 72% on monosyllabic words and sentences, respectively. The majority of subjects in both studies used and scored better with the CIS strategy compared with CA. These subjects did not receive the S-series implant that incorporates enhanced bipolar coupling. Battmer (1997) reported initial experiences with 12 adults who consecutively underwent implantation of the S-series. Eleven of these subjects' implants could be programmed and tested with SAS and CIS. One subject could not be fit successfully with SAS and used only CIS. The 11 subjects used both strategies equally for 2 weeks. After 2 weeks, six preferred SAS and five preferred CIS. After 4 weeks of experience, half the group performed better with CIS and the other half with SAS. One subject's performance was equivalent. In this pilot study, subjects performed better with their preferred strategy. Additional controlled studies are underway to understand better the effects of these different strategies on patient performance.

Recent postoperative outcome data also are available for the Nucleus 24 system. Staller et al. (1998) summarized the North American clinical trial results for 67 adults with 6 months of experience. Subjects in this trial could have as much as 40% aided open-set sentence recognition preoperatively. The mean preoperative and 6-month postoperative performance on a variety of open-set tests is shown in Figure 15.4. All data were collected with the SPEAK strategy. Currently, investigations are underway with these subjects to compare their performance across SPEAK, CIS, and ACE strategies. Additionally, 36 subjects were fit with the ear-level ESPrit processor and their performance was compared with performance using the body-worn SPrint. Performance

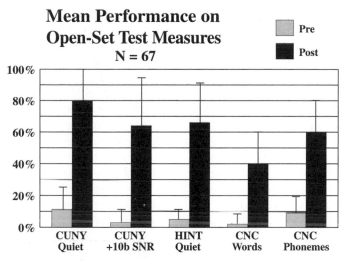

Figure 15.4. Preoperative and 6-month postoperative means and standard deviations for Nucleus 24 recipients on the following open-set measures: City University of New York (CUNY) Sentences, in quiet and at a +10 dB SNR; Hearing in Noise Test (HINT) Sentences in quiet; and Consonant-Nucleus-Consonant words and phonemes.

was equivalent between the two processors for all measures in both quiet and noise. In summary, these data suggest that adults with a postlinguistic onset of hearing impairment can achieve high levels of open-set speech recognition, although there remains a large amount of variability across individuals.

CHILDREN

The first FDA-approved clinical investigation to study the safety and effectiveness of a multichannel implant system in children began in 1986 and resulted in approval of the Nucleus 22 Cochlear Implant System in June 1990. Since that time, both the Clarion (June 1997) and the Nucleus 24 (June 1998) systems have gained regulatory approval. Multichannel cochlear implants, regardless of their design differences, should provide important information about sound so that children can use hearing through the implant to develop basic auditory skills. Historically, assessment of benefit derived from a cochlear implant has focused on the child's developing speech perception abilities using hearing alone. However, it is important to remember that the ultimate goal is for the child to develop useful hearing that allows him or her to learn speech and oral language for communication. Of course, many other

variables come into play that affect an individual's development of oral communication skills. Factors such as the child's age at implantation, the length of auditory deprivation, and the commitment of the family, educators, and therapists to maintain a strong auditory habilitation program can influence the final outcome.

Numerous researchers have shown that prelinguistically and postlinguistically deafened children using multichannel implants demonstrate significant improvement in the identification of words within a closed-set compared with their preoperative abilities with hearing aids. Many of these children also demonstrate some open-set word and sentence recognition. However, when compared to adults with postlinguistic onset of hearing impairment who demonstrate rapid acquisition of open-set abilities, this higher level of performance tends to be reached over time, in some cases several years (Staller et al., 1991b, 1994; Dawson et al., 1992; Gantz et al., 1994; Geers and Brenner, 1994). The majority of children with cochlear implants have a prelinguistic onset of deafness and may not have developed the cognitive, speech production, or linguistic skills required for many formal test measures. Some children who received their implants at an early age and have been educated in auditory-oral programs exhibit high levels of open-set speech recognition. This longitudinal research indicates that children who are born with profound hearing losses or are deafened very early in life can achieve these high levels of performance. However, the age at implantation seems to be a significant factor in predicting performance (Staller et al., 1994; Waltzman et al., 1994; Dowell and Cowan, 1997). This research finding is highly significant, because in the past many professionals questioned whether prelinguistically deafened children could gain enough auditory information through an implant to develop high levels of speech perception and oral language.

Questions also have been raised as to whether children who developed their speech perception and auditory memories based on sound processed by a given speech coding strategy would be able to take advantage of more sophisticated speech encoders. In the case of the Nucleus 22 system, most children who used the earlier MPEAK strategy and have had their devices reprogrammed using SPEAK have demonstrated improved speech perception abilities with SPEAK. Cowan et al. (1995) followed 7 children over 18 months after the change from MPEAK to SPEAK. Six of the seven children scored significantly higher when using SPEAK, especially when testing in background noise. Staller et al. (1997) studied 34 prelinguistically deafened children who changed from MPEAK to SPEAK after an average of 2.4 years of experience with MPEAK. After 6 months of experience with SPEAK, 77% of children achieved some open-set sentence recognition compared with 20% at the MPEAK baseline testing. These data suggest that even early deafened children can make use of the new information provided by a more advanced strategy. Thus, there is reason to believe that children receiving implants today will have the advantage of auditory learning with current implant technology but should also be able to take advantage of future technological advancements.

Pediatric speech perception data collected during the recent Clarion and Nucleus 24 clinical investigations provide evidence of improved speech perception compared with preoperative abilities, even with limited cochlear implant experience (Advanced Bionics Corporation, 1997a; Arndt, 1998). Figure 15.5 illustrates longitudinal changes in mean speech recognition by younger and older children who received the Clarion de-

Open-Set Sentence Recognition

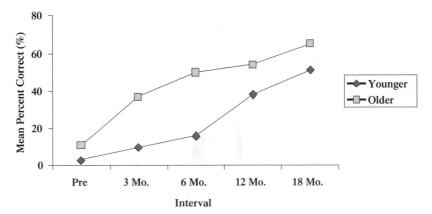

Figure 15.5. Longitudinal mean speech recognition for children who use the Clarion device. Younger children were administered the quasi open-set Mr. Potato Head task. Older children were administered the Common Phrases test.

vice. The younger children (mean age at implant, 3.4 years) were administered the open-set Mr. Potato Head task, and the older children (mean age at implant, 9.3 years) were given the Common Phrases test. Clinicians administered both tests monitored by live voice in the hearing-only condition. Although the older children made larger gains initially, the younger children exhibited a definite spurt in performance after 1 year of implant use. Both groups showed evidence of open-set speech recognition after limited exposure to the device, and there is a trend for improved performance with additional hearing experience (Osberger, 1997).

Figure 15.6 shows mean longitudinal performance on a variety of open-set measures for children 5 years and older (mean age at implant, 9.6 years) who received the Nucleus 24 implant. On average, the children demonstrated significant gains on all test measures after only 3 months, and improvements in performance were noted across all tests after 6 months of device use. The younger children in this study had a mean age at implantation of 2.9 years. Consistent with the data from children implanted with the Clarion device, these children showed smaller, although consistent gains

in auditory-only speech perception at the 3-month test interval, and their performance improved with additional experience.

In summary, the data gathered to date from children who have received the Nucleus and Clarion multichannel cochlear implant systems demonstrate significant improvements on both closed- and open-set speech perception measures. Continued monitoring of children's performance over time suggests that children improve as they gain more experience and training with the device. Many children, including congenitally and prelinguistically deafened children, will achieve some level of open-set speech recognition after sufficient listening experience.

SPEECH AND LANGUAGE DEVELOPMENT

The consequences of severe to profound hearing impairment include loss of the auditory feedback loop necessary for the development of normal segmental and suprasegmental feature production and general speech intelligibility. Multichannel cochlear implants transmit important spectral and temporal cues critical for the development of normal articulatory patterns. Children's

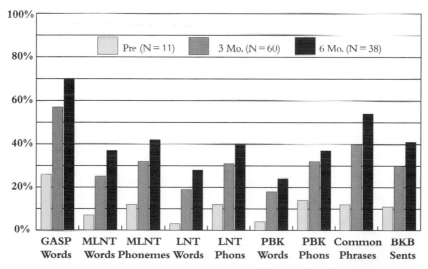

Figure 15.6. Longitudinal, mean open-set speech recognition for children 5 years and older who use the Nucleus 24 device. Data from the following measures are shown: GASP words, Multisyllabic Neighborhood (words and phonemes), Lexical Neighborhood Monosyllable Test (words and phonemes), Phonetically Balanced Kindergarten Monosyllable Test (words and phonemes), Common Phrases Test, and Bamford-Kowal-Bench Sentences.

imitated and spontaneous speech production and general speech intelligibility improve with cochlear implant use, provided they receive appropriate training (Tobey et al., 1991, 1994; Dawson et al., 1995). In addition, the communication mode (oral/aural or simultaneous communication) used with children appears to be a significant factor associated with speech intelligibility. Although children in both groups exhibit postoperative improvements and a range of intelligibility scores, on average children who rely on oral communication are more intelligible (Osberger et al., 1994; Geers et al., 1998).

The development of language and communicative function has been studied in children using multichannel cochlear implants. Geers and Moog (1994) and McConkey-Robbins et al. (1997) have reported significant improvements in receptive and expressive skills above what would be expected due to maturation alone. This means that with early intervention, some children have the opportunity to "catch up" to their normal-hearing peers with regard to language learning. In addition, children using cochlear implants progress faster in language and communication skills than profoundly hearing-impaired children matched on important variables who use other types of sensory aids (Geers and Moog, 1994; Nicholas, 1994). Geers et al. (1998) are studying the effects of communication mode (oral versus simultaneous communication) on the development of various speech and language skills. Preliminary results indicate a definite advantage in some areas for those children using oral communication. However, both groups use auditory input to increase receptive language skills that are important for the development of new vocabulary and sentence comprehension related to reading.

Much work remains to be done in the areas of speech and language acquisition. These studies highlight the importance of early intervention to decrease the gap that occurs in the rate of speech and language development between young children with normal hearing and children with severe to profound hearing impairment.

Future Directions

Within the past decade, improvements in cochlear implant design have led to increased benefit for individuals with severe to profound hearing impairment. As demonstrated by speech perception outcome measures, current multichannel implants provide access to acoustic information about speech and environmental sounds that was not available previously. For young children, implants significantly assist in the acquisition of speech and language. Implantation of very young children is increasingly more common. It is expected that this trend will enhance a child's chance of developing open-set speech perception and spoken language abilities. Studies demonstrate that implants significantly affect the lives of many adults and children (Wyatt and Niparko, 1996; Wyatt et al., 1996; Knutson et al., 1998). Such quality of life studies are relatively recent and represent an important area for future investigations.

Future improvements in electrode design and digital signal processing may result in more sophisticated speech-coding strategies. Improved noise reduction techniques may permit cochlear implant recipients to understand ongoing conversations better in difficult listening environments. Such innovations should increase levels of speech recognition, allowing for a broadening of audiologic criteria so that more individuals (including children) with severe hearing impairments may benefit from implantation.

Finally, one can anticipate that the external equipment will continue to be miniaturized and become even more cosmetically appealing. Ultimately, this process will result in fully implantable cochlear implant systems.

REFERENCES

Advanced Bionics Corporation. Clarion pediatric clinical study. Strategies: Pediatric use of Clarion, Spring 1997a; Spring(Suppl).

Advanced Bionics Corporation. Clarion S-Series, 1997b; Summer.

Allum DJ, ed. Cochlear implant rehabilitation in children and adults. San Diego: Singular, 1996.

American Speech-Language-Hearing Association. Aural rehabilitation: an annotated bibliography. 1990;1(Suppl)32.

Arndt P, Staller SJ, Beiter AL, et al. Initial pediatric results with the Nucleus 24 cochlear implant system. From 1997 NYU symposium, 1999 publication.

Balkany TJ, Dreisbach JN, Seibert CE. Radiographic imaging of the cochlear implant candidate: preliminary results. Otolaryngol Head Neck Surg 1986;95:592–597.

Balkany TJ, Dreisbach JN. Surgical anatomy and radiographic imaging of cochlear implant surgery. Am J Otol 1987;8:195–200.

Balkany TJ, Gantz BJ, Nadol JB. Multichannel cochlear implants in partially ossified cochleas. Ann Otol Rhinol Laryngol 1988;97(Suppl 135):3–7.

Battmer RD. Pilot study of CIS and SAS. Paper presented at the XVI world congress of otorhinolaryngology, head and neck surgery, Sydney, Australia, March 1997.

Beiter AL, Staller SJ, Dowell RC. Evaluation and device programming in children. In: Staller SJ, ed. Multi-channel cochlear implants in children. Ear Hear 1991;4(Suppl 12):25–33.

Beiter AL, Brimacombe JA. Cochlear implants. In: Alpiner JG, McCarthy PA, eds. Rehabilitative audiology: children and adults. 2nd ed. Baltimore: Williams & Wilkins, 1993:417–440.

Beiter AL, Staller SJ, Arndt P, et al. Implant performance in children with limited residual hearing. Paper presented at the 7th symposium on cochlear implants in children. Iowa City, IA, June 4–7, 1998.

Boothroyd A. Hearing aids, cochlear implants, and profoundly deaf children. In: Owens E, Kessler DK, eds. Cochlear implants in young deaf children. Boston: College Hill, 1989:81–100.

Boothroyd A, Geers AE, Moog JS. Practical implications of cochlear implants in children. In Staller SJ, ed. Multichannel cochlear implants in children. Ear Hear 1991;4 (Suppl 12)81–89.

Brackett D. Rehabilitation/education strategies for children with cochlear implants. Cochlear Corp Clin Bull 1991; November:.

Brimacombe JA, Beiter AL. The application of digital technology to cochlear implants. In: Sandlin RE, ed. Digital hearing aid systems. San Diego: Singular, 1994.

Brimacombe JA, Beiter AL, Barker MJ, et al. Comparative results with speech recognition testing with subjects who have used both a single-channel and a multichannel cochlear implant system. In: Fraysse B, Cochard N, eds. Cochlear implants: acquisitions and controversies. Toulouse: Paragraphic, 1989:427–444.

Clark GM. Historical perspectives. In: Clark GM, Cowan RSC, Dowell RC, eds. Cochlear implantation for infants and children. San Diego: Singular, 1997: 9–27.

Clark GM, Pyman BC. Preoperative medical evaluation. In: Clark GM, Cowan RSC, Dowell RC, eds. Cochlear implantation for infants and children. San Diego: Singular, 1997:71–82.

Clark GM, Blamey PJ, Brown AM, et al. The engineering of the receiver-stimulator and speech processor. In: Pfaltz CR, ed. The University of Melbourne-nucleus multielectrode cochlear implant. Adv Otorhinolaryngol 1987a; 38:63–84.

Clark GM, Blamey PJ, Brown AM, et al. The surgery. In: Pfaltz CR, ed. The University of Melbourne—Nucleus multi-electrode cochlear implant. Adv Otorhinolaryngol 1987b;38:93–112.

Clark GM, Cohen NL, Shepherd RK. Surgical and safety considerations of multichannel cochlear implants in children. In: Staller SJ, ed. Multichannel cochlear implants in children. Ear Hear 1991a;4(Suppl 12):15–24.

Clark GM, Franz BK-H, Pyman BC, et al. Surgery for multichannel cochlear implantation. In: Cooper H, ed. Cochlear implants: a practical guide. London: Whurr, 1991b: 169–200.

Clark GM, Pyman BC, Webb RL. Surgery. In: Clark GM, Cowan RSC, Dowell RC, eds. Cochlear implantation for infants and children. San Diego: Singular, 1997:111–124.

Cochlear Corporation. Promontory stimulation manual. Englewood: Cochlear Corporation, 1994.

Cochlear Corporation. Nucleus cochlear implant procedures manual. Englewood: Cochlear Corporation, 1998a.

Cochlear Corporation. Surgical procedure manual for the Nucleus 24 cochlear implant. Englewood: Cochlear Corporation, 1998b.

Cochlear Corporation. Parents' guide: a handbook for parents considering a Nucleus cochlear implant for their Child. Englewood: Cochlear Corporation, 1999a.

Cochlear Corporation. Teachers' guide to the Nucleus cochlear implant systems. Englewood: Cochlear Corporation, 1999b.

Cohen NL, Waltzman SB, Shapiro WH. Clinical trials with a 22-channel cochlear prosthesis. Laryngoscope 1985; 91:1448–1454.

Cowan RSC, Brown C, Whitford LA, et al. Speech perception in children using the advanced Speak speech-processing strategy. In: Clark GM, Cowan RSC, eds. International cochlear implant, speech and hearing symposium 1994. Ann Otol Rhinol Laryngol 1995;104(Suppl 166): 318–321.

Dawson PW, Blamey PJ, Rowland LC, et al. Cochlear implants in children, adolescents, and prelinguistically deafened adults: speech perception. J Speech Hear Res 1992; 35:401–417.

Dawson PW, Blamey PJ, Dettman SJ, et al. A clinical report on speech production of cochlear implant users. Ear Hear 1995;16:551–561.

Dorman MF, Hannley MT, Dankowski K, et al. Word recognition by 50 patients fitted with the Symbion multichannel cochlear implant. Ear Hear 1989;10:44–49.

Dowell RC, Cowan RS. Evaluation of benefit: infants and children. In: Clark GM, Cowan RSC, Dowell RC, eds. Cochlear implantation for infants and children. San Diego: Singular, 1997:205–222.

Elliott L, Katz D. Northwestern University children's perception of speech. St. Louis: Auditec, 1980.

Erber N. Auditory training. Washington, DC: Alexander Graham Bell Association for the Deaf, 1982.

Erber N, Alencewicz C. Audiologic evaluation of deaf children. J Speech Hear Disord 1976;41:256–267.

Estabrooks W, ed. Auditory-verbal therapy for parents and professionals. Washington, DC: Alexander Graham Bell Association for the Deaf, 1994.

Estabrooks W, ed. Cochlear implants for kids. Washington, DC: Alexander Graham Bell Association for the Deaf, 1998.

Fritze W, Eisenwort B. Statistical procedure for the preoperative prediction of the result of cochlear implantation. Br J Audiol 1989;23:293–297.

Fugain C, Ouayoun M, Monneron L, et al. Differences in postoperative management of postlingual and prelingual adults and children using cochlear implants. In: Allum DJ, ed. Cochlear implant rehabilitation in children and adults. San Diego: Singular, 1996:297–310.

Fujikawa S, Owens E. Hearing aid evaluation for persons with total postlingual hearing loss. Arch Otolaryngol 1978;104:446–450.

Fujikawa S, Owens E. Hearing aid evaluation for persons with postlingual hearing levels of 90 to 100 dB. Arch Otolaryngol 1979;105:662–665.

Gantz BJ. Iowa cochlear implant project. Presented at the Colorado Otology Audiology Conference, Breckenridge, Colorado, March 4, 1992.

Gantz BJ, Tyler RS, Knutson JF, et al. Evaluation of five different cochlear implant designs: audiologic assessment and predictors of performance. Laryngoscope 1988;98: 1100–1106.

Gantz BJ, Tyler RS, Woodworth GG, et al. Results of multichannel cochlear implants in congenital and acquired prelingual deafness in children: five year follow-up. Am J Otol 1994;15(Suppl 2):1–8.

Geers A, Brenner C. Speech perception results: audition and lipreading enhancement. In: Geers AE, Moog JS, eds. Effectiveness of cochlear implants and tactile aids for deaf children: the sensory aids study at Central Institute for the Deaf. Volta Rev 1994;96:97–108.

Geers AE, Moog JS. Evaluating speech perception skills: tools for measuring benefits of cochlear implants, tactile aids, and hearing aids. In: Owens E, Kessler DK, eds. Cochlear implants in young deaf children. Boston: College Hill, 1989:227–256.

Geers A, Moog J. Spoken language results: vocabulary, syntax and communication. In: Geers AE, Moog JS, eds. Effectiveness of cochlear implants and tactile aids for deaf children: the sensory aids study at Central Institute for the Deaf. Volta Rev 1994;96:97–108.

Geers A, Tobey E, Brenner C, et al. Factors associated with speech intelligibility in children with cochlear implants. Paper presented at the 7th symposium on cochlear implants in children. Iowa City, Iowa, June 4–7, 1998.

Gray RF. Cochlear implants: the medical criteria for patient selection. In: Cooper H, ed. Cochlear implants: a practical guide. London: Whurr, 1991:146–154.

Haskins J. Kindergarten phonetically balanced word lists (PBK). St. Louis: Auditec, 1949.

House WF, Berliner KK. Cochlear implants: from idea to clinical practice. In: Cooper H, ed. Cochlear implants: a practical guide. London: Whurr, 1991:9–33.

Jackler RK, Luxford WM, House WM. Congenital malformations of the inner ear: a classification based on embryogenesis. Laryngoscope 1987a;90(Suppl 40):2–14.

Jackler RK, Luxford WM, House WM. Sound detection with the cochlear implant in five ears of four children with congenital malformations of the cochlea. Laryngoscope 1987b;90(Suppl 40):15–17.

Jeffers J, Barley M. Speech reading "lipreading." Springfield: Charles C. Thomas, 1977.

Kessler DK, Schindler RA. Progress with a multi-strategy cochlear implant system: the Clarion. In: Hochmair-Desoyer IJ, Hochmair ES, eds. Advances in cochlear implants. Manz: Wien, 1994:354–362.

Kessler DK, Loeb GE, Barker MJ. Distribution of speech recognition results with the Clarion cochlear prosthesis. Ann Otol Rhinol Laryngol 1995;104(Suppl 166): 283–285.

Kileny PR, Kemink JL. Electrically evoked middle-latency auditory potentials in cochlear implant candidates. Arch Otolaryngol Head Neck Surg 1987;113:1072–1077.

Kileny PR, Zimmerman-Phillips S, Kemink JL, et al. The effects of preoperative electrical stimulability and historical factors on performance with multichannel cochlear implant. Ann Otol Rhinol Laryngol 1991;100:563–568.

Kileny PR, Zwolan TA, Zimmerman-Phillips S, et al. A comparison of round window and transtympanic promontory electric stimulation in cochlear implant candidates. Ear Hear 1992;13:294–299.

Kileny PR, Zwolan TA, Zimmerman-Phillips S, et al. Electrically evoked auditory brain-stem response in pediatric patients with cochlear implants. Arch Otolaryngol Head Neck Surg 1994;120:1083–1090.

Kirk KI, Pisoni DB, Osberger MJ. Lexical effects of spoken word recognition by pediatric cochlear implant users. Ear Hear 1995;16:440–481.

Knutson JF, Murray KT, Husarek S, et al. Psychological change over 54 months of cochlear implant use. Ear Hear 1998;19:191–201.

Lalwani AK, Larky JB, Wareing MJ, et al. The Clarion multi-strategy cochlear implant—surgical technique, complications, and results: a single institutional experience. Am J Otol 1998;19:66–70.

Lambert PR, Ruth RA, Hodges AV. Meningitis and facial paresis. Arch Otolaryngol Head Neck Surg 1987;113: 1101–1103.

Lerman J, Ross M, Mclauchin R. A picture-identification test for hearing-impaired children. J Auditor Res 1965;5: 273–278.

Lowell E, Stoner M. Play it by ear. Los Angeles: John Tracy Clinic, 1960.

Luxford WM, Brackmann DE. The history of cochlear implants. In: Gray RF, ed. Cochlear implants. San Diego: College Hill, 1985:1–26.

Mangham CA, Kuprenas SV. Open-set minimum auditory capability scores for House and Nucleus cochlear prostheses. Am J Otol 1989;10:263–266.

Martin EL, Burnett PA, Himelick TE, et al. Speech recognition by a deaf-blind multichannel cochlear patient. Ear Hearing 1988;9:70–74.

Mason SM, O'Donoghue GM, Gibbin KP, et al. Perioperative electrical auditory brain stem response in candidates for pediatric cochlear implantation. Am J Otol 1997; 18:466–471.

McConkey-Robbins A. Language acquisition paper for NYU meeting.

Mecklenburg DJ, Shallop JK. Cochlear implants. In: Lass NJ, McReynolds LV, Northern JL, et al., eds. Handbook of speech-language pathology and audiology. Toronto: B.C. Decker, 1988:1355–1368.

McConkey-Robbins A. Guidelines for the developing oral communication skills in children with cochlear implants. In: Geers AE, Moog JS, eds. Effectiveness of cochlear implants and tactile aids for deaf children: the sensory aids study at Central Institute for the Deaf. Volta Rev 1994; 96:75–84.

Mecklenburg DJ, Lehnhardt E. The development of cochlear implants in Europe, Asia, and Australia. In: Cooper H, ed. Cochlear implants: a practical guide. London: Whurr, 1991:34–57.

Millar JB, Blamey PJ, Tong YC, et al. Speech perception. In: Clark GM, Tong YC, Patrick JF, eds. Cochlear prostheses. Edinburgh: Churchill Livingstone, 1990:41–68.

Moeller MP. Hearing and speechreading assessment with the severely hearing-impaired child. In: Sims DG, Walter GG, Whitehead RL, eds. Deafness and communication assessment and training. Baltimore: Williams & Wilkins, 1982:127–140.

Moog JS, Geers AE. Early speech perception battery. St. Louis: Central Institute for the Deaf, 1990.

Moog JS, Biedenstein J, Davidson L, et al. Instruction for developing speech perception skills. In: Geers AE, Moog JS, eds. Effectiveness of cochlear implants and tactile aids for deaf children: the sensory aids study at Central Institute for the Deaf. Volta Rev 1994;96:61–74.

National Institutes of Health. Consensus statement cochlear implants in adults and children. 1995;2:13.

Nevins ME, Kretschmer RE, Chute PM, et al. The role of an educational consultant in a pediatric cochlear implant program. Volta Rev 1991;93:197–204.

Nicholas JG. Sensory aid use and the development of communicative function. In: Geers AE, Moog JS, eds. Effectiveness of cochlear implants and tactile aids for deaf children: the sensory aids study at Central Institute for the Deaf. Volta Rev 1994;96:181–198.

Osberger MJ. Clinical results in children with the Clarion multi-strategy cochlear implant. Personal communication, 1997.

Osberger MJ, Kessler DK. New directions in speech processing: patient performance with simultaneous analog stimulation (SAS) and the electrode connection. Paper presented at the 7th symposium on cochlear implants in children. Iowa City, Iowa, June 4–7, 1998.

Osberger MJ, Miyamoto RT, Zimmerman-Phillips S, et al. Independent evaluation of the speech perception abilities of children with the Nucleus 22 channel cochlear implant system. In: Staller SJ, ed. Multichannel cochlear implants in children. Ear Hear 1991;4(Suppl 12):66–80.

Osberger MJ, McConkey-Robbins A, Todd SL, et al. Speech intelligibility in children with cochlear implants. In: Geers AE, Moog JS, eds. Effectiveness of cochlear implants and tactile aids for deaf children: the sensory aids study at Central Institute for the Deaf. Volta Rev 1994;96:169–180.

Owens E, Raggio MW. Performance inventory for profound and severe loss (PIPSL). J Speech Hear Disord 1988; 53:42–56.

Owens E, Kessler DK, Raggio MW, et al. Analysis and revision of the minimal auditory capabilities (MAC) battery. Ear Hear 1985a;6:280–290.

Owens E, Kessler DK, Telleen CC, et al. The minimal auditory capabilities battery. St. Louis: Auditec, 1985b.

Patrick JF. Cochlear implants—future features and benefits. Paper presented at the 7th symposium on cochlear implants in children. Iowa City, Iowa, June 4–7, 1998.

Patrick JF, Clark GM. The Nucleus 22-channel cochlear implant system. In: Staller SJ, ed. Multichannel cochlear implants in children. Ear Hear 1991;4(Suppl 12):3–9.

Patrick JF, Seligman PM, Clark GM. Engineering. In: Clark GM, Cowan RSC, Dowell RC, eds. Cochlear implantation for infants and children. San Diego: Singular, 1997: 125–145.

Pollack MC, ed. Amplification for the hearing impaired. New York: Grune & Stratton, 1980.

Pope ML, Miyamoto RT, Myres WA, et al. Cochlear implant candidate selection. Ear Hear 1986;7:71–73.

Pyman BC, Brown AM, Dowell RC, et al. Preoperative evaluation and selection of adults. In: Clark GM, Tong YC, Patrick JF, eds. Cochlear prostheses. Edinburgh: Churchill Livingstone, 1990:125–134.

Rance G, Dowell RC. Speech processor programming. In: Clark GM, Cowan RSC, Dowell RC, eds. Cochlear implantation for infants and children. San Diego: Singular, 1997:147–170.

Robbins AM, Renshaw JJ, Berry SW. Evaluating meaningful auditory integration in profoundly hearing-impaired children. Am J Otol 1991;12(Suppl):151–164.

Roberts S. Speech-processor fitting for cochlear implants. In: Cooper H, ed. Cochlear implants: a practical guide. London: Whurr, 1991:201–218.

Rubenstein JT. New directions in signal processing. Paper presented at the 7th symposium on cochlear implants in children. Iowa City, Iowa, June 4–7, 1998.

Schindler RA, Kessler DK. State of the art of cochlear implants: the UCSF experience. Am J Otol 1989;10:79–83.

Schindler RA, Kessler DK. Preliminary results with the Clarion cochlear implant. Laryngoscope 1992;102:1006–1013.

Schindler RA, Kessler DK. Clarion cochlear implant: phase I investigational results. Am J Otol 1993;14:263–272.

Schuyler VS, Rushmer N, Arpan R, et al. Parent-infant communication. Portland: Infant Hearing Resource, 1985.

Shallop JK, Mecklenburg DJ. Technical aspects of cochlear implants. In: Sandlin RE, ed. Handbook of hearing aid amplification. San Diego: College Hill, 1987:265–280.

Shannon RV. Multichannel electrical stimulation of the auditory nerve in man: I. Basic psychophysics. Hear Res 1983;11:157–189.

Shapiro WH, Waltzman SB. Cochlear implant programming for children: the basics. In: Estabrooks W, ed. Cochlear implants for kids. Washington, DC: Alexander Graham Bell Association for the Deaf, 1998:58–68.

Sims DG. Hearing and speechreading evaluation for the deaf adult. In: Sims DG, Walter GG, Whitehead RL, eds. Deafness and communication assessment and training. Baltimore: Williams & Wilkins, 1982:141–154.

Simmons FB. Electrical stimulation of the auditory nerve in man. Arch Otolaryngol 1966;84:2–54.

Skinner MW. Hearing aid evaluation. Englewood Cliffs, NJ: Prentice Hall, 1988.

Skinner MW, Binzer SM, Fredrickson JM, et al. Comparison of benefit from vibrotactile aid and cochlear implant for postlinguistically deaf adults. Laryngoscope 1988;98: 1092–1099.

Skinner MW, Holden LK, Binzer S. Aural rehabilitation for individuals with severe and profound impairment: hearing aids, cochlear implants, counseling and training. In: Valente M, ed. Strategies for selecting and verifying hearing aid fittings. Thieme, 1994a.

Skinner MW, Clark GM, Whitford LA, et al. Evaluation of a new spectral peak coding strategy for the Nucleus 22 channel cochlear implant system. Am J Otol 1994b;15 (Suppl 2):15–27.

Staller SJ. Cochlear implant characteristics: a review of current technology. In: McCandless GA, ed. Cochlear implants, seminars in hearing. New York: Thieme-Stratton, 1985:23–32.

Staller SJ, Beiter AL, Brimacombe JA. Children and multichannel cochlear implants. In: Cooper H, ed. Cochlear implants: a practical guide. London: Whurr, 1991a: 283–321.

Staller SJ, Dowell RC, Beiter AL, et al. Perceptual abilities of children with the Nucleus 22-channel cochlear implant. In: Staller SJ, ed. Multichannel cochlear implants in children. Ear Hear 1991b;4(Suppl 12)34–47.

Staller SJ, Beiter AL, Brimacombe JA. Use of the Nucleus 22 channel cochlear implant system with children. In: Geers AE, Moog JS, eds. Effectiveness of cochlear implants and tactile aids for deaf children: the sensory aids study at Central Institute for the Deaf. Volta Rev 1994; 96:15–40.

Staller SJ, Menapace C, Domico E, et al. Speech perception abilities of adult and pediatric Nucleus implant recipients using the spectral peak (SPEAK) coding strategy. Otol Laryngol Head Neck Surg 1997;117:236–242.

Staller SJ, Arndt P, Brimacombe JA. Nucleus 24 cochlear implant: adult clinical trial results. From NYU 1997 symposium, 1999 publication.

Starr A, Picton TW, Sininger Y, et al. Auditory neuropathy. Brain 1996;119:741–753.

Steenerson RL, Gary LB, Wynens MS. Scala vestibuli cochlear implantation for labyrinthine ossification. Am J Otol 1990;11:360–363.

Stein L, Tremblay K, Pasternak J, et al. Brainstem abnormalities in neonates with normal otoacoustic emissions. Semin Hear 1996;17:197–213.

Stout G, Windle J. Developmental approach to successful listening. Houston: DASL, 1986.

Strauss-Schier A, Rost U. Rehabilitation in adult cochlear implant patients. In: Allum DJ, ed. Cochlear implant rehabilitation in children and adults. San Diego: Singular, 1996:254–265.

Tobey EA, Angelette S, Murchison C, et al. Speech production performance in children with multichannel cochlear implants. Am J Otol 1991;12(Suppl):165–173.

Tobey E, Geers A, Brenner C. Speech production results: speech feature acquisition. In: Geers AE, Moog JS, eds. Effectiveness of cochlear implants and tactile aids for deaf children: the sensory aids study at Central Institute for the Deaf. Volta Rev 1994;96:109–129.

Tyler RS, Tye-Murray N. Cochlear implant signal-processing strategies and patient perception of speech and environmental sounds. In: Cooper H, ed. Cochlear implants: a practical guide. London: Whurr, 1991:58–83.

Tyler R, Preece J, Lowder M. The Iowa cochlear implant tests. Iowa City: University of Iowa, Department of Otolaryngology-Head & Neck Surgery, 1983.

Tyler R, Preece J, Tye-Murray N. The laser videodisc sentence test. Iowa City: University of Iowa, Department of Otolaryngology-Head & Neck Surgery, 1986.

Tyler RS, Moore BC, Kuk FK. Performance of some of the better cochlear implant patients. J Speech Hear Res 1989; 32:887–911.

Tyler RS, Gantz BJ, Woodworth GG, et al. Initial independent results with the Clarion cochlear implant. Ear Hear 1996;17:528–536.

Waltzman SB, Cohen NL, Shapiro WH. Use of a multichannel cochlear implant in the congenitally and prelingually deaf population. Laryngoscope 1992;102:395–399.

Waltzman SB, Cohen NL, Gomolin RH, et al. Long-term results of early cochlear implantation in congenitally and prelingually deafened children. Am J Otol 1994;15(Suppl 2):9–13.

Waltzman SB, Fisher SG, Niparko JK, et al. Predictors of postoperative performance with cochlear implants. In: Cohen NL, Waltzman SB, eds. Multicenter comparative study of cochlear implants: final reports of the Department of Veterans Affairs cooperative studies program. Ann Otol Rhinol Laryngol 1995;104(Suppl 165):15–18.

Webb RL, Pyman BC, Franz BK-H, et al. The surgery of cochlear implantation. In: Clark GM, Tong YC, Patrick JF, eds. Cochlear prostheses. Edinburgh: Churchill Livingstone, 1990:158–180.

White MW, Merzenich MM, Gardi JN. Multichannel cochlear implants. Arch Otolaryngol 1984;110:493–501.

Wilson BS, Finley CC, Lawson DT, et al. Better speech recognition with cochlear implants. Nature 1991a;352: 236–238.

Wilson BS, Lawson DT, Finley CC, et al. Coding strategies for multichannel cochlear prostheses. Am J Otol 1991b; 12(Suppl):56–61.

Wilson BS, Lawson DT, Zerbi M, et al. Recent developments in CIS strategies. In: Hochmair-Desoyer IJ, Hochmair ES, eds. Advances in cochlear implants. Manz: Wien, 1994:103–112.

Wyatt JR, Niparko JK. Evaluation of benefit of the multichannel cochlear implant in children related to cost. In: Allum DJ, ed. Cochlear implant rehabilitation in children and adults. San Diego: Singular, 1996:22–30.

Wyatt JR, Niparko JK, Rothman M, et al. Cost utility of the multichannel cochlear implant in 258 profoundly deaf individuals. Laryngoscope 1996;106:816–821.

Zwolan TA, Zimmerman-Phillips S, Ashbaugh CJ, et al. Cochlear implantation of children with minimal open-set speech recognition skills. Ear Hear 1997;18:240–251.

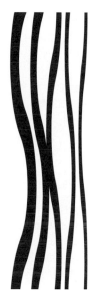

Assistive Technology for the Enhancement of Receptive Communication

Cynthia L. Compton, Ph.D.

Introduction

All people, including those who have hearing difficulty, have communication needs in four key areas: (1) face-to-face communication, (2) the enjoyment of broadcast or other media (radio, television, stereo, etc.), (3) telephone communication, and (4) communication of the occurrence of alerting signals and situations. Historically, the profession of audiology has depended on the personal hearing aid to meet these needs—and not always with success. In the past few years, however, technological advances in the personal hearing aid, coupled with improved fitting and rehabilitative techniques, have provided solutions to communication problems that could not have been resolved in the past. Hearing aid selection considerations now include a variety of electroacoustic parameters and innumerable special features such as microphone type (directional or omnidirectional), circuit type (various compression versus linear circuits), frequency-shaping, type of earmold plumbing, and programmability. Still, even today, this vast inventory of hearing aid technology cannot always be counted on to solve every client's receptive communication difficulties.

For example, it is common for a hearing aid user to experience difficulty understanding speech amidst noise and reverberation, from a distance, and on the telephone (where visual cues are unavailable and sound quality is decreased by band-pass filtering). A person with even a mild to moderate hearing impairment might be functionally deaf to a smoke alarm located down the hall and behind a closed door if he or she is in a deep sleep and has removed his or her hearing aids. The same person might miss the doorbell if listening to the television in a room located away from the doorbell chime, regardless of the fact that hearing aids are being worn. Finally, a child with normal hearing but with recurrent middle ear infections or a central auditory processing disorder is at a definite educational disadvantage when seated in a typical classroom characterized by excessive reverberation and ambient noise.

Numerous auditory and nonauditory technologies—assistive devices—are available to meet these communication needs. As important as the personal hearing aid, these devices may be used in addition to or in place of the personal hearing aid, cochlear implant, or tactile device. Audiologists must be prepared not only to fit and recommend personal amplification systems and assistive devices appropriately, but also to be able to evaluate their place within the larger framework of maximizing the communication skills of the person with a hearing problem in all aspects of his or her daily life. Accordingly, audiologists must also be prepared to provide the ongoing training and counseling necessary to assure successful use of the technology.

The purpose of this chapter is threefold: (1) to review the various types of assistive technologies, (2) to provide the reader with a framework for identifying the potential assistive device user and his or her specific equipment needs, and (3) to discuss the role of the professional in the procurement of assistive technology.

Assistive Devices: An Overview

Historically, both auditory and nonauditory devices have been grouped under the label "assistive listening devices"; however, not all communication involves listening, nor can all people with hearing impairment benefit from auditory technologies. Many people benefit from devices that convey information using visual and/or tactile stimuli. Thus, it is suggested that as a group, these technologies be referred to as "assistive devices" or even as "assistive technology for the enhancement of receptive communication." These labels not only are more precise but are also more acceptable by culturally deaf individuals who may find the term "listening" offensive. These labels also distinguish this technology from that used by persons with expressive communication difficulty (known as augmentative technology).

Assistive devices can be classified into four categories:

1. Systems to assist in face-to-face communication.
2. Systems to assist in the enjoyment of broadcast and other media.
3. Systems to assist in telephone communication.
4. Systems to assist in the awareness and identification of environmental sounds and situations (alerting devices).

Within each of these categories, auditory and nonauditory systems are available to accomplish these tasks. In the following paragraphs, the first two categories will be discussed jointly because they encompass similar technology.

SYSTEMS TO ASSIST IN FACE-TO-FACE COMMUNICATION AND THE RECEPTION OF MEDIA

Auditory devices (assistive listening devices)

Several factors affect a listener's access to auditory communication: the level of the sound source, the distance between the sound source and the listener, the amount and type of background noise in the room, the amount of room reverberation, and numerous linguistic and pragmatic factors.

Level of the Sound Source. For a person to understand speech, the sound source must be loud enough before it can be understood. Thus, at close distances (e.g., 1 meter), most people speak at conversational levels of approximately 50 to 65 dB SPL. However, it may not always be possible for two people to be close to each other. This is where the factor of distance comes into play.

Distance. Sound fades rapidly as distance increases. Even nominal distances can cause speech to become unintelligible for people with mild hearing loss. Asking someone to raise their voice or even shout may not always be a practical option because not only can a loud voice be annoying to other people, it can also be fatiguing to the speaker.

Background Noise. The masking effect of noise depends on its parameters—its long-term spectrum, how its intensity fluctuates in time, and its average intensity relative to the intensity of the speech. For example, classrooms and meeting areas tend to be noisy. This background noise can be generated from within the room (heating and cooling systems or movement of the occupants) or can originate from outside the room (hallway noise or traffic). It can be steady-state (e.g., a fan), quasi-steady-state (e.g., speech babble), or time-varying (e.g., airplanes taking off and landing). The overall effect of steady-state noise on speech recognition can be expressed by a metric called the speech-to-competition ratio, speech-to-noise ratio, or the signal-to-noise ratio (SNR). The signal is the desired stimulus (e.g., a teacher talking), and the noise is the undesired stimulus (e.g., cooling system noise). Most persons with normal hearing can communicate reasonably well at SNRs of approximately 7 to 11 dB. This means that the signal is 7 to 11 dB louder than the noise. However, persons with sensorineural hearing loss, children, elderly, and nonnative speakers need SNRs much larger than those required by those with normal auditory systems (Nabelek and Pickett, 1974; Finitzo-Hieber and Tillman, 1978).

Reverberation. In a room, the speech sound surrounds the talker. Part of the sound arrives at the listener's ears directly; the rest of the sound waves strike the walls of the room, forming reflections that reach the listener's ears some milliseconds after the direct sound. The strength and number of reflections depends on room characteristics— some rooms reflect sound more than others. The multiple reflections—or reverberation of sound disrupts speech understanding by causing multiple sound images or echoes to arrive at the listener's ears at slightly different times. These echoes cause speech sounds to "smear" and to become difficult to understand (Nabelek et al., 1989). The decrease in speech perception depends on the amount of reverberation (measured grossly as reverberation time), the distance between the talker and listener, and the level and type of noise in the room. Even in a quiet room, speech intelligibility for normal-hearing people gradually decreases with an increase of reverberation time (Nabelek and Pickett, 1974; Nabelek and Robinson, 1982; Helfer and Wilber, 1990). People with hearing loss, normal-hearing children, and the elderly cannot tolerate as much reverberation as can young adults with normal hearing (Nabelek and Robinson, 1982; Loven and Collins, 1988).

Noise and Reverberation. When noise and reverberation are combined (and they usu-

ally are), their effects on speech perception are multiplicative; that is, the combined effects of noise and reverberation are worse than the sum of both effects taken separately (Finitzo-Hieber and Tillman, 1978; Nabelek and Mason, 1981). Noise and reverberation affect the speech perception of people with hearing loss at levels that are acceptable for people with normal hearing. Thus, rooms designed for people with hearing loss should have stricter acoustic guidelines than rooms for listeners with normal hearing. Unfortunately, such rooms are not readily available to the public. In fact, poor room acoustics is such a large problem that the Architectural and Transportation Barriers Compliance Board received a petition for rule-making, requesting that it address architectural acoustics in schools and develop acoustic guidelines to ensure adequately low noise and reverberation to allow satisfactory communication and learning (*Federal Register,* June 1, 1998). In addition, the American National Standards Institute (ANSI) and the Acoustical Society of America (ASA) have established committees to develop a classroom acoustics standard.

Linguistic and Pragmatic Factors. The more redundant (e.g., familiar) the topic, the more a listener can tolerate noise and reverberation. It is also important that a speaker articulate clearly and at a rate that is neither too fast nor too slow. The speaker's emotional state or degree of stress can cause changes in vocal behavior and consequent changes in speech intelligibility.

In general, the importance of each of the above factors depends on the distance of the listener from the sound source, because the levels of direct and reflected sounds and background noise vary across the room. An important concept is that of the critical distance—the distance from the sound source where the intensities of direct and reflected sounds are equal. For a typical room, the critical distance is approximately 2 to 3 meters. However, the critical distance decreases with increase in room volume and increases with an increase in reverberation time. The critical distance is also the distance from the speaker beyond which the inverse square law breaks down. For example, if the critical distance in a room is 6 feet, then moving to within 3 feet of the sound source will increase its intensity by 6 dB. This "halving of the distance" will improve the SNR, for example, from 0 dB (speech and noise at same level) to +6 dB (speech 6 dB louder than noise). Closing the distance by one-half again (to within 1.5 feet of the speaker) will increase the sound source's intensity another 6 dB, thus improving the SNR to +12 dB. However, once the listener is beyond the critical distance (greater than 6 feet away), it does not matter where he or she is located in the room. The SNR will remain at 0 dB because the listener is now located in what is called the reverberant field (Fig. 16.1). Thus, halving the distance from 12 feet away from the sound source to 6 feet away will not improve the SNR (although it may assist with speechreading so it is still worth trying!).

The "take home message" from all of this is that poor listening environments are annoying to most people, but the effect they have on hearing-impaired listeners is much more severe. Hearing aids amplify not only desired sounds, but also noise and reverberation. Because the hearing aid's microphone is located at the listener's ear and not at the sound source, it is more likely to pick up background noise and reverberation as well as, or even better than, the desired sound—especially if the listener has no choice but to sit beyond the critical distance. Assistive listening devices (ALDs) are designed to reduce the effects of distance, background noise, and reverberation via an elegantly simple concept. The microphone on an ALD is positioned only a few inches from the desired sound source so that the listener hears the desired signal as if he or she were only a few inches from the sound source, rather than several feet away. Like binoculars for the ears, ALDs reach out and "grab" the desired sound source and send it directly to the listener's ear minus the deleterious effects of distance, background noise, and reverberation.

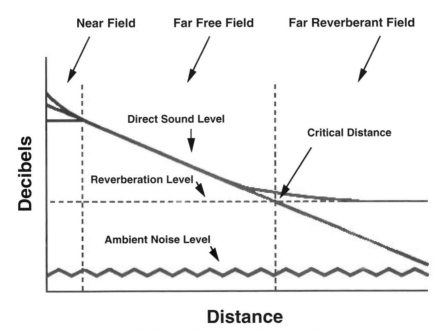

Figure 16.1. This figure illustrates how the intensity level of the direct sound (e.g., a person's voice) decreases in a predicted way (inverse square law) until the critical distance is achieved. Beyond the critical distance, the direct sound becomes "mixed in" with the room reverberation (reverberant field) so that further increases in distance do not affect the level of the direct sound. (Modified and reprinted with permission from editor is: Glen M. Ballou The handbook for sound engineers. 2nd ed. Carmel, IN: SAMS, a division of Macmillan Computer Publishing, 1991.)

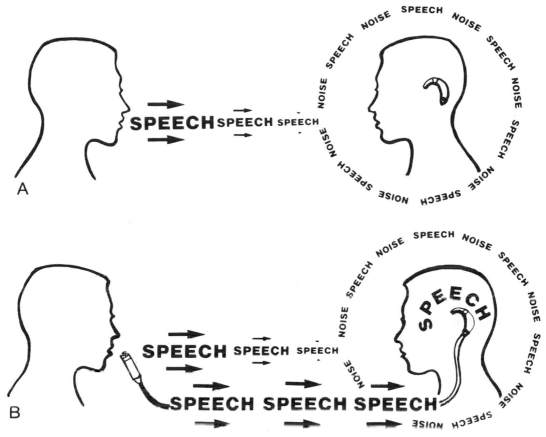

Figure 16.2. How assistive listening devices improve speech understanding. (Reprinted with permission from Compton CL. Assistive devices: doorways to independence. Annapolis, MD: Compton & Associates, 1991.)

As shown in Figure 16.2A, speech loses energy as it travels from the speaker's mouth to the listener's hearing aid, and there is confusion with the background noise. A hardwired remote microphone system attached to a hearing aid can preserve the loudness and the integrity of the speech signal (Fig. 16.2B). As speech leaves the speaker's lips, some of it travels through the air to the hearing aid, losing energy as in Figure 16.2A. However, with a remote microphone, most of the speech enters the microphone, travels through the cord as an electrical signal, and enters the hearing aid (or earphone) of the listener, where it is changed back to sound and sent to the ear without a loss of energy. Speech is therefore much louder than the surrounding noise, and understanding ability is improved. Studies have shown that ALDs can improve the

SNR for the listener by as much as 15 to 19 dB in moderate noise and reverberation (Hawkins, 1984, 1985). Modern directional microphone hearing aids also can significantly improve the SNR (Soede et al., 1993; Valente et al., 1995; Lurquin and Rafhay, 1996), although the amount of improvement is not as large as that seen with ALDs in which the remote microphone is placed within several inches of the sound source. The reader is referred to Chapter 11 for a discussion of directional microphone hearing aids.

Hardwired Systems. Hardwired systems physically tether the listener to the sound source (Figs. 16.3 and 16.4). The sound source (a person talking, a television, a radio) may be picked up via a remote handheld, lapel, or Velcro-attached microphone.

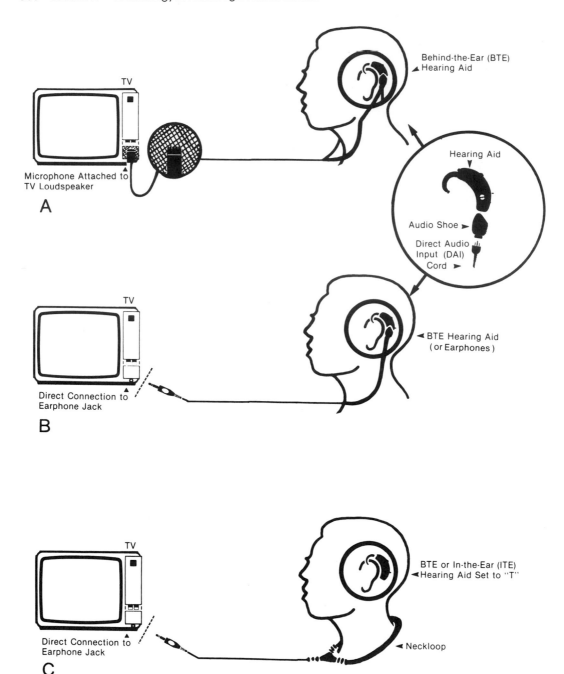

Figure 16.3. Use of a hearing-aid–dependent hardwired systems with television. (Reprinted with permission from Compton CL. Assistive devices: doorways to independence. Annapolis, MD: Compton & Associates, 1991.)

For electronic sound sources, an electrical plug-jack connection can also be used. The signal is then delivered to the listener's ears via a headset or earbuds or to a personal hearing aid via direct audio input (DAI) or inductive coupling (neckloop or silhouette inductor). Separation from the sound source is limited by the length of the cord (custom cords and extension cords can be ordered).

Hardwired systems are of two types: hearing-aid–dependent systems and hearing-aid–independent systems.

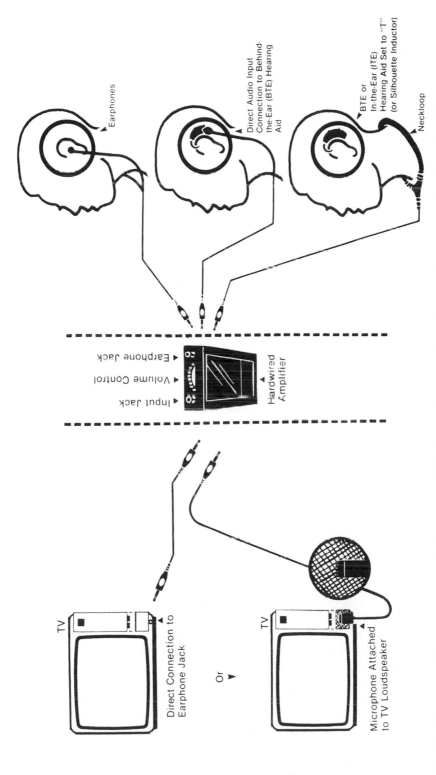

Figure 16.4. Use of a hardwired personal amplification system (PAS) with television. (Reprinted with permission from Compton CL. Assistive devices: doorways to independence. Annapolis, MD: Compton & Associates, 1991.)

Hearing-Aid–Dependent Systems. A hearing-aid–dependent system simply means that the listening system can be used only in connection with a hearing aid. This might occur in one of two ways: using DAI (Fig. 16.3A, B) or using inductive coupling (Fig. 16.3C).

DAI systems, available from most behind-the-ear (BTE) hearing aid companies, plug directly into hearing aids via an audio shoe (or boot). The technology is also available for cochlear implants, tactile aids, and some body-type hearing aids. Lightweight and inexpensive, these systems can be used to access broadcast or other media via a direct plug-in connection or remote microphone.

Currently, because of impedance variations, it cannot always be assumed that any DAI system can be used with any brand of hearing aid. Although there are exceptions and custom modifications are possible, in general, Brand "X" hearing aid must be used with its own audio shoe, cord, and microphone. Hearing-aid–dependent inductive systems also include plug-in neckloops and silhouette inductors that, like DAI, connect directly into the earphone jack of televisions, radios, tape players, dictation machines, hand-held VHF radios, and other electronic devices and are powered by the voltage from the device (Fig. 16.3). Connection to stereo television sets or VCRs also can be accomplished using the audio output jack on the back of such devices.

Hearing-Aid–Independent Systems. Also called personal amplification systems or stand-alone systems, these battery-powered hardwired systems have their own microphone, amplifier, and earphone headset. If desired, the system also can be used with hearing aids, via the use of a DAI cord, neckloop, or silhouette inductor (Fig. 16.4).

Stand-alone systems can serve as part-time or full-time amplification systems for those people who for one reason or another do not use a hearing aid. For those who do, stand-alone systems offer the only way a hearing aid equipped with a telecoil, but without a DAI connection, can be coupled to a remote microphone system (unless the hearing aids are of the canal type and worn far enough into the ear canal that feedback does not occur when a headset is used). Several brands of stand-alone systems are available, some with built-in telecoils that allow them to be used as induction loop receivers also (discussed later). Stand-alone amplifiers can be ordered with corded microphones and extension cords for use with neckloops or headphones to allow for remote microphone placement. Some brands do not have separate microphones that can be placed remotely at the sound source. Instead, the microphone and volume control are built into the amplifier. However, if an extension cord is added between the headset and the amplifier and the amplifier is placed close to the desired sound source, then an enhanced SNR can be provided—the purpose of an ALD. The problem with this arrangement is that the volume control is then located at the sound source (e.g., at the television) instead of in the listener's lap where it would be more convenient.

Wireless Systems. Wireless systems consist of a battery-powered or AC-powered transmitter that sends some type of radio signal to a battery-powered receiver, avoiding the need for a cord between the sound source and the listener. Although more expensive than hardwired systems, wireless systems are superior when mobility and versatility are concerns. Applications include large areas such as concert and lecture halls, classrooms, courtrooms, churches and temples, theaters, museums, theme parks, arenas, sports stadiums, ports of transportation, and retirement and nursing homes. They also work well in public transportation vehicles and tour buses. When used in these situations, the listening system is usually interfaced with a public address (PA) system. Wireless systems also can be used at home, in the car, at the office, at service counters, and in other situations involving small-group, one-to-one, or listening alone situations (e.g., television, radio, and stereo) when a hardwired system could be used but the user prefers not be tethered to the sound source. Each type of wireless system has its pros and cons. No one system is superior to the others in terms of sound quality, provided that the system itself is of good quality, is installed properly, and the electroacoustic transducers used with each system are equivalent in terms of output, frequency response, equivalent input noise level, and distortion (Nabelek et al., 1986). The system of choice depends on the situation in which it is to be used and many other factors such as available funding, maintenance and security requirements, presence of sources of interference, personal preference, and available technical expertise and service.

Induction Loop. Induction loop technology has been used in hearing assistance applications for more than four decades. Having its roots in Europe, it is now enjoying increased popularity in the United States. The basic component of an induction loop system is a loop of wire encircling a room and connected to the output of an audio power amplifier (Fig. 16.5).

The signal fed into the amplifier can originate from a microphone, a tape recorder, a television, or any sound source. Once sound enters the system, its electrical signal is amplified and sent through the loop, which broadcasts the signal to the entire room in the form of electromagnetic energy. This magnetic field varies in direct proportion to the strength and frequency of the signal being passed through the loop. The receiver for this system is the telecoil circuit in an individual's hearing aid (Fig. 16.6A, B). If a listener does not have a hearing aid or has a hearing aid not equipped with a telecoil, reception from a loop system is impossible unless the listener uses a special telecoil receiver (Fig. 16.6C).

There are three types of telecoil receivers. One is pocket-sized and equipped with earphones; another is encased in a hand-held wand (this type is often used at service counters, in museums, and in other public areas); and the third type is enclosed inside a plastic case that looks like a BTE, in-the-ear (ITE), or in-the-canal (ITC) type hearing aid.

Induction (or audio) loop systems range in price from a couple hundred dollars for a system to loop a den to several thousand dollars to loop a classroom or concert hall. A big advantage of loop systems is that they do not require maintenance of separate receivers, provided the listeners have telecoil-equipped hearing aids. With the other wireless systems, a separate receiver and maintenance program are required—even if the listener uses a hearing aid, it must be connected to an infrared or frequency mod-

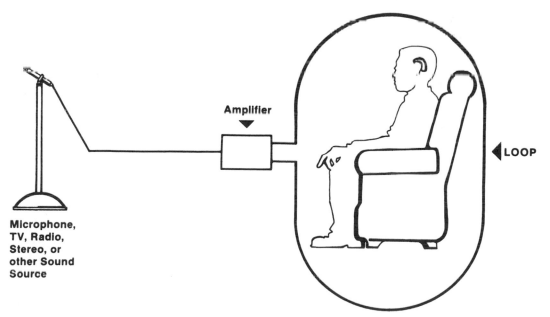

Figure 16.5. Use of an induction loop system with a behind-the-ear (BTE) hearing aid set to "T" (telecoil) position. (Reprinted with permission from Compton CL. Assistive devices: doorways to independence. Annapolis, MD: Compton & Associates, 1991.)

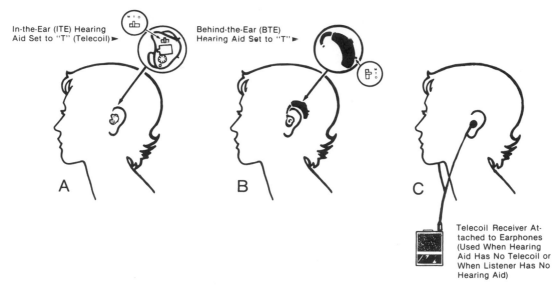

In-the-Ear (ITE) Hearing Aid Set to "T" (Telecoil) ►

Behind-the-Ear (BTE) Hearing Aid Set to "T" ►

A

B

C

Telecoil Receiver Attached to Earphones (Used When Hearing Aid Has No Telecoil or When Listener Has No Hearing Aid)

Figure 16.6. Methods of sound pickup from an induction loop system. (Reprinted with permission from Compton CL. Assistive devices: doorways to independence. Annapolis, MD: Compton & Associates, 1991.)

ulated (FM) receiver. Use of the hearing aid telecoil as a wireless receiver is also cosmetically appealing to many people. Another advantage is that the loop user does not need to borrow a separate receiver. In large-area applications such as movie theaters and airport terminals, this can save time and trouble both for the facility and the assistive technology user. Again, if a listener does not have a hearing aid or has a hearing aid without a telecoil, then a separate receiver can be used but must be maintained.

Induction loop systems are vulnerable to electromagnetic interference (60-cycle hum) from various sources such as fluorescent light, transformers, and electrical power wiring within a building. In addition, electromagnetic energy from a loop system can travel through solid surfaces, causing spillover of the signal into adjacent rooms. Another problem is that the strength of the magnetic signal decreases sharply with distance. Finally, sensitivity of hearing aid telecoil reception is often dependent on the spatial positioning of the coil within the hearing aid case. Reduction in output can occur simply by changing the plane of the telecoil in relation to the induction source. With a conventional room loop (or neckloop), it is best to mount the hearing aid telecoil in a verti-

cal position inside the hearing aid case so that it is perpendicular to the loop. In 1988, Oval Window Audio developed a three-dimensional induction system that consists of a prefabricated configuration of three audio loops, varying in amplitude and phase, embedded in a flexible foam mat that is placed under a carpet (Gilmore and Lederman, 1989). This design has resulted in signal uniformity throughout the room in which it is placed, irrespective of hearing aid telecoil positioning. In addition, spillover of the signal between rooms has been decreased to the point that in many cases, unlike with traditional loop systems, adjacent rooms can be looped.

If a person wants to use a loop system, he or she must sit within or next to the loop. Many times it is not practical or even possible to loop an entire room. Thus, the loop user may be required to sit within a designated looped area. If a portion of a room is looped, it usually will be toward the front of the room so that the listeners can take advantage of visual cues provided by the speaker. Because some people might not appreciate being required to sit within an assigned area, this issue should be addressed when deciding among wireless listening systems. Finally, it has often been said that the installation of a loop system can be difficult or impossible in some buildings because of the architectural characteristics and/or historic value of the buildings. Actually, although there are exceptions, it is possible to install a loop system in most buildings, regardless of their structure or historic value, without adversely affecting structural or aesthetic integrity. In Europe, for example, where loop technology has existed for many years, it is not uncommon for ancient churches and other structures to contain induction systems.

Infrared. Infrared systems transmit sound in the form of harmless light waves that are invisible to the human eye. An infrared system consists of four basic components: a pickup device (microphone or direct electrical connection), a transmitter (base station), an emitter, and a receiver. After the audio signal is picked up, it is conveyed onto a subcarrier in the base station and is then converted into infrared light by the emitter. The emitter sends the infrared light through the air via light emitting diodes (LEDs) that are distributed on the emitter panel. A photosensitive cell on the receiver picks up the infrared energy and converts it back into the original audio signal. The receiver can be worn connected to earphones or earbuds or can be used with a hearing aid via inductive pickup (neckloop or silhouette inductor) or DAI (Fig. 16.7).

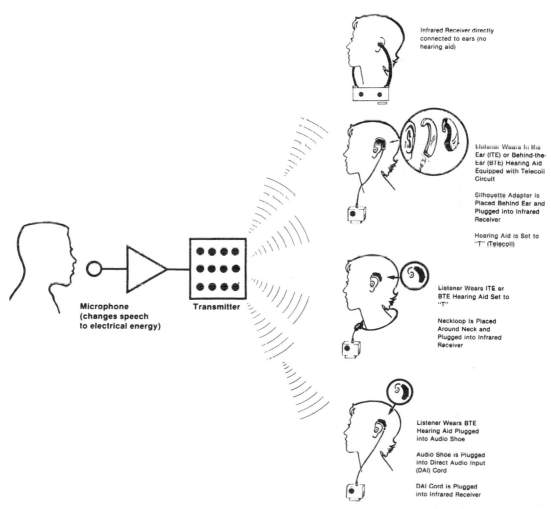

Figure 16.7. Use of an infrared transmission system. (Reprinted with permission from Compton CL. Assistive devices: doorways to independence. Annapolis, MD: Compton & Associates, 1991.)

There are no seating restrictions with infrared transmission, provided the room has a sufficient number of properly positioned infrared transmitters that will "bathe" the room with a sufficient amount of infrared light. In addition, because infrared light will not penetrate solid barriers, it can be used simultaneously in adjacent rooms without interference. Thus, it is ideal for use in the legitimate theater, courtrooms, larger conference rooms, cinema houses, and other areas where security of the signal is a concern. Infrared technology can be mono or stereo. Mono systems used to use 95 kHz as the de facto standard for transmission. Stereo systems used 96 kHz and 250 kHz. In the 1990s, the introduction of the electronic ballast for fluorescent lights caused severe interference with the 95 kHz systems, causing manufacturers to offer 250 kHz systems as standard or on a conversion basis. Because stereo infrared systems use two carriers, manufacturers of these types of systems have begun to use the transmission frequencies of 2.3 and 2.6 MHz to avoid interference from electronic ballasts used in the retrofitting of old and in new buildings. Most of the infrared systems sold to audiologists for use with persons with hearing loss are mono and transmit on a carrier frequency of 95 kHz. These small "home systems" are ideal for television listening at home as well as at business meetings and other small group or one-to-one situations. Because most systems still use a 95 kHz carrier frequency,[a] an infrared user can usually (but not always) take his or her receiver from home and use it at the theater to avoid waiting in line for the theater's receivers. However, if a stereo system is being used in the public area, the listener must realize that he or she will hear out of only one ear (because the headset will pick up only one of the two frequencies of transmission used in

stereo transmission). Most infrared transmitters require AC power, although some battery-powered (and thus more portable) transmitters are available.

The limitations of infrared technology are as follows. Infrared systems cannot be used outside because they are subject to interference from sunlight. Infrared light also travels in a straight line, meaning that the strongest and clearest signal is obtained when received from the direct line of transmission. In most applications, the infrared signal is also reflected by walls, ceilings, furnishings, clothing, and so on, and the reception of the signal is not completely directional. However, in large-area applications where the coverage area of the emitters may be pushed to its maximum, the infrared signal may prove to be more directional, requiring the user to face in the direction of the emitters to receive a clear signal.

The performance of an infrared transmitter is determined by the correlation between the number of transmitting diodes and the physical and lighting conditions in a given room. Attempting to use a personal transmitter in larger rooms without the addition of remote emitters may provide a limited signal and a potentially inferior performance.

Frequency Modulation. FM systems provide the greatest versatility of any of the wireless technologies. FM systems transmit the desired signal using an FM radio wave just like that used for commercial FM broadcast operating in the 88 to 108 MHz range. However, in the United States, personal and large-area FM systems are authorized by the Federal Communications Commission (FCC) to broadcast on two special-hearing assistance bands: 72 to 76 MHz and 216 to 217 MHz. For auditory assistance purposes, no license is required; however, users must accept the interference caused by licensed users sharing the same band.

As with the other two wireless systems, the FM transmitter can be coupled directly to a sound source via a plug/jack connection or can pick up sound by means of a microphone. At the transmitter, the signal is changed into an electrical signal and then

---

[a]Infrared systems used in locations for language translation (e.g., United Nations) or in studio recording may use up to 12 different frequencies, or channels, of transmission. Stereo infrared systems are also available for home use by persons who want to listen to music or stereo television with wireless headphones. These broadcast on two frequencies, 95 kHz and 250 kHz.

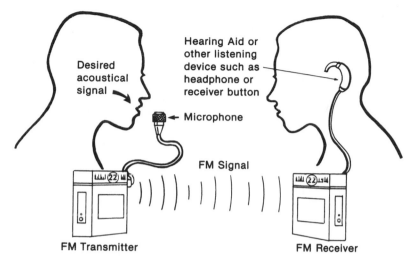

Figure 16.8. Use of an FM transmission system. (Reprinted with permission from Compton CL. Assistive devices: doorways to independence. Annapolis, MD: Compton & Associates, 1991.)

into an FM radio wave that is broadcast through the air. To receive the desired signal, the FM receiver used by the listener must be tuned to the same frequency as that of the FM transmitter. As with infrared, each listener must wear a receiver that picks up the radio transmission, demodulates it, and sends it to earphones or a hearing aid (via induction or DAI[b]) (Fig. 16.8).

The frequency range from 72 to 76 MHz can be divided into 10 wide-band (WB) channels or into 40 usable narrow-band (NB) channels. Channelization of the 72 to 76 MHz band was dropped in 1989; thus, there are currently no standards for assignment of carrier frequencies and bandwidths. Typically, NB systems in the 72 to 76 MHz band are spaced only 50 kHz apart, with a maximum allowed frequency deviation of ±10 kHz. The maximum bandwidth permitted for the 216 to 217 MHz band is 50 kHz.

Some manufacturers have chosen to divide the band into 20 channels spaced 50 kHz apart, whereas others have chosen 40 channels spaced 25 kHz apart. Therefore, it is important to understand that the labels "narrow band" and "wide band" are not necessarily expressions of audio performance, but are describing the bandwidth technology for a specific product line by a manufacturer. Sometimes manufacturers will state that wide band is of higher fidelity. This is true, but it does not really make a difference for our purposes because the earphones and hearing aids that we connect to the FM system have narrower bandwidths than either WB or NB FM transmission.

WB TRANSMISSION. Most WB frequencies are spaced 200 kHz apart, with an allowed maximum frequency deviation of ±75 kHz. Because channels for WB systems were standardized before channelization was dropped, most companies making WB systems use the same 10 carrier frequencies. Each of the 10 frequencies have been assigned a letter between A and H. In traditional WB systems, tuning an oscillator inside the transmitter to the desired frequency makes the selection of a carrier frequency. The receiver is also tuned to the same frequency. There are two types of frequency control. The first is called field tunable. This means that individual users can adjust or

---

[b]A unique boot receiver, the TMX TeleMagnetix boot attachment, is manufactured by Phonic Ear, Inc. Designed to receive a pulse-width modulated 40 kHz signal from a neckloop attached to a special FM receiver, the system reportedly has several advantages over conventional FM boot systems and neckloop/telecoil systems. It is not susceptible to inductive disturbances, has a broad audio frequency range (10 kHz), has an SNR as good as that obtained with DAI, is not sensitive to head movements, and has low current consumption and long receiving distance (as opposed to the newer FM boot receivers that snap on to the bottom of BTE hearing aids).

"tune" the transmitter and receiver to a different channel to avoid outside radio interference or to listen to another channel. However, the electronic components in this type of system are often sensitive to voltage and temperature changes, which can cause the transmitter or receiver to "drift" in frequency. Receivers can be equipped with an automatic frequency control circuit to control for this drift.

Another method used for stabilizing the frequency is the use of crystal control. In these systems, both the transmitter and receiver incorporate a crystal that oscillates at a specific frequency and is not sensitive to voltage or temperature changes. Crystal-controlled devices use plug-in modules that are labeled A to H. The user can change from one frequency to another by simply changing out the module. In general, there is full compatibility among different manufacturers using this letter coding.

NB TRANSMISSION. The bandwidth of true NB systems must always be less than 50 kHz, as opposed to 200 kHz for WB systems, so that all 40 channels may be used without interference from adjacent channels. In practical terms, this means that NB systems are significantly less susceptible to radio interference than are WB systems. Additionally, this means that NB systems are a better choice for educational institutions and multiplex movie houses where more than 10 systems may be operating at the same time. The author believes that NB systems are a good choice for metropolitan areas where interference from radio devices (e.g., police cars, ambulances, hospitals, etc.) is more of a concern.

NB systems are always crystal-controlled because the demands for frequency stability and selectivity are much greater than for WB systems. NB systems are available with fixed crystals (that have to be changed at the factory), interchangeable crystals (plug-in), and channel selector switches that may allow the user to select up to 40 different channels in one FM system. Systems using channel selection used "phase-lock loop" technology. This crystal-controlled digital frequency synthesis technology allows the FM receiver to "lock on to" the closest FM transmitter of the same frequency to prevent channel drift. In the 72 to 76 MHz band, most NB systems used a two-digit channel numbering system, although one company uses a color code system. In the 216 to 217 MHz band, single digits are used to code channels. For NB systems in general, because each manufacturer's selected carrier frequencies and bandwidths may not be the same, there is not necessarily compatibility between two different systems labeled with the same channel number. However, each manufacturer can provide a "frequency compatibility chart" so that if necessary, the individual can match a transmitter from one company to a receiver from another.

FM systems are perhaps the most versatile of all listening systems. Easy to install, they can be used indoors or outdoors, in large areas or in small groups, in one-to-one listening situations, or while listening to media. Through the use of separate frequencies, several groups of FM users can function in the same room without interfering with each other's transmission. The transmission range of FM systems range from 50 to 200 feet, but more powerful systems (transmission range of up to 1000 feet) are available for large areas such as auditoriums and outdoor stadiums. As with loop and infrared systems, FM systems can be connected to existing PA systems to provide communication access for people with hearing difficulties. FM technology is also being used in the education of children with hearing loss as well as children with central auditory processing disorders and recurring otitis media. Like all ALDs, FM systems are also becoming popular with adults to assist in communication at home, in the workplace, and while recreating.

Some FM systems contain hearing aids and some do not, and the term "inology" traditionally used to describe these two types of systems can be confusing. Historically, the term auditory trainer has been used to refer to FM systems used in educational settings with children who have hearing loss. Typically, the FM receiver of these systems also contained a hearing aid.

Older hardwired group amplification systems were also known as auditory trainers. The term personal FM came along later and refers to an FM system that does not contain a hearing aid, although it certainly can be used with one (via inductive coupling or DAI). Because all ALDs, hardwired and wireless, can be used in educational and clinical settings for auditory training and all are worn on the body, the terms auditory trainer and personal FM can be applied equally. Thus, when discussing FM systems, it might make more sense to refer to them as "FM systems" versus "FM systems with built-in hearing aids." However, this semantic problem is not so easily solved due to the emergence of some new FM systems. The reader is referred to Chapter 5 for further discussion of how FM systems are used with children.

BTE HEARING AIDS WITH BUILT-IN/SNAP-ON FM BOOT RECEIVERS (NB). As of this writing, there are several companies that offer combination FM/BTE hearing aid systems. Some systems consist of hearing aids that contain FM receivers that are permanently built into the hearing aid case. Others consist of tiny FM "boot receivers" that look like audio shoes and simply snap onto the bottom of a hearing aid. Some systems are used with traditional body-worn FM transmitters, whereas others can be used with both traditional FM transmitters and hand-held versions. For example, Phonak's (Naperville, IL) system, the MicroLink, can be ordered with the MicroVox (Fig. 16.9A), a traditional body-worn transmitter (available with a lapel omnidirectional or directional microphone), or with the Handy Mic TX3 (Fig. 16.9B), a hand-held FM transmitter whose microphone directivity can be switched from omnidirectional to supercardioid to hypercardioid.

The major advantages of these systems are their ease of use and cosmetic appeal. Some BTE FM systems use the 72 to 76 MHz band, whereas others use the newer 216 to 217 MHz band.

Limitations of FM systems include the fact that they can be expensive to maintain and are subject to sporadic interference from other radio transmissions that are allowed to use the same broadcast bands (pagers, etc.). Although the addition of the 216 to 217 MHz channel by the FCC has increased the total number of channels available for FM transmission, interference can still be a problem in some areas. Another problem involves the fact that NB and WB systems operate on different channels from each other, use different frequency spacing, and possess different transmission characteristics. Because of these differences, they are essentially incompatible with each other. For example, the signal produced by an NB transmitter may not be detected by a WB receiver or may not produce the same output signal as when used with the complementary NB receiver. Conversely, depending on the channel used, a small portion of the signal produced by a WB transmitter might align with an NB receiver. However, depending on the selectivity of the NB receiver, reception could be distorted. Because of this, it is not necessarily true that a user of FM transmission at home can necessarily use his or her personal FM receiver in a public area equipped with an FM system.

Selection and Use of Remote and Environmental Microphones. At the beginning of this section on ALDs, the importance of placing the remote microphone at the desired sound source was stressed. This is crucial for the successful use of all ALDs, hardwired or wireless. However, it is not always possible, or desirable, to clip a microphone to just one speaker. Although this may be possible and appropriate for a lecture situation, various types of communication situations lend themselves to a variety of microphone applications. Microphones of various types (omnidirectional, directional, pressure zone [PZM], noise cancellation) may be used when listening in one-to-one or group conversations.

For example, a meeting facilitator in front of a group of employees in a quiet room with negligible reverberation might use an omnidirectional microphone clipped to his or her lapel. However, a teacher in a noisy, reverberant classroom should choose a direc-

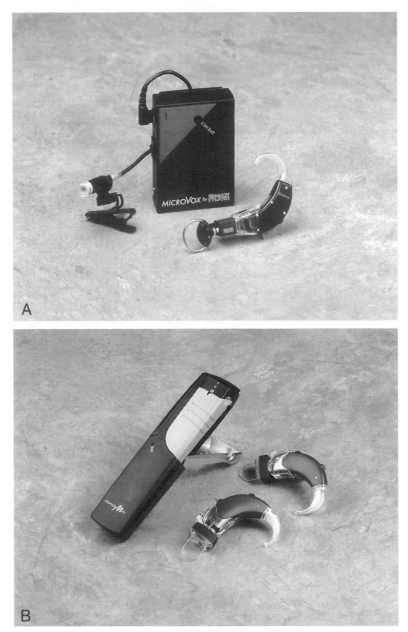

Figure 16.9. Behind-the-ear (BTE) hearing aids as used with FM boot receivers. Two FM transmitter options are shown. **A.** The traditional body-worn FM transmitter. **B.** The hand-held switchable omnidirectional versus directional microphone transmitter. Photograph courtesy of Phonak, Inc.

tional lapel type microphone because, if worn properly, it will do a better job of picking up just the teacher's voice and not the competing noise and echo (Hawkins and Yacullo, 1984). In a business meeting in which people are seated around a table, a PZM can be conveniently placed in the center of the table (on the table itself, not a tablecloth or other soft surface) and used with any of the assistive listening systems (Fig 16.10). As long as participants take turns talking and the conversation occurs in a quiet room, there is usually no need to pass a microphone around. This speeds up conversation and is less intrusive than asking each person to take turns using and pass-

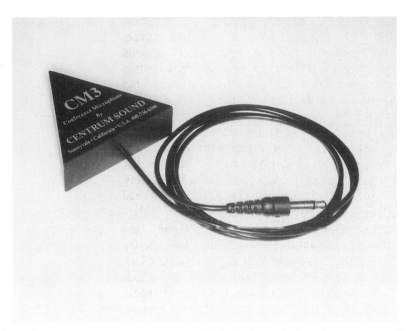

Figure 16.10. Example of a pressure zone microphone (PZM). This type of microphone can be attached to most assistive listening systems and placed in the center of a table in a meeting situation. Additional PZMs can be added for larger coverage (e.g., boardroom table). Photograph courtesy of Centrum Sound.

ing a microphone. Additional PZMs can be added and placed around a larger table such as that used in a boardroom.

Hand-held supercardioid and hypercardioid directional microphones are designed to reject sound from the sides and to therefore pick up sound mostly from the front (hypercardioid providing the most rejection) (Fig. 16.11). These types of microphones would appear to be a good choice for meetings or parties. However, they require that the listener maintain control of the microphone, pointing it directly at the person he or she desires to hear. More research in rooms with various acoustics is needed so that a fitting protocol can be developed for the various types of directional microphones. In extremely noisy situations such as on a motorcycle or in a factory, a noise cancellation microphone might be the best choice (Fig. 16.12). The microphone is designed to pick up the speaker's voice only when he or she talks and is not activated by the surrounding noise. In this situation, it would be best for the hearing aid/ALD user to make sure that his or her hearing aid environmental microphones (EM) are also

turned off to prevent interference and possible noise-induced hearing loss.

As mentioned above, when used with hearing aids, ALDs can be used with the hearing aid's EM activated or deactivated. Depending on the manufacturer's philosophy, control of the EM is accomplished via a switch on the FM receiver, hearing aid, or the audio shoe. Sometimes it is desirable to keep the hearing aid's EM on and sometimes it is not. For example, when people are listening to television using an infrared system, they might also want to be able to hear their spouse's comments. However, at a noisy party, users of hand-held directional microphones might want to deactivate their hearing aids' microphones and rely on the hand-held microphones to pick up the desired sound. Children developing speech and language skills need to hear teachers or parents as clearly as possible (via the FM transmitter microphone), yet they also need to hear their own voices for speech monitoring purposes (via the hearing aid or FM system's EM). Even adults need to be able to monitor their own voices. As an experiment, try switching a client's hearing aid to the

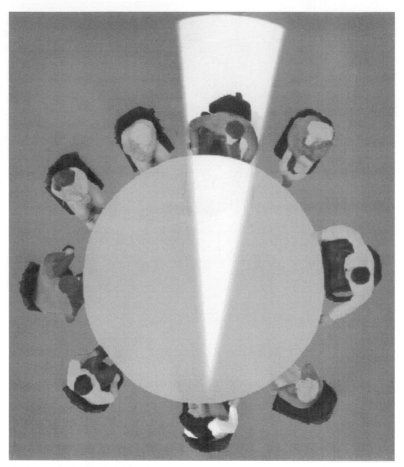

Figure 16.11. Simulation of the demonstration of the directivity of a supercardioid microphone. Illustration courtesy of Phonak, Inc.

telecoil-only mode and talk into an FM system. As the client begins to talk back, he may raise his voice in an attempt to hear it and will usually comment that it sounds strange not to be able to hear his own voice. When selecting an FM system for a given individual, it is important to maintain as much of an FM advantage as possible while keeping the EM signal audible to the listener (Lewis et al., 1991).

Monotic, Diotic, and Dichotic Signals. Most of the ALDs on the market provide either monotic or diotic signals, not stereo (dichotic). That is, one signal is presented to one ear (monotic) or one signal is split between two ears (diotic). If a client desires to hear true stereo sound, then the audiologist needs to recommend a system that will allow this to be accomplished. If, for example, the

practitioner plans to hardwire a binaural fitting of hearing aids to a portable stereo tape player, then a stereo DAI system must be used. Two cords (one for each hearing aid) terminate in a stereo plug (male connector), designated by two black connection rings (channels 1 and 2) on the plug itself. If a client prefers to use a neckloop, then he or she must be counseled that stereo sound is not possible because a neckloop is a mono device. Using it with two hearing aids will create a diotic signal at best. The neckloop should be attached to the stereo device using a stereo-to-mono adapter (the stereo male end [the plug] plugs into the stereo device, while the mono female end [the jack] plugs into the neckloop). If the client uses only one hearing aid, then what is confusingly marketed as a "stereo" cord should be ordered. The plug on the cord will be of a stereo type,

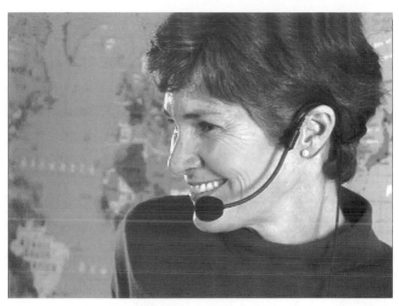

Figure 16.12. Head-worn noise cancellation microphone. Photograph courtesy of Phonic Ear, Inc.

but this is so that both channels of the recording will be transmitted into one ear. The client will not hear a dichotic signal, but at least will hear both channels of the recorded music. If a mono cord (one black ring on the plug) is used, the client will hear only one channel. For example, if the music was recorded such that the guitar is on channel one and the piano is on channel two, then the listener will hear only the guitar. Mono DAI cords are fine for nonstereo sound sources and can be ordered for monaural (monotic) or binaural (diotic) hearing aid fittings. Examples of when to use these types of cords include hardwiring hearing aids to dictation machines, mono televisions, etc.

Most wireless ALDs are not stereo (except for some infrared systems that are mostly used in large area settings). Because of this, binaurally fitted clients must be warned that wireless ALDs used with stereo television, etc. will not transmit a stereo (dichotic) signal. A stereo-to-mono adapter must be used when coupling an FM, infrared, or loop system to a stereo television. This adapter takes channel one and channel two of the television's audio output jacks and combines them into one mono output cord that is connected to the FM or infrared transmitter or to the amplifier of the loop

system. Adapters can be found at Radio Shack and other electronics stores.

Finally, if the practitioner fits a mono FM or infrared receiver using a headset, the headset must be mono. If a stereo headset is plugged into a mono device, only one earphone will work. To transmit mono sound to both stereo earphones, a mono-to-stereo adapter must be placed between the receiver and the headset. The adapter takes the mono signal from the ALD receiver and splits it in two so that it is delivered to each earphone.

Visual devices

Visual devices for face-to-face communication and for television reception are used by both deaf and hard-of-hearing people and may be used in conjunction with auditory technology, speechreading, or signed, oral, or cued speech interpreters.

Real-Time Captioning. Captioning of live lectures has grown in popularity in recent years and will continue to do so. As with live captioning of television, real-time captioning of lectures can be done in two ways. In the first, a transcript of the person's speech is fed into a computer system and then displayed on a projection screen. In the second method, verbatim captioning of unscripted material is done by a trained court reporter, using a special computerized system that can generate the full text of the proceedings with only slight time delays. With both methods, the captioning can be displayed either alone or along with a live picture of the lecturer (with the captioning as subtitles or surtitles).

Real-time captioning services can be purchased from a captioning vendor or provided by organizations that have purchased the necessary captioning systems. Costs of real-time captioning include the cost of the equipment plus the hourly fee of the captioner (Harkins, 1991; Compton, 1992). Remote real-time captioning services also are available that allow, for example, a classroom teacher's voice to be transmitted via telephone to an off-site caption writer. The captions are then transmitted via another telephone line (or on the same ISDN line) to a monitor in the classroom.

Projection Techniques for Note-Taking. Whereas real-time captioning provides a full, verbatim text of the proceedings of meetings, less expensive technologies can provide a lower level of output that may suffice in certain situations.

Note-Taking. A copy of a person's speech might be obtained ahead of time, transferred onto a transparency, and then projected on a screen during the actual lecture. An assistant can indicate with a pointer the speaker's place in the text. This technique is very inexpensive and can be helpful, particularly to hard-of-hearing people and late-deafened adults who are using auditory technologies and speechreading but who may still have difficulty understanding what is being said. If a script is not available, a competent notetaker can sit at an overhead projector and write notes as the speech is spoken. This helps the listener keep track of the topic at hand and can be especially helpful when the listener desires to take lecture notes (which, of course, requires the listener to move her eyes momentarily from the speaker and the speechreading cues).

Computer-Assisted Note-Taking. Using computer technology and a skilled typist, the same

process can be carried out with even more satisfactory results. When displaying notes for a large group, the necessary equipment includes a laptop or personal computer (PC), an LCD projector, and a projection screen or wall. The LCD projector is connected to the computer so that what is being typed is also projected onto the screen or wall. A typist takes notes during the lecture that then appear on the screen for the audience to read. As with real-time captioning, high-resolution projection systems are available, as is software that allows the use of various font sizes. For smaller groups, the notes can be displayed on a computer monitor. This technique is quickly gaining in popularity for meetings involving deaf and hard-of-hearing persons.

An important side benefit of both real-time and computer-assisted note-taking is that a hard copy of the lecture can be saved to a disk for editing and subsequent dissemination.

Note-Writing. Many times, situations occur during which a person desires to communicate with a deaf or hard-of-hearing person who cannot understand spoken language. If, for whatever reason, an interpreter is not used, some low-tech, common sense methods can be used to facilitate communication.

One option is for both people to simply write notes back and forth to each other. Another is to use a TTY or computer keyboard to speed up the process of note-writing.

Closed Captioning. Closed-captioned decoders provide television access to deaf and hard-of-hearing individuals. For many hard-of-hearing individuals, closed captioning can fill in the gaps of comprehension that amplification and speechreading cannot.[c] Even people who have more severe hearing loss and use amplification for awareness only can often enjoy the music tracks of movies, music videos, and other shows by

---

[c]Clients who plan to use captioning as well as speechreading and audition to receive television programming should be warned that captioned and spoken words do not occur simultaneously. This may create confusion and frustration for the television viewer.

using an ALD along with the decoder. The Television Decoder Circuitry Act of 1990 (Public Law No. 101-431) requires that all new televisions with screens 13 inches and larger contain decoder circuitry. This eliminates the need for a separate decoder box and has made captioning accessible to millions of Americans.

SYSTEMS TO ASSIST IN TELEPHONE COMMUNICATION

Auditory telephone devices

ALDs for the voice telephone can be used with or without a hearing aid. When used with a hearing aid, they can be used in conjunction with the hearing aid's microphone circuit (acoustic coupling) or with the hearing aid's telecoil circuit (inductive coupling). The appropriateness of each coupling method is largely dependent on the individual's hearing impairment.

Replacement Handsets. Available with round (G-style or 500-type) or square (K-style) ear and mouth pieces, these devices can be used with modular handset telephones only and must be matched electronically to the telephone to avoid distortion and to provide adequate gain. Replacement handset amplifiers can be used with or without a hearing aid, depending on the user's preference and particular hearing impairment. When used with a hearing aid telecoil, the handset must, of course, be hearing aid compatible. A person with even profound hearing impairment can often use a voice telephone successfully if fitted with a hearing aid with an adequate telecoil and a hearing-aid–compatible amplified replacement handset. Handsets are available with rotary volume controls and volume controls that turn themselves down on hang-up. Noise-canceling microphones or mute switches are also available on some handsets. These devices make telephone listening amid background noise easier.

In-Line Amplifiers. As with replacement handsets, in-line amplifiers must be used with modular phones. These devices attach between the body of the telephone and the curly cord of the handset. On some electronic (as opposed to carbon bell ringers) telephone systems, line-powered, in-line amplifiers will reduce the loudness of the user's voice to the person on the other end of the line because of power drain. In this case, a transformer- or battery-powered in-line amplifier can be used to alleviate the problem.

Portable Amplifiers. The Telecommunications for the Disabled Act of 1982 (Public Law No. 97-410) requires all "essential" telephones to be hearing aid compatible. In addition, the Hearing Aid Compatibility Act of 1988 (Public Law No. 100-394) mandates that all telephones manufactured or imported for use in the United States after August 16, 1989, be hearing aid compatible. Over the past decade, the FCC, charged with implementing these pieces of legislation, has gradually broadened the requirements for hearing aid compatibility. Although neither of the above acts or their implementing regulations require homeowners to replace their non-hearing-aid–compatible telephones with compatible models, within the first few years of the new millennium, virtually all wireline telephones in workplaces, confined settings (e.g., hospitals, nursing homes, and prisons) and hotels and motels will need to be hearing aid compatible. Additionally, Section 255 of the Telecommunications Act of 1996 (Public Law No. 104-104), which requires that telecommunications equipment and services be accessible where access is "readily achievable," requires wireless telephone manufacturers to make their telephones hearing aid compatible. Finally, an FCC ruling released in July 1997 also requires that telephones manufactured or imported into the United States after January 1, 2000, provide volume control (K. Peltz Strauss, personal communication, 1998).

There are two types of battery-powered portable amplifiers—those that couple magnetically to the telephone and those that couple acoustically. Magnetically coupled amplifiers can be used only on hearing-aid–compatible telephones. Although the above legal requirements will require most telephones in the public domain to be hearing aid compatible during the next few years, there will still be telephones that fall into the gaps left by these legal mandates. To ensure consumer telephone access (while traveling) for the next few years, it is prudent to recommend a portable amplifier that couples acoustically. As of this writing, there are two devices that couple to the telephone acoustically and can be used without a hearing aid (up to a moderate loss) or with a hearing aid's microphone or telecoil: the AT&T Portable Amplifier (New York, NY) and the Ameriphone (Garden Grove, CA) PA-25 Portable Amplifier.

Portable Induction Systems. Currently, three battery-powered, acoustic-to-magnetic (A/M) adapters are available that couple acoustically to any telephone. The Oticon TA-80 (Oticon, Inc., Somerset, NJ) is an A/M adapter that attaches to the telephone handset's earpiece, picks up an acoustic telephone signal, and changes it to electromagnetic energy for pickup by a hearing aid's telecoil. It also can be ordered with a monaural cord terminating in a silhouette inductor (TA-80C). By switching both hearing aids to "T" and by holding the handset and adapter to one hearing aid and placing the silhouette over the ear next to the other hearing aid, the listener can use both hearing aids for diotic telephone reception (Fig. 16.13). This device also can be used as a remote microphone system by wearing the silhouette on one ear and

holding out the microphone or attaching it to a television or other sound source using an extension cord. Having no loudspeaker, this device can only be used with a hearing aid's telecoil. The AT&T Portable Amplifier and the Ameriphone PA-25 mentioned previously can be used inductively and acoustically.

DAI-Only Devices for Telephone Communication. A unique device, the Phonak TC-100 (Phonak, Inc., Naperville, IL), consists of a disk-shaped microphone that is attached to the earpiece of a telephone handset. The listener picks up the sound from the telephone by using a DAI connection from his or her hearing aid to the device. This device can also be used as a remote microphone. Although it looks similar to the Oticon TA-80C, this device is not inductive. Oticon offers a DAI system for the telephone that plugs directly into the telephone and can be used with any of their DAI-equipped BTE hearing aids. In fact, any brand of hearing aid equipped with DAI can be connected directly to the telephone, provided impedance matching is performed. Each manufacturer's engineering department can help in this process. DAI devices are the systems of choice in situations in which the use of the hearing aid's telecoil for telephone listening is rendered useless because of electromagnetic interference from computers, fluorescent lighting, heating and cooling equipment, and other devices.

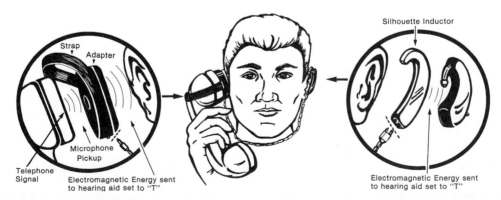

Figure 16.13. Use of Oticon TA-80C system for diotic telephone reception. (Reprinted with permission from Compton C, Assistive Devices Center, Department of Audiology and Speech-Language Pathology, School of Communication, Gallaudet University, Washington, DC, 1989.)

Interpersonal ALDs With Telephone Interfaces. Several hardwired and wireless interpersonal ALDs can be used for monotic or diotic telephone reception via DAI or inductive coupling (e.g., Williams Sound PockeTalker [Williams Sound, Minnetonka, MN], Audex SounDirector [Audex, Longview, TX], Comtek FM [Comtek, Salt Lake City, UT]). These devices must be used with modular telephone interfaces and thus are not practical for payphones, etc. In addition, this type of device is not recommended for everyday use on the telephone unless the device can be dedicated to the telephone (otherwise the user would constantly be connecting and disconnecting the device for use in both conversations and telephone communication).

All the devices mentioned in this section can be particularly useful for people who rely on heavy telephone usage for occupational reasons; these devices can make the difference between retaining or losing such employment.

Acoustic Telepads/Couplers. The feedback that occurs when coupling a custom ITE hearing aid acoustically to the telephone can often be eliminated through the use of an inexpensive foam telepad or plastic coupler that slips over the telephone receiver speaker. A shortened Styrofoam cup minus its bottom can also be used for this same purpose in an emergency situation.

Telephones Designed Specifically for Persons With Hearing Loss. As of this writing, three companies (Ameriphone, Walker [Walker Equipment, a division of Plantronics, Inc., Santa Cruz, CA], and Williams Sound) market hearing aid compatible telephones that provide significantly increased amplification over that of traditional telephone amplifiers via an adjustable gain-control built into the body of the telephone. These telephones also can provide enhanced high-frequency responses, much like a hearing aid. Some of the telephones have a jack to allow the connection of a neckloop or DAI cord. Some are available in both one-line and two-line telephones. All the telephones have low-frequency ringers and some have visual alerting signals. However, in the author's opinion, these built-in flashing lights are not bright enough to be seen from every angle and should be supplemented with an add-on alerting device (discussed later).

Nonauditory telephone devices

TTYs. The primary means of telephone communication by people who cannot understand even amplified speech on the telephone is the TTY. Descendants of teletypewriters (hence the abbreviation TTY), today's TTYs are small terminals approximately 9×12 inches in size (or smaller) and weighing between 2 and 5 pounds. TTYs are sometimes referred to as telecommunications devices for the deaf (TDDs), although this term has fallen out of favor with the culturally deaf community. In addition, the term is not completely accurate because TTYs also are used by people who are hard of hearing and/or speech impaired. In 1992, the FCC adopted the term text telephone (TT), but TTY seems to be the term of choice.

Standard TTYs transmit letters and numbers in a Baudot code that uses a five-bit character and transmits at 45.45 baud. There is normally no difficulty in communication between standard TTYs. The maximum rate of transmission is approximately 60 words per minute, which is consistent with a reasonable typing speed. More advanced TTYs incorporate Turbo Code technology. This technology saves time and money on telephone calls because it allows the user to type as fast or as slow as he or she can and also allows each TTY user to interrupt the other—a welcome feature in an emergency. Turbo TTYs communicate with all TTYs and with TTY services such as Relay and 911.

TTYs are available as "bare bones" models equipped with LCD screens only to high-end models containing features such as memory, various type sizes, a printer, a built-in answering machine, etc. Portable battery-powered TTYs are available for use when traveling and can be used with payphones and cellular phones.

Many people now use PCs at home and in the workplace. PCs can communicate with each other over telephone lines, making them useful as visual telephone devices. However, PCs use the American Standard Code for Information Interchange (ASCII), which is not compatible with the Baudot code used by traditional TTYs. That is, the TTY and the PC "speak" different languages at different speeds. TTYs are available with both Baudot and ASCII capability. ASCII TTYs can communicate at a faster rate (300 baud) with another similarly equipped TTY. However, the real advantage of an ASCII TTY is that it will allow the TTY user to communicate directly with any PC that is equipped with a modem and appropriate telecommunications software.

Computers as TTYs. PCs can be equipped with "smart" modems and software that allow them to communicate with both Baudot and ASCII TTY systems. Two excellent systems are Futura TTY and NexTalk (NXi Communications, Inc., Salt Lake City, UT). For TTY users who already have computers, the addition of a smart modem and TTY software provides a very powerful and flexible telephone communication system for less cost than a high-end stand-alone TTY.

Telecommunications Relay Services (TRS). As a result of the Americans with Disabilities Act (Public Law No. 101–336), all telephone companies have been providing intrastate and interstate TRS since 1993. TRS allow the user of a voice telephone to communicate with a person using a TTY or computer. For example, a normal-hearing person can call a state TRS and place a call to a TTY user. The TRS's communication assistant types everything said by the person using the voice telephone so that the TTY user can read it. As the TTY user types back, the communication assistant reads the message and voices it to the voice telephone user. Several companies and Gallaudet's Technology Assessment Program (TAP) have excellent Web sites for information on TTYs and TRS. Addresses are listed in Appendix 16.1.

Voice Carry Over (VCO) and Hearing Carry Over (HCO). VCO and HCO are two helpful features available through TRS and are accessed via special telephones. VCO allows individuals who cannot understand speech on the telephone but whose speech can be understood by others (e.g., severely hard-of-hearing or late-deafened individuals) to continue to use their voices over the telephone. Both Ultratec (Madison, WI) and Ameriphone offer VCO telephones. Ultratec's Uniphone 1140 is three telephones in one: a voice phone, a TTY, and a VCO phone. If two parties have a Uniphone, they can call one another and have a regular voice telephone conversation, switching to TTY mode for clarification (e.g., spellings, numbers, etc.). If one person has a Uniphone, he or she can use the TRS to place a call to another party. The other party simply talks back through the communication assistant, who types the comments that then appear on the first party's Uniphone screen. The first party can simply talk back to the second party by using the Uniphone handset. The Ameriphone is both a voice telephone and a VCO telephone, but not a TTY. It contains an LCD display (like the Uniphone) so that VCO can be used.

HCO is used by persons who can understand speech over the telephone but are speech impaired. The best solution for this need would be the Uniphone 1140, because it allows the first party to call a second party directly (provided they have a Uniphone phone) or via the TRS. The first party would "speak" by typing and would listen in the regular manner.

Facsimiles, E-mail, Pagers, and Video Phones. Many people who are deaf or hard-of-hearing use faxes or E-mail for verification of important information. Alphanumeric paging systems also have been a welcome technology. Most pagers today allow the wearer to be alerted via a beep or a vibrate mode, thus making them useful for deaf and hard-of-hearing people as well as for people with normal hearing who want privacy.

The first "alpha" pagers allowed deaf and hard-of-hearing users to receive text messages. This was thought to be quite rev-

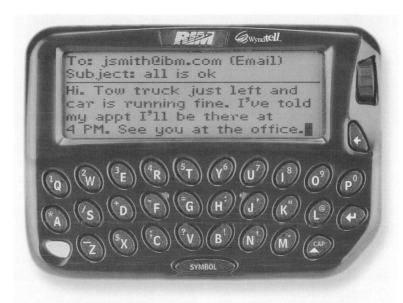

Figure 16.14. Example of a two-way pager that allows transmission and reception of E-mail and pages. Photograph courtesy of Wynd Communications, Inc.

olutionary because it allowed unprecedented communication freedom. However, the most recent generation of pagers are even more sophisticated. For example, Wynd Communications' (San Luis Obispo, CA) Model 950 system looks like a small pager but with a keyboard. It allows the user to not only send but also to receive E-mail and pages (Fig. 16.14). The system provides speech-to-text and text to speech communication. This means that a voice message can be changed to text and sent to the pager and that a text message can be typed into the pager and received as computer-generated voice mail at the other end. Thus, the system can be used instead of a TTY, computer, or fax, making it very convenient for travel and allowing deaf and hard-of-hearing people unparalleled communication access.

Perhaps by the time this chapter is read, video phones will be readily available, not only to businesses for conferencing but to anyone with a regular telephone line. As the technology improves, the use of sign language, cued speech, and speechreading will become commonplace on the telephone.

SYSTEMS TO ASSIST IN THE AWARENESS AND IDENTIFICATION OF ENVIRONMENTAL SOUNDS AND SITUATIONS

Electronic

Alerting devices are often thought of as being used only by people with severe to profound hearing loss. However, this technology is gaining in popularity with people who are hard-of-hearing who want to function independently and by normal-hearing individuals who may need assistance in detecting warning sounds amidst background noise and architectural barriers.

The first alerting devices developed focused on common signals to be monitored such as the telephone ring, the doorbell ring, the fire alarm, the wake-up alarm, and the baby's cry. Today, people with mild hearing loss or even normal hearing may need assistance in monitoring the increasing number of soft auditory signals. These include microwave timers, telephone ring "chirps," computer prompts, intercom prompts, and apartment intercom buzzers.

Because of the great variety of sounds used in our environment, the audiologist is often involved in the recommendation of an appropriate signaling system. In many instances, hearing aids enable a person to hear most sounds. What if a person is not wearing his or her hearing aids (e.g., while sleeping), is in another room, is amidst background noise, or is hooked up to the television with ALD? It is at these times that a visual or vibrotactile alerting systems may serve as a backup system to hearing aids.

Alerting devices monitor sounds using a microphone, a direct electrical connection, or inductive pick-up. Signal transmission occurs using hardwired or wireless technology. Types of alerting stimuli include visual (bright incandescent light, strobe light), auditory (signal that is louder and frequency-shaped for best reception), kinesthetic (vibration as in bed shakers, pocket pagers), or air stream (e.g., fan). Table 16.1 summarizes the various options available for monitoring, transmitting, and receiving information about environmental events.

Wireless systems can monitor various signals in an entire home or office from within any room of the building. They are much less expensive to install in existing buildings than are hardwired systems. How-ever, inexpensive hardwired systems make sense for some situations. For example, a hardwired device that plugs into a telephone jack along with the telephone cord (using a twin adapter) and flashes a light may be appropriate for an office desk or studio apartment, provided the user can see the light from any position in the room. If not, then a strobe light should be tried. A wireless system that allows more than one light to be positioned around the room can also be used. Waist-worn vibrotactile pagers are also available for home or office use. Some of these pagers transmit over short distances (100 feet), whereas others can reach out thousands of miles using sophisticated telecommunications systems composed of telephone lines, satellite down-links, and local pager antennas. Most newer paging systems alert the wearer via sound or vibration and display a numeric or alphanumeric message. For example, the Silent Call (Waterford, MI) Coordinator System uses several monitors that transmit to a transceiver that then communicates with a body-worn pager (Fig. 16.15). The pager vibrates in the same way for every signal, but displays a specific number corresponding to each monitoring device so that the user knows exactly what happened (for example, "1" always means

Table 16.1
Alerting systems: sound sources and methods for pickup, transmission, and stimulation

Sound Source	Pickup Method	Transmission Method	Stimulus (Alerting Signal)
Doorbell	Microphone	Hardwired (sound	Incandescent light
Fire alarm	Direct electrical connection to:	pickup and stimulus	Fluorescent light
Telephone ring	Telephone jack	are tethered)	Vibrotactile (e.g.,
Baby's cry	Doorbell chime	Wireless (airborne	bed shaker pager)
Appliance	Fire alarm system	radio waves or line	Fan
timer	Alarm clock	carrier current)	
		Transmitter built	
		into or attached	
		to sound pickup	
		portion of system	
		Receiver built into or	
		attached to stimulus	
		portion of system	

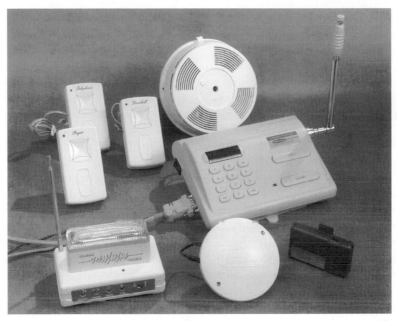

Figure 16.15. Example of wireless alerting system for home or office. Photograph courtesy of Silent Call Corporation.

that the smoke detector was activated).[d] A totally vibrotactile version of this system is available for use with deaf-blind individuals. Sonic Alert (Troy, MI) manufactures a system that does not use a pager but instead uses flashing lights that are coded for each sound. For example, when the doorbell is activated, the lights attached to receivers around the home or office will flash five to six times, whereas activation of the telephone will cause the lights to flash in cadence with the telephone ring. Ameriphone's system uses uncoded flashing lights that plug into receivers placed around the home or office. Each receiver contains a series of LEDs placed over icons that indicate the various sounds monitored (e.g., door, telephone, etc.). When the light flashes, the user simply looks at the receiver and notes which one of the LEDs is lit. Which type of system is best? This will be discussed in the needs assessment section.

Wake-up systems include small, portable, battery-powered clocks that can be placed inside a pillow and will vibrate the pillow to awaken the user. AC-powered clocks can be connected to a lamp, a strobe light, a bed shaker, or a fan. Some systems provide a multi-media event by shaking, flashing, and buzzing the heavy sleeper awake! A homemade system fashioned from a lamp, a lamp timer, and a flasher button (used to make the light flash on and off) placed in the lamp socket also can be recommended. This type of device can be used as an inexpensive teaching tool for parents of deaf children. Children should be exposed to alerting devices at an early age to learn cause and effect (e.g., "Why did Mommy open the door?") and to develop independence.

The monitoring of computer prompts can be accomplished through the use of hearing aids or special visual displays that can be programmed to appear on the monitor. DAI can also be used for this purpose.

Alerting technology that meets National Fire Protection Association (NFPA) criteria is available to warn deaf and hard-of-hearing people in the event of a fire or other emergency. This life-saving protection is accomplished using fire notification appliances

---

[d]Cellular pagers with numeric and text messages can be used to warn a group of deaf or hard-of-hearing employees in the event of a fire or other emergency. These systems can be ordered with an in-house transmitter so that the hospital or factory does not have to transmit through regular telephone lines.

such as strobe lights, fans, or vibration units with various intensities, often combined with compatible smoke detectors. The required signal intensity of these devices is determined by local fire protection authorities having jurisdiction. Two types of standards must be complied with when recommending fire-alerting technology: (1) installation standards and (2) performance standards. NFPA provides installation standards (The National Fire Alarm Code) that are used by local authorities and provides information as to the proper use and installation of these products. Underwriters Laboratories (UL) evaluates the product for its performance (i.e., applicable safety requirements and signal intensity rating only) (F. DeVoss, personal communication, 1998). All new strobe lights, fans, and vibrators must comply with a UL performance standard called UL#1971. If the device meets this standard, it should be marked with the round UL label, the standard number (1971), and the word "listed." If a product is found to comply with the applicable safety requirements, the company name and product identification is shown in one of UL's Product Directories. In the case of fire alarm signaling equipment, UL has a Fire Protection Equipment Directory (the "Brown Book") that lists the different product categories and the products listed within them. The directory is used by inspection authorities to confirm that the product has been evaluated in the category that addresses its intended use (F. DeVoss, personal communication, 1998). By reviewing the installation standard (NFPA) and the listing information provided in the UL products directory, an inspection authority can determine the acceptability of the final field installation. The NFPA committee responsible for the installation requirements for visual and audible signal appliances is referred to as the Committee on Notification Appliances for Signaling Systems. Work is constantly underway by both UL and NFPA to improve and clarify requirements for signaling devices used by people with hearing loss. This is extremely important because many fire warning systems currently being marketed do not meet NFPA and UL standards, yet are

being purchased and are giving a false sense of security to consumers. Clearly written standards will enable professionals who work with the deaf and hearing impaired, as well as other professionals in related fields, to recommend safe and effective products.

Several companies manufacture single-station smoke detectors with built-in horns and strobe lights that are UL 1971 and NFPA Fire Alarm Code approved. These may be used in situations in which the occupant is in the same room as the detector/alarm (e.g., a one-room studio). In an apartment building, single-station devices should be wired to the rest of the fire alarm system so that when a fire triggers the local single-station device, the device communicates that fact to a panel of lights connected to the central fire alarm system for the building. Fire officials can then inspect the panel to determine where the fire originated. Further, if the apartment's local smoke detector/alarm is connected to the general fire alarm system, the occupant is alerted when there is a fire elsewhere in the building, not only when it occurs in his or her living area. Systems are also available for private homes.

Before recommending any fire notification device, the practitioner must make sure it meets UL 1971 performance standards as well as NFPA installation standards and the local fire code. Fire safety experts should be consulted to protect the practitioner from potential liability (see Appendix 16.1 for fire safety consultants).

Mammalian

The hearing ear dog is a viable alternative to electronic alerting technology. Warm and fuzzy, a hearing ear dog is powered by food, water, and love and can provide important companionship as well as communication access and safety to its owner. Hearing ear dogs are professionally trained to alert their owners to various pertinent sounds. Some companies train specific breeds (such as German shepherds) and others visit local SPCAs and will train any breed (or multibreed) of dog that passes a series of tests designed to measure its potential as an assistance dog. Almost all states have hearing dog legislation. Although the vast majority of states may give legal status equivalent to seeing eye dogs, many require some form of certification and have some limitations. For more information, contact the National Information Center on Deafness (NICD) at Gallaudet University, 800 Florida Avenue, Washington, DC 20002-3695 (202-651-5051).

SUMMARY OF OVERVIEW

As discussed, a person's communication needs may not necessarily be met through hearing aids. In addition to personal hearing aids, there are numerous auditory and non-auditory technologies available to help deaf and hard-of-hearing people communicate. For a more detailed, generously illustrated review of these technologies, a monograph (Harkins, 1991) and videotape and companion book (Compton, 1991) are recommended. The Internet is also an excellent source of information; helpful Web sites are listed in Appendix 16.2.

Needs Assessment/ Selection Process

Audiologic assessment and the selection of appropriate technology must occur within the context of a comprehensive, individualized, reality-based communication needs assessment that looks at lifestyle, hearing level, speech recognition, and numerous other factors before determining which type or types of technologies are best for a client. Knowledge of the technology, coupled with thorough case history focusing on these factors, will determine not only whether a hearing aid and/or assistive devices are necessary, but what specific type of technology should be recommended.

LIFESTYLE

A patient's lifestyle plays a crucial role in deciding which type of technology is best or whether technology is needed at all. Analysis of interpersonal, telephone, and alerting communication needs should be carried out in every situation the client may encounter. These situations commonly include communication at home (private or group [e.g., retirement home]), at work, while traveling, while recreating, and at school. These situations will be examined individually, as technology requirements often vary with each one.

Communication needs at home

Communication needs at home include the following:

- Communicating via the telephone.
- Watching/listening to television.
- Listening to the radio or stereo.
- Participating in one-to-one conversations.
- Participating in group conversations (family, relatives, friend, associates).
- Receiving warning signals (e.g., telephone ring, doorbell/door knock, fire alarm, wake-up alarm, appliance signals, monitoring of children's or mate's activities from another room, security signals).

Communication at home will necessitate technologies that are compatible with the client's habits and the habits of other family members. For example, an amplified handset that turns itself down after hang-up is a prudent recommendation when normal-hearing family members will also be using that telephone. Television listening devices plugged into the audio output jack(s) of a television might be desired over models that plug into the earphone headset jack, so that all family members can enjoy the program (plugging into an earphone jack will usually turn off the television speaker; plugging into the audio output jack[s] will not).

Communication needs in a group home

Communication needs in a group home situation (retirement home, nursing home, half-way house) may be similar to those in a single-family home with the addition of the following:

- Receptive conversations in common dining areas, game rooms, media rooms, and chapel as well as in conferring with medical personnel and other care givers.

- Reception of warning signals also applies unless the client is under 24-hour supervision (wherein group home personnel would be responsible for the client's safety and security and for the admission of visitors to the client's room or apartment).

In addition to hearing aids and ALDs, acoustic treatment of common areas, especially dining rooms, can do much to reduce the negative effects of noise and reverberation on communication.

Communication needs in the workplace

When querying a client about communication at his or her workplace, it is important to look for possible needs in the following areas:

- Telephone communication (in office, while traveling).
- Office conversation (one-to-one, meetings within office).
- Lectures/seminars within or outside the office.
- Casual conversations with colleagues, clients (office, staff lounge, car, restaurants).
- Speech recognition from a dictation machine or telephone answering machine.
- Reception of important warning signals in the office and while traveling (e.g., fire alarm, telephone ring, pager, doorbell/door knock, computer prompts).

Selecting an amplifier for an office telephone is usually more difficult than selecting one for a home telephone. Numerous types of office telephones are available. Most of these are electronic and cannot be used with just any amplified handset. One must be aware of which handsets will work which phones as well as the availability of externally powered in-line amplifiers that work with most office telephones. Further, the use of a hearing aid's telecoil with the telephone might prove to be impossible in an office beset with electromagnetic interference from computers and fluorescent lighting. In this case, it might be more appropriate to couple the hearing aid to the telephone using its microphone and a telepad (if loss is mild enough) or by using DAI.

The need to listen to a dictation machine or to synthesized speech from a computerized speech-to-text program (e.g., Dragon Dictate) may point out the need for a hearing aid equipped with a DAI connection. Difficulty hearing incoming messages on an answering machine (even with a hearing aid) can be ameliorated via use of voice mail. A good solution for the home as well, voice mail allows the listener to retrieve messages using an amplified, hearing-aid–compatible telephone and avoids poor sound quality often provided by taped messages. Wireless listening devices such as FM, infrared, and induction loop systems are more appropriate for long-distance listening (e.g., seminars and group meetings) than would be hardwired systems that limit movement and distance from the sound source. If a client works in a high security area, infrared or hardwired systems may be the only technologies allowed.

Communication needs in educational settings

Communication needs here may include the following:

- Speech recognition in classrooms, lecture halls.
- Speech-language therapy.
- Auditory training.
- Meetings with teachers and other personnel.
- One-to-one or group conversation in dormitory, apartment, etc.
- Telecommunications in dormitory, apartment, on and off campus.
- Reception of warning signals as mentioned previously including local (client's room, apartment) and general (hallway and common areas) fire alarm systems in dormitory and/or apartment.

Reception of speech and music (e.g., microphone/transmitter on teacher, transmitter plugged into VCR) can be improved through the use of ALDs. Traditionally, FM systems have been used from kindergarten through grade 12 in the United States for the education of children with hearing impairment. However, this technology is also finding popularity in higher education and in the education of children with central auditory processing problems. FM systems lend themselves nicely to classroom usage in a college setting, allowing the listener complete freedom of movement and the added advantage of being able to tape record the lecture as it is being given. The tape recording can then be reviewed and compared with notes at a later date. Induction loop systems are also becoming more popular in education due to their low maintenance, low cost, and cosmetic acceptability (for classroom teaching, wireless microphones can be added so that the teacher is free to move around the room).

Amplified classrooms are gaining favor with educators. An amplified classroom is simply a portable PA system. The teacher uses a wireless microphone (FM) that transmits his or her voice to a receiver/amplifier that powers several speakers placed around the room. Classroom amplification systems are available from several companies. These so-called "sound field systems" can be used with normal-hearing children learning in classrooms characterized by poor room acoustics. In addition, children with central auditory processing difficulties, unilateral hearing loss, and recurrent otitis media can benefit from the enhanced SNR provided by these systems. Finally, because the transmitter broadcasts on an FM frequency, individual FM receivers also can be used to pick up the teacher's voice directly by those students who have more severe hearing difficulties and are using FM receivers with earphones or hearing aids.

All schools and colleges should be equipped with hearing-aid–compatible, amplified telephones and TTYs so that students have access to each other, their parents, and others. The use of TRS should also be taken advantage of when needed.

Communication needs while recreating and traveling

Recreational and travel activities include:

- Telephone conversations (payphone, hotel, car).
- One-to-one, small or large group conversations in hotels, lecture halls, restaurants.
- Speech recognition while on indoor and outdoor tours (bus, train, plane, boat, on foot, bicycles, horses, skis).
- Instruction (any type of hobby or activity during which the hearing-impaired person must be able to hear the instructor/guide).

Access to the telephone while traveling can be provided through the use of portable amplifiers and small, battery-powered TTYs or pagers that transmit and receive. As more and more theaters, movie houses, houses of worship, and other large areas install wireless listening systems, accessibility to these locations increases. However, it becomes even more important that hearing aid users be fitted with hearing aids that can be used in conjunction with these large area systems. Regardless of how well a hearing aid is fitted, if it does not contain a telecoil, it cannot be used with a large area listening system. This is not to say that all clients will need telecoils in their hearing aids. For example, a good-fitting canal hearing aid may allow acoustic coupling of the ALD or telephone without feedback. Nevertheless, when fitting personal amplification, it must be ensured that the client can benefit from large area listening systems in his or her community via a telecoil circuitry, acoustic coupling without feedback, or by removing the hearing aid and using a headset.

It is also important that people are encouraged to use the large area listening systems in their community. For example, movie theater companies who have spent corporate funds on Americans with Disabilities Act (ADA)-mandated technology often find very few consumers coming in to request it. This should not be happening.

Many people with hearing problems can benefit from ALDs when engaging in recreational activities. The type of activity can determine the listening device of choice. For example, skiing, horseback riding, hiking, and golfing occur outdoors and are mobile activities. Therefore, a personal FM system would be a convenient and effective choice for the transmission of an instructor's voice to the hearing-impaired person (or vice versa). On the other hand, quilting, usually an indoor and stationary activity, could be handled with an infrared or induction loop system. One-to-one instruction in a foreign language might be handled with a less-expensive hardwired system. This activity is stationary and could occur across a table with no danger of the student's hands becoming tangled in the cord connecting the teacher's microphone to the student's personal amplifier (as might occur with quilting).

Alerting devices also may be needed in all the communication situations mentioned. Wireless alerting devices for various sounds around the home or office can be monitored from any room in the home or office having a receiver. Paging systems can be beneficial at home and especially on the job. Systems that alert someone to the doorbell or door knock are important in all situations. Wake-up devices are important for home use as well as for business and pleasure travel. Visual, vibrotactile, or enhanced audio time reminders can be used for cooking, performing chemical experiments, taking tests, or participating in sports competitions. Emergency alerting devices, such as smoke detectors, are a must in all situations. Proper installation of UL approved alerting systems must be carried out in private homes, retirement homes, office buildings, schools, dormitories, hotels, and other accommodations. Alerting stimuli (enhanced auditory, visual, or vibrotactile stimuli or a combination thereof) must be chosen with the needs of the occupants in mind. These stimuli must be effective whether the person is awake or sleeping and must be detected regardless of where the person is located. For example, a flashing strobe light, no matter how bright, will not alert a deaf-blind person to danger. Accordingly, a sighted deaf person would not be able to detect a bright strobe light located in the person's office while he or she is in the restroom. Appropriately placed re-

mote signalers must be installed in all locations that building occupants could possibly be, or occupants must be provided with effective body-worn emergency pagers.

COUNSELING

Following a thorough communication and audiologic assessment, the audiologist should have a good foundation on which to base specific decisions concerning the need for personal amplification, assistive devices, and audiologic rehabilitation. Unfortunately, currently there are no empiric data (related to degree of hearing loss, speech recognition scores, etc.) on which to base decisions concerning personal hearing aids and assistive technology. However, based on the author's experience at the Gallaudet Audiology Clinic, some clinical observations are offered that might be helpful in the decision-making process:

- Often, clients with pure-tone averages of 40 dB HL or more may require telecoil circuitry if feedback due to telephone and ALD coupling cannot be controlled via the use of a canal aid. Telephone listening is probably the biggest concern of clients, next to one-to-one communication and television listening. To decide on whether to install a telecoil, the practitioner should observe how well the client performs on the telephone, both without and with an amplifier. If the client experiences difficulty without a telecoil, even with an amplifier, a telecoil should be installed (improvement of telecoil sensitivity will be discussed later in this chapter).
- There is not always a positive correlation between degree of hearing impairment and the need for ALDs. Although this is generally true, lifestyle often determines the need for an ALD. For example, clients with very mild hearing impairment who are employed may need the assistance of a remote microphone in staff meetings or in other difficult listening situations. On the other hand, a retired person with a very mild hearing impairment and a quiet lifestyle may not even require a hearing aid (as-

suming that the quiet lifestyle is not the re-sult of compensation for the hearing loss!).
• In general, there is a negative correlation between the need for ALDs and speech recognition ability. Nevertheless, lifestyle plays an important role here, too. An active lifestyle seems to call for ALDs more often, even for people with better speech recognition scores. Clients with mild high-frequency hearing impairment with good aided speech recognition scores can sometimes benefit from the use of a hearing aid coupled to a remote microphone system in staff meetings. Furthermore, clients who use hearing aids for speech awareness only can sometimes find ALDs beneficial, as in the case of deaf clients who use DAI and neckloop interfaces with portable tape players to enjoy music.
• In general, there is a positive correlation between degree of hearing impairment and the need for alerting devices. However, even people with mild hearing impairment may need enhanced auditory or visual signaling systems when their hearing aids are not being worn or when they are using an ALD to listen to media (television, stereo, etc.)

HEARING AID/ASSISTIVE DEVICE EVALUATION

If a hearing aid is to be recommended, it must be determined whether it will need to be used with an assistive device. This decision will be based on the communication needs assessment and the performance of the hearing aid. A Communication Needs Questionnaire can be helpful in equipment selection process. A copy of the questionnaire developed by the author (and used in Gallaudet's Audiology Clinic) can be found in Appendix 16.3.

Although final decisions do not always need to be made during the hearing aid evaluation, it has become increasingly necessary due to the integration of the hearing aid, directional microphone, and FM technology into one package (e.g., Phonak's MicroLink HA/FM system with hand-held switchable omni/directional microphone transmitter). The client should be shown models of BTE,

ITE, and ITC hearing aids with the pros and cons of each style (and circuitry) explained. If ALDs appear to be needed, this should be discussed at this time. It is also important to address the fact that, as in life, there are always trade-offs. For example, telecoil circuitry and DAI can be readily incorporated into some types of hearing aids but not others. Unfortunately, as of this writing, many hearing aids with more sophisticated programmable circuitry often have weak telecoils. Clients need to be aware of the trade-offs so that they can be empowered consumers. In the author's experience, clients are often willing to sacrifice cosmetics for better hearing once they truly understand the advantages and disadvantages of the various hearing aid technologies. This is also a good time to give the client a quick "ears-on" demonstration of an ALD (e.g., by allowing the client to listen to an FM system, the practitioner can demonstrate dramatically what is meant when it is said that ALDs can improve listening in situations with poor acoustics). By effectively demonstrating a device and by training a client about how to use it, the practitioner will greatly increase the chances that the client will accept and successfully use the device in the real world.

Selection of appropriate hearing aid(s)

Although it is not always possible to achieve, it goes without saying that hearing aids should be selected with the goal of solving as many of the client's communication difficulties as possible. One of the most common difficulties experienced by hearing aid users is listening amidst background noise. This problem may be partially or totally solved using directional microphones (how well it is solved depends on the person's hearing loss and lifestyle). If not, then the hearing aids should be equipped with features to allow them to be coupled to ALDs. Telecoil circuitry may also be needed specifically for telephone communication.

Use of Hearing Aid(s) With the Telephone. A client's ability to recognize speech through a telephone should be a major concern during the hearing aid selection process. For many people, the telecoil is the single most important hearing aid option, allowing access to not only the telephone but also to interpersonal and large-area ALDs. Some considerations for each type of hearing aid include:

1. BTE hearing aids offer stronger telecoil circuits and more sophisticated switching systems than do other hearing aids. They are therefore easier to use with ALDs and the telephone and provide many more listening options than do ITE hearing aids (there are exceptions, of course).
2. ITE hearing aids may be more cosmetically acceptable and may be the only hearing aid of choice in certain cases due to pinna malformation, activity level (e.g., participation in sports), etc.

   If an ITE hearing aid is chosen, the clinician must decide whether to install a telecoil circuit. Depending on the degree of the hearing impairment, the ITE may be coupled to the telephone in one of two ways, inductively or acoustically.

   A. Inductive coupling
      Inductive coupling is recommended for clients with moderate to severe hearing impairment due to the occurrence of feedback with acoustic coupling and because the installation of a telecoil circuit will allow for ALD interface in large areas such as theaters. When installing a telecoil, proper strength and orientation must be considered.

      Telecoil performance in ITE hearing aids can be improved by several methods: by adding a preamplifier circuit, by adding additional coils of wire to the telecoil, by wiring two telecoils together, by increasing the size of the telecoil's ferriferous core, and by orienting the telecoil perpendicular to the magnetic field it is trying to receive. If the hearing aid is to be used with an ALD, the telecoil should be mounted vertically inside the hearing aid case to allow for

the best reception from a room loop, neckloop, or silhouette inductor. If the hearing aid's telecoil is to be used to pick up electromagnetic leakage from the telephone only, then the telecoil should be mounted horizontally (one end facing the eardrum and the other end facing the outside world) (Fig. 16.16). If the telecoil is to be used with both ALDs and the telephone, then a compromise must be made. A vertical mount (Fig. 16.17), coupled with the addition of a preamplifier chip (Fig. 16.18) should be ordered. For telephone use, the client can be taught to compensate for reception.

      One must also consider whether switch modifications are necessary (e.g., does the client need a combination microphone/telecoil [M/T] switch?). It is never a good idea to sacrifice the microphone-only mode (M) to obtain an M/T mode. A client using M/T constantly will be annoyed by stray electromagnetic interference. The client must also be instructed on proper use of the telecoil.

   B. Acoustic coupling
      Acoustic coupling may be necessary when small ear size precludes telecoil installation in an ITE hearing aid or when a canal aid is worn. If feedback occurs when the hearing aid microphone is held next to the telephone handset, a foam telepad, plastic acoustic coupler, or handset amplifier (amplifier turned up, hearing aid microphone turned down) may provide relief. If not, then the client may have to remove the hearing aid and use a telephone amplifier. If this is the only option, the practitioner must make sure that the hearing loss allows it and that the client accepts it.

      If acoustic coupling (with or without a hearing aid) does not result in satisfactory telephone performance, then a hearing aid with an appropriate telecoil must be considered.

   C. Direct audio input
      It is also possible to install a DAI

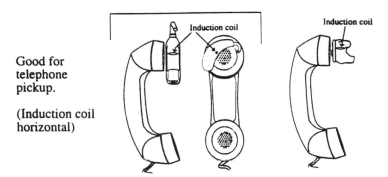

Figure 16.16. A horizontally mounted telecoil. (Reprinted with permission from David Preves, Ph.D., Micro-Tech, Minneapolis, MN.)

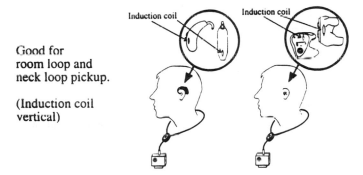

Figure 16.17. A vertically mounted telecoil is best for coupling to a room or neckloop. However, a vertical mount is a good compromise when the hearing aid user desires to use the telecoil for both the telephone and loop systems. (Reprinted with permission from David Preves, Ph.D., Micro-Tech, Minneapolis, MN.)

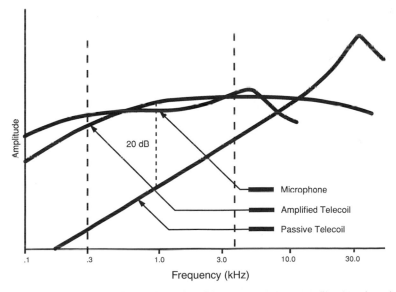

Figure 16.18. Comparison of passive and amplified telecoil frequency responses with a hearing aid's microphone response. (Reprinted with permission from David Preves, Ph.D., Micro-Tech, Minneapolis, MN.)

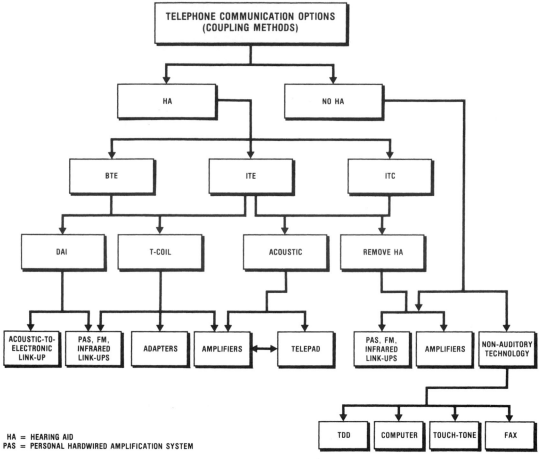

Figure 16.19. Telephone communication options (coupling methods). (Reprinted with permission from Compton C, Assistive Devices Center, Department of Audiology and Speech-Language Pathology, School of Communication, Gallaudet University, Washington, DC, 1989.)

circuit on some brands of ITE hearing aids, allowing them to be coupled to ALDs that can then be interfaced to the telephone. This might be warranted in the rare case of a cosmetics-conscious ITE user who cannot couple his or her hearing aid to the telephone—either inductively (due to magnetic interference) or acoustically (due to feedback, etc.)—and who cannot use the naked ear with the telephone.

Figure 16.19 illustrates the various ways the ear can be coupled to the telephone. Note that the use of a hearing aid telecoil increases one's telephone listening options.

Use of Hearing Aids With ALDs. If it appears that a client's interpersonal communication difficulties will not/are not being solved through the use of a personal hearing aid only, then interfacing the hearing aid with an ALD must be considered. In fact, the needs of some clients may be best met through the use of an ALD only, as in the case of an elderly, hospital-bound person. Figure 16.20 illustrates the communication options provided by using an ALD with and without a hearing aid as well as with the various types of hearing aids.

Some issues to consider are as follows:

1. BTE hearing aids provide the most flexibility with ALDs. Switching systems of-

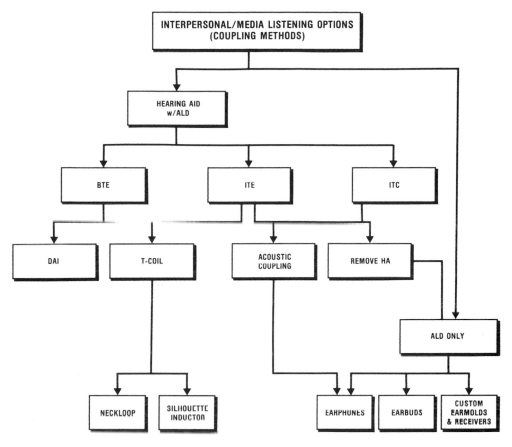

Figure 16.20. Interpersonal listening options (coupling methods). (Reprinted with permission from Compton C, Assistive Devices Center, Department of Audiology and Speech-Language Pathology, School of Communication, Gallaudet University, Washington, DC, 1989.)

fer various modes for control of the hearing aid EM. Due to the larger hearing aid case, stronger telecoils are available for use with large-area induction loops, neck loops, and silhouette inductors.

2. If an ITE hearing aid is chosen, it should be equipped with a proper telecoil. If not, the client should also be counseled concerning his or her future ability to hear and understand speech in face-to-face and broadcast media listening situations. The following questions must be asked:
   - If the client continues to have difficulty listening in noise and from a distance, how will he or she use the hearing aid with an ALD?
   - Will it be possible for the person to re-move the hearing aid and use a hard-wired ALD or wireless ALD receiver with earphones, earbuds, or custom earmold receivers?

3. Does the client need a way of controlling the hearing aid's external microphone? BTE hearing aids allow for more flexible manipulation of the hearing aid's external microphone. A combination M/T or M/DAI mode is desired for people who want to maintain contact with outside world while using ALDs. T-only and DAI-only modes are desired for especially noisy situations or for people whose speech recognition ability deteriorates significantly in presence of any background competition.

ITE hearing aids can be ordered with M-T toggle switches or combination M/T switches (or programmable modes). As mentioned previously, telecoil performance in ITE hearing aids can be improved. Adjustments must be made on a case-by-case basis by consulting with each manufacturer's engineering department.

Finally, as mentioned in the section on using hearing aids with the telephone, DAI is also available from some manufacturers.

Selection of appropriate assistive devices

Often, the hearing aid is fitted and the client is given an opportunity to use it in the "real world" before a final decision is made concerning the need for assistive devices. During the hearing aid trial, the needs assessment process can be repeated. If the client continues to experience difficulty in certain listening situations, then assistive devices may be indicated. In addition to the lifestyle considerations already discussed, several other issues need to be weighed when selecting appropriate assistive technology. Each issue is addressed below.

Effectiveness. Clients should be fitted with technology that is effective. Although this may seem obvious, all too often technology is recommended that is too complicated for the client to use. In other cases, the client has not received sufficient instruction in the use of the technology to make it effective.

Affordability. Affordability of technology will always be an issue, especially if the client has been instructed to purchase hearing aids in addition to assistive devices. However, it is important to present the assistive device(s) and the hearing aid(s) as a total communication system. If the client understands that, for example, the hearing aid by itself cannot be expected to solve the four basic communication needs, then he or she will be more accepting of the need to purchase additional technology. Sometimes it is helpful to have the client prioritize his

or her communication needs. This helps in selecting the most versatile system and also effectively involves the client as an active participant in the solution of his or her communication problems.

Training in the use of recommended equipment also figures into the affordability issue. Training and counseling in the use of the equipment must be offered to the client. However, this service and the time it commands must be built into the audiologist's fee structure.

Operability. Is the system too complicated for the client to manage? If so, then another system should be considered. Physical design of the device is also important. Are the batteries easy to remove/replace? Is a raised volume control wheel needed? Can the device be recharged without removing the batteries?

Quality/Dependability. Clients demand technology that will perform for them when needed and will last. Prices for technology vary, and each client should be counseled regarding which is the best technology for the money. In this day and age of slick advertising, clients should be made aware that, in most cases, dependable technology will cost more. Dependability becomes an even more important issue in the area of emergency alerting systems such as smoke detectors.

Portability. Some systems are easier to carry around than others. For example, a DAI remote microphone system is lighter in weight and easier to set up than is an FM system (although an FM system is more versatile). A battery-powered portable telephone amplifier is easier to put in one's pocket or purse than is a replacement handset amplifier (which can be used only with a modular telephone).

Versatility. Some systems are more versatile than others. Although they may cost more, they avoid the need for a different system for each application—and the training that goes with it. For example, FM is more versatile than other interpersonal listening systems. It works well indoors or outdoors, can be used for television or telephone listening, or for listening to a lecture or meeting. If, however, a client has only TV listening needs, then an inexpensive hardwired system might be the system of choice. All interpersonal listening systems can be equipped with various types of microphones, making them applicable to a variety of listening situations. Similarly, some alerting systems allow the user to select the most effective way of alerting him or her to the sound.

Mobility. Distance and mobility needs will often determine the choice between hardwired and wireless systems. For example, short-distance and immobile activities (e.g., TV listening, one-to-one, small group conversation) can be performed with both hardwired and wireless systems. Short-distance, mobile, indoor, and outdoor activities (e.g., sports, hobbies) can best be performed with FM technology, although some short-distance, mobile activities such as "working a room" at a party can be met via a hardwired remote microphone system. For example, a DAI directional boom microphone or even hearing aids with highly directional microphones could be used in this situation. Long-distance, immobile, indoor, or outdoor (e.g., lectures) needs can best be met with FM or loop technology (although infrared and loop technology would be appropriate for indoor activities). A wireless system such as FM would be most appropriate for a person with both mobile and immobile receptive communication needs. A person with a limited budget and mostly indoor, immobile needs might be best served with hardwired technology, provided that his or her large-area listening needs can be met with wireless systems available in the community.

Durability. Clients want technology that will last, especially if they have paid a significant amount of money for it.

Compatibility. If a person must wear hearing aids all the time, care should be taken to assure they are compatible with telephones and with personal ALD receivers in the home and community. This is most easily accomplished by including a telecoil circuit, although DAI circuitry can be added if necessary. In some cases, acoustic coupling of the hearing aid to the telephone can be successfully carried out and the use of ALDs can be accomplished by removing the hearing aid and using earphones.

Compatibility of TTYs with each other and with computers is also an issue that must be addressed.

Cosmetics. Clients may require reassurance and even assertiveness training to use certain ALDs. In general, it is best to first demonstrate the equipment before discussing cosmetics. Often the client is so impressed with the assistance provided by the technology that the issue of cosmetics becomes less important. Sometimes "more is less" (i.e., equipment such as an FM system can be less obvious than a small, hardwired DAI remote microphone due to the ability to hide the FM receiver and neckloop under clothing [or to the tiny size of FM boot receivers]). Audio loop systems are particularly cosmetically acceptable because they allow the listener to use his or her hearing aid telecoil as the ALD receiver. Some people may associate hardwired amplifiers and wireless receivers with portable radios or tape players and may therefore not be adverse to using assistive listening technology.

Previous Experience. Previous experience with technology and/or hearing health care professionals can have a positive, negative, or neutral effect. It is important to find out where the patient is "coming from" so that his or her preconceptions can be understood and handled in a positive way.

Need for Nonauditory Telecommunications Systems. TTYs, computers, captioning, pagers, and other nonauditory technologies may be needed to augment or even replace auditory devices. One must consider what standard and optional features are necessary based on the client's communication needs in various living situations.

Need for Alerting Devices. Alerting devices can augment or replace hearing aids. Alerting devices might be needed in the home or office while the client is using an ALD to couple to a desired sound source (e.g., dictation machine or television). They can also be indicated when hearing aids are used in noise, reverberation, from a distance, in another room, or are not being used at all, as when sleeping. Whereas vibrotactile devices can maintain privacy, some people consider them an intrusion into their physical space and might prefer to use flashing lights. Others might prefer a vibrotactile pager for work and lights for home.

Alerting devices should not be recommended unless they have an appropriate UL listing and meet safety and housing codes. Coverage and mobility needs must also be addressed. For example, if the sender and the receiver must be mobile, then a telephone-activated alphanumeric pager might be best. If both the sender and the receiver are confined to a particular building, then an AC- or battery-powered interoffice paging system might work, depending on the transmission range required and the amount of metal support beams in the building. Alerting devices offer various options in terms of the way they monitor, transmit, and signal. The advantages and disadvantages of hard-wired and wireless systems should be considered and explained.

When selecting a device for a client's home, office, or other setting in which the device(s) will be used, a floor plan is very helpful. It does not have to be fancy. The purpose of the floor plan is to inform the practitioner where the electrical outlets and telephone jacks are located so that the best location for the various transmitters and receivers can be discerned. The more open the floor plan, the more likely it is that fewer receivers will need to be used (e.g., one flashing light may be visible in an L-shaped living room/dining room versus two completely separate rooms). As the system is discussed with the client, the floor plan can be marked with the locations of the recommended transmitter and receivers. By using actual model numbers or created symbols, the practitioner can coordinate the locations with the actual products illustrated and listed in the product literature and the practitioner's report. This will make installation much easier, because clients will usually end up installing the devices themselves or will hire an electrician to do so.

Cultural Issues. Although hearing impairment is commonly treated from a medical model point of view, many people with hearing loss also view it from a cultural perspective. Cultural orientation can have an important effect on a person's acceptance or rejection of technology. Clients who have lost their hearing gradually usually consider themselves "hard of hearing" and from an auditory world. Consequently, they may be reticent, and even fearful, to use nonauditory technologies representative of deaf culture (TTYs, decoders, and visual and vibrotactile alerting devices). Similarly, clients who, despite their significant auditory skills, identify themselves with the deaf culture, are often fearful of using auditory technologies. This may be due to negative past experiences and current conceptions that the use of auditory technology will cause them to be labeled by their peers as "hearing minded."

It is essential that clients be provided with a comfortable, supportive, and nonjudgmental atmosphere in which he or she can examine technology options. It is important to communicate to the client that assistive devices are simply tools for communication access and that the use of these tools does not suggest that one must abandon his or her cultural identity.

The support of the client's family, friends, and colleagues is often instrumental in the successful use of assistive devices. Thus, it is important to involve them in counseling sessions.

Everyone wants to feel like he or she is "part of the gang," especially when something new is tried. Introducing clients to support groups such as Self Help for Hard of Hearing People (SHHH), the Alexander Graham Bell Association for the Deaf (AG Bell), and the Association for Late Deafened Adults (ALDA) is very helpful in this regard. These organizations provide invaluable consumer information, advocacy, and the opportunity to develop new and lasting friendships.

Demonstration/evaluation of equipment

Behavioral Evaluation. When demonstrating assistive technology, it is important to provide the client with "ears-on" and "hands-on" experience so that he or she can gain an appreciation and a comfort level for it. The demonstration should be made as relevant as possible to the client's real life communication needs. Some examples follow.

- If a client is experiencing difficulty on the telephone, then the hearing aid telecoil, telephone amplifier, or other device should be demonstrated using telephone recordings or actual telephone conversations.
- A client desiring to once again enjoy music can be shown how to connect his or her hearing aid to a portable stereo tape player via a binaural, stereo DAI cord or a neckloop connected to a stereo-to-mono adapter.
- Demonstration of television as played through an ALD or closed-captioned decoder can be made using recordings of interesting programs. A library of relevant audio and video tapes can be developed. For example, music may include classical to jazz, and television may include "Sesame Street" for kids, music videos for teens, and "Wall Street Week" for investors.
- The use of an FM system at a meeting or card party can be demonstrated by having the audiologist, client, and his or her family sit around a table with the FM system in use. The use of a lapel versus a PZM microphone can be demonstrated.
- If desired, a hardwired or wireless remote microphone system can be demonstrated in a test booth in background noise or in a room set aside for assistive device demonstrations. This room can be equipped with a loudspeaker system through which various types of background noise can be played.

A display of selected alerting devices is helpful in explaining their setup and usage.

Objective Measurement. Choosing an ALD for a client involves an analysis of that client's hearing impairment and listening needs in a variety of relevant everyday situations. Once the type of device is determined, then a brand must be selected. A serious impediment to the objective selection of ALDs is the lack of standardized protocols for electroacoustic and probe tube measurement.

Although electroacoustic measurement procedures have been suggested (Van Tasell and Landin, 1980; Sinclair et al., 1981; Gravel and Konkle, 1982; Hawkins and Van Tasell, 1982; Lewis et al., 1991; Thibodeau, 1990a), until there is a national standard we will not see unity of measurement across the various brands of products, thus making it difficult to judge the quality of the various types of systems. Clinical test equipment and protocols are also needed for electroacoustic evaluation of telephone amplifiers, adapters, and specialty telephones. Finally, although the current standard for the electroacoustic measurement of hearing aids with telecoils (ANSI S3.22, 1996) was designed "specifically to provide an indication of how well hearing aids pick up inductive signal emanating from telephone receivers" and neckloops (independent of telecoil position) and is a significant improvement over the former standard (ANSI S3.22, 1987), it should be emphasized that this standard does just that—it simply indicates how well a telecoil might perform with a hearing-aid–compatible telephone receiver or neckloop. It does not necessarily indicate how well a hearing aid telecoil will perform with a neckloop, or what the telecoil response will be in the real ear when the hearing aid is being worn.

If probe tube measurement is considered important in the hearing aid fitting process, then a comparable protocol must be developed for the evaluation of ALDs. ALDs can be used alone or in conjunction with a personal hearing aid. Either way, objective measurement of the system (ALD and/or hearing aid telecoil) must be made if one is to ascertain that an appropriate frequency response (without the risk of excessive harmonic distortion, uncomfortable and/or overamplification, or underamplification) is being provided.

Research has shown that when hearing aids are coupled to FM systems, the hearing aid characteristics are not necessarily maintained (Hawkins and Schum, 1985; Thibodeau et al., 1988, Thibodeau, 1990b). Currently, there are very limited assessment techniques being developed to look at the real-ear performance of ALDs (Hawkins, 1987; Lewis et al., 1991; Thibodeau, 1990a; Grimes and Mueller, 1991). The establishment of a national measurement protocol is essential for clients to be fitted in a scientific and safe manner. This is particularly important for young children or others who cannot provide subjective feedback regarding potentially inappropriate fittings.

Speech Perception Testing. Once appropriate coupling method and settings have been chosen, speech recognition or discrimination testing as well as quality ratings may be carried out to determine the performance of the ALD or to compare performance between the personal hearing aid and the ALD in the sound field. Lewis et al. (1991) provide a step-by-step method for documenting the advantage of an FM system. This protocol could also be adapted for other ALDs as well. Holmes and Frank (1984) and Wallber et al. (1987) have developed formalized behavioral assessment procedures for documenting telecoil performance with the telephone.

Documentation of the ALD performance may be needed for educational purposes, for third-party and/or employer financial support for ALDs, or to simply prove to a client that he or she can be assisted by the technology.

Follow-up/aural rehabilitation

Just as with personal hearing aid fittings, follow-up counseling and evaluation is essential after the recommendation of assistive technology. Additional orientation and training may also be necessary. For example, some clients may require repeated instruction on how to use their hearing aid telecoil circuit with the telephone and ALDs. Others may need intensive practice in setting up, using, trouble-shooting, and maintaining auditory and nonauditory assistive devices. Speechreading, auditory training (face-to-face and telephone), training in the use of communication/environmental strategies, and counseling may also be needed. Furthermore, assertiveness training may be required as the use of assistive technology often requires the cooperation of others. For example, it can be especially anxiety-producing to have to ask a lecturer to wear an FM transmitter, to request that colleagues at a staff meeting take turns talking into a microphone, or to ask a speaker to slow down for the real-time caption writer. For these reasons, it is important to assist the client, via instruction and role-playing, in developing the skills and psychological stamina necessary to assure successful, long-term assistive device usage.

The Role of the Professional

In the past 15 years, the area of assistive technology has matured from an academic curiosity to a legitimate clinical specialty. Several forces have contributed to this transformation, with two being the most influential—consumer activism and legislative mandates. Consumers who have hearing difficulty are becoming increasingly aware of their rights to communication access. Third-party providers are beginning to recognize and pay for this technology. What does all this mean to the audiologist in training?

It is critical that future audiologists be able to recognize when assistive technology is needed, be able to evaluate it, to recommend it, to advocate for it, to secure funding for it, and to train clients to use it. This training will extend to school officials, employers, and others who affect the lives of persons with reception communication problems. Work in the area of assistive technology will also demand excellent networking skills. Audiologists must be prepared to work effectively with consumers, acoustic engineers, attorneys, employers, teachers, state and local government officials, and managers of public accommodations.

Audiologists should have a good working knowledge of the various types of auditory and nonauditory assistive technologies and when they are appropriate. With proper training, it may be appropriate for both audiologists and speech-language pathologists to recommend nonauditory technology (alerting and visual telephone and television systems). However, the fitting and recommending of ALDs (as with hearing aids and cochlear implants) fall within the scope of practice of an audiologist. In many cases, an audiologist should be consulted before nonauditory technology is recommended so that it can be determined whether auditory technology might be more appropriate in some instances. For example, the author once received a call from a hearing aid user who wanted to investigate closed captioning because he was "deaf" and could not understand the television. Actually, all he needed was a tone control adjustment.

Because both audiologists and speech-language pathologists engage in aural rehabilitation training, both should be familiar with the use of telecoils, remote microphones, amplified handsets, and auditory as well as nonauditory technology used in this process. Furthermore, practitioners in both professions should be comfortable in including assistive technology in individual educational plans for children.

Summary

A variety of auditory and nonauditory technology is available to assist in removing the communication barriers that can prevent people with hearing problems from leading independent and productive lives.

By carefully evaluating clients' communication needs and by having a good working knowledge of today's hearing aids and other equally important assistive technologies, audiologists can select systems to meet clients' needs effectively. When audiologists incorporate all these factors into ap-

propriate and comprehensive rehabilitative programs, clients' communication skills can be improved and clients themselves can be empowered to function in today's society with independence and dignity. To do less would be a disservice to our clients and to our profession.

REFERENCES

American National Standards Institute. ANSI S3.22–1996. Specification of hearing aid characteristics. Revision of ANSI S3.22–1987.

Compton CL. Assistive devices: doorways to independence Videotape: Washington, DC: Gallaudet University, 1991. Book: Annapolis, MD: Compton & Associates, 1991.

Compton C. Assistive listening devices: videotext displays. Am J Audiol 1992;1:19–20.

Finitzo-Hieber T, Tillman TW. Room acoustics effects on monosyllabic word discrimination ability for normal and hearing-impaired children. J Speech Hear Res 1978;21: 440–458.

Gilmore R, Lederman N. Induction loop assistive listening systems: back to the future? Hear Instr 1989;40:3.

Gravel J, Konkle D. Electroacoustic hearing aid performance with neckloop inductive coupling. Presented at the American Speech-Language-Hearing Association Convention, Toronto, Canada, 1982.

Grimes AM, Mueller HG. Using probe-microphone measures to assess telecoils and ALDs. Hear J 1991;44:16–21.

Harkins JE. Visual devices for deaf and hard of hearing people: state-of-the-art. GRI monograph series. Washington, DC: Gallaudet Research Institute, series A, no 2, 1991.

Hawkins DB. Comparisons of speech recognition in noise by mildly-to-moderately HI children using hearing aids and FM systems. J Speech Hear Disord 1984;49:409–418.

Hawkins DB. Methods of improving speech recognition in the presence of noise and reverberation. Audiol Acoust 1985;9:124–142.

Hawkins DB. Assessment of FM systems with an ear canal probe tube microphone system. Ear Hear 1987;8: 301–303.

Hawkins DB, Schum DJ. Some effects of FM coupling on hearing aid characteristics. J Speech Hear Disord 1985; 50:132–141.

Hawkins D, Van Tasell D. Some effects of FM-system coupling on hearing aid characteristics. J Speech Hear Disord 1982;47:355–362.

Hawkins D, Yacullo W. Signal-to-noise ratio advantage of binaural hearing aids and directional microphones under different levels of reverberation. J Speech Hear Disord 1984;49:278–286.

Holmes A, Frank T. Telephone listening ability for hearing impaired individuals. Ear Hear 1984;5:96–100.

Helfer KS, Wilber LA. Hearing loss, aging, and speech perception in reverberation and noise. J Speech Hear Res 1990;33:149–155.

Lewis D, Feigin J, Karasek A, et al. Evaluation and assessment of FM systems. Ear Hear 1991;12:268–280.

Loven FC, Collins MJ. Reverberation masking, filtering, and level effects on speech recognition performance. J Speech Hear Res 1988;31:681–695.

Lurquin P, Rafhay S. Intelligibility in noise using multimicrophone hearing aids. Acta Otorhinolaryngol Belg 1996;50:103–109.

Nabelek AK, Mason D. Effect of noise and reverberation on binaural and monaural word identification by subjects with various audiograms. J Speech Hear Res 1981;24: 375–383.

Nabelek AK, Picket JM. Monaural and binaural speech perception through hearing aids under noise and reverberation with normal and hearing-impaired listeners. J Speech Hear Res 1974;17: 724–739.

Nabelek AK, Robinson PK. Monaural and binaural speech perception in reverberation for listeners of various ages. J Acoust Soc Am 1982;71:1242–1248.

Nabelek A, Donahue A, Letowski T. Comparison of amplification systems in a classroom. J Rehabil Res 1986;23: 41–52.

Nabelek AK, Letowski TR, Tucker FM. Reverberant overlap and self-masking in consonant identification. J Acoust Soc Am 1989;86:1259–1265.

Sinclair JS, Freeman BA, Riggs DE. Appendix: the use of the hearing aid test box to assess the performance of FM auditory training units. In: Bess FH, Freeman BA, Sinclair JS, eds. Amplification in education. Washington, DC: A.G. Bell Association, 1981:381–383.

Soede W, Bilsen F, Berkhout A. Assessment of a direc-tional microphone array for hearing impaired listeners. Journal of the Acoustical Society of America 1993; 94:785–798.

Thibodeau L. Clinical considerations in using classroom amplification systems. Paper read at the second annual meeting of the American Academy of Audiology, New Orleans, Louisiana, April 1990a.

Thibodeau L. Electroacoustic performance of direct-input hearing aids with FM amplification systems. Lang Speech Hear Serv Schools 1990b;21:49–56.

Thibodeau L, McCaffrey H, Abrahamson J. Effects of coupling hearing aids to FM systems via neckloops. J Acad Rehabil Audiol 1988;21:49–56.

Valente M, Fabry D, Potts L. Recognition of speech in noise with HAs using dual mics. J Am Acad Audiol 1995; 6:440–449.

Van Tasell D, Landin D. Frequency response characteristics of FM mini-loop auditory trainers. J Speech Hear Disord 1980;45:247–258.

Wallber M, MacKenzie D, Clyme E. Telecoil evaluation procedure. National Technical Institute for the Deaf, RIT, Rochester, New York. By agreement with the U.S. Department of Education. St. Louis: Auditec, 1987.

APPENDIX 16.1   *Selected Web Sites, Other Resources, and Teaching Materials*

Websites

HTTP://WWW.ACCESS-BOARD.GOV

Home page for the U.S. Architectural and Transportation Barriers Compliance Board (nickname: U.S. Access Board). Excellent source for information on scoping requirements of Americans with Disabilities Act (ADA), petitions for rule-making, etc. It also has links to other resources such as the Equal Employment Opportunity Commission (EEOC) and the Department of Justice (DOJ).

HTTP://WWW.MCSQUARED.COM

This is a real find. The Mc Squared System Design Group, Inc. is an audio engineering firm in Vancouver, B.C. This site is an excellent place for students and practitioners to learn more about room acoustics, microphone directivity, etc.

HTTP://WWW.GALLAUDET.EDU/~ASLPWEB/BUSINESS/ALD/ALD DESC.HTML

This is the web site for Gallaudet University's Assistive Devices Center as well as the entire Department of Audiology and Speech-Language Pathology. The site provides general information about assistive technology. Plans are in development to provide links to other sites.

HTTP://WWW.IAP.GALLAUDET.EDU

Another office on Galludet's campus, the Technology Assessment Program (TAP) is an excellent source for information on visual telecommunications devices, cell phones, and legislation.

Other Resources

LEGAL ASSISTANCE FOR CONSUMERS

Law Center
National Association of the Deaf (NAD)
814 Thayer Avenue
Silver Spring, MD 20910
V: 301-587-1788
TTY: 301-587-1789
Fax: 301-587-1791

FIRE SAFETY CONSULTANTS

Donald E. Sievers (Fire Safety Consultant to the National Association of the Deaf [NAD])
Donald E. Sievers & Associates, LTD
6309 Bradley Boulevard
Bethesda, MD 20817-3243
V/TYY: 301-469-0278
Fax: 301-469-7541

George J. Elwell
Silent Call Corporation
2950 Sashabaw Road Suite B
Waterford, MI 48329
V: 313-673-0221
TTY: 313-673-6069
Fax: 313-673-5442

UL LISTING INFORMATION AND RESEARCH RESULTS RELATED TO VISUAL AND VIBROTACTILE FIRE NOTIFICATION DEVICES

Underwriters Laboratories, Inc.
Publications Stock
333 Pfingsten Road
Northbrook, IL 60062
708-272-8800
Web site: www.ul.com

INFORMATION ON REAL-TIME REPORTING

National Court Reporters Association
8224 Old Courthouse Road
Vienna, VA 22182
703-556-6272
Website: www.ncraonline.org
Contact: Stephanie Davidson
Referral source for certified real-time reporters in each state

Teaching Materials

ASSISTIVE DEVICES: DOORWAYS TO INDEPENDENCE

This 65-minute open-captioned videotape and booklet discuss assistive devices in-depth and are appropriate for those interested in learning more about the various technologies for receptive communication. Designed to be used in waiting rooms, professional libraries, graduate training programs, senior centers, and nursing homes, the extensively illustrated booklet serves as a detailed reference for topics discussed in the video and contains a comprehensive section on large area ALD applications and nonauditory technologies, topics often overlooked. To order, call 202-651-5326.

APPENDIX
16.2 *Manufacturers and Distributors of Assistive Technology*

- When available, Web sites (and E-mail addresses) have been included. Some of these sites are extremely well done and contain not only product information, but also links to other sites and lists of research papers, etc.
- When consulting the lists, please note the following:

1. A hearing aid company is listed as a manufacturer or distributor of assistive technology if it produces and/or sells on FM system (traditional body-worn or BTE) or other assistive technology. Some of these companies may manufacturer the FM receiver but not the transmitter (which they purchase from another company and relabel with their own company's name). Relabeling is a common occurrence for both auditory and nonauditory devices.
2. Many hearing aid companies sell the various DAI cords necessary for coupling their hearing aids to various sound sources and ALDs; however, these companies are not listed due to space considerations. Audiologists can find out who they are by checking with their representative and consulting their hearing aid specifications book.
3. Several hearing aid companies manufacture the Telepin system for use with Phonic Ear's TMX FM receiver (body-worn).

Manufacturers of Assistive Technology[a]

Ameriphone, Inc.
7231 Garden Grove
  Boulevard, Suite E
Garden Grove, CA 92641
Voice: 800-874-3005
TTY: 800-772-2889
www. ameriphoneic.com
Ameriphone@ameriphone.
  com
(TTYs, alerting devices,
  phone amps)

Audex
710 Standard Street
Longview, TX 75601
800-237-0716
www.audex.com
vbeatty@iamerica.net
Contact: Mr. Charles Beatty
(IR, hardwired devices;
  hearing aid compatible
  cell phones)

AVR Sonnovation, Inc.
7636 Executive Drive
Eden Prairie, MN 55344
800-462-8336
Fax: 612-934-3033
www.avrsono.com
sonous@bitstream.net
(BTE FM systems)

Comtek
3572 700 South
Salt Lake City, UT 84115
Voice: 801-466-3463
Fax: 801-484-6906
www.comtek.com
sales@comtek.com

Oval Window Audio
33 Wild Flower Court
Nederland, CO 80466
Voice, TTY, Fax: 303-447-
  360
Contact: Mr. Norman
  Lederman
(Audioloops)

Phonak
PO Box 3017
Naperville, IL 60566
Main number: 800-777-7333
FM: 888-777-7316
www.@phonak.com
(Hearing aids; directional
  microphones; BTE, FM]

Phonic Ear, Inc.
3880 Cypress Drive
Petaluma, CA 94954-7600
800-227-0735
www.phonicear.com
rick steighner@phonicear.
  com
Contact: Mr. Rick Steighner
(FM; IR)

**Plantronics/Walker
  Equipment**
345 Encinal Street
Santa Cruz, CA 95060
408-426-5858
www.plantronics. com
(Telephone amplifiers,
  headsets, etc.)

Radio Shack
300 One Tandy Center
Fort Worth, TX 76102
(Consult your local store)
(Do-it-yourself ALDs,
  alerting devices; phone
  amps)

Sennheiser
6 Vista Drive
PO Box 987
Old Lyme, CT 06371
860-434-9190
www.sennheiser.com
Contact: Laurie DeConte
(Infrared)

Silent Call Corporation
2220 Scott Lake Road
Waterford, MI 48328
Voice: 313-673-0221
TTY: 313-673-6069
Fax: 313-673-5442
Silentcall@ameritech.com
(Alerting devices; custom
  work)

Sonic Alert, Inc.
1050 East Maple Road
Troy, MI 48083
Voice/TTY: 800-566-3210
Fax: 248-577-5433
www.Sonicalert.com
info@sonicalert.com
(Broad selection of alerting
    devices)

**Telex Communications,
    Inc.**
9600 Aldrich Avenue, South
Minneapolis, MN 55420
800-328-3102
Fax: 612-884-0043
www.telex.com
[FM]

Ultratec, Inc.
6442 Normandy Lane
Madison, WI 53719
800-482-2424
www.ultratec.com
(TTYs; Alerting devices)

Unitron Industries, Inc.
3555 Walnut Street, PO
    5010
Port Huron, MI 48061
800-521-5400
Fax: 810-987-2011
www.unitron.com
(Unicom System [BTE FM])

Wheelock, Inc.
273 Branchport Avenue
Long Branch, NJ 07740
800-631-2148
Fax: 732-222-8707
www.wheelockinc.com
info@wheelockinc.com
(Auditory and visual fire
    notification devices)

**Whelen Engineering
    Company**
Route 145, Winthrop Road
Chester, CT 06412-0684
860-526-9504
Fax: 860-526-4078
www.whelen.com
whelen@connix.com
(Auditory and visual fire
    notification devices)

**Williams Sound
    Corporation**
5929 Baker Road
Minnetonka, MN 55345-
    5997
800-843-3544
Fax: 612-943-2174
www.williamssound.com
info@williamssound.com
(FM, hardwired)

**Wynd Communications
    Corporation**
75 Higuera Street, Suite 240
San Luis Obispo, CA 93401
TTY: 800-549-2800
Fax: 805-781-6001
Voice: 800-549-9800
www.wyndtell.com
wyndtell@wynd.com
Contact: Mr. Joe Karp
(Innovative paging system)

Distributors of Assistive Technology[a]

American Loop Systems
43 Davis Road Suite 2
Belmont, MA 02178
617-776-5667
Fax: 617-666-5228
Contact: Mr. Robert Gilmore
(Oval Window Loop
    Systems; exclusive
    distributor of 3-D
    Induction System)

Audio Enhancement
1748 West 12600 South
Riverton, UT 84065
800-383-9362
Fax: 801-254-3802
Contact: Claudia Anderson
(Comtek FM; IR; etc)

www.audioenhancement.
    com
claudia@audioenhancement.
    com

Centrum Sound
572 LaConner Drive
Sunnyvale, CA 94087
408-736-6500
Fax: 408-736-6552
Members.aol.com/centrum
    web/centrum
Centrumweb@aol.com
Contact: Peter Bengtsson
(TA-80, CM-3 PZM and all
    types of large-area ALDs;
    consultation and
    installation services)

Duartek Inc.
11150 Main Street, Suite
    105
Fairfax, VA 22030
Voice: 703-352-2285
TTY: 703-352-2286
Fax: 703-352-2287
(Broad selection of auditory
    and nonauditory
    technology)

**Global Assistive Devices,
    Inc.**
4950 N. Dixie Highway
    Suite 121
Ft. Lauderdale, FL 33334
Voice: 888-778-4237
Fax: 305-563-9770

www.globalassistive.com
info@globalassistive.com
Contact: Peggy or Brian
    Hewitt
(Manufacturer and
    distributor of UL-listed
    wakeup devices; Li'l Ben
    shaker, etc.)

Hal-Hen Co.*
35-53 24th Street
Long Island City, NY 11106
718-392-6020
(Broad selection of auditory
    and nonauditory
    technology)

HARC Mercantile, Ltd.*
111 West Centre Avenue
Kalamazoo, MI 49002
Voice: 800-445-9968
TTY: 800-413-5245
Fax: 800-413-5248
www.harcmercantile.com
Contact: Mr. Ron Slager or
    Ms. Joyce Thorsom
(Broad selection of auditory
    and nonauditory
    technology; technology
    displays; marketing
    assistance)

HITEC Group Int'l., Inc.*
8160 Madison
Burr Ridge, IL 60521
800-288-8303
Fax: 888-654-9219
www.hitec.com
webmaster@hitec.com
Contact: Richard Uzuanis
(Broad selection of auditory
    and nonauditory
    technology)

NFSS*
8120 Fenton Street
Silver Spring, MD 20910
Voice: 888-589-6671
TTY: 888-589-6670
Fax: 301-589-5153
www.nfss.com
info@nfss.com
Contact: Mr. Paul Haines
(Broad selection of
    nonauditory; some
    auditory technology)

Phone TTY*
202 Lexington Avenue
Hackensack, NJ 08701
Voice/TTY: 973-299-6627
phonetty@aol.com
(TTYs, interfaces for
    computers as TTYs (lo/hi
    baud rate modems and
    Futura Software, alerting
    devices)

Potomac Technology*
1 Church Streeet Suite 101
Rockville, MD 20850
Voice/TTY: 800-433
www.potomactech.com
info@potomactech.com
Contact: Ms. Patricia Relihan
(Broad selection of auditory
    and nonauditory
    technology)

Audiology Sales & Service
3861 Oakcliff Industrial
    Court
Atlanta, GA 30340
Voice/TTY: 800-241-2465
Contact: Ms. Rebecca
    Lindsey
(Broad selection of auditory
    and nonauditory
    technology)

**Siemens Hearing
    Instruments, Inc.***
16 East Piper Lane, Suite
    128
Prospect Heights, IL 60070-
    1799
800-333-9083
Fax: 847-808-1299
www.siemens-hearing.com
dfuller@siemens-
    heawring.com
(Broad selection of auditory
    and nonauditory
    technology, technology
    displays; marketing
    assistance)

Silent Call Corporation*
2950 Sashabaw Road, STE B
Waterford, MI 48329
Voice: 800-572-5227
TTY: 313-673-6069
Fax: 313-673-5442
Silentcall@ameritech.com
Contact: Mr. George Elwell
(Mfgr./distrib. broad
    selection of alerting
    devices, including fire
    safety technology, e.g.,
    Shake-Up System;
    custom work)

---

*Catalog available.

ªInclusion or exclusion of companies in
this list does not reflect endorsement or
lack thereof.

APPENDIX 16.3 *Communication Needs Assessment Questionnaire*

The Compton Assistive Technology Questionnaire

Client's Name _____   ID # _____

Date _____   Audiologist _____

Whether you use hearing aids or not, you may hear fairly well in some situations while having to strain to hear in others. Your answers on this questionnaire will help point to ways to help you hear better in as many situations as possible.

Read the statements and questions below. Place a check mark by the statements that are true for you and answer the questions. You may have to complete some of the statements by filling in information in the middle or at the end of the statement. PLEASE FEEL FREE TO MAKE COMMENTS OR ASK QUESTIONS **ANYWHERE** ON THE QUESTIONNAIRE.

HEARING AIDS

_____I DO NOT OWN HEARING AIDS; I AM INTERESTED IN FINDING OUT IF ONE
            CAN HELP ME

_____I DO NOT OWN HEARING AIDS; I AM NOT INTERESTED IN GETTING HEAR-
            ING AIDS AT THIS TIME BECAUSE (Write in the reason you are not interested
            in obtaining hearing aids at this time.):

_____I OWN HEARING AIDS NOW BUT DO NOT USE THEM BECAUSE (Write in the
            reason you don't use your hearing aids.):

_____I OWNED HEARING AIDS AT ONE TIME; I QUIT USING THEM BECAUSE
            (Write in the reason you stopped using your hearing aids.):

[IF YOU **DO NOT** USE HEARING AIDS NOW, SKIP TO THE NEXT SECTION
CALLED "PROBLEM LISTENING SITUATIONS".]

I USE (1) (2) HEARING AID(S)
  (circle "1" if you use 1 hearing aid; circle "2" if you use one in each year.)

I OWN _____BEHIND-THE-EAR (BTE) HEARING AID(s).
            _____IN-THE-EAR HEARING (ITE) AID(s).
            _____IN-THE-CANAL (ITC) HEARING AID(s).
            _____BODY HEARING AID(s).
            _____EYEGLASS HEARING AID(s).
            _____OTHER (Explain)

_____I USE MY HEARING AID(S) (Mark how often you use the hearing aid(s):
            _____all day long every day.
            _____off and on during the day.
            _____only a few times a week.
            _____only on special occasions.

_____I WOULD USE MY HEARING AIDS MORE OFTEN IF (Write in ways you think your hearing aids could work better for you.):

_____I USE MY HEARING AIDS WHEN LISTENING ON THE TELEPHONE BY:
   _____using the "T" (telecoil switch).
   _____holding the telephone receiver next to the hearing microphone. My hearing aid _____does/_____ does not squeal or whistle when I use it this way with the phone.
   _____other (explain)

IF YOU HAVE PROBLEMS USING YOUR HEARING AID ON THE TELEPHONE, EX-PLAIN WHY:

_____I DON'T USE MY HEARING AID WHEN TALKING ON THE TELEPHONE BE-CAUSE (Write in the reason you don't use your hearing aid on the telephone.):

PROBLEM LISTENING SITUATIONS

I WOULD LIKE TO HEAR BETTER IN THE FOLLOWING SITUATIONS: (CHECK ALL THAT APPLY.)

Face-to-face communication

One-to-One:
_____at home, sitting with one other person (Circle all those that apply: den, living room, dining room, meal time, watching television, other (list).
_____at work, with my employer, employees, co-workers, other (list)
   while riding or driving in the car
   while people with whom I transact personal business (doctor, nurse, attorney, banker, insurance or real estate agent, etc.)
_____with one or two other people in social situations (visiting, playing cards or board games, etc.)
_____eating out (restaurant, cafeteria, etc.)

Groups:
_____at home, in a small family group (5 people or less)
_____at work, school, or other, in a small discussion group (5 people or less)
_____at work, school, or other in a large discussion group (5 people or more)
_____at a meeting where there is one main speaker at a time
_____at a meeting where there is a panel discussion
_____at a lecture/presentation where there is audience participation
_____in a small recreation/leisure group (cards, boardgames, handiwork, etc.)
_____at a small dinner party
_____at a large dinner party/cocktail party
_____in a place of worship (church, synagogue, meeting room)
_____in a movie theater
_____at the theater (live play)
_____at concerts or other live musical/dramatic programs
_____OTHER situations in which I would like to be able to hear better (Write in your answer(s)):

Telephone communication
_____at home
_____at work

_____when I am traveling (hotel rooms)
_____pay phone
_____at other people's homes

Televison, radio, stereo, etc.

_____home television
_____home radio or stereo
_____car/truck radio, cassette or CD player
_____home telephone answering machine
_____work television (e.g., staff lounge)
_____classroom television (live or videos)
_____television while traveling (e.g. hotels)
_____work telephone answering machine
_____dictation machine
_____"Walkman" type radio/tape player
_____two-way radio or CB
_____I cannot understand public address system announcements (at school, work, at airports, etc.)
_____other? Explain.

Alerting needs

(1) Check those sounds that you have difficulty hearing. (2) For each sound you check, circle whether you experience the difficulty –**with** or **without** your hearing aid on. Circle **both** if appropriate.

At home, I have difficulty hearing:

_____my telephone ring *with* or *without* my hearing aid on
_____my doorbell *with* or *without* my hearing aid on
_____a door knock *with* or *without* my hearing aid on
_____my alarm clock *with* or *without* my hearing aid on
_____my smoke or burglar alarm *with* or *without* my hearing aid on
_____a baby or child calling me from another room *with* or *without* my hearing aid on
_____an adult calling me from another room *with* or *without* my hearing aid on
_____a stove or microwave oven timer *with* or *without* my hearing aid on
_____my washer, dryer, or other appliance *with* or *without* my hearing aid on
_____OTHER (explain)

At school, I have difficulty hearing:

_____the smoke alarm or other emergency signals *with* or *without* my hearing aid on
_____computer prompts *with* or *without* my hearing aid on
_____status/warning sounds from machinery (e.g., woodshop) *with* or *without* my hearing aid on
_____timers (e.g., for chemical experiments, timed tests, etc.) *with* or *without* my hearing aid on
_____OTHER (explain)

I live in a dormitory or campus apartment and have difficulty hearing:
_____my telephone ring *with* or *without* my hearing aid on
_____the telephone in the hallway ring *with* or *without* my hearing aid on
_____the smoke alarm in my quarters *with* or *without* my hearing aid on

_____the smoke alarm for the entire building (hallway bells, etc.) *with* or *without* my hearing aid on

_____the doorbell/door knock for my quarters *with* or *without* my hearing aid on

_____the doorbell/door knock for the front door to the building *with* or *without* my hearing aid on

_____OTHER (explain)

At work, I have difficulty hearing:

_____my telephone ring *with* or *without* my hearing aid on

_____a doorbell *with* or *without* my hearing aid on

_____a door knock *with* or *without* my hearing aid on

_____the office smoke or other emergency alarm *with* or *without* my hearing aid on

_____a supervisor or colleague calling me in my office *with* or *without* my hearing aid on

_____a supervisor or colleague calling me from another room *with* or *without* my hearing aid on

_____my pager go off *with* or *without* my hearing aid on

_____computer prompts *with* or *without* my hearing aid on

_____status/warning sounds from machinery *with* or *without* my hearing aid on

_____OTHER (explain)

While traveling, I have difficulty hearing:

_____door knocks in hotels, friends' homes, etc. *with* or *without* my hearing aid on

_____alarm clocks in hotels, friends' homes, etc. *with* or *without* hearing aid on

_____my wristwatch alarm after I set it for a nap on a subway train, etc. *with* or *without* my hearing aid on

_____wake up calls (via telephone) in hotels *with* or *without* my hearing aid on

_____smoke alarms in hotels, etc. *with* or *without* my hearing aid on

_____public address system pages and/or alerts in airports, public buildings, etc. *with* or *without* my hearing aid on

_____the blinker signal on my car/truck *with* or *without* my hearing aid on

_____announcements on airplanes, trains, buses, etc. *with* or *without* my hearing aid on

_____OTHER (explain)

Three of the most difficult listening situations for me are:

(Feel free to add more.)

1)

2)

3)

SPECIAL COMMUNICATION DEVICES I ALREADY USE

Place an asterisk (*) by each device you currently use. If you do not use any special communication devices now, skip ahead to the next section titled "SPECIAL LISTENING DEVICES AVAILABLE IN MY COMMUNITY".

I already own and/or use the following devices (fill in or circle brand names if you don't know the generic name of the device):

Telephone Devices:

_____amplified handset for the telephone

_____in-line telephone amplifier (connects between receiver and body of phone)

_____portable telephone amplifier (AT&T, Ameriphone, Radio Shack, Plantronics, Walker, etc.)

_____portable telephone adapter for "T" switch (AT&T, Oticon, etc.)

_____DAI: direct plug-in hearing aid to phone (hearing aid audio shoe connected to cord that connects into body of telephone).

_____Williams Sound Pocket Talker, Audex SoundDirector, or Comtek FM receiver connected to phone and used with earphones, neckloop (hearing aid on T) or DAI (hearing aid and audio shoe).

_____TTY (also called TT or TDD)

_____OTHER (Please name or describe any other special telephone listening devices you use.):

Face-to-Face/Media Communication Devices:

_____direct earphone connection to TV, radio, tape player, dictation machine

_____remote microphone which plugs into hearing aid

_____personal hardwired listening device (Pocket Talker, Audex, RadioShack)

_____AM/FM/TV Band radio:

    _____next to chair and turned up

    _____next to chair with neck loop and hearing aid on "T"

    _____hearing aid plugged directly into radio earphone jack

_____infrared listening system for TV (Sennheiser, Audex, SoundPlus, other)

_____FM listening system (Comtek, Phonak, Phonic Ear, Siemens, Telex, Williams Sound, etc.)

_____loop system for TV (using hearing aid on "T")

_____loop system for classroom or meeting room (using hearing aid on "T" or special telecoil receiver w/earphones)

_____Closed captioned decoder or TV with built-in captions

_____Computer-assisted note taking

_____Computer-assisted real time captioning

_____OTHER (Please name or describe any other special listening devices you use.):

IF YOU USE COMMUNICATION DEVICES, USE THIS SPACE (or other side) TO EXPLAIN HOW OFTEN YOU USE THEM AND HOW MUCH THEY HELP YOU. ALSO, BE SURE TO INCLUDE PROBLEMS YOU HAVE EXPERIENCED WHILE USING THESE SYSTEMS:

SPECIAL COMMUNICATION SYSTEMS AVAILABLE IN MY COMMUNITY

A SPECIAL LISTENING DEVICE IS AVAILABLE AT THE FOLLOWING PLACES I GO TO: (FOR EACH PLACE, INCLUDE THE TYPE OF DEVICE INSTALLED, IF YOU KNOW IT: I = infrared; F = FM; L = audio loop; H = hardwired. For example:

F Church/Synagogue means that an FM system is located at your church or synagogue. If you do not know the type of system installed, just place a checkmark.)

    _____CHURCH/SYNAGOGUE

    _____THEATER (LIVE PLAYS AND CONCERTS)

    _____MOVIE THEATER

    _____COMMUNITY THEATER

    _____COURTROOM

_____WORKPLACE
_____OTHER (Write in other places that have special listening devices):
_____check here if you have attended a community function where computer-assisted
　　　note taking or captioning has been used. What did you think?

_____I <u>HAVE</u> TRIED TO USE ONE OR MORE OF THESE DEVICES.

_____I <u>HAVE NOT</u> TRIED TO USE ANY OF THESE DEVICES BECAUSE:

　　_____I do not know how to find out about using the device.
　　_____I hear well enough with my own hearing (and hearing aid).
　　_____I do not think it will help.
　　_____I do not know if it will help.
　　_____I feel self-conscious about using the device in public.
　　_____OTHER (Write in any other reason you may not have used these devices.):

ADDITIONAL COMMENTS

Did you know that legislation exists that requires employers, state and local governments, and public accommodations (stores, banks, hotels, and any other public place) to provide you with assistive technology and other reasonable accommodations, upon request? If you would like more information on this, please indicate so on back on this questionnaire. Finally, please feel free to add any information you feel would be important in helping us to understand your communication needs. Thank you.

CHAPTER

17

Computer Applications in Audiologic Rehabilitation

Donald G. Sims, Ph.D., and Linda Gottermeier, M.A.

During our initial audiologic interviews with college-age deaf students, we found the case histories to be remarkably the same. Deafness was discovered at age 2, and a y-cord body hearing aid was fitted. Speech and language therapy was started during the preschool years, but memory of it is unclear. During elementary mainstreamed school years, once- or twice-a-week group therapy was performed for a class period. Therapy and possibly hearing aid use were discontinued in junior high school when social forces emphasized the need to appear "normal."

However, when we see an orally proficient student, the story is different. First, the student clearly recalls Mom spending hours each day teaching speech and language. While in elementary and secondary schools, individual communication disorders therapy support was provided. In addition, parents often provided years of private, individual speech therapy. In other words, these children with hearing loss probably spent thousands of hours on the task of learning spoken English supported by knowledgeable professionals and parents.

Summerfield (1987) states that a typical 100 hours per year of aural rehabilitation (AR) is not enough to achieve mastery of the complex skills of speech production and perception. He describes an analogy of the time necessary to become skilled in music performance. Studies have shown that music skills must be practiced for 1000 to 2000 hours for

an enjoyment level of proficiency, but 5000 to 10,000 hours of practice are necessary for one to be admitted to a college-level music school. Assuming a 12-year practice period window (beginning at age 6 and continuing to age 18), a conservative estimate of the practice needed would be 2 to 3 hours per day, 5 days a week, 50 weeks per year, for 12 years!

As clinicians for hearing-impaired children, we probably do not assume that developing speech with severe or profound deafness would require less sustained practice and instruction than that of a hearing musician. However, resource allocation of that magnitude has not been frequently available. What then are some practical ways that the amount of guided practice time given to AR can be increased? The reader may have surmised that the authors believe that computer-assisted aural rehabilitation (CAAR) may be a partial answer. Current laptop, computer-multimedia technology is within the economic reach of many more families for this purpose; in addition, it can allow learning to take place beyond the school building by encouraging interaction with parents, advisors, student peers, and community support individuals.

GENERAL BENEFITS OF COMPUTER-ASSISTED INSTRUCTION

Fox (1998) describes three major advantages of quality computer-based instruction

(CBI) that apply to all educational circumstances and content material to be learned. First, CBI is second only to one-on-one instruction for providing individualized, self-paced interactive instructional delivery. This is important because a lockstep pace or a traditional group or classroom situation overlooks students' need to process the information for different amounts of time until comprehension occurs. Second, CBI also maximizes the time that the student spends engaged in meaningful learning activities while not being interrupted by the teacher's need to respond to the differing needs of other students or manage the classroom. Third, the present educational system relies on the teacher to evaluate the individual's progress by collection, collation, and analysis of all of a student's records. After these data are collected they should allow comparisons, identify areas of weakness, and document prescriptions for future progress. This is an administrative task for the purpose of aligning curriculum instruction and enabling superior guidance. However, completion of these tasks typically exceeds the time available in most schools. CBI can easily include this important but seldom accomplished administrative activity.

COMPUTER-ASSISTED INSTRUCTION PROVEN EFFECTIVE

Summative research has demonstrated that in schools, educational technology (such as multimedia computer applications) has a significant positive impact. Students feel more successful, are more motivated to learn, and have increased self-confidence and self-esteem when using CBI. Positive effects have been found for all major subject areas, in preschool through higher education, and for both regular education and special needs students. Evidence suggests that interactive video is especially effective when the skills and concepts to be learned have a visual component and when the software incorporates a research-based instructional design.

If the use of computers in schools has proven beneficial, then relative to AR, what is the evidence that it can be beneficial for hearing-impaired children and adults? This chapter describes current ideas and activities in CAAR. Commercial products and laboratory projects will be discussed. The reader will appreciate the variety of approaches and, in a few cases, review the supporting efficacy data. Over the next few years, this information may help readers to design and perhaps construct their own CAAR applications.

State of the Art in Computer-Based AR

Binnie predicted in 1994 that "By the year 2000, computer based instruction in the form of interactive video and multimedia presentations will assume a significant role in audiologic rehabilitation by increasing the availability of information, counseling, and skill-building exercises for adults with hearing impairment." However, therapeutic application of computer-based AR is not widespread. One reason for this may have been the expense and complexity of producing lessons that had the required interactive audio and video stimuli. When these lessons were produced, a federal grant was needed to cover the expense of a short series of programs. However, the current human resource and equipment costs have plummeted while the capability of computers to capture and playback audio and video has slowly grown to the point where the clinician may now easily record and playback video with smooth motion and good image size. The technical reason for the slow development of full motion-full screen video was the one megabyte-per-second video data throughput required. Until recently, many compromises in picture quality and image size had to be made if the computer was storing and playing back the video. Earlier interactive video lessons used videotape or videodisc to store the video action, and the computer simply enabled random access to the prerecorded video. Thus, it is now more feasible, practical, and possible for interactive CAAR to be created by the clinician in the field for the AR session.

Today's commercially available computer-assisted instruction for communication disorders is just beginning to use some of these capabilities. The majority of today's lessons use the computer to manage instructionally a series of therapy exercise materials that would otherwise be presented via live-voice with current therapy processes. Thus, software companies are producing what clinicians are doing in therapy. Current lessons use digitized voice stimuli and animated graphics to enhance the lessons' interest and motivation for children. In our view, a clinician paradigm shift is needed that considers the expanding number of computer-assisted multimedia possibilities and, in this way, fundamentally changes therapeutic activities. In other words, the multimedia computer allows therapy to take on new dimensions and use techniques that have not been possible or practical in the past. This chapter explores CAAR lessons now in development that have enhanced adaptive interaction with clients and use full-motion video as well as high-quality audio to provide training stimuli and reinforcement. Use of the word "adaptive" in this context means that these lessons will be able to change instructional strategies during the lesson by analysis of the client's performance.

As a brief introduction to this advanced CAAR, consider that at the Tucker Maxon School for the Deaf, speech and language lessons are supplemented by a three-dimensional, graphic image of a talking head known as "Baldi." Baldi accurately articulates speech and then recognizes whether individual word responses by the students are correctly spoken. In addition, consider the use of digitally processed auditory training stimuli that provide acoustic emphasis of specific phonetic features (e.g., lengthened formant transitions or vowel segments). Modifying natural speech in this way has enhanced speech perception for persons with severe hearing loss and has been used instructionally for persons with central auditory processing disorders (Tellal et al., 1996).

We begin with a review of the elements of past CAAR applications that are noteworthy and merit consideration for inclusion in future CAAR development. A "dream" lesson that includes the summed creativity and expertise from these authors would result in an ideal, intelligent, interactive computerized AR learning experience. Later sections of this chapter review computer applications that support AR (i.e., handicap assessment and hearing aid evaluation).

PAST CAAR PROJECTS

Nickerson et al. (1976) were among the first to build a multimedia self-instruction program with a mainframe computer for teaching speech to deaf children. The laboratory mainframe computer was equipped with a speech recognition unit that analyzed students' verbal responses. The computer monitor provided visual feedback on the children's phonologic productions with a cartoon face. Voicing was indicated by the appearance of an Adam's apple, and loudness level was indicated by the size of the mouth. Their work included many of the concepts currently in use with state-of-the-art CAAR (see also Rushakoff [1984] for a review of early communication disorders computer-assisted applications).

Computer-aided speechreading training (CAST)

Pinchora-Fuller and Benguerel (1991) described a computerized speechreading assessment and training system that simulates face-to-face intervention. It is highlighted in this chapter to model what may be included in CAAR for preretirement adults with acquired mild to moderate hearing loss. Eight training lessons were available that focused on a particular viseme group. Each of the texts was primarily narrative, but some descriptive passages were used. A variety of syntactic structures and sentence lengths were also included. The text for each lesson was constructed on a particular topic, so within each lesson the materials were semantically related. For each trial the student received stimuli that made the answer successively easier to obtain. This was done by using a version of the target stimulus with a slower talker rate and/or adding auditory cues. For example, the first showing of the stimulus was fast-rate, visual-only. If the student did not give the correct answer, the second replay was at a slow rate by the visual modality only. If the student was still having difficulty, then a fast-rate and audiovisual version of the target was shown; finally, before the answer was revealed, a slow-rate audiovisual version of the item was presented.

Pinchora-Fuller and Benguerel (1991) found that it was possible to categorize students' response errors according to whether they seemed to be visually appropriate and/or linguistically appropriate. A response was categorized as "incomplete" when it contained no errors other than omission (e.g., "and sauce" for "and orange sauce"). Because incomplete responses contained no errors, they were considered to be both linguistically and visually appropriate. If the source of the error could not be inferred it was categorized as "unknown." By analysis of the error types, a student's strategies could be examined. Examination of their clients' tracking rates varied as a function of the types of errors made and learning styles. Some were slow but accurate, others were fast responders with higher error rates and stimulus repetition requirements. The authors suggested that future applications could incorporate other types of repair strategies, including word-by-word or syllable-by syllable recordings by multiple speakers, or paraphrase and spelling options. Such repair options could be predetermined by the instructor or selected by the learner.

Compared with face-to-face discourse tracking procedures, the authors stated that CAST tracking had the advantage of allowing easy measurement and analysis of speechreading performance. Such precise analysis allowed for a quick adjustment in instruction on the part of the audiologist.

Another useful feature of CAST was phonemic scoring when open-set, keyboarded, sentence-length responses were used. Their method allowed feedback on the basis of the visemic match between response and target. The learner was given credit for within-viseme errors while drawing attention, as might be done in live therapy, to confusions in the response. In addition, the answer character

strings were scored according to what visemes had been previously taught and according to word boundaries in the target sentence. For example, if the stimulus was "in particular" and the response was "aperture," the feedback correction was "__ particular" or with a response "payoff" for the stimulus "post office"; feedback to the student was "po__ _ff__.". Thus, credit was given for all vowels and the consonant visemes related to the target.

Bernstein and Demorest (1994) and Demorest and Bernstein (1991) have used a similar but more exacting approach to machine answer analysis by using (1) DECtalk (Educational Services Dept., Digital Equipment Corp., 1984) phonetic recoding, (2) viseme similarity data, and (3) a stimulus versus response alignment algorithm. Demorest and Bernstein (1991) state that this scoring procedure allows a "comparison of characteristics of words that tend to be partially correct with those that elicit an all-or-none pattern of performance [which] may provide insights regarding whole-word versus phonemic-level processing of the visual stimulus." They also suggest that individual subject's performance can be better described using their visual distance score because from a statistical standpoint, the visual distance score is "equally sensitive to individual differences throughout the performance range."

Aside from these details of scoring responses, Pinchora Fuller and Benguerel (1991) suggest that computer simulations of face-to-face interventions by using an expert systems approach requiring explicity in the specification of training procedures may offer a useful tool to fine-tune rehabilitative techniques. CAST can be used as a tool by the audiologist to extend rather than replace existing rehabilitative techniques (see also Gagné et al. [1991] for a detailed evaluation of the effectiveness of CAST).

Computer-assisted speech perception evaluation and research (CASPER)

Boothroyd and others (Boothroyd, 1987; Boothroyd and Hanath-Chisolm, 1988; Hanin et al., 1988) designed a system to assist with continuous discourse tracking (CDT) as a method to evaluate tactile and cochlear implant sensory aids in or for lip-reading. In their approach, the live therapy session was supported with computer-controlled, videodisc sentence materials. Other analytic exercises have included detection/identification of speech contrasts in nonsense syllables, words, and phrases; recognition of phonemes in consonant-vowel-consonant (CVC) words; and recognition of words in carrier phrases and sentences. In one study (Boothroyd et al., 1987), five adults with cochlear implants benefited most from the CASPER sentence training compared with the analytic exercises. One subject who participated in 26 hours of the semiautomated CDT with and without a tactile aid demonstrated no pre-post test performance improvements in visual-only word recognition scores but substantial gains in performance with the tactile aid (Boothroyd and Hanath-Chisolm, 1988).

The use of digitized, prerecorded stimuli in face-to-face therapy facilitates research in clinical endeavors because some variables associated with the teacher are controlled. Further, real-time data collection within the therapy session is made practical.

ALVIS

Kopra and colleagues at the Austin Veterans' Hospital (Kopra et al., 1986; Sims et al., 1985) developed CAAR with the unique approach that presented 300 training sentences that had been studied previously for difficulty level. Training proceeded from easy to difficult sentences. If learners could not type the text of the target sentence after viewing it without sound twice, the next presentation was visual plus auditory at 2 dB SL. Additional 2-dB increments were added for each subject requesting repetition until the sentence was typed correctly.

Tye-Murray

Tye-Murray et al. (1988) prepared a PC-based CAAR videodisc along conventional analytic and synthetic training protocols but also included assertiveness training exercises for adults and school-age children. Training with video simulations (Tye-Murray, 1992) is an engaging CAAR activity and can provide a safe environment to practice psychologically uncomfortable activities like assertiveness training or conflict resolution.

CURRENT CAAR IN THE UNITED STATES

AR for adults in the United States often consists only of fitting hearing aids and some postfitting counseling individually or in small groups. Children with hearing loss are typically seen by the educator of the deaf and the speech-language therapist, with the audiologist playing a consultative role regarding hearing assessment and amplification. Traditional auditory and speechreading training have been occasionally described as ineffective and tedious for the clinician and client alike. Also, the deemphasis of drill and practice AR methods has been rationalized according to the argument that the client may have missed the developmental "critical period" for language learning and/or suffered neural atrophy due to a lack of auditory stimulation. We also have "justification" for the notion that speechreading skills cannot be taught because they are "innately limited by speed of lexical access" (Lyxell and Ronnberg, 1991, 1992) and by the invisibility of speech sounds (Clouser, 1977). However, recent functional magnetic resonance imaging findings have shown that neural plasticity of the human brain is not lost with age or with lack of neural stimulation (Weinberger, 1999). Once stimulation and intensive training begins, the brain slowly reorganizes and makes use of the input, even if the input is impoverished. However, the addition of practical CAAR to provide the requisite, adaptive drill and practice or problem-solving tasks in an interesting, game-like fashion has been proven effective in the programs described below.

Dynamic audio visual interactive device (DAVID)

This project at the National Technical Institute for the Deaf (NTID) began in 1973 and is a good illustration of the synergy between computers and AR. The prototype lesson was to train auditory discrimination of the four telephone signals with a multiple-choice task. We used the Institute's $1.5 million IBM mainframe with 32K of memory running eight learning stations! It took the programmer 70 hours to write the FORTRAN code. By 1982, we had "progressed" to the DAVID system on a $3,000 Apple II with a $15,000 random access VCR controller to perform multiple-choice and open-set speechreading sentence recognition. It took the programmer 9 months to write the code for the first version (there have been at least 12 major revisions since). For the past 8 years, we have been using a $1500 Macintosh and $1000 videodisc player. Soon we will be moving to a $200 CD-ROM on a laptop computer. The trend for computers is clear: costs and complexity have come down and capabilities have gone up. What follows is a brief review of the lesson strategies and the evidence for its effectiveness.

DAVID presents a prerecorded target sentence via the videodisc. The sentences have been recorded by speakers with good articulatory visibility as rated by hearing and deaf colleagues. There are many sets of 100 to 200 sentences about topics such as job interviews or college life (e.g., "RIT social,") or activities of daily living (e.g., "Survival"). These sets and the original paper-and-pencil videotape lessons were developed by Jacobs (1982). The sentences of a set are all topical but they are not related as from connected discourse (the advantage of this is discussed below). The student views a sentence and then responds on the keyboard. The instructor has many options regarding assignment of training task difficulty and modality (auditory, visual, or auditory plus visual). For example, the easiest training task is four alternative choices. Students using this method can usually identify a sentence if they are able to recognize one or two content words of the target sentence. At the intermediate difficulty level, we use a semi-open set response. The semi-open set response provides the learner (1) with a key word from the sentence (e.g., a noun or verb) or (2) with the functor/structure words supplied and the key words eliminated. This second method enables the speech-reader to

focus on the content words and thus speed the practice toward comprehension rather than word-for-word transcription. This is helpful for students with limited written English skills. The final level of difficulty is open-set in which the learner views a sentence and must enter all words correctly. This is a lesson in speechreading, spelling, and written English.

The program prevents frustration by tracking the student strategies and suggesting the use of an array of "help" alternatives. Helps consist of stimulus repetition. Within the "repeat" option the student can choose (1) front or 45° azimuth views; (2) "normal," "slow," or "slowest" replay speeds (without audio); or (3) individual word repetition (all individual words of the sentence set were recorded a second time in isolation with clear speech). The student can request help via "hints" about the topic in general or ask for a fill-in of a missing or incorrect letter or word in the current response attempt. The use of the help alternatives is also monitored by the program, and perseveration in an unproductive help strategy is detected and alternative strategies suggested.

Response time (in seconds) required to achieve a 100% correct response is used to evaluate student strategies, examine training items' difficulty level, and document learning. Longer than average response times for individual sentences are reported to the instructor via a printout of the student's learning trajectory with that target sentence. Student learning performance is also reported in terms of the history of response time for sentences of equal difficulty. As student skill improves, the response time required for the 100% correct response decreases. The key to the use of this metric is identifying equivalent difficulty target sentences to use as probes of student skill. This was accomplished by presenting the sentences in random order to a group of students and then identifying individual sentences that had average response times similar to the mean for the set of sentences. These probe sentences then were used to determine skill change of the course of the CAAR intervention. In this way, performance is assessed during training, and the pitfalls of pretesting and post-testing are avoided (Sims et al., 1979, 1982; Sims and Clymer, 1986).[a]

Sims and Zhwei (1993) suggested a normative approach to identifying probe sentences of equivalent difficulty within a set of sentences to be learned and then documenting training effects with response time measures of performance with these probe sentences. No separate testing is required to do this, that is, assessment of learning (decreased response time) takes place during the course of training. To do this, the difficulty level of the training stimuli must be well known in advance. This was accomplished for DAVID lessons by presenting the training sentences in random order to a sample population and obtaining Z-score transformations of response time for each sentence item. Performance could then be examined with the probe training items which were distributed evenly across the normal training sequence. They were able to demonstrate improved response times for the probe sentences as a function of the order in which they occurred within the lesson. That is, response times were slower for probes at the beginning of the lesson and then faster at the end. A key assumption for this procedure is that each sentence is an independent measure of performance. Clearly, if connected discourse is used as the stimulus material, that assumption is violated. Thus, there is a trade-off between the ability to measure performance within a lesson (with DAVID response time) versus performance between lessons (as with CDT).

Speechreading challenges on CD-ROM

This computer application (Bloomsburg University, Bloomsburg, PA) is the only interactive video for speechreading currently on the market. The CD has 150 different speakers ages 4 to 70 years, whose faces and lips are seen from a variety of angles. Some of the speakers chew gum, wear mustaches, or talk with accents. Training stimuli are words, sentences, and stories on a variety of everyday topics. There are 10 progressively difficult lesson "Chapters" recorded with audio (which can be turned off for visual-only study). Word and sentence drills are in multiple-choice format, and the paragraph exercises ask comprehension-type questions. Each chapter contains 30 to 40 vocabulary words, 20 sentences, and a short story that can be viewed in either glossary mode or a "learn" mode depending on student preference. Thus, the student chooses to read the text or the words or sentences spoken by the talent before seeing the speaker (glossary mode), or attempts to speech-read the video segments with a multiple-choice answer task. A pretest and a posttest of 20 sentences with words from the chapter are administered with a novel speaker.

Evaluation of this program was reported on an earlier videodisc version and consisted of surveys of student opinion and pre- and posttest assessment with the Costello Word and Sentence Tests as well as the program-related pretests and posttests. Both exact and gist correct scoring were used. Seventy-four normally hearing college age students completed the course. These data clearly show that ". . . subjects' speechreading performance improved following the videodisc instruction, and that their scores were significantly better on all tests." Survey results were also positive, with 97% of the subjects giving ". . . good to excellent rating(s) of the program overall" (Slike et al., 1995).

The current CD-ROM version images are compromised somewhat (compared with videodisc), with nearly full motion (smooth action) and an image size on the computer screen of approximately 2 × 3 inches. To help the lip-reader, there is an inserted, simultaneous 45° angle enlarged view of the talent's lips to which the student can refer when repeating the stimulus for closer study. A Macintosh 120 MHz processor, with 64 MB RAM and 2.0 or better Quick Time software, are required to see an

---

[a]The current DAVID application is not available for distribution because it has a limited life span regarding newer operating systems and hardware. NTID (Rochester, NY) is planning to record DVD versions for home use by students and for general distribution.

acceptable image and have lip and voice synchronized. Since this application has been on the market, CD-ROM and computer capabilities for handling video have improved and larger images with full motion are possible with high-end, laptop computers. Allen (1995) and Ijsseldijk (1992) have shown that video must be digitized at a frame rate of at least 10 to 15 per second, but with higher rates (e.g., normal television is 30 FPS), image motion is smooth and the picture is sharp. A complete description of the technology associated with current lip-reading research is available in Massaro (1998).

INDIRECT APPLICATION SOFTWARE

Most of the computer applications for communication disorders are written for child language and phonologic stimulation by speech-language pathologists in the schools (e.g., Laureate Inc., www.LaureateLearning.com, or TheraSimplicity www.therasimplicity.com). Because these programs use lively graphics, text, and voice, they may be useful for hearing-impaired children if the hearing loss is not too great. Use of hearing aids' direct audio-input boot connected to the earphone jack of a computer may be useful in this circumstance. Fast ForWord and Earobics, described below, are good examples of potential reusable application software for AR.

Fast ForWord®

One can assume that hearing-impaired children and adults have at least the same incidence of attentional deficit disorders and related learning disabilities as do normal-hearing children. However, little has been done to diagnose these complicating fac-tors when hearing impairment is present (Samar and Parasnis, 1998; see also www.rit.edu/~468www/LD.html) A study by Jutras and Gagné (1999) demonstrated no significant differences in matched hearing-impaired and normal-hearing children on auditory memory and sequencing tasks that were nonverbal. However, some verbal memory and sequencing tasks were per-formed more poorly by hearing-impaired children. The authors suggest that the verbal stimuli were not as audible to the hearing-impaired children. We suspect that a fruitful area of research and development for hearing-impaired children needing AR might follow Tellal et al.'s work (Tellal et al., 1996; Miller et al., 1997). Their Fast ForWord (Scientific Learning Corporation, Berkley, CA) auditory training program for time-related auditory processing, phonologic analysis, and language processing skills might also benefit children with hearing impairment who also have processing problems. Further, if there are no processing problems, the enhanced acoustic cues may facilitate discrimination of some phonetic features.

The basic auditory processing research began with the discovery that children with reading delays had some striking deficits in studies of auditory temporal processing. Computer-based therapeutic training was begun with perceptual tasks that "would be sensitive to the phonological decoding deficits at the root of language and reading difficulties. They devised cognitive-linguistic tasks that would address problems with planning, sequencing and working memory that are found to be frequent sequelae of language problems . . . then based on the acoustic properties of speech that children with language problems need to successfully process speech sounds, the researchers augmented brief consonantal portions of all the stimuli by increasing the duration and loudness of the brief segments only" (Burns, 1998). For example, when 40-msec stop consonants such as [ba / da] were expanded digitally to 80 msec, language-learning–impaired children were able to discriminate this minimal contrast. During the adaptive training, the digital expansion was reduced for speech (and nonspeech) stimuli. Research data on more than 500 children at 35 sites to date have indicated its effectiveness across a number of objective and subjective measures. For example, with a 6- to 8-week daily training program, children have 1.5 years' growth in receptive language skills, and longitudinal studies have shown continued improvement 6 months after training

(Tellal and Merzenich, 1997). The success of this auditory training protocol is encouraging, and it is hoped that it helps to stimulate more CAAR development. In our opinion, the success of the program is importantly related to the demand for significant time on the training task (8 weeks of daily work). It remains to be studied as to whether the specific training stimuli of Tellal et al. would be useful for children with abnormal hearing (all of the subjects had normal hearing). The data showing changes in several measures of language competence, as well as data showing changes in electrophysiologic and brain function (fMRI), are exciting objective evidence that sustained CAAR is successful (see Weinberger [1999] for a review of auditory neural plasticity studies).

CURRENT WORLDWIDE CAAR

Canadian

The Speech Assessment and Interactive Learning System (SAILS, AVAAZ Innovations London, Ontario, Canada) approach emphasizes training and listening skills to help children develop an accurate perceptual representation for the correct production of target sounds. Each module is an interactive computer game that presents the child with carefully selected auditory stimuli representing correct and incorrect articulations of the target sound in a single-word context. These stimuli are recorded from adults and children and are naturally occurring misarticulations of the target sounds, not simulations. For example, in 1 of the 16 modules a child who misarticulates /k/ would be asked to listen to digitized recordings of "cat." The child's task is to identify the correctly produced versions of "cat" by pointing to a picture of a cat when "cat" is heard and by pointing to an "X" when any mispronunciation of "cat" is heard. Cartoon images reward the child for correct judgments with visual feedback.

The SAILS approach to therapy is based on the work of Rvachew and Jamieson (1989), who found that many misarticulating children have difficulty with perceiving the sounds that they misarticulate (see also Broen et al. [1983] and Hoffman et al. [1985]). Subsequent work has demonstrated that improving children's perception of such speech stimuli produces concomitant improvements in speech production abilities, with or even without explicit articulation therapy (Jamieson and Rvachew, 1992; Rvachew, 1994).

AVAAZ Innovations, Inc., argues that the auditory stimuli used in SAILS are critical to the success of the approach: "You might think that an experienced speech-language pathologist could speak words like "cat" and "tat" to clients and not bother with using pre-selected sounds in a computer program like SAILS. However, experience shows that this is not the case. Most of the more than one hundred children involved in the research described above have had no difficulty with live-voice, adult-produced stimuli. In fact, adult simulations of phonological errors do not typically reproduce key acoustic characteristics of children's misarticulations" (Avaaz Innovations Inc., 1998). They suggest that examination of spectrograms illustrates the importance of using children's speech for assessment and speech perception training. For example, most adults, including speech-language pathologists, find it virtually impossible to produce the word "shoe" with the same acoustic characteristics of a child's defective speech production. However, such ambiguous productions are quite common in children's speech, reflecting their tendency to focus on formant transition cues rather than on noise frequency cues to fricative identity. The inclusion of such sounds in the training set helps children to shift their attentional focus to the more reliable noise frequency cue.

Avaaz Innovations Inc. (1998) indicates that SAILS has been used as an assessment tool to help identify children who are most likely to benefit from a phonology group therapy program. Pretreatment perceptual performance, as measured by SAILS, may emerge as a good predictor of treatment progress. They found that neither performance on a pretreatment production probe nor degree of stimulability for the target sound predicted the amount of treatment progress. SAILS performance was the only reliable predictor of treatment progress for these children. "As a consequence of these findings, all children referred to the phonology groups treatment program now receive three weeks of treatment using SAILS before beginning group therapy" (Avaaz Innovations Inc., 1998).

Sweden

The KTH, Speech, Music and Hearing Lab of Stockholm has had a long and distinguished research and development interest in rehabilitative technology for deaf persons. Cook and Haneklou (1998) have used interactive videodiscs and now CD-ROM for laboratory investigations and in clinical practice. Their applications are now being used clinically for lipreading, lipreading with tactile aid, and sign-supported speech. Instruction uses analytic drill and assessment for vowel, consonant, "global training (numbers), and memory training." KTH is also working on the use of a computer to present DeFilippo's CDT as a method for training hearing-impaired persons to use tactile cues for speech perception.

Finland

Majaranta (1998) describes a personal computer (PC), CD-ROM lipreading tutoring program called HyperLips ("HyperHuulet" in Finnish). It has four types of exercises: words, similar words, compound words, and sentences (Lonka, 1995). The user tries to lip-read the video stimulus and gives his or her response by selecting the answer from given choices or by typing his or her response into the answer field. The program analyzes the user's response by checking for correct words and letters. The feedback is given in a separate dialog that opens after the user has clicked the "Check" or "Give Hint" button. The strategy for supplying the hints has been derived from a careful pedagogy that reveals the answer bit by bit. For example, there is an analysis and feedback system for homophenous words and logical control over the sequence of hints provided to the student on the syllable, word, and topic levels. The ability to play the video in slow motion was also added.

A second prototype lesson was tested on four normal-hearing volunteers with no previous lipreading training. Majaranta (1998) indicated that all test users were "fairly good lipreaders." Feedback from the volunteers indicated that when word-by-word hints were given, the first and last words in a sentence should be given special consideration. Apparently for the hearing lip-readers, these words were the easiest to recognize and provided a great deal of contextual information. They also indicated that in instances in which the lip-reader did not understand any of the sentence, a contextual clue would be helpful before revealing the sentence syllable by syllable. Majaranta concluded that the test piloting on hearing subjects has helped to eliminate major flaws in the feedback system.

AR Computer Application Tools

Aside from computer applications for instructing and training hearing-impaired persons, the daily use of computer support to assist the clinician in assessment and management is now commonplace. Large databases are used for interpretation of patient handicap and treatment outcomes. Computer-supported complex computations are now a required part of many hearing aid fittings. Some examples of these applications are mentioned below. The future will bring many more that will sharpen and amplify our clinical skills and knowledge. We should acknowledge and actively produce applications that also have a goal of instruction for the professional clinician who will be using the program. As our need to become more efficient in the health care system grows, the computer applications that we use can play a role in professional development. These applications are designed to bring research findings to the front lines of treatment as quickly as possible.

HANDICAP ANALYSIS

CAAR is also important in the assessment of the needs of hearing-impaired clients and in the documentation of the benefit outcomes of therapy (see Chapter 18). Hearing handicap scales now include national normative populations to assist in interpretation of results (see Chapters 10 and 14). Computer support for administrating and grading these scales are available and helpful. However, the administration of the handicap scale can be influenced by whether it is administered face-to-face or via a computer screen. The clinician should follow the test administration protocol strictly to take advantage of any normative data associated with the test (Palmer, 1992). Recently, Newman et al. (1997) set up the Hearing Handicap Inventory for Adults (HHIA) and the Hearing Handicap Inventory for the Elderly (HHIE) (Newman et al., 1990, 1991) for reporting test results via computer-generated "macro statements." Each statement describes the clinical impression and the functional implications of answering "yes" or "sometimes" to specific inventory items. Thus, it is possible to develop personalized hearing handicap profiles based on a patient's responses with a few keystrokes. The generated report can be used to answer questions about the following:

1. What is the probability of benefiting from amplification?
2. Is audiologic intervention warranted?
3. What are the probabilities for compliance with recommendations?

HEARING AID BENEFIT MEASURES

Scaled measures of the client's perceived benefit from a given hearing aid fitting have enjoyed some success when the client is involved in the description of his or her problem areas when using a hearing aid (see Gatehouse's results as summarized in Chapter 14). The Client-Oriented Scale of Improvement (COSI) has been incorporated into hearing aid manufacturers' computer-based software applications for fitting. The clinician can thus document the perceived improvements in the final fitting compared with the previous fitting for five priority areas for problem resolution. The Abbrevi-

ated Profile of Hearing Aid Benefit (APHAB) (Cox and Alexander, 1995) is a normed, hearing aid benefit measure that is shareware. The client's unaided versus aided benefit is assessed with 25 questions that can be administered via paper and pencil or via computer screen. Computer-scored results graph the percentage improvement provided by the hearing aid in relation to normative data.

ERBER'S DISCOURSE FLUENCY ANALYSIS

When one first conceptualizes computer-assisted learning, the assumption is that the computer will take over and provide the AR. This is appropriate for the drill and practice components of AR but it does not obviate the need for live therapy (which, by definition and all accounts, is far superior when available). However, the computer can assist in the process of live therapy by providing technical support for media presentation and response data collection. Boothroyd's CASPER and the CAST applications were designed in this way to semiautomate De-Filippo's CDT technique (see above). Erber's Dialog therapeutic techniques (Erber, 1996) have been assisted by a PC application tool that simply records the percentage of time spent in repair versus fluent diad conversation. The clinician pushes the space bar during conversational breakdown and repair activities. In this way, the efficiency of communication can be measured easily before and after strategy training.

HEARING AID FITTING

Hearing aid fittings have been improved by bringing research findings to the process through computer applications for hearing aid selection and adjustment (see Chapters 5 and 11). Indeed, modern hearing aids' flexibility demanded computer support to provide fitting recommendations from the thousands of possible combinations of control settings. The following is a very brief listing of some of the computer applications. The first describes NOAH, which is designed to be a macro program to host proprietary fitting software and databases from hearing aid manufacturers. A standard interface box is available to enable direct hearing aid programming. The second section describes stand-alone hearing aid fitting applications.

NOAH

Gitlin (1995) indicates that more than 90% of dispensing audiologists have PCs in their offices. The dispenser's office typically has an office management database coupled with a clinical database. NOAH is a "software database" or "group of fields" that can be shared by compatible software on a computer. Conceived by the Hearing Instrument Manufacturers Software Association (HIMSA, Minneapolis, MN), the goal in development of NOAH was to keep costs down for dispensers by eliminating parallel software development. NOAH allows the audiologist to program a hearing aid by importing the client's audiogram and/or other relevant information such as MCL/UCL measures and speech discrimination results.

Stand alone programs

DeJonge (1996) outlines hardware requirements, the theoretical basis and application interactions for several free-standing computer programs that can be used to facilitate the selection and verification of hearing aids, for example:

1. The Memphis State University Hearing Aid Prescription, Cox and Bisset (1992),
2. Desired Sensation Level (DSL 4) (Seewald, 1997).
3. FIG6 (1996).
4. National Acoustic Laboratories' (Sydney, Australia) NAL-R & Non Linear (Byrne and Dillon, 1986) Hearing Aid Selection Procedure, and
5. the IHAFF protocol (Independent Hearing Aid Fitting Forum [see Valente and VanFliet, 1997]).

While the clinician's fitting philosophy dictates a hearing aid prescription, the client may have more confidence in the opinions of hearing aid dispenser if he/she can see the reasoning to support the recommendations pictured on the computer screen. The use of consistent, computer-based fitting algorithms allow for the clinician to add more science and objectivity to the art of hearing aid fitting (DeJonge, 1996).

Research and Development in CAAR

This section highlights some laboratory work that is currently being applied in the field on an experimental basis.

MASSARO

A three-dimensional computerized talking head nicknamed "Baldi" is being used by deaf children at the Tucker-Maxon Oral School. The image on the computer screen "talks" when text is typed in. When a student speaks single words, Baldi "listens" by combining input from a camera that tracks the student's lip movements and the acoustic utterances of the child. The value of the animated, synthetic speech is that it provides the critical visual cues for speech perception by allowing students the opportunity to observe facial movements closely and even to strip away the "skin" of the face and study a half sagittal view that mimics the speech organs underlying the production (Cohen et al., 1998). Baldi can be programmed to speak in any voice, including the teacher's or student's voice; in the future, his image will be able to be substituted with any face.

It will be important to assess how well the learning transfers outside the instructional situation. Another issue is whether instruction should be focused on the visible speech or whether it should include auditory input. If speech production mirrors speech perception, then we expect that multimodal training should be beneficial, as suggested by Summerfield (1987). The child could learn multimodal targets, which would provide more resolution than either modality alone. Another issue concerns whether the visible speech targets should be illustrated in static or dynamic presentations. An NSF Grant is planned to evaluate both types of presentation and it is expected that some combination of modes would be optimal.

With regard to speechreading, software is being developed to capture and interpret the student's facial movements during speech production. Visual speech information will be combined with the acoustic signal to help deaf students learn the temporal characteristics of speech. Baldi will reproduce the child's visual speech using the child's voice. A juxtaposed image of Baldi will then produce the utterance correctly. The child will be able to play these sequences at different speeds to observe the differences and practice the correct pronunciation. The importance of having visual feedback in learning speech and speechreading has been demonstrated by van Uden (1983) and DeFilippo et al. (1995).

Table 17.1
Useful World Wide Web sites and materials

Nordic Interactive Video for speechreading and sign-supported speech
Cook@speech.kth.se or
robert@macoriginal.se
Three-dimensional graphic talking head for speechreading, machine recognition for speechreading
http://mambo.ucsc.edu/psl/lipr.html
http://www.oraldeafed.org/schools/tmos/news
Learning disabilities and deafness
www.rit.edu/~468www/LD.html
Sources for applications and support
CD-ROM Speechreading
Speechreading Challenges on CD-ROM
Graduate School Box V
Bloomsburg University
Bloomsburg, PA 17815

WORLD WIDE WEB (TABLE 17.1)

The Web is helpful for clinicians, but more and more, it is being used by consumers as well. For example, forums (e.g., www.ASHA.org and www.audiology.org) are helping clinicians and hearing-impaired persons find professional resources and advice. Web sites offer downloads of applications such as IHAFF hearing aid fitting formulas (www.frye.com//news) and APHAB patient benefit surveys (www.ausp.memphis.edu/harl). Formal distance learning via the Web is growing fast, especially for the attainment of the Au.D. degree. For the consumer, there are informational sites (e.g., www.boystown.org) that offer good advice about hearing loss and what to do about it. One site is delivering a 21-day hearing aid adjustment instruction set (www.minfox.com/synthesis/homepage; see also www.audiology.org/proflink/auralhab for other AR links).

When wide bandwidth on the Web becomes generally available, there will be no technical reason why components of AR cannot be provided via Web transmission of audio/video training materials (e.g., drill and practice for speechreading, cued speech, or sign language instruction in the home) (see Chapters 1 and 2).

Development Advice

The following is a listing of characteristics of successful computer-based learning programs and the necessary conditions for successful implementation of computer-based learning in schools.

CHARACTERISTICS OF GOOD LESSON DESIGN

The level of effectiveness of educational technology is influenced by the specific student population, software design, teacher's role, how the students are grouped, and level of student access to technology. Specific software design elements that are highly desirable include the following:

1. Students should be offered some control over the amount, review, and sequence of instruction. This can result in higher achievement. However, low-achieving students and students with little prior content knowledge are likely to require more structure.
2. In tutorial and practice software, programs that provide students with knowledge of correct responses are superior to programs that require students to answer until they are correct.

3. When informational content is to be learned, software that includes repetition and rehearsal of content, paraphrasing, outlining, cognitive mapping or diagramming, drawing analogies and inferences, and generating illustrative examples will provide better achievement.

4. Animation and/or video will enhance learning when the skills or concepts to be learned involve motion or action (e.g., speech production and perception).

5. Fantasy contexts may be advantageous to young children learning abstract concepts.

IMPLEMENTATION IN SCHOOLS

A critical element of the success on any new instructional technology lies in how the persons providing the instruction are included in the process of design and revision of the lessons provided by a computer. Involvement at the school district level and the leadership of a school-level computer coordinator are key factors in developing a school environment conducive to effective use of technology. Once a program is developed, teachers are more effective after receiving extensive training in integrating computer technology with the curriculum. In addition, a social network of other computer-using teachers at their school is an important source of daily support for the devilish details of day-to-day use. In the best of all worlds, a full-time programmer-systems analyst specialist(s) are available for support with application development, revision, and implementation. In general, positive changes in the learning environment brought about by technology are more evolutionary than revolutionary. These changes occur over a period of years as teachers become more experienced with technology.

Evaluation Methods

Assessment of the outcome of an AR intervention relative to improved performance for the understanding of speech has been traditionally stated in terms of pre- and postmeasures of speech recognition. However, clinicians are now examining the time taken by the client to respond correctly as a measure of learning/skills acquired. This metric enables training to continue until a high criterion performance level is reached (e.g., 95 to 100% correct), as would be required in everyday life. Once achieved, the question becomes how long did it take to get all the information. Time-to-criterion performance measures can be a words-per-minute value for Connected Discourse Tracking, a conversational fluency measure as with Erber's Dylog (Erber, 1998) measurement or a simple response time as in Sims' DAVID application. A great benefit of time-based performance measures is that they are gathered during the training with the training stimuli. Thus, the pre/posttest conundrum of measurement errors are avoided (see Montgomery and Demorest, 1988). The assumption of the metric is that all training stimuli that are used for response time assessment are of equal (or known) difficulty level. Consequently, a significant sample of 100 learners should train with the stimuli in random order, then an item analysis can be completed, and the select, equivalent-difficulty, probe training items can be placed periodically in the instructional sequence of events. Once the probes are in place, the computer program can use the probe's normative values to change the trajectory of the course according to individual needs (Sims and Zhwei, 1993).

REFERENCES

Allen MJ. Evaluation of computers for learning lipreading. Honors thesis for Bachelor of Arts (Communication Studies), School of Communication and Information Studies, University of South Australia, 1995.

Avaaz Innovations Inc. SAILS: the speech assessment and interactive learning system. 1998. www.avaaz.com/flyer.htm

Bernstein L, Demorest M. A computational approach to analyzing sentential speech perception: phoneme-to-phoneme stimulus-response alignment. J Acoust Soc Am 1994;95:3617–3622.

Binnie C. The future of audiologic rehabilitation: An overview and forecast. In: Gagné JP, Tye-Murray N, eds. Research in audiological rehabilitation: Current trends and future directions. Monograph Suppl J Acad Rehab Audiol 1994;27:19.

Boothroyd A. CASPER: a computer-assisted system for speech-perception testing and training. Proceedings of the 10th annual conference of the Rehabilitation Society of North America. 1987:734–736.

Boothroyd A, Hnath-Chisolm T. Spatial, tactile, presentation of voice fundamental frequency as a supplement to lipreading: results of extended training with a single subject. J Rehabil Res Dev 1988;25:51–56.

Boothroyd A, Hanin L, Waltzman S. Development of speech perception skills in cochlear implantees. Proceeding of the 10th annual conference of the Rehabilitative Society of North America 1987:428–430.

Broen P, Strange W, Doyle S, et al. Perception and production of approximate consonants by normal and articulation delayed preschool children. J Speech Hear Res 1983; 26:601–608.

Burns M. Scientific disciplines unite to identify causes and improve outcomes for children with language and reading problems. Scientific Learning Corp., Berkeley, CA,1998.

Byrne D, Dillon H. The National Acoustic Laboratories' (NAL) new procedure for selecting the gain and frequency response of a hearing aid. Ear Hear 1986;7: 257–265.

Clouser R. Relative phoneme visibility and lipreading performance. Volta Rev 1977;79:27–34.

Cohen MM, Beskow J, Massaro DW. Recent developments in facial animation: an inside view. AVSP '98, Sydney, Australia, December 4–6, 1998. http://mambo.ucsc.edu/psl/avsp98/11.doc

Cook B, Haneklou R. Computer-based interactive video training in lipreading and sign-supported speech [ISAC proceedings abstract]. 1998. E-mail: cook@kth.se or robert@macoriginal.se

Cox R, Alexander G. The Abbreviated Profile of Hearing Aid Benefit (APHAB). Ear Hear 1995;16:176–186.

Cox R, Bisset J. Prediction of preferred listening levels for hearing aid gain preselection. Ear Hear 1982;3:66–71.

DeFilippo C, Sims D, Gottermeier L. Linking visual and kinesthetic imagery in lipreading instruction. J Speech Hear Res 1995;38:244–256.

DeJonge R. Microcomputer applications for hearing aid selection and fitting. Trends Ampl 1996;1:86–113.

Demorest M, Bernstein L. Computational explorations of speechreading. J Acad Rehabil Audiol 1991;24:97–111.

Educational Services Department, Digital Equipment Corporation. DECtalk DTCOI Programmer Reference Manual, Digital Equipment Corporation, Maynard, MD, 1984.

Erber N. Communication therapy for adults with sensory loss. San Diego: Singular, 1996.

Erber N. DYLOG: A computer-based measure of conversational performance. J Acad Rehab Audiol 1998; 31:69–76.

FIG6: Hearing aid fitting protocol manual. Etymotic Research, Elk Grove, IL, 1996

Fox R. Technology-based systems in education. Soc Appl Learn Tech Newsletter 1998;Fall.

Gagné J, Dinon D, Parsons J. An evaluation of CAST: a computer-aided speechreading training program. J Speech Hear Res 1991;34:213–221.

Gitlin R. Software-driven audiology powers hearing professionals. Hear Instr 1995;May.

Hanin L, Boothroyd A, Hnath-Chisolm T. The presentation of voice fundamental frequency as an aid to the speechreading of sentences. Ear Hear 1988;9:335–341.

Hoffman P, Daniloff R, Bengoa D, et al. Misarticulating and normally articulating children's identification and discrimination of synthetic [r] and [w]. J Speech Hear Dis 1985;50:46–53.

Ijsseldijk F. Speechreading performance under different conditions of video image, repetition and speech rate. J Speech Hear Res 1992;35:418–429.

Jacobs M. Speechreading training for severely and profoundly hearing impaired young adults. In: Sims D, Walter G, Whitehead R, eds. Deafness and communication: assessment and training. Baltimore: Williams & Wilkins, 1982.

Jamieson DG, Rvachew S. Remediating speech production errors with sound identification training. J Speech Lang Pathol Audiol 1992;16:201–210.

Jutras B, Gagné JP. Auditory sequential organization among children with and without a hearing loss. J Sp Lang Hear Resh 1999;42:553–567.

Kopra L, Kopra M, Abrahamson J, et al. Development of sentences graded on difficulty for lipreading practice. J Acad Rehabil Audiol 1986;19:71–86.

Lonka E. Speechreading instruction for hard-of-hearing adults: effects of training face-to-face and with a video program. Scand Audiol 1995;24:193–198.

Lyxell B, Ronnberg J. Visual speech processing: word-decoding and word-discrimination related to sentence-based speechreading and hearing impairment. Scand Psychol 1991;32:9–17.

Lyxell B, Ronnberg J. The relationship between verbal ability and sentence-based speechreading. Scand Audiol 1992;21:76–72.

Majaranta, P. Stepwise tutoring in teaching lipreading. Department of Computer Science report. Tampere, Finland: University of Tampere, Department of Computer Science, 1998. E-mail: curly@cs.uta.fi

Massaro DW. Perceiving talking faces: from speech perception to a behavioral principle. Cambridge: MIT Press, 1998.

Miller S, Merzenich G, Jenkins W, et al. Improvements in language abilities with training of children with both attentional and language impairments. Soc Neurosci Reprint Series 1997;23:490.

Montgomery A, Demorest M. Issues and developments in the evaluation of speechreading. In: De Filippo C, Sims D, eds. New reflections on speechreading. Volta Rev 1988; 90:189–214.

Newman C, Weinstein B, Jacobson G, et al. The hearing handicap inventory for adults: psychometric adequacy and audiometric correlates. Ear Hear 1990;11: 430–433.

Newman C, Weinstein B, Jacobson G, et al. Test-retest reliability of the Hearing Handicap Inventory for Adults. Ear Hear 1991;5:355–357.

Newman C, Jacobson G, Weinstein B, et al. Computer-generated hearing disability/handicap profiles. Am J Audiol 1997;6:17–21.

Nickerson R, Kalikow C, Stevens K. Computer aided speech training for the deaf. J Speech Hear Disord 1976;41: 120–132.

Palmer C. Computer administration of hearing performance inventories. Am J Audiol 1992;1:13–14.

Pinchora-Fuller M, Benguerel A. The design of CAST (computer-aided speechreading training). J Speech Hear Res 1991;34:202–212.

Rushakoff G. Clinical applications in communication disorders. In: Schwartz M, ed. Handbook of microcomputer applications in communication disorders. San Diego: College Hill, 1984.

Rvachew S. Speech perception training can facilitate sound production learning. J Speech Hear Res 1994; 37:347–357.

Rvachew S, Jamieson DG. Perception of voiceless fricatives by children with a functional articulation disorder. J Speech Hear Dis 1989;54:193–208.

Samar V, Parasnis I. Learning disabilities, attention deficit disorders and deafness. In: Marschark M, Clark D, eds. Psychological perspectives on deafness. Hillsdale, NJ: Lawrence Erlbaum, 1998;2.

Seewald RC. Amplification: A child-centered approach. Hear J 1997;50:61.

Sims D, Clymer W. Computer-assisted instruction for the hearing impaired. In: Northern J, ed. The personal computer for speech, language, and hearing professionals. Boston: Little Brown, 1986;11:157–176.

Sims D, Zhwei X. An ecological method for response time to measure interactive video speechreading training. Presented at the Academy of Rehabilitative Audiology summer institute, Orlando, Florida, 1993.

Sims D, Von Feldt J, Dowaliby F, et al. A pilot experiment in computer assisted speechreading instruction utilizing the DAVID. Am Ann Deaf 1979;127:545–563.

Sims D, Scott L, Myers T. Past, present and future computer assisted communication training at the National Technical Institute for the Deaf. J Acad Rehabil Audiol 1982; 15:103–115.

Sims D, Kopra L, Dunlop R, et al. A survey of microcomputer applications in aural rehabilitation. J Acad Rehabil Audiol 1985;18:9–26.

Slike S, Thornton N, Hobbis D, et al. The development and analysis of interactive videodisc technology to teach speechreading. Am Ann Deaf 1995;140:346–351.

Summerfield AQ. Some preliminaries to a comprehensive account of audio-visual speech perception. In: Dodd B, Campbell R, eds. Hearing by eye: the psychology of lipreading. Hillsdale, NJ: Lawrence Erlbaum, 1987:3–51.

Tellal P, Merzenich M. Fast ForWord© training for children with language-learning problems: national field trial results. Presented at the annual meeting of the American Speech-Language-Hearing Association, Boston, Massachusetts, 1997.

Tellal P, Miller S, Bedi G, et al. Language comprehension in language-learning impaired children improved with acoustically modified speech. Science 1996;271:81–84.

Tye-Murray N. Laser videodisc technology in the aural rehabilitation setting: good news for people with severe and profound hearing impairments. Am J Audiol 1992;1:33–36.

Tye-Murray N, Tyler R, Bong B, et al. Computerized laser videodisc programs for training speeechreading and assertive communication behaviors. J Acad Rehabil Audiol 1988;21:143–152.

Valente M, Van Vliet D. The independent hearing aid fitting forum (IHAFF) protocol. Trends in amplification 1997;2:1–30.

van Uden A. Diagnostic testing of deaf children: the syndrome of dyspraxia. Lisse: Swets and Zeitlinger, 1983.

Weinberger N. Music and the auditory system. In: Deutsch D, ed. The psychology of music. San Diego: Academic, 1999:47–87.

SUGGESTED READINGS ON AUDITORY AND VISUAL SPEECH RECOGNITION

DeFilippo C. Tracking for speechreading training. In: DeFilippo C, Sims D, eds. New reflections on speechreading. Volta Rev Monogr 1988;90:215–240.

Ludvigsen C, ed. Operation Helen. Auditive, visual and audio-visual perception of speech. Copenhagen: Stougard Jensen, 1981.

Massaro D, Stork D. Speech recognition and sensory integration. Amer Scientist 86:236–244.

Massaro DW, Cohen MM, Daniel S, et al. Developing and evaluating conversational agents. In: Hancock, PA, ed. Human performance and ergonomics. Handbook of perception and cognition. 2nd ed. San Diego: Academic Press, 1999:173–194.

Stork D, Hennecke M. eds. Speechreading by humans and machines. NATO ASI Series, series F, computers and systems science. Berlin: Springer-Verlag, 1996;150.

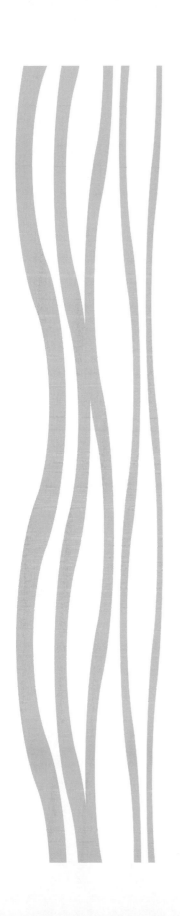

FUTURE
DIRECTIONS

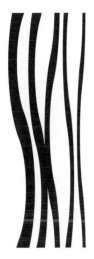

18

Outcome Measures in Rehabilitative Audiology

Barbara E. Weinstein, Ph.D.

In this era of managed care, health care professionals in general and audiologists in particular must identify and quantify the positive benefits of what they do (Kane, 1997). The quality of care delivered is an important issue to consumers and providers alike. The definition of quality must be understood before it can be assessed and promoted (Weitzman, 1995). This chapter begins with some operational definitions of quality of care in health care settings and proceeds to a discussion of methods for measuring quality. As demands for outcome data are most prevalent in the health care system, the discussion focuses on settings in which hearing health care delivery takes place. The goal is to offer the reader strategies and incentives for initiating quality of care measurements as a routine part of audiologic practice, especially practices that emphasize rehabilitation of those with handicapping hearing impairments.

Defining Quality of Care

According to Webster's *Seventh Collegiate Dictionary,* quality refers to a degree of excellence. It refers to the extent to which improvements in health status, which are in fact possible, are actually realized (Weitzman, 1995). Health care providers interested in delivering quality care are guided by the common goals of promoting, preserving, and restoring health (Weitzman, 1995).

Contemporary theorists in the area of quality improvement, most notably Donabedian (1988), hold that the quality of health care must be defined in terms of the attributes of care provided, including the technical and interpersonal aspects of care as well as criteria for what comprises good care (e.g., the amenities of care) (Cleary and McNeil, 1988). Further, when defining quality it is important to consider from whose perspective it will be measured. The author's review of the literature on outcomes in rehabilitation suggests that quality of care should be considered from two different perspectives: the provider and the consumer. Above all, consumers/clients play an important role in defining what values and outcomes define quality care. Their internal perceptions are an important criterion against which quality is judged (Cleary and McNeil, 1988). Clinical experience suggests that each participant in health care emphasizes different attributes of care. The practitioner tends to be concerned with the technical aspects (e.g., real-ear measures), whereas the client is more concerned with interpersonal aspects of care, namely patient-practitioner interactions (Weitzman, 1995).

According to Donabedian (1981), three variables including structure, process, and outcome should be assessed. Structure denotes the attributes of the setting in which care occurs and the characteristics of the care providers, the tools, and the resources at their disposal (Weitzman, 1995). Structure indicators include practitioner certification, waiting time for an appointment, staff characteristics, and adequacy of technology. An important indicator that must always be kept in mind is ensuring that care is delivered according to the ethical practices of the profession, in this case as defined by the American Speech-Language-Hearing Association or the American Academy of Audiology (Donabedian, 1988). According to Weitzman (1995), structure is an indirect indicator of quality in that it is useful to the extent that it affects the direct provision of services.

Process denotes what is actually done in giving and receiving care. That is, what is actually going on between the patient and the practitioner? Process measures assess various aspects of the care such as the manner in which a case history is taken, the manner in which the patient is counseled, or the appropriateness of a given test procedure. In addition, process measures ask whether the patient was given sufficient information to make a choice/decision or whether care was implemented in a timely fashion. Although process can be viewed as what is done to patients, outcomes are what actually happens to the patient. Outcome refers to change(s) in the patient's behavior or health status as a result of an intervention. Here the internal perceptions of the client and family members are critical, and respect for client/patient preferences and expressed needs is of utmost importance (Donabedian, 1988).

An underlying premise of quality assessment studies is that structure influences the process of care, which in turn has an effect on the outcome of care (Weitzman, 1995). That is, judgments about quality are based on the relationship between structure and process of care and their effect on the health of the patients. Process is the most direct indicator of quality, whereas structure is a crude measure of quality in that it only addresses trends (Weitzman, 1995). According to Donabedian's (1988) teachings, process and outcomes are inextricably intertwined. It should be obvious to most clinicians that the set of activities that take place between the audiologist and the hearing-impaired patient (i.e., process) will affect outcome (Frattali, 1998).

The term outcome refers to the measurable effect, either real or perceived, of a particular intervention on the individual's disability or handicap. Hence, an outcome is the result of an intervention; it refers to a characteristic under scrutiny such as a treatment goal, an indicator of progress in rehabilitation, or an indicator of the effect of care on health status or educational performance. An outcome can be positive or negative, that is, an individual may experience a decrease or increase in their disability or handicap as a result of intervention (Humes, 1999).

Outcome measures are the interface between the health care professional's goals for rehabilitation and the client's response to specific clinical procedures (Montgomery, 1994). Selection of an outcome measure indicates what the professional considers to be the goal of a given intervention for a particular patient/client (Boston Working Group on Improving Health Care Outcomes, 1997). Clinicians should gather data on process outcomes, program outcomes, or some combination of the above (Donabedian, 1988; Robertson and Colborn, 1997). Process outcomes are those changes in performance that clients experience during rehabilitation (Robertson and Colborn, 1997). They are highly individualized and depend in large part on the client's social, psychological, cognitive, and physical skills. Process outcomes that are the most subtle indicators of progress are typically demonstrated through nonverbal communication, statements, and behaviors (Robertson and Colborn, 1997). According to Robertson and Colborn (1997), process outcomes help the clinician to establish clinical concepts of function. Process outcomes can be client defined (e.g., satisfaction with service) and/or clinician defined. Audiologists have become accustomed to describing outcomes in terms of impairment, disability, and handicap. They should now be ready to embrace the schema described by Wilson and Cleary (1995). This model proposes that clinicians categorize patient outcomes according to the underlying health concept they represent (Frattali, 1998)—in terms of the effect of an intervention on quality of life, health status, or presenting symptoms. In a sense, the latter consequences can be subsumed under the category of handicap or disability.

Program outcomes produce data that pertain to the administration of a facility, including patient demographics, number of treatment sessions, and length of stay. An example of program evaluation data may be the proportion of clients who received hearing aids who experienced a reduction in the extent of disability or handicap. Hence, these data may reveal information about practices, services, etc. Unlike process outcomes, which address the how and why of practice, program outcomes rarely address causal factors in changing behavior (Robertson and Colborn, 1997). Agencies are likely to infer quality from process outcomes underlining their importance in this era of managed care (Robertson and Colborn, 1997). According to Robertson and Colborn (1997), the real strength of any rehabilitation program is the link between process and program outcomes. Hence, the two should be interrelated. That is, studies on the how and why of practice (process outcomes) should take into consideration quantitative data about programs (e.g., personnel, resources used). This approach will ensure that outcomes specific to the rehabilitative process are clear (Robertson or Colborn, 1997).

Audiologists usually select outcome measures that will enable them to demonstrate that in fact, the client and the clinician have been successful in changing a target behavior, hence influencing functional performance in whatever domains they function (e.g., school, home, work, health care setting). Potential outcomes achieved during rehabilitation are quite numerous depending in large part on the nature of the disability, the client's age, and lifestyle considerations. For example, when working with older adults with communication problems, the professional strives to give the patient a subjective sense of well-being, improve communication ability, improve participation in social and recreational activities, reduce the extent of communication handicap, and enable the client to return to the community. For younger adults, the ability to work effectively and interact in a host of social roles is important, and hearing aids can promote function in these areas.

Another key issue in this era of changing health care is whether a patient's health improves as a result of a given treatment, with the net benefit measured using health-related quality of life assessment measures. That is, change in physical, social, mental, and functional health is used to evaluate the human benefits and financial value of selected programs and interventions. The term efficacy refers to the probability that individuals in a particular population will benefit from a well-defined treatment applied for a given problem or predicament (Hyde and Riko, 1994). The client's predicament is the sum of all pertinent aspects of his or her state and situation including disorders, impairment disabilities, and handicapping situations (Hyde and Riko, 1994). The efficacy of a given treatment is defined in terms of the extent to which it reduces or eliminates the client's predicament in one or more domains of function. Typically, the amount of change in predicament experienced by the patient defines the benefit or advantage conferred by the treatment (Gagne et al., 1994). Stated differently, benefit refers to the difference between a patient's predicament before and after a given intervention. Benefit expresses the magnitude or degree of change from an unaided to an aided condition (Humes, 1999). When studying benefit, the clinician may obtain a difference score that actually reflects what happened as a result of the intervention. At least two measures are taken, a measure before and after intervention or aided or unaided performance (Cleary and McNeil, 1988) As will become apparent in this chapter, objective and subjective metrics can be used when quantifying benefit. Irrespective of the metric, the information comes from the patient and is quantitative; hence, the measures should be robust psychometrically (i.e., high in test-retest reliability and validity).

An important component of quality of care is patient satisfaction with service outcomes. Quantifying satisfaction is important in rehabilitation in that the data shed light on how to improve services and accountability as well as how to make initiating and terminating services more attractive to the client (Simon and Patrick, 1997). Patient satisfaction, a subjective phenomenon, can be defined as the client's reaction to salient aspects of the context, process, and results of service experience (Pascoe, 1983). Satisfaction consists of both a cognitive evaluation and an emotional reaction to the structure, process, and outcome of services. Thus, the experience of consumer satisfaction involves a subjective reaction to some external reality. Satisfaction with dimensions of health care is an effect that results from social and psychological determinants including perceptions, evaluations, and comparisons (Simon and Patrick, 1997). Hence, professionals must measure both the external reality and the individual's perceptions (Simon and Patrick, 1997).

The measurement of satisfaction is a complex issue as it too requires clinicians to measure the full service spectrum including personal aspects of care, accessibility and availability of care, continuity of care, patient convenience, physical setting, financial considerations, and efficacy of satisfaction with the clinical service delivered (Simon and Patrick, 1997). A number of variables exogenous to the service influence satisfaction ratings. Age influences ratings in that older people tend to report higher levels of satisfaction than do their younger counterparts. Gender also influences satisfaction; women tend to be more satisfied then men (Cleary and McNeil, 1988). Satisfaction relates to perceptions of technical skills and to interpersonal and communication skills. Past experience, word of mouth, external communications, and personal needs also influence judgments of satisfaction (Brown et al., 1993). The latter are important considerations for the audiologist in private practice.

Patterns of expectations in part shape satisfaction judgments as well. In short, clients/patients compare their expectations (i.e., what they anticipate will take place) against their perceptions of the clinical encounter. Overall, individuals tend to be more satisfied with care if their expectations are met. This is in keeping with expectations performance theory, which holds that experience + needs + communications = expectations (Brown et al., 1993). When perception exceeds expectations, the client is satisfied; if expectations are less than perceptions, dissatisfaction ensues irrespective of the clinical outcome. It is important to emphasize that satisfaction is a unique personal state that depends on factors over which clinicians may have limited control, including patient needs, external communication, and previous experience (Brown et al., 1993). In light of the latter, management of factors over which clinicians have some control is critical. For example, it is incumbent on audiologists to spend some time setting realistic expectations. Dispensing audiologists must provide their patients with realistic expectations regarding what they can expect from hearing aids and assistive listening devices.

In addition to client expectations being critical to quality service, client involvement in decision-making is integral to satisfaction. Clients who are more involved in their care tend to be more satisfied, are more likely to comply with treatment regimens, and are more likely to return for care (Cleary and McNeil, 1988). Hence, levels of satisfaction may be explained in terms of the degree to which specific service experiences that are deemed as important by clients are perceived as present or absent during the total service experience (Simon and Patrick, 1997).

Finally, characteristics of the provider or the organization that make care more personal are associated with higher levels of satisfaction. These personal skills include good communication skills, empathy, and caring. Table 18.1 lists some steps to be taken to maximize satisfaction. Kochkin (1997) explained that satisfaction occurs through the blending of science and art and ensues from the correct application of technology and counseling based on the unique

Table 18.1
Strategies for promoting client satisfaction with the delivery of audiologic rehabilitation services

Make sure the client is the focus of your practice
Get to know your client's expectations
Empower your staff to help instill your clients with realistic expectations
Have a system in place for measuring how well you are meeting client expectations
Make sure your staff understands and shares your practice's mission
Have a system in place for measuring how well you meet the needs of other health professionals
  who refer clients to you
Consider people and technical skills when you hire
Make sure your practice is patient-centered and quality-service–oriented

Adapted from Brown S, Nelson A, Bronkesh S, et al. Patient satisfaction pays. Rockville, MD: Aspen, 1993.

needs of the client. He suggested that assessing satisfaction following the delivery of services is important, as this demonstrates that the professional cares about what the client thinks. He emphasized that when setting expectations, it is important to make sure that the objectives/goals of intervention are useful, understandable, obtainable, and agreed on in advance. Kochkin (1997) concluded his article by suggesting that one way of ensuring client satisfaction is to assure that the energy one expends in terms of service and time exceeds the energy the client expends in terms of money and time. Kochkin's approach to measuring satisfaction with hearing aids is the most extensively studied, and results can be quite useful to the audiologist. He considers satisfaction to be a function of three important variables including satisfaction with the physical features of the instrument dispensed, satisfaction with the unit's performance in a variety of listening situations, and satisfaction with the quality of services. The consumer merely applies a satisfaction rating to items that contribute to satisfaction in each of these areas, and satisfaction scores emerge.

Having provided an extensive philosophical review of the variables to consider when assessing outcomes, this chapter proceeds with a review of approaches to assessing outcomes, followed by some examples from the literature that demonstrate how useful outcome measures can be in practice. Because emphasis will be placed on outcomes during audiologic rehabilitation and the hearing aid fitting, the author's philoso-

phy regarding the latter must be enumerated before proceeding with a discussion of outcome measures.

Goals of Audiologic Rehabilitation

Audiologic rehabilitation is a problem-solving process engaged in to resolve or alleviate situations of handicap rather than to eliminate or reduce hearing impairment or disorders (Gagne et al., 1999). Hence as an outcome, clinicians and client want to know whether the intervention was successful in alleviating the specific difficulties experienced by the client in everyday listening situations (Gagne et al., 1999). It is critical from the outset that the client is involved in each stage of the rehabilitative process, including the recognition and identification of the problem, the description of the difficulties, the selection of the intervention strategy, and the evaluation of the effects of the intervention (Gagne et al., 1999). From the outset, defining the goal of the intervention process sets a tangible criterion against which to judge outcome and ensure that the client's needs are met (Liang, 1997). Because a key component of problem-solving is defining the intended goal of the intervention, normed outcome measures are integral to the process. The goal of the hearing aid fitting is to select hearing aid circuitry, which will achieve some or all of the ends listed in Table 18.2. In the author's view, the hearing aid is the treatment—it is the nucleus of the rehabilitative process. In whatever form it takes, rehabilitation reinforces

Table 18.2
Goals of the hearing aid fitting

Impairment oriented
    Enable reasonably good aided audibility across a broad frequency region without simultaneously
        making average and loud speech too loud
    Place amplified speech above threshold and below discomfort level
    Restore normal loudness impression
    Restore normal loudness growth
Disability/Handicap oriented
    Minimize the communicative disability
    Reduce the psychosocial handicap
    Improve functional status

the success of the hearing aid fitting (Mc-Carthy, 1996). Hence, rehabilitation (in the form of counseling, speechreading, etc.) assists the professional in achieving the goals of the hearing aid fitting. These include (1) ensuring that the variety of speech inputs to which the client is exposed are audible, comfortable, and tolerable across as wide a frequency range as possible; (2) ensuring that the eletroacoustic characteristics necessary to achieve the target produce maximum speech recognition and sound quality; and (3) addressing the communication/psychosocial handicap associated with hearing loss so that the intervention minimizes the individual's presenting problems. The first two goals are impairment oriented, whereas the final goal is oriented toward the handicap/disability.

Researchers, clinicians, and third-party representatives have begun to focus on how well the dispenser is realizing his or her fitting outcomes. As discussed above, measures of hearing aid benefit are the objective data adopted by audiologists to verify the adequacy of the hearing aid fitting. Specifically, the nature and severity of the predicament (hearing impairment) is defined objectively using threshold- or suprathreshold-based measures or subjectively using subjective performance measures such as quality judgments, loudness judgments, or perceived disability or handicap.

These data serve as a baseline against which the adequacy of both the signal processing and hearing aid fitting are judged. Thus, change in the predicament or im-

provement in performance on clinical measures is seen as synonymous with benefit. As discussed in more depth later in this chapter, the author views hearing aid benefit as a multidimensional rather than unidimensional measure; thus, the hearing aid outcomes should be assessed accordingly. For example, a hearing aid can provide reasonably good aided audibility across a broad frequency region as evidenced by the aided audibility or articulation index (AI), but the residual auditory disability or psychosocial handicap may remain considerable. Conversely, a hearing aid may make only a small percentage of speech audible, yet the extent of perceived disability or handicap may be dramatically reduced. The imperfect relation between objectively measured outcomes and those based on client self-perceptions has led to the development of a variety of subjective and objective approaches to measuring benefit.

With regard to subjective benefit, the client's perception of the overall advantage conferred by a hearing aid (e.g., the extent to which a hearing aid is perceived to facilitate communication and reduce psychosocial handicap) is increasingly used by audiologists to prove the value of the hearing aid fitting. That is, the centrality of the consumer's perspective as the ultimate arbiter of efficacy is gaining acceptance as research continues to demonstrate a link between therapeutic intervention with hearing aids and meaningful short-, medium-, and long-term quality of life changes (Cox et al., 1991b; Gatehouse, 1994). In turn, health care policy planners can use these quality of life treatment effects to justify the inclusion of audiologic rehabilitation with hearing aids as a benefit for the increasing number of adults and older adults with handicapping hearing impairments.

Subjective Outcome Measures

The most widely used tools available for measuring outcomes in the disability and handicap domains are listed in Table 18.3. According to a review of available outcome studies in the area of hearing aid fittings, the Hearing Handicap Inventory for the Elderly (HHIE) (Attachment 22) is a widely used clinical tool for measuring self-reported outcomes with hearing aids in the handicap domain. Its simplicity, reliability, and validity (as well as the fact that benefit in the handicap domain can be measured quickly and efficiently) may account in part for the acceptance of the HHIE. The HHIE provides insight into the relationship between hearing loss and psychological/emotional and social/communication variables more than other self-report measures (Etienne, 1996).

The 25-item HHIE is a self-administered questionnaire that quantifies the emotional (13 items) and social/situational (12 items) problems associated with hearing loss in older adults. The Hearing Handicap Inventory for Adults (HHIA) (Attachment 6) is a companion version appropriate for adults younger than 65 years of age. A "no" response to an item is awarded a "0," a "sometimes" scores a "2," and a "yes" scores a "4." Scores for the HHIE range from 0 to 100, with higher values representing greater perceived handicap. The HHIE was shortened from the full version (25 items) to a 10-item screening tool for which sensitivity and specificity values have been determined to be adequate (Ventry and Weinstein, 1982; Newman et al., 1997). The 95% confidence interval (CI or critical difference values) associated with the HHIE is 18.7 using a face-to-face administration, whereas the 95% CI for the screening version of the Hearing Handicap Inventory for the Elderly (HHIE-S) (Attachment 23) is 10. Test-retest reliability diminishes and the 95% CI increases slightly as one moves to a face-face/paper-pencil administration (95% CI = 19.2) or paper-and-pencil administration on each occasion (95% CI = 36.0). For the HHIA, the 95% CI using a face-to-face administration is 11.9.

The Abbreviated Profile for Hearing Aid

Table 18.3
Approaches to measuring impairment, disability, and handicap

Impairment domain
    Real-ear measures
    Functional gain
    Speech recognition measures
Disability domain
    Measure disadvantage with the auditory activities of daily living
        Abbreviated Profile for Hearing Aid Benefit (APHAB)
        Hearing Performance Inventory (HPI)
        Hearing Aid Performance Inventory (HAPI)
        Shortened Hearing Aid Performance Inventory (SHAPI)
        Client-Oriented Scale of Improvement (COSI)
Handicap domain
    Measure nonauditory problems resulting from diminished auditory capacity and the auditory
        demands of real-life situations (Gagne et al., 1995)
    Hearing Handicap Inventory for the Elderly (HHIE)
    Hearing Handicap Inventory for Adults (HHIA)
    Screening version of the HHIE (HHIE-S)
    Screening version of the HHIA (HHIA-S)
    Communication Profile for the Hearing Impaired (CPHI)

Benefit (APHAB) (Attachment 24) consists of 24 items with four 6-item subscales including ease of communication (EC), background noise (BN), reverberation (RV), and aversiveness of sound (AV). It is considered a measure of disability (Mueller, 1996). The response format entails indicating the percentage of time the individual experiences problems hearing in situations described in the questionnaire. According to the instructions detailed in the normative study, respondents complete the APHAB under both aided and nonaided conditions following the hearing aid fitting. Hearing aid benefit in the disability domain is operationally defined as a change score indicative of hearing problem reduction. The difference between aided and unaided scores on each of the four subscales serves as the index of benefit in the particular situations sampled by the subscale items. Further, a respondent's score on each scale can be compared with equal percentile profiles for APHAB subscales developed by Cox and Alexander (1995) on a sample of successful hearing aid users. When scoring the APHAB, unaided scores on the four subscales are first reported. Scores for example may range from 80.8% on the subscale that assesses speech understanding in BN to 97.0% on the EC subscale. Thus, in the above case, the client reports that when listening in a noisy environment (BN), he or she has problems understanding speech nearly 81% of the time. Next, responses to the same four subscales are elicited according to how the client feels after having had the opportunity to use the hearing aid(s) for a brief period, usually 3 to 4 weeks. A hearing aid user may report that now problems related to understanding speech in noise occur only 2.8% of the time. The difference between scores obtained on each of the subscales is computed. The difference between aided and unaided responses reflects the amount of problem reduction attributable to hearing aid use. In the above case, the difference translates into a benefit score of 78.%.

According to the norms provided by Cox and Alexander (1995), a benefit score of 78.% places this client's score in greater than the 95th percentile. Hence, for this patient, reported benefit with the hearing aids, when listening in noise, was greater than the benefit reported by 95% of the successful users of linear amplification (Cox and Alexander, 1995). The test-retest reliability of the APHAB in the unaided and unaided conditions has been established for experienced hearing aid users; thus, the applicability of the normative data (e.g., percentile scores) to new hearing aid users remains unknown as of this writing. When using the APHAB, unaided and aided performances can be assessed either at one point in time after hearing aid use or at two different points in time (namely, before and after hearing aid use).

Another approach to measuring subjective benefit is to ask the user to judge how much benefit the hearing aid is providing. The Hearing Aid Performance Inventory (HAPI) (Attachment 25) developed by Walden et al. (1984), one of the few available tools specifically designed for use in the hearing instrument verification process, allows for such an approach. It consists of 64 items that quantify hearing aid benefit in everyday life. The four types of listening situations surveyed include noisy listening situations, quiet situations with speaker in close proximity, situations with reduced signal information, and situations with nonspeech stimuli. The HAPI is somewhat different from the HHIE and the APHAB in that it provides a post-fit assessment of subjective hearing aid benefit. The client is presented with a particular communication situation and/or environment and is asked to rate the amount of help afforded by the hearing aid ranging from "very helpful" to "hinders performance." The lower the client's score, the better the hearing aid performance.

The HAPI was recently shortened to include 38 items and 4 subscales that assess speech understanding in quiet, in noise, and in situations that are low in redundancy (Schum, 1992). As with the 64-item version, the respondent rates the benefit of the hearing aid in each of the 38 situations sampled. The Hearing Performance Inventory (HPI) (Attachment 26), developed by Giolas et al.

(1979), assesses hearing performance in everyday life. The entire inventory includes 158 questions that sample the following areas: understanding of speech, intensity of speech, response to auditory failure, social communication difficulties, personal communication difficulties, and occupational difficulties. Additional scales used to assess outcomes with hearing aids include the Hearing Handicap Scale and the Communication Profile for Hearing Impaired Individuals (CPHI) (Attachment 27) (Demorest and Erdman, 1986). The former has been shown to be sensitive to hearing aid benefit in the disability domain; the latter, although quite lengthy, is also a sensitive outcome measure in both the disability and handicap domains.

The Client-Oriented Scale of Improvement (COSI) (Attachment 28) is the most recent scale to be described for subjectively measuring hearing aid performance (Dillon et al., 1997). It differs from other measures in that the client decides on the listening situations in which help with hearing is required. Stated differently, the client and the audiologist work together at the beginning of the fitting process to identify specific goals for the fitting. Open-ended scale items are tailored to each individual's particular listening needs and experiences (Dillon et al., 1997). Specifically, the patient nominates up to five situations in which he or she would like to cope better. The patient is asked to rank each situation in order of importance. At the follow-up appointment, the patient is asked to judge the degree of change attributable to the hearing aid. For each situation, the patient is asked how much better he or she can now hear relative to before hearing aid use and how ably he or she can hear with the device. Degree of change is ranked on a five-point scale ranging from "worse" to "slightly better" to "much better," or from "hardly ever" to "occasionally" to "almost always." A "5" corresponds to "much better/almost always," whereas a "1" corresponds to "worse/hardly ever." Hence, with the COSI, it is not simply the amount of benefit provided in a communication situation that is important, but the importance of the situation to the individual. The COSI can be very helpful as audiologists work with their clients to try to shape the course of rehabilitation. Clearly, some of the above scales are disability measures and some are measures of perceived handicap. Some of the earliest studies in the area of outcomes assessment have used measures of disability to quantify short-term benefit with hearing aids. Some of these studies combined audiologic rehabilitation with hearing aids to document the benefits of hearing aids in various communication situations.

The findings from a number of investigators who have used a variety of disability measures to assess the functional benefits of hearing aids are presented below. Bentler et al. (1993) evaluated the efficacy of hearing aids on a sample of 65 adults with mild to moderate sensorineural hearing loss. The majority of subjects were new hearing aid users. All subjects completed the 38-item HPI at baseline, 6 months, and 12 months after the initial fitting. The most notable finding was a substantial improvement in scores on the scales that measure speech understanding in a fairly quiet background. Improvements were notable after 6 months and 1 year of hearing aid use. Beneficial treatment effects were not apparent on the subsections that assessed speech understanding in the presence of background noise or in performance on the Nonsense Syllable Test (NST) and the Speech in Noise Test (SPIN), irrespective of the type of noise circuitry. Using the HPI, Dempsey (1986) also noted a significant decrease in hearing handicap for the speech understanding subsection of the HPI. These studies confirm client reports that hearing aids improve speech understanding in optimal listening situations.

Cox et al. (1991a) demonstrated benefit in the disability domain using the Profile of Hearing Aid Benefit (PHAB) (Attachment 29). The data that emerged from their study revealed that short-term hearing aid benefit is demonstrable in easy listening situations, yet the magnitude of benefit in the disability domain decreases as the listening situation becomes more difficult. Similarly, Cox and Alexander (1995) demonstrated that hearing aids provide statistically significant benefit in a variety of listening situations according to improvements in scores on selected scales of the Abbreviated Profile of Hearing Aid Benefit (APHAB) following hearing aid use. However, it was notable that in their sample of 22 new hearing aid users, a number of subjects still chose to return their hearing aids despite significant improvement in communication ability in various daily life situations. Specifically, all subjects who kept their hearing aids showed significant benefit according to difference scores on the APHAB. Similarly, most of the individuals who chose to return their hearing aids showed significant benefit in the disability domain according to difference scores on the APHAB. In light of their findings, the authors tentatively concluded that the amount of reported benefit in the disability domain (i.e., difference scores on the APHAB) is not always enough to make the hearing aid purchase worthwhile for the hearing-impaired individual. In a sense, this conclusion and their preliminary findings tend to suggest that hearing aid satisfaction does not necessarily correlate with hearing aid benefit in the disability domain.

Ebinger et al. (1995) reported on the benefit experienced by 90 adults with varying degrees of sensorineural hearing loss who obtained completely-in-the-canal (CIC) hearing aids. Subjects completed the APHAB 2 to 10 months after the initial hearing aid fitting. Approximately half the subjects were new users, and half were previous hearing aid users. It was reported that the CIC fitting reduced the percent of aided problems to below the 50th percentile of the norms (Cox and Alexander, 1995). Humes et al. (1996) followed a sample of 20 older adults fit with binaural multiple memory in-the-ear hearing aids. A close match to National Acoustic Laborataies–Revised (NAL-R) target was achieved for the majority of subjects. Subjects completed the HAPI at several intervals including 20, 40, 60, 80, and 180 days after the fitting. Depending on the subscale, subjects experienced significant amounts of benefit in the disability domain from hearing aids after a brief interval of use. Between 45 and 65% of

subjects demonstrated significant benefit according to absolute scores on the HAPI subscales. A study conducted by Kricos and Holmes (1996) demonstrated that 4 weeks of active listening training (i.e., training in the recognition of message meaning), coupled with hearing aid use, can reduce the extent of self-perceived communication disability in adverse listening conditions, as shown by change in scores on the CPHI. Their finding underlined the importance of some form of listening training when self-perceived speech understanding in adverse situations fails to improve with hearing aid use.

The above studies clearly demonstrate that when using disease-specific measures of auditory disability, hearing aids have been proven to be effective means of reducing the extent of self-perceived speech understanding difficulties in various listening situations. The study by Kricos and Holmes (1996) is among the first using a disability measure to show the value of listening training as a means of enhancing benefit of hearing aids in adverse listening situations. As would be expected, listening training had little effect on psychosocial handicap according to difference scores on the HHIE. Their finding makes a case for measuring benefit in a variety of domains, as benefit in the disability domain is not necessarily related to benefit in the handicap domain. Further, the form of intervention (namely, listening training) may not affect psychosocial adjustment to communicative disability. The fact that benefit may be a multidimensional phenomenon will be discussed in a later section of this chapter.

A number of studies have been conducted using the HHIE/HHIE-S as a measure of subjective benefit in the handicap domain. The studies have attempted to measure short-term, medium-term, and long-term benefits from hearing aid use with different hearing aid technologies. It is evident from the variety of studies conducted on samples of subjects drawn from Veterans Administration (VA) Medical Centers, private practices, and hospital-based clinics that hearing aids do lower handicap after even 2 to 3 weeks of hearing aid use. Malinoff and

Weinstein (1989) studied a sample of 45 subjects with mild to moderate bilateral sensorineural hearing loss who were fit with in-the-ear hearing aids. Subjects were recruited from the hearing aid dispensary at an eye, ear, and throat hospital in a major metropolitan area. Following a rather brief period of hearing aid use, there was a statistically and clinically significant reduction in self-perceived hearing handicap in the emotional and social domains of function. Nearly 80% of subjects in this study had mean scores differing by more than 18%, the value which reflects the 95% CI for a true change attributed to intervention (Malinoff and Weinstein, 1989).

In a large-scale study (n = 91), Newman et al. (1991) explored the short-term benefits of hearing aids. Once again, the majority of subjects had mild to moderate sensorineural hearing loss. Mean scores on the total, emotional, and social subscales of the HHIE-S improved dramatically and significantly after short-term hearing aid use. Using 10 points as the 95% CI for computing a true change in HHIE-S scores, 78% of subjects demonstrated a true change/reduction in perceived hearing handicap, whereas 7% of subjects did not reach the criterion for a significant change in handicap (Newman et al., 1991). The remaining proportion of subjects (i.e., 15%) had total handicap scores that were less than the 95% CI of 10 and thus were not eligible to be included in this computation. The authors concluded that these data confirm the beneficial effects of hearing aid use among older adults.

Primeau (1997) reported on the efficacy of hearing aids worn by a population of 233 veterans ranging in age from 27 to 97 years (mean age, 65.5 years). The majority of subjects had mild to moderately severe, adult-onset, bilaterally symmetric, sensorineural hearing loss and were fit binaurally with in-the-ear hearing aids. Before obtaining the hearing aid(s) and 6 weeks after the initial fitting, patients completed the screening version of the Hearing Handicap Inventory for Adults (HHIA-S) (Attachment 30) or the HHIE-S to determine the short-term benefit of hearing aids. Of the 233 individuals obtaining hearing aids, 181 (77.7%) experienced a significant reduction in self-perceived handicap with hearing aid use. Young and older adults were similar in the amount of perceived psychosocial handicap experienced before and after hearing aid use and hence in the magnitude of benefit in the psychosocial domain. In addition, new and experienced hearing aid users were comparable in terms of the magnitude of perceived benefit in the psychosocial domain.

The most comprehensive randomized, controlled clinical trial of the numerous benefits derived from hearing aids was conducted on a sample of male veterans (Mulrow et al., 1990). One hundred ninety-four older adults with mild to moderately severe sensorineural hearing loss participated. Half the subjects were assigned to a hearing aid group and the other half to a waiting list group. Each group was matched on important demographic and clinical characteristics. Ninety-eight percent of individuals in the hearing aid group received monaural in-the-ear hearing aids. Hearing aid benefit was defined as a multidimensional phenomenon, according to the amount of improvement in scores on a variety of quality-of-life measures. The domains of function that were tapped included social, emotional, cognitive, physical, and psychological. Responses to items on the HHIE provided data on the perceived emotional and social effects of hearing loss. The other disorder-specific outcome measure was the Denver Scale of Communication Function (DSCF) (Attachment 3), which provided an estimate of perceived communication function. Subjects completed each of these disorder-specific quality-of-life measures at baseline and at 6-week and 4-month follow-up visits. Mean scores on each of these measures were comparable between the control (waiting list) and experimental (hearing aid recipients) groups at baseline.

According to scores on the HHIE, 63% of subjects perceived their hearing handicap in the psychosocial domain to be severe and 20% perceived it to be mild to moderate. Moderate communication difficulties were reported by 85% of subjects on the DSCF (Mulrow et al., 1990). Hearing aid treatment effects were noted on each of the disorder-specific quality-of-life outcome measures for the experimental group at both the 6-week and 4-month follow-up visits. Although dramatic improvements in social and emotional function as assessed by the HHIE emerged in the hearing aid group, mean scores for the control group remained the same. Similarly, the hearing aid group demonstrated significant improvement in communication function as measured on the DSCF, whereas no change in communication function was noted for the waiting list group. Of interest was the finding that benefit, according to the difference between unaided and aided responses to items on the HHIE and the DSCF, emerged 6 weeks after receipt of the hearing aid and was sustained at the 4-month follow-up visit (Mulrow et al., 1990). That is, hearing aid benefit after 4 months of hearing aid use was comparable to that obtained as early as 6 weeks after the initial fitting. The authors concluded that their study established that hearing aids do in fact improve the quality of life for persons with hearing loss and that their short- and medium-term effects are most pronounced when using disorder-specific quality-of-life instruments.

Newman et al. (1993a) evaluated the benefit of hearing aids as measured by the HHIE over 6 months. Subjects ranged in age from 65 to 85 years and were new hearing aid users with essentially mild to moderate sensorineural hearing loss. Subjects experienced a dramatic reduction in self-perceived hearing handicap after 3 weeks of hearing aid use and continued to experience benefit up to 6 months after first obtaining the hearing aids. However, the mean HHIE score at 6 months postfit was slightly higher than that obtained at 3 weeks, albeit still significantly better than the mean baseline HHIE score. This trend suggests that a type of psychosocial acclimatization may take place, wherein following exposure to varied listening experiences, the client experiences some of the limitations inherent in hearing aid technology but continues to feel the advantage in the psychosocial domain over their unaided hearing.

Mulrow et al. (1992) conducted a longitudinal study of hearing aid benefit, with the goal being to determine whether it can be sustained as long as 1 year following the initial fitting. Subjects were new hearing aid users with mild to moderate sensorineural hearing loss. Approximately half the subjects were assigned to an experimental group and fit with monaural in-the-ear hearing aids, whereas the other half comprised the control or waiting list group. Groups were matched for hearing loss, age, physical status, and educational level. The majority of subjects in the experimental group wore their hearing aids for more than 4 hours daily at 4-month, 8-month, and 12-month follow-up visits. In general, 70 to 80% of the 162 subjects reported being quite satisfied with their units during the 1 year during which they participated in follow-up. Mean scores on the HHIE improved after 6 weeks of hearing aid use and were sustained at 4, 8, and 12 months, concluding that the benefits of hearing aids in the psychosocial and communicative domains of function are sustainable over 1 year. In their study, absolute and relative benefit in the psychosocial domain at 6 weeks was comparable to that at 4 months, 8 months, and 1 year.

Taylor (1993) also conducted a longitudinal study of change in self-perceived hearing handicap following 3 weeks, 3 months, 6 months, and 1 year of hearing aid use. The majority of the 58 subjects were older first-time hearing aid users, with mild to moderate sensorineural hearing loss. Subjects were fit with in-the-ear hearing aids. In general, the majority of subjects (78%) demonstrated statistically and clinically significant reductions in HHIE scores after 3 weeks of hearing aid use. Taylor (1993) found significant differences in HHIE scores at baseline, 3 weeks, 3 months, 6 months, and 1 year after the hearing aid fitting. The most dramatic reduction in social and emotional function emerged just 3 weeks after hearing aid use. The mean score on the HHIE rose significantly after 3 months of hearing aid use but stabilized after 6 months and 1 year, suggesting some form of acclimatization in the psychosocial domain. These data once again demonstrate the medium- and long-term benefit of hearing aids on the emotional and social domains of function. Although subjects' scores on the HHIE varied somewhat over time, functional gain estimates and aided word recognition scores remained stable over time, failing to reflect acclimatization effects noted on responses to the HHIE.

The data of Malinoff and Weinstein (1989) confirmed the findings of Taylor (1993), namely the potential for some form of psychosocial acclimatization with new hearing aid use. As noted above, subjects in their study were older adults with mild to moderate sensorineural hearing loss. They reported that the initial benefit from hearing aids, which emerged at 3 weeks (mean difference score, 29.6), was more dramatic than that which emerged at 3 months and 1 year (difference score, ~15 points). It appears that in their sample—as in that of Taylor (1993)—benefit may stabilize at 3 months such that it is comparable and sustainable after 1 year of use. The longitudinal study of Malinoff and Weinstein (1989) corroborated the data of Taylor (1993) as well as did the findings of Newman et al. (1993a). Based on the pattern of findings described above, it appears that a period of accommodation, adaptation, or acclimatization may occur within the first several months of hearing aid use such that the magnitude of benefit in the psychosocial domain may change somewhat over time, with reality and exposure to a variety of listening situations moderating the initial enthusiasm some people feel after the initial hearing aid fitting. The findings from the longitudinal studies on benefit in the psychosocial domain concur with the observations made by Gatehouse (1991), in that stabilization appears to take place approximately 3 months after the initial fitting. This trend underlines the importance of following clients over time (at least for 3 months) as problems arise that can probably be remedied through counseling and/or hearing aid modification. The psychological literature is replete with studies demonstrating that 3 months is a key time frame for adaptation or acclimatization in a variety of domains.

In sum, it is clear from the above review that the benefit derived from hearing aids can be quantified using subjective measures of hearing aid outcome. These tools enable the audiologist to demonstrate short-term, medium-term, and long-term benefits from traditional hearing aid technologies. A number of factors have been found to influence findings on the self-assessment scales and are noteworthy, as they have implications for interpretation of outcomes and for conducting hearing aid fittings in the context of audiologic rehabilitation.

VARIABLES INFLUENCING OUTCOMES WITH HEARING AIDS ON SELF-REPORT MEASURES

One myth surrounding hearing aids is that older adults use their hearing aids less consistently and derive less benefit from them than do younger adults. A series of studies have demonstrated that this conclusion cannot be substantiated empirically. Bender and Mueller (1984) compared younger and older adults in their subjective judgments of hearing aid use, satisfaction, and benefit. After 1 year of hearing aid use, the responses of older adults were comparable to those of younger adults. In fact, the vast majority of older adults reported more than a moderate degree of benefit and satisfaction with amplification. Kochkin (1992) also reported that there were no statistically significant differences by age group in overall mean satisfaction ratings. Ebinger et al. (1995) found that older and younger adults reported comparable benefit in the disability domain from CIC hearing aids. Specifically, according to responses to the APHAB, the percentage of aided problems in various listening conditions was comparable for older and younger adults. Further, the CIC units reduced the percentage of listening problems experienced by older and younger adults to below the 50th percentile of the norms established by Cox and Alexander (1995). Finally, Primeau (1997) reported that older and younger adults were comparable in the magnitude of perceived benefit in the psychosocial domain that emerged on the HHIE/HHIA. Cox et al. (1999) recently reported that in their sample of 83 older adults who were experienced hearing aid users, older subjects reported less unpleasant reactions to amplified sounds than did younger individuals.

Cost is another factor that has been considered a variable influencing hearing aid benefit. Newman et al. (1993a) explored the effects of financial outlay on self-perceived hearing aid benefit. As noted above, the older adults comprising the sample had essentially mild to moderate sensorineural hearing loss. Individuals who paid privately for their hearing aids who had comparable hearing levels and prefitting HHIE scores were age-matched to the group of subjects whose health insurance paid for the hearing aid. The magnitude of hearing aid benefit at 3 weeks and 6 months was comparable for the insured and uninsured groups. That is, each group demonstrated a statistically and clinically significant reduction in perceived emotional and social handicap following short- and long-term hearing aid use. These data suggest that financial outlay for a hearing aid does not appear to influence perceived hearing aid benefit in the psychosocial domain.

Three other potential variables that may influence hearing aid outcomes include the perspective of significant others, expectations regarding the value of hearing aids, and personality. Chmiel and Jerger (1996) evaluated the effect of hearing aids on the quality of life of older adults with or without a central auditory processing disorder. Subjects who had primarily high-frequency sensorineural hearing loss were classified into two groups according to scores on the dichotically presented synthetic sentences (DSI) test. The DSI normal group (n = 42) had comparable audiograms to those in the DSI abnormal group (n = 21). The subjects who were closely matched for age (with a mean age of 72 years for the former group and 70 years for the latter group) were fit monaurally with either a Siemens Triton 3000 or a 3M Memory Mate digital/analog hybrid instrument. Their data suggested the treatment effects varied as a function of group membership. Persons in the DSI nor-

mal group derived significant benefit from their hearing aids as evidenced by the reduction in HHIE scores after 6 weeks of hearing aid use. Subjects in the DSI abnormal group, namely those considered to have central auditory processing disorder (CAPD), did not derive clinically significant benefits from hearing aids in the psychosocial domain of function as evidenced by the comparability of scores on the HHIE at baseline and after 6 weeks of hearing aid use. The apparent central auditory deficit appeared to attenuate the self-perceived improvement in quality of life afforded by amplification. Informal caregivers, however, perceived benefits in the psychosocial domain attributable to hearing aid use in older adults with CAPD. Caregiver ratings of psychosocial handicap experienced by subjects with CAPD revealed statistically significant reductions in scores on the Hearing Handicap Inventory for the Elderly for Significant Others (HHIE-SO). That is, even when the patient with CAPD did not report a reduction in hearing handicap with hearing aid use, the significant other often reported a reduction in handicap as a result of hearing aid use. The latter finding suggests that hearing aids may reduce the stress on communication partners even though the respondent with CAPD does not necessarily judge hearing aids to be effective in reducing their psychosocial handicap. Hence, the HHIE-SO as a prefitting and postfitting measure is sensitive to short-term and long-term differences achieved with hearing aid use (Newman and Weinstein, 1988). Information from significant others can also be helpful during counseling sessions to help formulate the content to be discussed with the audiologist.

Schum (1999) speculated that level of need of the hearing aid user may influence the level of perceived benefit in the disability domain. That is, do client expectations regarding hearing aid use influence the ultimate outcome? A sample of 82 adults participated in their study. The mean bilateral hearing level across frequencies of subjects in his sample was 46.3 dB HL. The majority of subjects had sensorineural hearing loss and approximately 30% had previously used hearing aids. Subjects completed the HAPI and the Hearing Aid Needs Assessment (HANA) (Attachment 31). The HANA was designed as a companion scale to the HAPI and the shortened HAPI (Schum, 1992). It consists of 11 questions drawn from the HAPI. The client is asked to rate each of 11 situations on 3 criteria, namely how often he or she is in the situation, how much difficulty he or she currently experiences, and how much benefit is expected from the new hearing aids (Schum, 1999). Forty-two subjects completed the HANA before the hearing aid fitting, were monitored over time, and completed the HAPI approximately 2 to 3 months after the fitting. Overall expectations were higher than the benefits ultimately achieved. However, expectations and achieved benefit did coincide on the questions requiring rating of nonspeech sounds. The match between expectations and benefit was higher for quiet situations than it was for noisy situations. The finding that client expectations were higher than the actual benefit achieved is in keeping with expectations performance theory, which suggests that satisfaction with a device or service is achieved when performance matches expectations. Hence, before fitting individuals with hearing aids, the audiologist must make sure to instill realistic expectations in keeping with what hearing aids can reasonably provide (Schum, 1999).

Cox et al. (1999) attempted to examine the relationship between self-reported hearing aid outcomes and aspects of personality that might influence responses to self-perceived hearing aid benefit. Eighty-three older adults who had previous experience with hearing aids participated in their study. Subjects had audiograms typical of individuals as they age, namely mild to moderate hearing loss that was more pronounced in the high frequencies. Subjects completed the APHAB and three measures of personality including the State-Trait Anxiety Inventory (STAI) (which quantifies anxiety level), the Myers-Briggs Type Indicator (MBTI) (which assesses extroversion-introversion dimensions of personality), and a measure of locus of control (Cox et al., 1999). Although the con-

tribution was not that large, the extroversion-introversion dimension of personality was found to contribute significantly to hearing aid benefit in reverberant conditions, noisy situations, and relatively quiet situations. Extroversion appeared to account for approximately 10 to 20% of the variance in APHAB benefit scores regardless of extent of hearing impairment. Hence, they found that outgoing individuals tend to report significant speech communication benefit from their hearing aids (Cox et al., 1999). They also found that people who feel that others are more in control of situations than they are reported amplified sounds to be unpleasant; hence, benefit scores were low. The variance in APHAB scores accounted for by the locus of control measure was, however, quite minimal (~10%). Gatehouse (1994) also found that aspects of personality (including anxiety level, affect, and attitudes toward and expectations of hearing aid use) effect the eventual reduction in disability due to and satisfaction achieved with hearing aids.

Finally, a question that surrounds much of audiologic practice is whether counseling influences outcomes with hearing aids as measured using self-report data. Abrams et al. (1992) demonstrated that benefit from hearing aids, namely improvements in emotional and social function, can be enhanced when a hearing aid is dispensed in the context of a counseling-based audiologic rehabilitation program. Abrams et al. (1992) divided their sample of older adults with mild to moderate sensorineural hearing loss into three treatment groups. Treatment group I received a hearing aid and participated in 3 weeks of counseling-based audiologic rehabilitation. The counseling-based audiologic rehabilitation included an overview of the anatomy of the ear, an overview of hearing and communication, discussions about speechreading, and an overview of assistive listening devices. Treatment group II received the hearing aid accompanied by a brief counseling session. Treatment group III served as the control group, merely completing the HHIE at baseline and at the 2-month follow-up visit. Mean HHIE scores for each group were comparable at baseline.

Two months after the hearing aid fitting, there was a clinically and statistically significant reduction in HHIE scores for treatment groups I and II, but not for the control group. Subjects obtaining the hearing aid and counseling-based audiologic rehabilitation experienced more significant reductions in psychosocial handicap than those who obtained the hearing aid without rehabilitation. Furthermore, self-perceived psychosocial handicap was reduced in 45% of participants in treatment group I versus 18% of subjects in treatment group II. This study demonstrates that the self-perception of hearing handicap can be reduced significantly in persons who have used hearing aids and have participated in a counseling-based audiologic rehabilitation program. Hence, it underlines the value of counseling-based audiologic rehabilitation in the hearing aid delivery process.

In sum, contrary to popular belief, age and cost may not influence outcomes with hearing aids as has previously been assumed. Further, as would be expected, expectations and personality do influence responses to self-assessment scales and ultimate outcomes with hearing aids. Finally, counseling is an important adjunct to the hearing aid fitting because it can positively influence outcomes.

USE OF SUBJECTIVE OUTCOME MEASURES IN COMPARING DIFFERENT HEARING AIDS

In addition to widespread use of subjective outcome measures in quantifying absolute benefit from hearing aids, investigators have begun to use these instruments for contrasting different hearing aids in a clinical trial paradigm. Newman and Sandridge (1998) evaluated the effectiveness of three commercially available behind-the-ear hearing aids representing the continuum of hearing aid technology including a linear unit; a two-channel, mini–behind-the-ear hearing aid; and a seven-band, two-channel digital signal processing (DSP) hearing aid. All subjects wore each hearing aid for a 4-week interval. Outcomes with the hearing aids were assessed using objective speech mea-

sures (SPIN), two self-report measures including the APHAB and the HHIE, and the Knowles Hearing Aid Satisfaction Survey. The low and high predictability sentences of the SPIN were effective in distinguishing between the three different types of hearing aids; however, the differences were quite small (on the order of 8 to 10 points). Hearing aid benefit according to difference scores on the APHAB did not differ significantly across the three different hearing aids. Similarly, benefit scores did not appear to differ across hearing aids on the HHIE, nor did satisfaction scores on the Knowles Hearing Aid Satisfaction Survey. Hearing aid use patterns did not differ across hearing aids either. The authors concluded that the large variability in responses to the various questionnaires may have accounted for the fact that these measures did not differentiate among hearing aids. Nevertheless, each of the questionnaires did demonstrate that the subjects derived benefit from the various hearing aids, judging from the difference between aided and unaided scores on the questionnaires with each device. The COSI, which enables the individual to hand-pick the listening situations that are problematic, may be more sensitive to differences among hearing aids.

Finally, Humes et al. (1999) attempted to compare the benefits of two-channel, wide-dynamic-range compression hearing aids (D2) fit binaurally and housed in an in-the-canal assembly with the binaural performance of a linear circuit using subjective measures of benefit as well as tests of speech recognition ability in quiet and noise. Subjects were adults with mild to severe hearing loss. Evaluation of benefit from hearing aids was assessed after a minimum of 2 months of hearing aid use, this time frame being predetermined by the authors to be the adjustment period necessary for maturation of hearing aid benefit or acclimatization to set in. Stated differently, an adjustment period (i.e., 2 to 3 months following the initial hearing aid fitting) is necessary to allow for plateau performance wherein a new hearing aid user is given the opportunity to make maximum use of the newly amplified information (Humes et al., 1999). As was the case with the study of Newman and Sandridge (1998), subjects demonstrated significant benefit from both sets of hearing aids over the unaided condition according to difference scores on the speech recognition tests and subjective benefit ratings on the HAPI. Subjects also reported that hearing aids made listening easier. The authors reported that observed differences between devices were not noted frequently on the measure of subjective benefit (HAPI), although differences did emerge when speech recognition ability was assessed at lower speech presentation levels. The authors also found that the objective measures of benefit (e.g., scores on the Connected Speech Test [CST] and the NU-6 word lists) coupled with quality ratings were predictive of the circuit selected by the majority of subjects in the study. The vast majority of subjects preferred the new D2 circuit over the linear hearing aids.

Multidimensional Assessment of Hearing Aid Benefit

Assessing hearing aid outcomes is a complicated endeavor because it is unclear as to how outcomes should be defined. No one model for measuring outcomes has emerged. The author's view, which is in keeping with the philosophy of Gagne et al. (1994), is that outcomes should be considered along a continuum of the consequences of disease which incorporates impairment, disability, and handicap (Weinstein, 1996, 1997). Impairment, of course, is any loss or abnormality of structure or function that can be measured audiometrically using speech recognition measures, functional gain, or real-ear measures. In contrast, disability is the functional consequence of the impairment manifested in inability to perform some routine activities of daily living. Responses to such subjective measures as the HAPI and the APHAB are considered to be indices of disability. Handicap is seen as the social consequence of the impairment or disability and limits the individual from fulfilling social roles. The HHIE has evolved as a measure of subjective handicap (WHO, 1980).

Changes in impairment (e.g., aided speech recognition performance), changes in disability (e.g., change in APHAB scores aided versus unaided), and changes in handicap (e.g., difference between HHIE scores aided and unaided) have become the markers for measuring outcomes in audiologic rehabilitation. When audiologists first began to assess outcomes, one measure was chosen as the index of treatment effectiveness. Disagreement arose over which was the best measure of treatment effects, and some investigators suggested that possibly hearing aid outcomes is not a unidimensional construct but rather has several independent dimensions associated with it (Humes, 1999). Weinstein et al. (1995) were among the first investigators to conceptualize hearing aid outcomes as having several related and sometimes unrelated dimensions. Weinstein et al. (1995) reported on the results of a pilot study of seven subjects fit with linear hearing aids. In all cases, real-ear insertion gain values met the NAL-R prescribed target with slight deviations at 4000 Hz. Functional gain ranged from 15 to 25 dB depending on hearing loss severity and hearing aid gain. Seventy-one percent of subjects were reportedly satisfied with their hearing aids and experienced statistically and clinically significant reductions in perceived handicap on the HHIE/HHIA. The remaining 29% of subjects met the target but were not satisfied and felt that the hearing aid did not alleviate their handicap. Benefit in the disability domain, as evidenced by change in APHAB scores before and after fitting, was more difficult to achieve because of the large critical differences necessary to conclude that the hearing aid is in fact beneficial (Cox and Alexander, 1995; Cox and Alexander, 1991b). According to responses to the Knowles Satisfaction Survey, subjects who experienced a reduction in the extent of handicap on the HHIE/-HHIA also expressed satisfaction with features of their hearing aids. This preliminary study underlines the importance of combining measures of outcome because even when target values are met, benefit in one domain (e.g., disability) does not necessarily signify benefit in another domain (e.g., handicap). Their conclusions suggest that there are several dimensions of outcome that clinicians should consider.

Humes (1999) presented a theoretical principal components factor analysis of hearing aid outcomes. He incorporated measures of subjective benefit (e.g., HAPI, HHIE, hearing aid satisfaction, hours of use) and measures of objective benefit (e.g., aided speech recognition) into the equation. A total of 13 measures of hearing aid outcome were analyzed to determine the factors that contributed most substantially to the variability in hearing aid outcomes. His data support the notion that hearing aid outcomes are multidimensional rather than unidimensional (Humes, 1999). He concluded that hearing aid outcomes have a well-defined underlying structure, with aided speech recognition performance emerging as a major factor and subjective satisfaction and benefit ratings emerging as less of a factor in outcome measures. The theoretical study by Humes (1999) and the findings of Weinstein et al. (1995) suggest that perhaps an ideal model for assessing outcomes with hearing aids has emerged. Data-driven methods are important given the context of health care of the 1990s and the new millennium.

An Ideal Approach to Measuring Outcomes in Audiologic Rehabilitation

It is clear from the above review that outcomes assessment is moving out of its infancy into the toddler stage, and with such growth comes a lack of complacency and numerous questions. To date, there is not a best way for measuring outcomes in audiologic rehabilitation, nor is there one approach that meets everyone's needs. It is the author's belief that a multiple-attacks approach, wherein hearing aid outcomes are seen as a multidimensional phenomenon, is the best way to proceed at this point in the evolutionary process of outcomes assessment (Frattali, 1998). Audiologists should consider outcomes assessment as a tool designed to help the patient, provider, and third-party payer (when appropriate) make

more informed decisions regarding the impact of a particular treatment on the client's/patient's life and lifestyle (Frattali, 1998). Outcomes must be defined operationally depending on the change in behavior that is being measured. Ultimate outcomes are those that demonstrate the social validity of audiologic interventions such as social integration, positive affect, independence, and functional communication (Frattali, 1998). The client in consultation with the audiologist is the ultimate arbiter of the outcome that is most important. Hence, it is difficult to prescribe an approach to outcomes assessment. Based on the data that have emerged, the author advocates that audiologists incorporate an objective measure of benefit, a subjective measure of benefit, and a preference judgment that can emerge from comparative trials even with one instrument and various settings. The latter should tap into the client's expectations because these influence ultimate choice and outcomes. It appears that aided speech recognition performance at a challenging rather than optimal presentation level, some measure of subjective benefit such as the APHAB or HHIE, and an estimate of the client's preference that can emerge through the COSI in combination with informal conversations is effective. When a discrepancy emerges between the measures, the decision should rest with the client's judgments as research seems to support the notion that the client often knows best.

An important issue that one must address before moving down the outcomes assessment path is to make sure to measure outcome at an optimal time. It is critical that the time interval between the fitting and the outcome assessment be long enough to allow for adjustment or acclimatization but not too long so that discontent and frustration predominate. Data from a number of studies suggest that 2 to 3 months after the fitting is the optimal time frame. This allows for the client to return several times after the initial fitting for some counseling and hearing aid adjustments before the actual assessment of hearing aid outcomes takes place. In the author's view, outcomes data should be an integral part of practice as an invaluable tool for assisting the audiologist to better serve hearing-impaired consumers. Although currently the debate is over which assessment tool is best (not unlike the debate in the 1970s over which speech recognition test [if any] was best for differentiating among hearing aids), audiologists should be proactive and test the available measures to decide which one works best for the particular setting and client base served. If audiologists are to remain viable players in this current service delivery environment, outcomes data should be collected as a routine part of daily practice.

REFERENCES

Abrams H, Chisolm T, Guerreiro S, et al. The effects of intervention strategy on self perception of hearing handicap. Ear Hear 1992;13:371–377.

Bender D, Mueller G. Factors influencing the decision to obtain amplification. ASHA, 1984;26:120.

Bentler R, Niebuhr D, Getta J, et al. Longitudinal study of hearing aid effectiveness. I: objective measures. J Speech Hear Res 1993;36:808–819.

Boston Working Group on Improving Health Care Outcomes through Geriatric Rehabilitation. Med Care 1997;35(Suppl):JS4–JS20.

Brown S, Nelson A, Bronkesh S, et al. Patient satisfaction pays. Rockville, MD: Aspen, 1993.

Chmiel R, Jerger J. Hearing aid use, central auditory disorder, and hearing handicap in elderly persons. J Am Acad Audiol 1996;7:190–202.

Cleary P, McNeil B. (1988). Patient satisfaction as an indicator of quality of care. Inquiry 1988;25:25–36.

Cox R, Alexander G. The Abbreviated Profile of Hearing Aid Benefit. Ear Hear 1995;16:176–186.

Cox R, Gilmore C, Alexander G. Comparison of two questionnaires for patient assessed hearing aid benefit. J Am Acad Audiol 1991a;2:134–145.

Cox R, Gilmore C, Alexander G. Objective and self-report measures of hearing aid benefit. In: Studebaker G, Bess F, Beck L, eds. The Vanderbilt hearing aid report, II. Parkton, MD: York, 1991b.

Cox R, Alexander G, Gray G. Personality and the subjective assessment of hearing aids. J Am Acad Audiol 1999;10:1–13.

Dempsey J. The Hearing Performance Inventory as a tool in fitting hearing aids. J Acad Rehabil Audiol 1986;19:116–125.

Demorest M, Erdman S. Scale composition and item analysis of the Communication Profile for the Hearing Impaired. J Speech Hear Res 1986;29:515–535.

Dillon H, James A, Ginis J. Client oriented scale of improvement (COSI) and its relationship to several other measures of benefit and satisfaction provided by hearing aids. J Am Acad Audiol 1997;8:27–43.

Donabedian A. Criteria, norms and standards of quality: what do they mean? Am J Public Health 1981;71:409–412.

Donabedian A. The quality of care: how can it be assessed. JAMA 1988;260:1743–1748.

Ebinger K, Holland S, Holland J, et al. Using the APHAB to assess benefit from CIC hearing aids. Poster session presented at the American Academy of Audiology annual meeting, Dallas, Texas, 1995.

Etienne J. Quantifying a hearing handicap. Hear Rev 1996;3:26–34.

Frattali C. Outcomes measurement: definitions, dimensions and perspectives. In: Frattali C, ed. Measuring outcomes in speech-language pathology. New York: Thieme, 1998.

Gagne J, McDuffy S, Getty L. Some limitations of evaluative investigations based solely on normed outcome measures. J Am Acad Audiol 1999;10:46–62.

Gatehouse S. Acclimatization to amplified speech. Paper presented at the International Hearing Aid Conference, Iowa City, Iowa, 1991.

Gatehouse S. Components and determinants of hearing aid benefit. Ear Hear 1994;15:30–49.

Giolas T, Owens E, Lamb S, et al. Hearing Performance Inventory. J Speech Hear Disord 1979;44:169–195.

Humes L. Dimensions of hearing aid outcome. J Am Acad Audiol 1999;10:26–39.

Humes L, Halling D, Coughlin M. Reliability and stability of various hearing aid outcome measures in a group of elderly hearing aid wearers. J Speech Hear Res 1996;39:923–935.

Humes L, Christensen L, Thomas T, et al. A comparison of the aided performance and benefit provided by a linear and two channel wide dynamic range compression hearing aid. J Speech Lang Hear Res 1999;32:65–79.

Hyde M, Riko K. A decision-analytic approach to audiological rehabilitation. In: Gagne JP, Murray NT, eds. Research in audiological rehabilitation: current trends and future directions. J Am Acad Rehabil Audiol Monogr 1994;27.

Kane R. Improving outcomes in rehabilitation: a call to arms. Med Care 1997;35, JS4–JS7.

Kochkin S. MarkeTrak III. Higher hearing aid sales don't signal better market penetration. Hear J 1992;45:47–54.

Kochkin S. MarkeTrak IV. What is the viable market for hearing aids? Hear J 1997;50:31–39.

Kricos P, Holmes A. Efficacy of audiologic rehabilitation for older adults. J Am Acad Audiol 1996;7:219–229.

Liang M. Response to disablement outcomes in geriatric rehabilitation. Med Care 1997;35:JS8.

Malinoff R, Weinstein B. Measurement of hearing aid benefit in the elderly. Ear Hear 1989;10:354–356.

McCarthy P. Hearing aid fitting and audiologic rehabilitation: a complementary relationship. Am J Audiol 1996;5:24–29.

Montgomery A. Treatment efficacy in adult audiological rehabilitation. In: Gagne JP, Murray NT, eds. Research in audiological rehabilitation: current trends and future directions. J Am Acad Rehabil Audiol Monogr 1994;27:317–337.

Mueller G. Hearing aids and people: strategies for a successful match. Hear J 1996;49:13–28.

Mulrow C, Aguilar C, Endicott J, et al. Quality of life changes and hearing impairment. Ann Intern Med 1990;113,:188–194.

Mulrow C, Tuley M, Aguilar C. Sustained benefits of hearing aids. J Speech Hear Res 1992;35:1402–1405.

Newman C, Jacobson G, Hug G, et al. Practical method for quantifying hearing aid benefit in older adults. J Am Acad Audiol 1991;2:70–75.

Newman C, Sandridge S. Benefit from, satisfaction with and cost-effectiveness of three different hearing aid technologies. Am J Audiol 1998;7:115–128.

Newman C, Weinstein B. The Hearing Handicap Inventory for the Elderly. Ear Hear 1988;9:81–85.

Newman C, Hug G, Wharton G, et al. The influence of hearing aid cost on perceived benefit in older adults. Ear Hear 1993a;14:285–289.

Newman C, Weinstein B, Jacobson G, et al. Test retest reliability of the Hearing Handicap Inventory for Adults. Ear Hear 1993b;12:155–157.

Ottenbacher K. Methodological issue in measurement of functional status and rehabilitation outcomes. In: Dittmar S, Gresham G, eds. Functional assessment and outcome measures for the rehabilitation health professional. Rockville, MD: Aspen, 1987.

Pascoe G. Patient satisfaction in primary health care: a literature review and analysis. Eval Progr Plan 1983;6:185–210.

Primeau R. Hearing aid benefit in adults and older people. Semin Hear 1997;18:29–36.

Robertson S, Colborn A. (1997) Outcomes research for rehabilitation: issues and solutions. J Rehabil Outcomes Measure Appl Methodol Technol 1997;1:15–24.

Schum D. Responses of elderly hearing aid users on the Hearing Aid Performance Inventory. Ear Hear 1992;6:354–356.

Schum D. Perceived hearing aid benefit in relation to perceived needs. J Am Acad Audiol 1999;10:40–45.

Simon S, Patrick A. Understanding and assessing consumer satisfaction in rehabilitation. J Rehabil Outcomes Measure Appl Methodol Technol 1997;5:1–15.

Taylor K. Self-perceived and audiometric evaluations of hearing aid benefit in the elderly. Ear Hear 1993;14:390–395.

Ventry I, Weinstein B. The Hearing Handicap Inventory for the Elderly: a new tool. Ear Hear 1982;3:128–134.

Walden B, Demorest M, Hepler E. Self report approach to assessing benefit derived from amplification. J Speech Hear Res 1984;27:49–56.

Weinstein B. Treatment efficacy: hearing aids in the management of hearing loss in adults. J Speech Hear Res 1996;39(Suppl):37–45.

Weinstein B. Outcome measures in the hearing aid fitting process. Trends Ampl 1997;2:117–137.

Weinstein B, Newman C, Montano J. A multidimensional analysis of hearing aid benefit. Paper presented at the first biennial Hearing Aid Research and Development conference, Bethesda Maryland, 1995.

Weitzman B. Improving quality of care. In: Kovner A, ed. Health care delivery in the United States. New York: Springer, 1995.

Wilson B, Cleary P. Linking clinical variables with quality of life: conceptual model of patient outcomes. JAMA 1995;273:59–65.

World Health Organization. International classification of impairments, disabilities and handicaps. Geneva: World Health Organization, 1980.

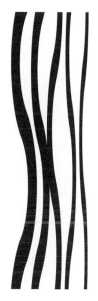

Future Directions for Research in Audiologic Rehabilitation

Nancy Tye-Murray, Ph.D.

In several of the foregoing chapters, the authors have explicitly considered four distinct population groups who have hearing loss and who require aural (re)habilitation services. These four populations represent the full spectrum of life stages: infancy (Chapters 4, 5, and 6), childhood (Chapters 7, 8, and 9), adulthood (Chapters 10, 11, and 12), and the later years (Chapter 13). Most practicing speech and hearing professionals will likely have an opportunity to provide services to members of each of these populations at some time in their career, to a greater or lesser extent.

The materials and information provided by this book's authors have equipped readers with a sound understanding of who their patients are, what patients' aural rehabilitation needs are likely to be, and how to design and implement an optimal aural rehabilitation plan for a particular individual. There is no doubt that future editions will contain some of the same information as is included in the current edition. Today's clinical practices and their theoretical underpinnings have emerged gradually over time, and most are based on sound scientific data. It is likely that much of what we do and what we know now will stand the test of time.

Even so, many scientists and clinicians are actively investigating new frontiers in the field of aural rehabilitation, and it is likely that much supplementary data and many new ideas will arise. Undoubtedly, some topics will receive different treatments in future texts. Quite simply, we will have learned more and tried more in the ensuing years.

The current chapter's purpose is twofold. The first purpose is to alert readers to those issues that they may learn more about in the future if they opt to become practicing speech and hearing professionals. The second purpose is to spark the interest of student scientists in possible research topics.

For each of the four populations, trends and/or developments in society are identified that have relevance to future research, and then a handful of important topics are considered. Questions and issues are outlined; for some topics, possible difficulties that may confound investigation are identified.

Infants With Hearing Loss

TRENDS AND DEVELOPMENTS

Advances in neonatology and critical care medicine have resulted in a greater survival rate of high-risk newborns and babies. Infants who might have died in earlier times now survive, often with more than one disability, including hearing loss. Families of babies who have hearing loss expect speech and hearing professionals to provide assistance and support that will enable their children to achieve their full potential. Public policy reflects these trends. Universal screening of newborns is becoming commonplace in hospitals across the United States. Public Laws 94-142 and 99-452 stipulate that public resources be funneled toward early identification and service provision for young children who have hearing loss.

Two important research topics that are likely to receive much attention in the near future relate to early intervention procedures for infants. Specifically, these questions are, "How do we best diagnose the degree of hearing loss in infants and fit appropriate listening devices?" and "What is the value of various early intervention efforts?"

Diagnosing degree of hearing loss and fitting listening devices

The issues of how to diagnose degree of hearing loss and how to fit listening devices will likely receive much attention by researchers and clinicians, regardless of whether the listening device under consideration is either a hearing aid or a cochlear implant.

Hearing Aids. According to Seewald (1998), many audiologists do not use systematic approaches or current technologies when working with the young pediatric patient. For instance, one difficulty in fitting amplification to babies is that audiologists typically desire to provide amplification shortly after identification, which may be at 6 months or younger. However, the most common procedures for assessing hearing loss (i.e., aided thresholds and word recognition tests) and selecting and fitting amplification devices are not age-appropriate. Moreover, 2-cc coupler specifications that are often used to select hearing aid output limitations are inappropriate because there may be a 30-dB difference in what is found in a coupler versus an infant. An important direction for future research is to develop optimal fitting strategies and optimal service delivery models. For instance, fitting babies with hearing aids requires specialized professional expertise. It may be that in the fu-

ture, only certain hearing centers will be designated as facilities qualified to fit infants with hearing aids.

Cochlear Implants. The issue of how to assess degree of hearing loss in infants and how to fit a listening device is especially germane when a baby is a possible candidate for cochlear implantation. In 1998, the Food and Drug Administration approved the Cochlear Corporation's (Englewood, Colorado) cochlear implant for children as young as 18 months of age. Some centers currently provide cochlear implants on a limited basis to children who are even younger than 18 months. It is highly likely that the age at which implantation may occur will continue to retreat toward birth. A major impetus for this trend is the fact that children who receive implants at younger ages have been shown to outperform children who receive implants later on tests of speech production and speech perception (Tye-Murray et al., 1995; Fryauf-Bertschy et al., 1997).

It is essential that diagnostic procedures be developed that permit the determination of whether a baby has usable residual hearing and the determination of whether the child would benefit more from a hearing aid or a cochlear implant. For example, if a baby has moderate to severe hearing loss, he or she is not a candidate for a cochlear implant under today's guidelines. Thus, determining the degree of hearing loss becomes a critical issue for selecting the optimal listening device.

Procedures for mapping a cochlear implant for an infant must also be developed. Mapping procedures entail establishing electrical thresholds and maximum comfort levels for the electrodes in the electrode array as well as loudness balancing the electrodes.

Finally, it is important to develop means for documenting progress with a cochlear implant. Many traditional measures, such as those obtained with tests of speech production and speech recognition, are inappropriate for this population because babies probably do not have the necessary baseline skills to take the tests. Thus, we may have to rely on nonverbal measures, such as nonverbal communicative intents (Nicholas and Geers, 1997), to monitor whether a baby is making satisfactory progress with the device. Nonverbal communicative intents occur during the prelinguistic stages of language development and include a wide variety of vocal, gestural, facial, and even verbal signals that are intended to convey meaning. Preliminary research with a group of 13 36-month-old deaf and normal-hearing children suggest that early communicative attempts relate to later verbal language development (Nicolas and Geers, 1997); therefore, attention to these behaviors may indicate whether the child is progressing with the cochlear implant.

Efficacy of early intervention

An increasing body of data suggests that children whose hearing losses are identified by 6 months of age are likely to develop better receptive and expressive language skills than children whose hearing losses are identified after 6 months of age (Yoshinaga-Itano et al., 1998). Findings such as these have underscored the importance of early screening for hearing loss and early intervention.

The growing advocacy for universal screening has led to new questions about the outcome of intervention. Researchers are now addressing such questions as "What is good intervention?" "How do different intervention strategies compare?" "How much progress should we expect over a given period?" "Are we closing gaps between chronologic and language age over time?" "Is the quality of a baby's life made better by early intervention?" (Moeller, 1998).

These questions are difficult to address experimentally for several reasons (Calderon and Greenberg, 1993; Moeller, 1998), and discussion in this section will focus primarily on those difficulties. The first difficulty is that hearing loss has a low incidence, and the population of infants who have hearing loss is heterogeneous. This state of affairs has many ramifications for experimentation. For instance, it is hard to obtain a sufficient number of subjects to par-

ticipate in an experiment, and it is almost impossible to implement random assignment and selection. Ordinarily, a researcher would opt to select subjects randomly from a pool of possible subjects and then randomly assign them to one of the possible comparison treatments. With few available subjects, it is not easy to assign children randomly to different treatments for comparison purposes. The heterogeneity of the population also poses problems. Extraneous variables, such as co-occurring medical conditions or cognitive impairment in some subjects, are likely to confound results. It is often difficult to separate outcomes that are due to hearing loss alone and outcomes that are due to hearing loss coupled with other medical, cognitive, home, or environmental conditions.

A considerable obstruction to experimentation relates to ethical considerations. It may not be ethical either to assign an infant to a no-treatment group for comparison purposes or to assign an infant to a treatment that is thought a priori to be inferior to an alternative treatment. For example, a researcher might be interested in determining whether children who eventually become good readers have families who received more professional support than children who eventually became poor readers (e.g., Schlesinger and Acree, 1984). However, it would not be appropriate to withhold support purposefully from parents to test the hypothesis that early support leads to higher reading achievement. This kind of question would probably have to be addressed with a retrospective experimental design.

Another difficulty in conducting research with infants lies in the fact that most intervention programs are multidimensional and complex. For instance, a program's success may vary as a function of the clinician who is primarily involved in the implementation of a program or as a function of the family and the baby, or even as a function of the kind (and appropriateness) of the amplification device used. Therefore, it is possible that the same experimental question may give way to very different experimental results on different occasions.

Finally, there is the difficulty of defining outcome (Moeller, 1998) and the issue of how to define success and how to measure it. For instance, do we define success in terms of a baby's subsequent language development? If so, what is the optimal way to measure progress and at what point in the child's life does one measure it? Other parameters of a child's performance that might be used as benchmarks for success include the child's speech development, self-concept and personal adjustment, and academic achievement. What constitutes success in one parent's or researcher's eye may not necessarily constitute success in another's.

There are important questions to be asked concerning early intervention programs and formidable hurdles to leap to provide answers. The next few years will bring more research activity in this area.

Young and School-Aged Children

TRENDS AND DEVELOPMENTS

Two major trends relevant to young children and school-aged children are apparent. First, since the passage of U.S. Public Law 94–142 (the Education for All Handicapped Children Act) in 1975, more and more children remain in their home communities and receive a public education. Moores (1992) reported that enrollment in residential programs has declined by 6945 students, whereas enrollment in public day classes increased by 8163 students since 1975. This trend suggests that many decisions about a child's intervention program are made by the families and professionals available in the family's locale. The intervention plan is often implemented within the purview of educational settings primarily designed for children who have normal hearing.

The second apparent trend is that many children who are of school age and who have profound (and even severe to profound) hearing loss use cochlear implants. This trend will only continue to grow. Some professionals have suggested that children who use cochlear implants may be served better by somewhat different curricula, particularly for language instruction.

The following section considers how decisions about intervention are made and the development of appropriate instructional curricula.

Decisions about intervention

Three important decisions that parents and educators must make about the intervention program are communication mode, classroom placement, and listening device(s). Many years of experience and research point to the conclusion that no single route is appropriate for all children. A set of decisions that is optimal for one child might be inappropriate for another. For example, a child with significant residual hearing might excel in an oral-aural program and might be a candidate for mainstreaming in elementary school. A child with minimal hearing and reduced cognitive skills may benefit more from a program that uses manual communication to some extent and placement in a self-contained classroom.

A major challenge for researchers and clinicians is to develop procedures for placing children into appropriate intervention programs as early as possible. For example, some researchers have developed metrics to help families choose among communication modalities. Northern and Downs (1991) developed the Deafness Management Quotient (DMQ). This formula factors in residual hearing, central intactness, intellectual factors, family constellation, and socioeconomic situation. Moeller et al. (1990) devised a system that bases this decision on both family- and child-centered measures in addition to the progress a child makes during a 6-month period in a program conducted by speech and hearing professionals. This program is called the Diagnostic Early Intervention Project (DEIP).

In the future, researchers, clinicians, and educators might develop similar strategies for making decisions about other aspects of a child's intervention plan. For instance, a metric might indicate whether a child is best served in a self-contained classroom, part-time self-contained classroom and part-time mainstream classroom, part-time mainstream classroom and part-time resource room, or full-time mainstream classroom.

Curricula

Another area that deserves attention pertains to efficacy of various curricula and the development of new instructional routines. Few systematic studies have evaluated or compared curricula that are in use with children who have significant hearing loss. Carney and Moeller (1998), for instance, list several auditory training programs that have been designed for use with children who have cochlear implants (Robbins, 1990; Tye-Murray, 1992; Vergara and Miskiel, 1994). They lament that "specific performance data comparing curricula or testing their efficacy have not been published" (Carney and Moeller, 1998, p. 75).

Perhaps an area of curriculum development most in need of research is that of reading. Children who have significant hearing loss often are delayed and/or deviant in their reading skills compared with children who have normal hearing. The average reading level of deaf high school students is about at the third or fourth grade level (Allen, 1986), and rarely does a child exceed the 7.5 grade level (Trybus and Karchmer, 1977). Such poor performance is unacceptable, and a major effort must be launched to develop more effective reading programs. The need for research in this area is further underscored by this fact: there has been little improvement in the average reading performance of children who have significant hearing loss, relative to their normal hearing classmates, over the past 80 years (LaSasso and Mobley, 1997; Paul, 1997). What we have been doing, and what we are now doing, is not very effective.

Not all children who have significant hearing loss read poorly. For instance, some children in oral programs or model programs that use simultaneous communication perform better than average. Paul (1997) suggests that one direction for future research is to examine why these students perform better than others. In addition, we might develop a better description of the

reading process, so there are metatheoretical and theoretical frameworks on which to base curriculum design. The well-designed reading curriculum should take into account test-based, reader-based, and task-based variables (Paul, 1997).

Another issue in curriculum development pertains to those children who use cochlear implants. With the advent of these electronic devices, many deaf children are hearing more and speaking better than ever before in the history of deaf education. Some of our curricula that have been developed for previous generations may be inadequate for the present generation.

Many clinicians and educators believe that auditory training and speech-language therapy curricula for children who use cochlear implants can have content and organization similar to those that are appropriate for children who use hearing aids. For example, the same techniques and hierarchies of auditory training objectives may be appropriate for children who use hearing aids and children who use cochlear implants. The greatest difference might be that children who use cochlear implants progress faster and further in their skill acquisition than children who use hearing aids. Therefore, a child who uses a cochlear implant may someday perform comprehension-level exercises in an auditory-training program (Tye-Murray, 1992, 1998), whereas a child who uses a hearing aid may only advance to exercises that require closed-set identification.

Although some curricula may be appropriate for both groups, some may have to be revised. For instance, children who use cochlear implants may have more incidental learning of language than children who use hearing aids. They may require less structured language teaching techniques, and instead may progress with more naturalistic, real-world language instruction than their counterparts who use hearing aids (Tye-Murray, 1998, p. 499). However, this is speculation, and research is necessary to determine the optimal educational strategies for children who have more functional hearing than deaf children historically have demonstrated.

Adults With Hearing Loss

TRENDS AND DEVELOPMENTS

A major trend in society that may influence future research pertaining to adults who have hearing loss relates to noise exposure. Noise is a pervasive problem in the United States and has been increasing during the past 25 years. As technology advances, so do noise levels (Merry and Franks, 1995). In today's world, many professions create work environments that have sound levels above damage risk criteria (e.g., farmers, factory workers, car mechanics, professional musicians), and many people engage in leisure activities that expose them to noisy environments, such as target shooting or attending rock concerts (see Clark, 1998). This state of affairs points to at least two areas for future research, feasible noise protection devices and the development of effective noise-related education programs, such as communication strategies and hearing protection training.

Hearing protectors

One direction for research relates to types of hearing protection. In situations in which noise cannot be eliminated, individuals may wear ear protection such as earplugs or muffs. However, many workers do not do so because of safety reasons. They worry that they may not hear warning signals or shouts from coworkers. Thus, it would be valuable to develop noise protection devices that could permit warning signals to be intercepted while preventing reception of hazardous sound signals.

Communication strategies training programs tailored for noisy listening environments

In addition to not wanting to miss warning signals, some individuals do not use noise protection because they desire to communicate with coworkers and others in their environments. For these individuals, there is a need to develop communication strategies training programs. The goal of such programs would be to encourage persons who use ear protection to use facilitative strategies and repair strategies to promote con-

versational interactions. Facilitative and repair strategies are summarized in Tables 19.1 and 19.2.

When their hearing acuity is attenuated, an individual might use a facilitative strategy to influence speech recognition skills (e.g., the individual may make a concerted effort to focus on the talker's mouth movements to enhance his or her speechreading performance), the communication environment (e.g., the individual may suggest, "Let's walk over to the hall way where it is quieter"), the manner by which communication partners speak the messages (e.g., "Please face me when you speak"), and the message proper (e.g., using closed-set questions instead of open-set questions; e.g., "Did you say hammer or the ladder?" as opposed to, "What did you say?"). The individual may use a repair strategy to provide explicit instruction to the communication partner following a communication breakdown (e.g., "You said the boss is doing what?").

To develop effective communication strategies training programs, three directions of research might be addressed. The first direction is to identify ways that we can evaluate how well a particular person implements communication strategies. This information indicates particular training needs. This assessment must cover the following issues: (1) communication demands placed on the individual in a noisy environment, (2) how the inability to hear (because of ear protectors) may affect the person's activities, (3) how well the individual uses communications strategies, and (4) the patient's employment responsibilities. Assessment instruments for obtaining information about individuals' communication needs and behaviors currently include procedures for assessing performance in optimal listening conditions and not necessarily noisy (work) environments. They include interviews, questionnaires such as the Communication Profile for the Hearing Impaired (Demorest and Erdman, 1987), informal conversations (Erber, 1988), case histories, and simulated conversations such as Topicon (Erber, 1988). One future need for research is to develop means for assess-

Table 19.1
Facilitative strategies used by employees to influence speech recognition performance, the communication environment, the communication partners' presentation of a message, and the message

Facilitative strategies are meant to influence
1. Speech recognition performance
   a. Attending strategies: The employee pays attention to the situation or a particular word in a message to deduce a partially understood message
      Example: The employee approaches a snack bar and recognizes the word "candy" spoken by a concession stand woker. By combining the situational cues and the word "candy," the employee might guess that the message was, "Do you want candy?"
   b. Anticipatory strategies: The employee anticipates a topic of conversation and the related vocabulary before the communication interaction
      Example: The employee predicts the response or responses before approaching a coworker with a question
2. The communication environment
   a. Constructive strategies: The employee manipulates the environment to ensure optimal speech-reading and listening conditions
      Example: The employee asks a coworker to move away from a noisy fan in order to converse
3. The communication partner
   a. Instructive strategies: The employee informs the communication partner of appropriate speaker behaviors
      Example: The employee says, "I can't follow you. Could you please speak slower?"
4. The message
   a. Message-tailoring strategies: The employee informs the communication partner of appropriate message organization
      Example: The employee asks the communication partner to speak short, simple sentences

Adapted from Tye-Murray N, Witt B. Communication strategies training. Semin Hear 1997;18:153–165.

ing performance in real-world environments in which noise levels are high.

A second need related to communication strategies training is to develop effective training procedures. Optimal program length and optimal training activities must be determined. It may be that many persons in the workplace are not motivated to participate in a communication strategies training program, so methods for developing motivation may also need to be developed. Marketing models designed to increase motivation for a service or a product, such as those described by Kotler and Andreasen (1996), may provide guidance (see Tye-Murray 1998, p. 278, for application of this model). Finally, to create viable programs, methods of evaluating benefits of intervention must be developed. Many businesses will not support employee training without objective evidence of benefit.

Education programs about prevention of noise-induced hearing loss

A final area for research related to noise exposure and adults pertains to prevention of noise-induced hearing loss. Many members of the general population do not realize that exposure to noise throughout their daily lives can lead to significant hearing loss, whether they are at work, play, or home. The good news is that noise-induced hearing loss is preventable. The bad news is that increasing numbers of people experience this kind of hearing impairment, some because they are not aware of the dangers of noise exposure and some because they are unwilling to take preventive measures. There is a great need to identify "strategies to prevent hazardous exposures, to protect the hearing of individuals who must or choose to be exposed, and to offer methods of rehabilitation for those who must communicate in a noisy environment or cope with a noise induced

Table 19.2
Repair strategies and examples of each

1. Repeat: say the message again
     Original utterance: The hammer is still in the shed.
     Repair strategy: The hammer is still in the shed.
2. Simplify: use fewer words or more commonplace words
     Original utterance: Let's break for a bite to eat at about 12:00 or so.
     Repair strategy: Let's break at noon.
3. Rephrase: use different words
     Original utterance: I'm out of nails here.
     Repair strategy: I need more nails.
4. Keyword: repeat one important word
     Original utterance: Will you please bring the ladder over here?
     Repair strategy: Ladder.
5. Elaborate: provide additional information
     Original utterance: Tom is going to join us.
     Repair strategy: Tom will join us soon. Tom is going to help put up the fume hood.
6. Delimit: ask a question that requires a limited answer from a closed set
     Original utterance: What color is this going to be?
     Repair strategy: Yellow or white?
7. Build from the known: present information that can be recognized easily
     Original utterance: please put the pen in the box.
     Repair strategy: please put the pen (point to the pen) in the tool box (gesture toward the tool box).

Adapted from Tye-Murray N, Witt B. Communication strategies training. Semin Hear 1997;18:153–165.

hearing loss" (Axelsson and Clark, 1995, p. 347).

One important venue for research is the development of effective educational programs. Although education programs are often provided to employees exposed to hazardous noise levels, this is not universally true. Moreover, few adults receive information about the hazards of recreational noise exposure. There is a need to develop education programs for the prevention of noise-induced hearing loss that concern all individuals who are exposed to potentially harmful noise levels, and to extend topics of instruction beyond those relevant to the work place to encompass other areas of individuals' lives (Clark, 1998).

The Elderly (Persons Aged 65 Years and Older)

TRENDS AND DEVELOPMENTS

The elderly are the fastest growing segment of the U.S. population. There are more than 30 million persons older than 65 years of age today, and demographers project that this number will swell to more than 39 million by 2010 (U.S. Department of Commerce, Bureau of the Census, 1986). By 2020, the elderly will comprise 13 to 18% of the U.S. population compared with 12% in 1988.

Two factors contribute to the boon that is occurring. First, the members of the "baby boom," which began after World War II and hit a peak in 1961, are aging. Individuals born in this era are fast approaching the 65-year mark. Second, co-occurring with the baby boom, an immigration wave occurred in the United States from 1978 to 1991. A large percentage of those individuals were approximately 30 years of age when they entered the United States. Thus, the peak in immigration of individuals who were about 30 years at the time of U.S. entry corresponds with the peak in the baby boom children at the time that they reached age 30 (Dent, 1998). Obviously, those individuals are also approaching the 65-year mark.

Older persons often refuse, and rightly so, to sit on the sidelines of life because they may have incurred a hearing loss. Many have a high demand for audiologic services and a great desire for unencumbered communication with their families, friends, and/or coworkers. Many desire to participate in community activities, and some postpone retirement far beyond the traditional age of 65 years. The advent of preventive medicine routines has resulted in more people living longer and with a better quality of life. Apart from hearing loss, many older persons have few other health problems that curtail their everyday functioning.

The upcoming surge in the number of older persons in the near future, and the increased demand for geriatric audiologic services that should accompany this surge, likely means that a great deal of research effort will be directed toward this population. It may be that we learn more about this segment of society than any other segment in the next few years. A decade from now, we will know more about how age interacts with speech perception and recognition skills and more about how to best deliver optimal aural rehabilitation services than we know today.

Speech recognition skills

To serve the elderly population and to potentiate successful everyday communication even in the presence of hearing loss, it is critical to obtain a clear understanding of their speech perception skills in three conditions: audition-only, vision-only, and audition-plus-vision. A better understanding of how these skills change with age may lead to advances in every stage of the aural rehabilitation process. These advances may range from how speech recognition skills are assessed, to the kinds of listening devices and assistive devices recommended, and finally to the kinds of follow-up support and counseling provided to patients and their families after the individual receives appropriate amplification.

Many older persons with hearing loss often demonstrate a greater decline in their speech recognition performance when listening in challenging conditions versus ideal conditions. For example, speech recognition difficulties are exacerbated when an older person attempts to listen in a noisy environment, more so than is the case for younger listeners (Pederson et al., 1991; Plath, 1991). Older persons may be especially susceptible to temporal distortions of the speech signal. They have greater difficulty than younger listeners in recognizing speech that is time-compressed (Stitch and Gray, 1969; Divenyi and Haupt, 1997) or reverberated (Harris and Reitz, 1985). Such findings may reflect age-related changes in speech processing abilities that are not due to hearing loss alone.

Much research has been conducted to determine whether auditory-only speech recognition difficulties stem primarily from peripheral cochlear pathology or primarily from central auditory changes in the central nervous system and central auditory processing. This is a complex issue, and much research remains to be done before a clear understanding is gained. It is known that the brain demonstrates a number of age-related changes. These changes may include a loss of neurons, a reduction in the number of synaptic connections between neurons, changes in the excitatory and inhibitory neurotransmitter systems, changes in neural transmission along the auditory pathway, and a decrement in long-term memory. In addition, the aging brain may also, possibly, demonstrate changes in cognitive processing of the acoustic signal. Such changes may include changes in information processing, labeling, retrieval, and storage. Such global changes in brain functioning may decrease an older person's ability to comprehend rapid streams of speech information.

However, although factors such as those just mentioned may affect speech recognition, some researchers have argued that decreased word recognition is related primarily to changes in the cochlear periphery. In particular, hearing sensitivity for the higher frequencies relates to speech recognition performance. Indeed, an older person's average hearing loss at the frequencies 1000, 2000, and 4000 Hz appears to be the single best predictor of a variety of different speech recognition test scores (Humes, 1996). One direction for future research is to explore this issue in depth and to determine to what extent listening difficulties are of peripheral origin and to what extent they are of more central origins.

It may be that older persons also experience declines in their abilities to recognize the visual speech signal, and that these declines may have either peripheral (relating to the eyeball) or central origin. However, few studies have specifically compared older and younger adults' ability to recognize speech using only the visual signal, and even fewer have examined vision-only speech recognition performance in challenging conditions. Some research suggests that lipreading ability decreases with age, even when visual acuity is not an issue (Farrimond, 1959; Middleweed and Plomp, 1987; Lyxell and Ronnberg, 1991). Hefler (1998) suggests that this decline may be related to changes in older persons' decreased abilities to process temporally changing visual information. Older persons are more likely to experience greater visual persistence (i.e., the duration of time in which a visual image is maintained) than younger persons and are more likely to experience backward masking for visual images (Kline and Orme-Rogers, 1978; DiLollo et al., 1982). These age-related changes may relate to decreased lipreading performance. Again, only further study will elucidate how age interacts with vision-only speech recognition performance.

Finally, little is known about the multimodal integration skills of older persons. We do know that even when individuals receive the complete signals, the perception of the auditory and visual signals may interact. For example, McGurk and MacDonald (1976) presented individuals with conflicting auditory and visual information and found that subjects perceived a fusion of information from the two modalities. When their subjects saw a talker speak /gi/ and simultaneously heard the syllable /bi/, they often reported hearing /di/ (which in terms of articulation is midway between /gi/ and /di/). If they closed their eyes, their perceptual experience was a clear /bi/. Other evidence suggesting the importance of visual enhancement for speech recognition is found when individuals are asked to repeat unfamiliar phrases. Reisberg et al. (1987) asked subjects to shadow passages from Kant's *Critique of Reason.* Performance was significantly better when subjects saw and heard the talker compared with when they only listened. Such findings underscore the fact that speech recognition is multimodal: individuals integrate different channels of speech information early in the speech analysis process to achieve a unified percept of the incoming signals (Braida, 1991; Massaro, 1987).

The issues of audiovisual speech integration may be especially relevant for the older segment of our society, given their growing numbers. Unfortunately, although this group has a high incidence of co-occurring hearing loss and impaired vision (Vinding, 1989), there are few studies describing changes in audiovisual speech recognition as a function of age.

Hefler (1998) conducted one of the few studies to examine auditory-visual speech recognition and speechreading enhancement in both ideal and less-than-ideal conditions. Fifteen older individuals were asked to recognize 200 nonsense sentences spoken with clear and conversational speech. Clear speech is speech that is spoken slowly with precise articulation. A signature characteristic of conversational speech is that it is spoken more quickly than clear speech, often with a shortening of phonemes (Picheny et al., 1986). Helfer found that age was negatively correlated with speechreading enhancement in the conversational but not the clear speech condition. That is, the older the subject, the more poorly he or she was able to recognize speech visually in a conversational test condition and the less speechreading enhancement (defined as the difference between speech recognition performance in a vision-only condition and an audition-plus-vision condition) received. This finding suggests that speechreading enhancement may decrease with age, especially in challenging test conditions. The small sample size used in this study and the absence of information about the performance of younger subjects for comparison purposes make these conclusions tentative.

In sum, the data reviewed here suggest that

older persons may experience decreased auditory and visual word recognition abilities, although the extent and source of such difficulties remain to be delineated. Very few studies have focused on the ability of older persons to integrate the auditory and visual speech signals or have focused on the issue of their speechreading enhancement. Thus, we do not have a clear understanding of whether older persons experience declines in their abilities to integrate multimodal information. Moreover, we do not know how they perform in challenging conditions. Thus, future research should be directed at determining whether speech recognition declines.

Service delivery

Now that the theoretical issue of perceptual processing has been considered, the sector of more applied research can be discussed. An important area for research related to older persons who have hearing loss pertains to service delivery. A number of factors influence the effects of hearing loss on older persons. These factors are shown in Figure 19.1.

Economically, many older persons have a modest income, and a significant number live below the poverty line. Women in particular tend to be disadvantaged economically (U.S. Department of Commerce, Bureau of the Census, 1986). One area for research relates to how economic circumstances interact with older patients' willingness and ability to obtain aural rehabilitation services. Garstecki and Erler (1996) have begun preliminary work in this area.

Problems associated with hearing loss can be compounded by an older person's social milieu, which is defined by the individuals that a hearing-impaired person interacts with and the listening environments in which the interactions occur. Many hearing-impaired persons interact with individuals who do not know how to maximize face-to-face communication success by using communication strategies. Moreover, the listening environments that comprise the social milieu of the older listener may be noisy and/or poorly lit. They may not be equipped with appropriate assistive devices, or individuals in the environments (e.g., nursing home employees) may not know how to operate existing devices (as has been reported by Roper, 1975).

Speech and hearing professionals have become increasingly convinced that a comprehensive hearing rehabilitation program

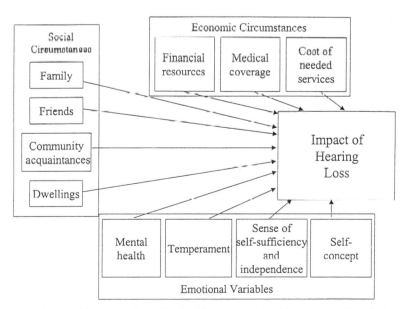

Figure 19.1. Some factors that influence the effects of hearing loss in older persons. (Reprinted with permission from Tye-Murray N. Foundations of aural rehabilitation: children, adults, and their family members. In addition to those depicted in this figure, physical status may also have an influence. San Diego: Singular, 1998:306.

for an older clientele must factor in the social milieu (Hull, 1995; Kricos and Holmes, 1996). Although much lip service has been paid to the importance of providing counseling and communication strategies training to the communication partners of hearing-impaired persons (Tye-Murray and Schum, 1994), very few data have been collected to validate its effects. Indeed, little attention has been paid to evaluating and comparing the effectiveness of various training programs. Perhaps the reason for this dearth of research lies in the fact that it is very difficult to assess benefit. For example, how do you assess whether a health care worker is a better communicator with an older adult after participating in a communication strategies training class (e.g., with a written examination? with real-world observation? by use of a simulated conversation?).

Emotional variables that may influence the effect of hearing loss include one's mental health, temperament, sense of self-sufficiency and independence, and self-concept. For example, mental conditions such as anxiety, obsessive-compulsiveness, and neuroticism may increase the communication difficulties associated with an older person's hearing loss (Eriksson-Mangold and Carlsson, 1991). Such temperament traits as introversion versus extroversion, assertiveness versus passiveness, and optimism versus pessimism also relate to the effects of hearing loss (e.g., Knutson and Lansing, 1990). One area of research that has received attention in recent years, and is likely to receive more, is the degree to which emotional variables portend success in an aural rehabilitation program.

Finally, physical variables may influence the impact of hearing loss in older persons. Three common physical conditions are especially relevant to the older population. These are reduced vision, arthritis, and dementia. Here, we will consider dementia.

The symptoms of dementia may include gradual memory loss, disorientation, loss of language skills, and a decline in the ability to perform everyday tasks. Individuals who have dementia commonly have hearing loss. Current research suggests that aural rehabil-

itation may be particularly important for these persons. For instance, Mulrow et al. (1990) showed that use of hearing aids often improved cognitive functioning. The means to support hearing aid use in this population, including the means to provide instruction and assistance to care givers and family members, need to be developed.

Final Comments

This chapter considered future directions in aural-rehabilitation–related research for the four life stages highlighted: infancy, childhood, adulthood, and the golden years. This is an exciting time to be interested in research about aural rehabilitation. Advances in hearing measurement, signal processing, and listening device technology (in addition to increased interest and understanding in sociolinguistics, psychology, speech acquisition, and speech perception) have opened the door to many new vistas of exploration. New developments in both the understanding of hearing loss and the delivery of aural rehabilitation services is limited only by the imagination of researchers and clinicians who will be working in the upcoming years.

REFERENCES

Allen T. Patterns of academic achievement among hearing impaired students: 1974 and 1983. In: Schildroth AN, Karchmer MA, eds. Deaf children in America. San Diego: College-Hill, 1986:161–206.

Axelsson A, Clark W. Hearing conservation programs for nonserved occupations. In: Morata TC, Dunn DE, eds. Occupational hearing loss, occupational medicine: state of the art reviews. Philadelphia, PA: Hanley and Belfus, 1995;10:657–663.

Braida L. Crossmodal integration in the identification of consonant segments. Q J Exp Psychol 1991;43:647–677.

Calderon R, Greenberg M. Considerations in the adaptation of families with school-aged deaf children. In: Marschark M, Clark MD, eds. Psychological perspectives on deafness. Hillsdale, NJ: Lawrence Erlbaum, 1993:27–48.

Carney A, Moeller M. Treatment efficacy: hearing loss in children. J Speech Lang Hear Res 1998;41(Suppl):61–84.

Clark W. Effects of noise on hearing and communication. In: Tye Murray N, editor. Foundations of aural rehabilitation: children, adults, and their family members. San Diego: Singular, 1998:327–352.

Demorest M, Erdman S. Development of the communication profile for the hearing impaired. J Speech Hear Disord 1987;52:129–143.

Dent H. The roaring 2000s. New York: Simon & Schuster, 1998.

Divenyi P, Haupt K. Audiological correlates of speech understanding deficits in elderly listeners with mild-to-moderate hearing loss. I. Age and lateral asymmetry effects. Ear Hear 1997a;18:42–61.

Divenyi P, Haupt K. Audiological correlates of speech understanding deficits in elderly listeners with mild-to-moderate hearing loss. II. Correlation analysis. Ear Hear 1997b;18:100–113.

Divenyi P, Haupt K. Audiological correlates of speech understanding deficits in elderly listeners with mild-to-moderate hearing loss. III. Factor representation. Ear Hear 1997c;18:189–201.

Erber N. Communication therapy for hearing-impaired adults. Melbourne, Australia: Clavis, 1988.

Eriksson-Mangold M, Carlsson S. Psychological and somatic distress in relation to hearing disability, hearing handicap, and hearing measurements. J Psychosom Res 1991;35:729–740.

Farrimond T. Age differences in the ability to use visual codes in auditory communication. Lang Speech 1959;2:179.

Fryauf-Bertschy H, Tyle R, Kelsay D, et al. Cochlear implant use by prelingually deafened children: the influences of age at implant and length of devise use. J Speech Hear Lang Res 1997;40:183–199.

Garstecki D, Erler S. Older adult performance on the Communication Profile for the Hearing Impaired. J Speech Hear Res 1996;39:28–42.

Harris R, Reitz M. Effects of room reverberation and noise on speech discrimination by the elderly. Audiology 1985; 24:319–24.

Hefler KS. Auditory and auditory-visual recognition of clear and conversational speech of older adults. J Am Acad Audiol 1998;9:234–242.

Hull R. Hearing in aging. San Diego: Singular, 1995.

Humes L. Speech understanding in the elderly. J Am Acad Audiol 1996;7:161–176.

Kline D, Orme-Rogers C. Examination of stimulus persistence as the basis for superior visual identification performance among older adults. J Gerontol 1978;33:76–81.

Knutson J, Lansing C. The relationship between communication problems and psychological difficulties in persons with profound acquired hearing loss. J Speech Hear Disord 1990;55:656–664.

Kotler P, Andreasen A. Strategic marketing for nonprofit organizations. 5th ed. Upper Saddle River, NJ: Prentice-Hall, 1996.

Kricos P, Holmes A. Efficacy of audiologic rehabilitation for older adults. J Am Acad Audiol 1996;7:219–229.

LaSasso C, Mobley R. National survey of reading instruction for deaf or hard-of-hearing students. Volta Rev 1997; 99:31–56.

Lyxell B, Ronnberg J. Visual speech processing: word-decoding and word-discrimination related to sentence-based speechreading and hearing-impairment. Scand J Psychol 1991;32:9–17.

Massaro D. Speech perception by ear and eye: a paradigm for psychological inquiry. Hillsdale, NJ: Lawrence Erlbaum, 1987.

McGurk H, MacDonald J. Hearing lips and seeing voices. Nature 1976;264:746–748.

Merry C, Franks J. Historical assessment and future directions in the prevention of occupational hearing loss. In: Morata TC, Dunn DE eds. Occupational hearing loss, occupational medicine: state of the art reviews. Philadelphia, PA: Hanley and Belfus, 1995;10:669–683.

Middleweerd M, Plomp R. The effect of speechreading on the speech reception threshold of sentences in noise. J Acoust Soc Am 1987;82:2145–2147.

Moeller M. Effectiveness of early intervention. Paper presented at the Academy of Rehabilitative Audiology Summer Institute, Fontana, Wisconsin, 1998.

Moeller M, Coufal K, Hixson P. The efficacy of speech-language intervention: hearing-impaired children. Semin Speech Lang Pathol 1990;11:227–241.

Moores D. An historical perspective on school placement. In: Kluwin TN, Moores DF, Gaustad MG, eds. Toward effective public school programs for deaf students: context, process and outcomes. New York: Teachers College Press, 1992.

Mulrow C, Aguilar C, Endicott J. Association between hearing impairment and the quality of life of elderly individuals. J Am Geriatr Soc 1990;38:45–50.

Nicholas J, Geers A. Communication of oral deaf and normally hearing children at 36 months. J Speech Lang Hear Res 1997;40:1314–1327.

Northern J, Downs M. Hearing in children. 4th ed. Baltimore, MD: Williams & Wilkins. 1991.

Paul P. Reading for students with hearing impairment: research review and implications. Volta Rev 1997;99:73–88.

Pederson K, Rosenhall U, Moller M. Longitudinal study of changes in speech perception between 70 and 81 years of age. Audiology 1991;30:201–211.

Picheny MA, Durlach NL, Braida LD. Speaking clearly for the hard of hearing II: Acoustic characteristics of clear and conversational speech. J Speech Hear Res 1986;29:434 446.

Plath P. Speech recognition in the elderly. Acta Otolaryngol 1991;476(Suppl):127–120.

Reisberg D, McLean J, Goldfield A. Easy to hear but hard to understand: A lipreading advantage with intact auditory stimuli. In: B. Dodds, R. Campbell, Eds. Hearing by eye. Erlbowm, NJ 1987:97–113.

Robbins A. Developing meaningful auditory integration in children with cochlear implants. Volta Rev 1990;92:361–370.

Schlesinger H, Acree M. Antecedents to achievement and adjustment in deaf adolescents: a longitudinal study of deaf children. In: Anderson GB, Watson D, eds. The habilitation and rehabilitation of deaf adolescents. Washington, DC: The National Academy of Gallaudet College, 1984: 18 61.

Seewald R. Update on the fitting of amplification in infants and young children. Presented at the Academy of Rehabilitative Audiology Summer Institute, Fontana, Wisconsin, 1998.

Stitch R, Gray B. The intelligibility of time compressed words as a function of age and hearing loss. J Speech Hear Res 1969;12:443–448.

Trybus R, Karchmer M. School achievement scores of hearing-impaired children: national data on achievement status and growth patterns. Am Ann Deaf 1977; 122:62–69.

Tye-Murray N. Cochlear implants and children: a handbook for parents, teachers, and speech and hearing professionals. Washington, DC: A. G. Bell Association, 1992.

Tye-Murray N. Foundations of aural rehabilitation: children, adults and their family members. San Diego: Singular, 1998.

Tye Murray N, Schum L. Conversation training for frequent communication partners. J Acad Rehabil Audiol 1994;27 (Suppl):209–222.

Tye-Murray N, Witt B. Communication strategies training. Semin Hear 1997;18:153–165.

Tye-Murray N, Spencer L, Woodworth G. Acquisition of speech by children who have prolonged cochlear implant experience. J Speech Hear Res 1995;38:327–337.

U.S. Department of Commerce, Bureau of the Census. Statistical abstract of the U.S. 106th ed. Washington, DC: Government Printing Office, 1986.

Vergara K, Miskiel L. CHATS: the Miami cochlear implant, auditory and tactile skills curriculum. Miami: Intelligent Hearing Systems, 1994.

Vinding T. Age-related macular degeneration: macular changes, prevalence, and sex ratio. Acta Ophthalmol 1989;67:609–616.

Yoshinaga-Itano C, Sedey A, Coulter D, et al. Language of early—and late—identified children with hearing loss. J Pediatr 1998;102:1161–1171.

ATTACHMENTS: SELF-ASSESSMENT TOOLS FOR AUDIOLOGIC REHABILITATION

ATTACHMENT 1
Self-Assessment of Communication (SAC)

Name _____

Date _____   Raw Score ____ × 2 = ____ − 20 = ____ × 1.25 ____%

Please select the appropriate number ranging from 1 to 5 for the following questions.
Circle only one number for each question. If you have a hearing aid, please fill out the form according to how you communicate when the hearing aid <u>is not</u> in use.

Disability

<u>Various Communication Situations</u>

1. Do you experience communication difficulties in situations when speaking with one other person? (for example, at home, at work, in a social situation, with a waitress, a store clerk, with a spouse, boss, etc.)

   1) almost never (or never)   2) occasionally (about ¼ of the time)   3) about half of the time   4) frequently (about ¾ of the time)   5) practically always (or always)

2. Do you experience communication difficulties in situations when conversing with a small group of several persons? (for example, with friends or family, co-workers, in meetings or casual conversations, over dinner or while playing cards, etc.)

   1) almost never (or never)   2) occasionally (about ¼ of the time)   3) about half of the time   4) frequently (about ¾ of the time)   5) practically always (or always)

3. Do you experience communication difficulties while listening to someone speak to a large group? (for example, at a church or in a civic meeting, in a fraternal or women's club, at an educational lecture, etc.)

   1) almost never (or never)   2) occasionally (about ¼ of the time)   3) about half of the time   4) frequently (about ¾ of the time)   5) practically always (or always)

4. Do you experience communication difficulties while participating in various types of entertainment? (for example, movies, TV, radio, plays, night clubs, musical entertainment, etc.)

   1) almost never (or never)   2) occasionally (about ¼ of the time)   3) about half of the time   4) frequently (about ¾ of the time)   5) practically always (or always)

5. Do you experience communication difficulties when you are in an unfavorable listening environment? (for example, at a noisy party, where there is background music, when riding in an auto or bus, when someone whispers or talks from across the room, etc.)

   1) almost never (or never)   2) occasionally (about ¼ of the time)   3) about half of the time   4) frequently (about ¾ of the time)   5) practically always (or always)

6. Do you experience communication difficulties when using or listening to various communication devices? (for example, telephone, telephone ring, doorbell, public address system, warning signals, alarms, etc.)

   1) almost never (or never)   2) occasionally (about ¼ of the time)   3) about half of the time   4) frequently (about ¾ of the time)   5) practically always (or always)

Handicap

<u>Feelings About Communication</u>

7. Do you feel that any difficulty with your hearing limits or hampers your personal or social life?

   1) almost never (or never)   2) occasionally (about ¼ of the time)   3) about half of the time   4) frequently (about ¾ of the time)   5) practically always (or always)

8. Does any problem or difficulty with your hearing upset you?

   1) almost never (or never)   2) occasionally (about ¼ of the time)   3) about half of the time   4) frequently (about ¾ of the time)   5) practically always (or always)

Handicap

<u>Other people</u>

9. Do others suggest that you have a hearing problem?

   1) almost never (or never)   2) occasionally (about ¼ of the time)   3) about half of the time   4) frequently (about ¾ of the time)   5) practically always (or always)

10. Do others leave you out of conversations or become annoyed because of your hearing?

   1) almost never (or never)   2) occasionally (about ¼ of the time)   3) about half of the time   4) frequently (about ¾ of the time)   5) practically always (or always)

Reprinted by permission from Schow RL, Nerbonne MA. Communication screening profile; use with elderly clients. Ear Hear 1982;3:135–147.

ATTACHMENT 2 *Significant Other Assessment of Communication (SOAC)*

Name _____
Form filled out with reference to _____ (client/patient)
Relationship to client/patient _____ (for example, wife, son, friend)
Date _____ Raw Score ____ × 2 = ____ − 20 = ____ × 1.25 ____%

Please select the appropriate number ranging from 1 to 5 for the following questions. Circle only one number for each question. If the client/patient has a hearing aid, please fill out the form according to how he/she communicates when the hearing aid is not in use.

Disability

Various Communication Situations

1. Does he/she experience communication difficulties in situations when speaking with one other person? (for example, at home, at work, in a social situation, with a waitress, a store clerk, with a spouse, boss, etc.)
   1) almost never (or never)   2) occasionally (about ¼ of the time)   3) about half of the time   4) frequently (about ¾ of the time)   5) practically always (or always)

2. Does he/she experience communication difficulties in situations when conversing with a small group of several persons? (for example, with friends or family, co-workers, in meetings or casual conversations, over dinner or while playing cards, etc.)
   1) almost never (or never)   2) occasionally (about ¼ of the time)   3) about half of the time   4) frequently (about ¾ of the time)   5) practically always (or always)

3. Does he/she experience communication difficulties while listening to someone speak to a large group? (for example, at a church or in a civic meeting, in a fraternal or women's club, at an educational lecture, etc.)
   1) almost never (or never)   2) occasionally (about ¼ of the time)   3) about half of the time   4) frequently (about ¾ of the time)   5) practically always (or always)

4. Does he/she experience communication difficulties while participating in various types of entertainment? (for example, movies, TV, radio, plays, night clubs, musical entertainment, etc.)
   1) almost never (or never)   2) occasionally (about ¼ of the time)   3) about half of the time   4) frequently (about ¾ of the time)   5) practically always (or always)

5. Does he/she experience communication difficulties when in an unfavorable listening environment? (for example, at a noisy party, where there is background music, when riding in an auto or bus, when someone whispers or talks from across the room, etc.)
   1) almost never (or never)   2) occasionally (about ¼ of the time)   3) about half of the time   4) frequently (about ¾ of the time)   5) practically always (or always)

6. Does he/she experience communication difficulties when using or listening to various communication devices? (for example, telephone, telephone ring, doorbell, public address system, warning signals, alarms, etc.)
   1) almost never (or never)   2) occasionally (about ¼ of the time)   3) about half of the time   4) frequently (about ¾ of the time)   5) practically always (or always)

Handicap

Feeling About Communication

7. Do you feel that any difficulty with his/her hearing limits or hampers his/her personal or social life?
   1) almost never (or never)   2) occasionally (about ¼ of the time)   3) about half of the time   4) frequently (about ¾ of the time)   5) practically always (or always)

8. Does any problem or difficulty with his/her hearing visibly upset them?
   1) almost never (or never)   2) occasionally (about ¼ of the time)   3) about half of the time   4) frequently (about ¾ of the time)   5) practically always (or always)

Handicap

Other People

9. Do others suggest he/she has a hearing problem?
   1) almost never (or never)   2) occasionally (about ¼ of the time)   3) about half of the time   4) frequently (about ¾ of the time)   5) practically always (or always)

10. Do you or others leave him/her out of conversations or become annoyed because of your hearing?
   1) almost never (or never)   2) occasionally (about ¼ of the time)   3) about half of the time   4) frequently (about ¾ of the time)   5) practically always (or always)

Reprinted by permission from Schow RL, Nerbonne MA. Communication screening profile; use with elderly clients. Ear Hear 1982;3:135–147.

ATTACHMENT 3 *Denver Scale of Communication Function*

Pre-Service _____ Post-Service _____

Date _____ Case No. _____

Name _____ Age _____ Sex _____

Address _____

_____
          (City)   (State)   (Zip)

Lives Alone _____ In Apartment _____ Retired _____
                                          (if no, specify)

Occupation _____

Audiogram (Examination Date _____ Agency _____)

Pure Tone:

	250	500	1000	2000	4000	8000	Hz
RE	____	____	____	____	____	____	
LE	____	____	____	____	____	____	dB (re: ANSI)

Speech:

<u>SRT</u>   <u>DISCRIMINATION SCORE</u> (%)

                           Quiet   Noise (S/N =   )

RE ____dB   RE ____

LE ____dB   LE ____

Aided ____   For How Long _____ Aid Type _____

Satisfaction _____

                                      EXAMINER:_____

Reprinted by permission from Alpiner, Chevrette, Glascoe, Metz, Olsen, unpublished study, the University of Denver, 1974.

The following questionnaire was designed to evaluate your communication ability as you view it. You are asked to judge or scale each statement in the following manner.

If you judge the statement to be *very closely related* to either extreme, please place your check mark as follows:

Agree __X__ _____ _____ _____ _____ _____ _____ Disagree

or

Agree _____ _____ _____ _____ _____ _____ __X__ Disagree

If you judge the statement to be *closely related* to either end of the scale, please mark as follows:

Agree _____ __X__ _____ _____ _____ _____ _____ Disagree

or

Agree _____ _____ _____ _____ _____ __X__ _____ Disagree

If you judge the statement to be only slightly related to either end of the scale, please mark as follows:

Agree _____ _____ __X__ _____ _____ _____ _____ Disagree

or

Agree _____ _____ _____ _____ __X__ _____ _____ Disagree

If you consider the statement to be irrelevant or unassociated to your communication situation, please mark as follows:

Agree _____ _____ _____ __X__ _____ _____ _____ Disagree

PLEASE NOTE: Check a scale for every statement.
Put only one checkmark on each scale.
Make a separate judgment for each statement.

ALSO: You may comment on each statement in the space provided.

1. The members of my family are annoyed with my loss of hearing.
Agree _____ _____ _____ _____ _____ _____ _____ Disagree
Comments:

2. The members of my family sometimes leave me out of conversations or discussions.
Agree _____ _____ _____ _____ _____ _____ _____ Disagree
Comments:

3. Sometimes my family makes decisions for me because I have a hard time following discussions.
Agree _____ _____ _____ _____ _____ _____ _____ Disagree
Comments:

4. My family becomes annoyed when I ask them to repeat what was said because I did not hear them.
Agree _____ _____ _____ _____ _____ _____ _____ Disagree
Comments:

5. I am not an "outgoing" person because I have a hearing loss.
Agree _____ _____ _____ _____ _____ _____ _____ Disagree
Comments:

6. I now take less of an interest in many things as compared to when I did not have a hearing problem.
Agree _____ _____ _____ _____ _____ _____ _____ Disagree
Comments:

7. Other people do not realize how frustrated I got when I cannot hear or understand.
Agree _____ _____ _____ _____ _____ _____ _____ Disagree
Comments:

8. People sometimes avoid me because of my hearing loss.
Agree _____ _____ _____ _____ _____ _____ _____ Disagree
Comments:

9. I am not a calm person because of my hearing loss.
Agree _____ _____ _____ _____ _____ _____ _____ Disagree
Comments:

10. I tend to be negative about life in general because of my hearing loss.
Agree _____ _____ _____ _____ _____ _____ _____ Disagree
Comments:

11. I do not socialize as much as I did before I began to lose my hearing.
Agree _____ _____ _____ _____ _____ _____ _____ Disagree
Comments:

12. Since I have trouble hearing, I do not like to go places with friends.
Agree _____ _____ _____ _____ _____ _____ _____ Disagree
Comments:

13. Since I have trouble hearing, I hesitate to meet new people.
Agree _____ _____ _____ _____ _____ _____ _____ Disagree
Comments:

14. I do not enjoy my job as much as I did before I began to lose my hearing.
Agree _____ _____ _____ _____ _____ _____ _____ Disagree
Comments:

15. Other people do not understand what it is like to have a hearing loss.
Agree _____ _____ _____ _____ _____ _____ _____ Disagree
Comments:

16. Because I have difficulty understanding what is said to me, I sometimes answer questions wrong.
Agree _____ _____ _____ _____ _____ _____ _____ Disagree
Comments:

17. I do not feel relaxed in a communicative situation.
Agree _____ _____ _____ _____ _____ _____ _____ Disagree
Comments:

18. I do not feel comfortable in most communication situations.
Agree _____ _____ _____ _____ _____ _____ _____ Disagree
Comments:

19. Conversations in a noisy room prevent me from attempting to communicate with others.
Agree _____ _____ _____ _____ _____ _____ _____ Disagree
Comments:

20. I am not comfortable having to speak in a group situation.
Agree _____ _____ _____ _____ _____ _____ _____ Disagree
Comments:

21. In general, I do not find listening relaxing.
Agree _____ _____ _____ _____ _____ _____ _____ Disagree
Comments:

22. I feel threatened by many communication situations due to difficulty hearing.
Agree _____ _____ _____ _____ _____ _____ _____ Disagree
Comments:

23. I seldom watch other people's facial expressions when talking to them.
Agree _____ _____ _____ _____ _____ _____ _____ Disagree
Comments:

24. I hesitate to ask people to repeat if I do not understand them the first time they speak.
Agree _____ _____ _____ _____ _____ _____ _____ Disagree
Comments:

25. Because I have difficulty understanding what is said to me, I sometimes make comments that do not fit into the conversation.
Agree _____ _____ _____ _____ _____ _____ _____ Disagree
Comments:

ATTACHMENT 4

Quantified Denver Scale

Name _____   Score: _____

Age _____   Raw score:_____

Date _____

		Strongly disagree				Strongly agree
1. The members of my family are annoyed with my loss of hearing.		1	2	3	4	5
2. The members of my family sometimes leave me out of conversations or discussions.		1	2	3	4	5
3. Sometimes my family makes decisions for me because I have a hard time following discussions.		1	2	3	4	5
4. My family becomes annoyed when I ask them to repeat what was said because I did not hear them.		1	2	3	4	5
5. I am not an "outgoing" person because I have a hearing loss.		1	2	3	4	5
6. I now take less of an interest in many things as compared to when I did not have a hearing problem.		1	2	3	4	5
7. Other people do not realize how frustrated I get when I cannot hear or understand.		1	2	3	4	5
8. People sometimes avoid me because of my hearing loss.		1	2	3	4	5
9. I am not a calm person because of my hearing loss.		1	2	3	4	5
10. I tend to be negative about life in general because of my hearing loss.		1	2	3	4	5
11. I do not socialize as much as I did before I began to lose my hearing.		1	2	3	4	5
12. Since I have trouble hearing, I do not like to go places with friends.		1	2	3	4	5
13. Since I have trouble hearing, I hesitate to meet new people.		1	2	3	4	5
14. I do not enjoy my job as much as I did before I began to lose my hearing.		1	2	3	4	5
15. Other people do not understand what it is like to have a hearing loss.		1	2	3	4	5
16. Because I have difficulty understanding what is said to me, I sometimes answer questions wrong.		1	2	3	4	5
17. I do not feel relaxed in a communicative situation.		1	2	3	4	5
18. I don't feel comfortable in most communication situations.		1	2	3	4	5
19. Conversations in a noisy room prevent me from attempting to communicate with others.		1	2	3	4	5
20. I am not comfortable having to speak in a group situation.		1	2	3	4	5
21. In general, I do not find listening relaxing.		1	2	3	4	5
22. I feel threatened by many communication situations due to difficulty hearing.		1	2	3	4	5
23. I seldom watch other people's facial expressions when talking to them.		1	2	3	4	5
24. I hesitate to ask people to repeat if I do not understand them the first time they speak.		1	2	3	4	5
25. Because I have difficulty understanding what is said to me, I sometimes make comments that do not fit into the conversation.		1	2	3	4	5

Modified from Denver Scale of Communication Function (Alpiner et al., 1974).

McCarthy-Alpiner Scale of Hearing Handicap (M-A Scale)

by
Patricia McCarthy, PhD. and Jerome G. Alpiner, PhD.

FORM A

NAME: _____ DATE: _____

AGE: _____ SEX: _____ TIME: _____

OCCUPATION: _____ PHONE: _____

ADDRESS: _____

HEARING AID: YES _____ NO _____   ONSET OF HEARING LOSS: _____

                TYPE _____

                HOW LONG _____

                SATISFACTION _____

AUDIOGRAM: DATE OF EXAMINATION _____

                EXAMINER _____

                CATEGORY OF HEARING LOSS _____

RIGHT EAR	250 Hz	500 Hz	1000 Hz	2000 Hz	4000 Hz	8000 Hz
AIR						
BONE						

LEFT EAR	250 Hz	500 Hz	1000 Hz	2000 Hz	4000 Hz	8000 Hz
AIR						
BONE						

SPEECH RECEPTION THRESHOLD:

RIGHT EAR _____ dB HL

LEFT EAR _____ dB HL

SPEECH DISCRIMINATION:

RIGHT EAR _____% @ _____ dB HL

LEFT EAR _____% @ _____ dB HL

DIRECTIONS

The following questionnaire will be used to help audiologists understand what it is like to have a hearing loss and the effects of a hearing loss on your life. You are asked to give your reaction to each of the statements included in the questionnaire. For example, you might be given this statement:

People avoid me because of my hearing loss.

		X		
ALWAYS	USUALLY	SOMETIMES	RARELY	NEVER

You are asked to mark your reaction to the statement with an X on the appropriate space. Please mark every item with only one answer as seen in the example.

In marking your answer, please keep in mind that ALWAYS means at all times or on all occasions. USUALLY refers to generally, commonly or ordinarily. SOMETIMES means occasionally or on various occasions. RARELY refers to seldom or infrequently. NEVER means not ever or at no time.

If you are not presently employed, please respond "N/A" for not applicable.

All answers will be kept strictly confidential and used only to help audiologists to understand what it is like to have a hearing loss and the effects of hearing loss on your life.

1. I get annoyed when people do not speak loud enough for me to hear them.

ALWAYS	USUALLY	SOMETIMES	RARELY	NEVER

2. I get upset if I cannot hear or understand a conversation.

ALWAYS	USUALLY	SOMETIMES	RARELY	NEVER

3. I feel like I am isolated from things because of my hearing loss.

ALWAYS	USUALLY	SOMETIMES	RARELY	NEVER

4. I feel negative about life in general because of my hearing loss.

ALWAYS	USUALLY	SOMETIMES	RARELY	NEVER

5. I admit that I have a hearing loss to most people.

ALWAYS	USUALLY	SOMETIMES	RARELY	NEVER

6. I get upset when I feel that people are "mumbling."

ALWAYS	USUALLY	SOMETIMES	RARELY	NEVER

7. I feel very frustrated when I cannot understand a conversation.

ALWAYS	USUALLY	SOMETIMES	RARELY	NEVER

8. I feel that people in general understand what it is like to have a hearing loss.

ALWAYS	USUALLY	SOMETIMES	RARELY	NEVER

9. My hearing loss has affected my life in general.

ALWAYS	USUALLY	SOMETIMES	RARELY	NEVER

10. I am afraid that people will not like me if they find out that I have a hearing loss.

ALWAYS	USUALLY	SOMETIMES	RARELY	NEVER

11. I tend to avoid people because of my hearing loss.

ALWAYS	USUALLY	SOMETIMES	RARELY	NEVER

12. People act annoyed when I cannot understand what is being said in a group conversation.

ALWAYS	USUALLY	SOMETIMES	RARELY	NEVER

13. My family is patient with me when I cannot hear.

ALWAYS	USUALLY	SOMETIMES	RARELY	NEVER

14. Strangers react rudely when I do not understand what they say.

ALWAYS	USUALLY	SOMETIMES	RARELY	NEVER

15. I ask a person to repeat if I do not hear or understand what he said.

| ALWAYS | USUALLY | SOMETIMES | RARELY | NEVER |

16. My hearing loss has affected my relationship with my spouse.

| ALWAYS | USUALLY | SOMETIMES | RARELY | NEVER |

17. I do not go places with my family because of my hearing loss.

| ALWAYS | USUALLY | SOMETIMES | RARELY | NEVER |

18. Group discussions make me nervous because of my hearing loss.

| ALWAYS | USUALLY | SOMETIMES | RARELY | NEVER |

19. People in general are tolerant of my hearing loss.

| ALWAYS | USUALLY | SOMETIMES | RARELY | NEVER |

20. I avoid going to movies or plays because of my hearing loss.

| ALWAYS | USUALLY | SOMETIMES | RARELY | NEVER |

21. I avoid going to restaurants because of my hearing loss.

| ALWAYS | USUALLY | SOMETIMES | RARELY | NEVER |

22. I enjoy social situations with considerable conversation.

| ALWAYS | USUALLY | SOMETIMES | RARELY | NEVER |

23. I am not interested in group activities because of my hearing loss.

| ALWAYS | USUALLY | SOMETIMES | RARELY | NEVER |

24. I enjoy group discussions even though I have a hearing loss.

| ALWAYS | USUALLY | SOMETIMES | RARELY | NEVER |

25. My hearing loss has interfered with my job performance.

| ALWAYS | USUALLY | SOMETIMES | RARELY | NEVER |

26. I cannot perform my job well because of my hearing loss.

| ALWAYS | USUALLY | SOMETIMES | RARELY | NEVER |

27. My co-workers know what it is like to have a hearing loss.

| ALWAYS | USUALLY | SOMETIMES | RARELY | NEVER |

28. I try to hide my hearing loss from my co-workers.

| ALWAYS | USUALLY | SOMETIMES | RARELY | NEVER |

29. I do not enjoy going to work because of my hearing loss.

| ALWAYS | USUALLY | SOMETIMES | RARELY | NEVER |

30. I am given credit for doing a good job at work even though I have a hearing loss.

| ALWAYS | USUALLY | SOMETIMES | RARELY | NEVER |

31. I feel more pressure at work because of my hearing loss.

| ALWAYS | USUALLY | SOMETIMES | RARELY | NEVER |

32. My employer understands what it is like to have a hearing loss.

| ALWAYS | USUALLY | SOMETIMES | RARELY | NEVER |

33. I try to hide my hearing loss from my employer.

| ALWAYS | USUALLY | SOMETIMES | RARELY | NEVER |

34. My co-workers speak loudly and clearly.

| ALWAYS | USUALLY | SOMETIMES | RARELY | NEVER |

ATTACHMENT 6
Hearing Handicap Inventory for Adults (HHIA)

Instructions: The purpose of the scale is to identify the problems your hearing loss may be causing you. Check Yes, Sometimes, or No for each question. Do not skip a question if you avoid a situation because of a hearing problem.

		Yes (4)	Some-times (2)	No (0)
S-1.	Does a hearing problem cause you to use the phone less often than you would like?	____	____	____
E-2.*	Does a hearing problem cause you to feel embarrassed when meeting new people?	____	____	____
S-3	Does a hearing problem cause you to avoid groups of people?		____
E-4.	Does a hearing problem make you irritable?	____	____	____
E-5.*	Does a hearing problem cause you to feel frustrated when talking to members of your family?	____	____	____
S-6.	Does a hearing problem cause you difficulty when attending a party?	____	____	____
S-7.*	Does a hearing prolem cause you difficulty hearing/understanding coworkers, clients, or customers?	____	____	____
E-8.*	Do you feel handicapped by a hearing problem?	____	____	____
S-9.*	Does a hearing problem cause you difficulty when visiting friends, relatives, or neighbors?	____	____	____
E-10.	Does a hearing problem cause you to feel frustrated when talking to coworkers, clients, or customers?	____	____	____
S-11.*	Does a hearing problem cause you difficulty in the movies or theater?	____	____	____
E-12.	Does a hearing problem cause you to be nervous?	____	____	____
S-13.	Does a hearing problem cause you to visit friends, relatives, or neighbors less often than you would like?	____	____	
E-14.*	Does a hearing problem cause you to have arguments with family members?	____	____	____
S-15.*	Does a hearing problem cause you difficulty when listening to TV or radio?	____	____	____
S-16.	Does a hearing problem cause you to go shopping less often than you would like?	____		
E-17.	Does any problem or difficulty with your hearing upset you at all?	____	____	____
E-18.	Does a hearing problem cause you to want to be by yourself?	____	____	____
S-19.	Does a hearing problem cause you to talk to family members less often than you would like?	____	____	____
E-20.*	Do you feel that any difficulty with your hearing limits or hampers your personal or social life?	____	____	____
S-21.*	Does a hearing problem cause you difficulty when in a restaurant with relatives or friends?	____	____	____
E-22.	Does a hearing problem cause you to feel depressed?	____	____	____
S-23.	Does a hearing problem cause you to listen to TV or radio less often than you would like?	____	____	____
E-24.	Does a hearing problem cause you to feel uncomfortable when talking to friends?	____	____	____
E-25.	Does a hearing problem cause you to feel left out when you are with a group of people?	____	____	____

Reprinted by permission from Newman CW, Weinstein BE, Jacobson GP, et al. Test-retest reliability of the Hearing Handicap Inventory for Adults. Ear Hear 1991;12:355–357.
*Items comprising the HHIA-S.

ATTACHMENT 7

California Consonant Test

Name _____   Date _____

List 1

Test Items

1 GAVE ____	11 PAGE ____	21 SHIN ____	31 VALE ____	41 KIT ____
GAME ____	PAID ____	SIN ____	DALE ____	KICK ____
GAZE ____	PAYS ____	THIN ____	JAIL ____	KISS ____
GAGE ____	PAVE ____	CHIN ____	BALE ____	KID ____

2 PAIL ____	12 KICK ____	22 MUFF ____	32 PEACH ____	42 PIN ____
SAIL ____	PICK ____	MUCH ____	PEAT ____	KIN ____
FAIL ____	TICK ____	MUSH ____	PEAK ____	TIN ____
TAIL ____	THICK ____	MUSS ____	PEEP ____	THIN ____

Sample Items

1 BACK ____	3 CUFF ____	13 LAUGH ____	23 REACH ____	33 RACK ____	43 BUS ____
BAG ____	CUP ____	LASH ____	REAP ____	RASH ____	BUT ____
BATCH ____	CUSS ____	LASS ____	REEF ____	RAT ____	BUCK ____
BATH ____	CUT ____	LAP ____	REEK ____	RAP ____	BUFF ____

2 RICE ____	4 MUSS ____	14 SHEEP ____	24 BACK ____	34 HAG ____	44 GATE ____
DICE ____	MUCH ____	SEEP ____	BAT ____	HAD ____	BAIT ____
NICE ____	MUSH ____	CHEAP ____	BATCH ____	HAVE ____	DATE ____
LICE ____	MUFF ____	HEAP ____	BATH ____	HAS ____	WAIT ____

3 SEEN ____	5 FAKE ____	15 GAVE ____	25 TAME ____	35 TICK ____	45 LAUGH ____
SEED ____	FATE ____	GAME ____	SHAME ____	SICK ____	LASS ____
SEAL ____	FACE ____	GAGE ____	FAME ____	THICK ____	LASH ____
SEAT ____	FAITH ____	GAZE ____	SAME ____	PICK ____	LAP ____

4 BAIL ____	6 TILL ____	16 BEACH ____	26 CORE ____	36 CHAIR ____	46 HIP ____
TALE ____	CHILL ____	BEEP ____	PORE ____	CARE ____	HIT ____
SAIL ____	PILL ____	BEAK ____	TORE ____	SHARE ____	HISS ____
DALE ____	KILL ____	BEET ____	SORE ____	FAIR ____	HITCH ____

5 LEAVE ____	7 LEASE ____	17 MASS ____	27 RAGE ____	37 BEACH ____	47 HICK ____
LEASH ____	LEASH ____	MAP ____	RAISE ____	BEAK ____	SICK ____
LEAN ____	LEAF ____	MAT ____	RAVE ____	BEET ____	THICK ____
LEAGUE ____	LEAP ____	MATH ____	RAID ____	BEEP ____	CHICK ____

6 RAIL ____	8 SEEP ____	18 PATH ____	28 FILL ____	38 BEAK ____	48 LEAF ____
JAIL ____	CHEAP ____	PATCH ____	PILL ____	BEEP ____	LEASE ____
TAIL ____	SHEEP ____	PACK ____	KILL ____	BEAT ____	LEASH ____
BALE ____	HEAP ____	PAT ____	TILL ____	BEEF ____	LEAK ____

9 FACE ____	19 GAZE ____	29 CHOP ____	39 CHEEK ____	49 CHEEK ____
FAITH ____	GAGE ____	POP ____	CHIEF ____	CHEAP ____
FATE ____	GAVE ____	TOP ____	CHEAT ____	CHEAT ____
FAKE ____	GAME ____	SHOP ____	CHEAP ____	CHIEF ____

10 BAYS ____	20 SICK ____	30 MUCH ____	40 CUP ____	50 RID ____
BABE ____	CHICK ____	MUTT ____	CUT ____	RIB ____
BALE ____	THICK ____	MUSS ____	CUSS ____	RIDGE ____
BATHE ____	TICK ____	MUFF ____	CUFF ____	RIG ____

51	THIN	____	61	TAN	____	71	THAN	____	81	MATCH	____	91	HIP	
	TIN	____		CAN	____		VAN	____		MAT	____		HICK	
	SIN	____		FAN	____		BAN	____		MATH	____		HIT	____
	SHIN	____		PAN	____		PAN	____		MAP	____		HISS	____
52	HIT	____	62	TORE	____	72	SHEATH	____	82	PATCH	____	92	TIN	____
	HIP	____		CORE	____		SHEEP	____		PAT	____		KIN	____
	HISS	____		PORE	____		SHEIK	____		PASS	____		PIN	____
	HITCH	____		CHORE	____		SHEET	____		PATH	____		THIN	____
53	PAYS	____	63	SIS	____	73	TAN	____	83	FAITH	____	93	CASH	____
	PAVE	____		SIP	____		PAN	____		FATE	____		CAT	____
	PAGE	____		SIT	____		CAN	____		FAKE	____		CAP	____
	PAID	____		SICK	____		FAN	____		FACE	____		CATCH	____
54	HIT	____	64	CUSS	____	74	BATCH	____	84	RID	____	94	HATCH	____
	HICK	____		CUP	____		BAT	____		RIB	____		HAT	____
	HITCH	____		CUT	____		BACK	____		RIG	____		HACK	____
	HIP	____		CUFF	____		BATH	____		RIDGE	____		HALF	____
55	SICK	____	65	RAP	____	75	PAIL	____	85	CHEAP	____	95	DIVE	____
	SIP	____		RACK	____		TAIL	____		CHEAT	____		DIED	____
	SIT	____		RASH	____		SAIL	____		CHEEK	____		DIES	____
	SIS	____		RAT	____		FAIL	____		CHIEF	____		DINE	____
56	BEET	____	66	KILL	____	76	BUG	____	86	SORE	____	96	SIN	____
	BEEP	____		PILL	____		BUDGE	____		CHORE	____		FIN	____
	BEACH	____		TILL	____		BUZZ	____		SHORE	____		THIN	____
	BEAK	____		FILL	____		BUD	____		FOR	____		SHIN	____
57	HATCH	____	67	SICK	____	77	SAIL	____	87	POP	____	97	RODE	____
	HACK	____		TICK	____		PAIL	____		TOP	____		ROBE	____
	HALF	____		PICK	____		TAIL	____		CHOP	____		ROVE	____
	HAT	____		THICK	____		FAIL	____		COP	____		ROSE	____
58	CHIN	____	68	PAGE	____	78	ROBE	____	88	MAP	____	98	BAIL	____
	SHIN	____		PAYS	____		RODE	____		MATCH	____		JAIL	____
	THIN	____		PAVE	____		ROSE	____		MATH	____		DALE	____
	PIN	____		PAID	____		ROVE	____		MAT	____		GALE	____
59	HAIL	____	69	TORE	____	79	LASS	____	89	DIES	____	99	LEAF	____
	TAIL	____		PORE	____		LAUGH	____		DIED	____		LEASE	____
	FAIL	____		CORE	____		LATCH	____		DIVE	____		LEACH	____
	SAIL	____		SORE	____		LASH	____		DINE	____		LEASH	____
60	SHUN	____	70	LEASH	____	80	FIN	____	90	PEAK	____	100	RAISE	____
	PUN	____		LEAK	____		PIN	____		PEACH	____		RAID	____
	SUN	____		LEASE	____		KIN	____		PEAT	____		RAGE	____
	FUN	____		LEAF	____		TIN	____		PEEP	____		RAVE	____

ATTACHMENT 8

Central Institute for the Deaf (CID) Everyday Speech Sentences

LIST A

1. Walking's my favorite exercise.
2. Here's a nice quiet place to rest.
3. Our janitor sweeps the floors every night.
4. It would be much easier if everyone would help.
5. Good morning.
6. Open your window before you go to bed!
7. Do you think that she should stay out so late?
8. How do you feel about changing the time when we begin to work?
9. Here we go.
10. Move out of the way.

LIST B

1. The water's too cold for swimming.
2. Why should I get up so early in the morning?
3. Here are your shoes.
4. It's raining.
5. Where are you going?
6. Come here when I call you!
7. Don't try to get out of it this time!
8. Should we let little children go to the movies by themselves?
9. There isn't enough paint to finish the room.
10. Do you want an egg for breakfast?

LIST C

1. Everybody should brush his teeth after meals.
2. Everything's all right.
3. Don't use up all the paper when you write your letter.
4. That's right.
5. People ought to see a doctor once a year.
6. Those windows are so dirty I can't see anything outside.
7. Pass the bread and butter please!
8. Don't forget to pay your bill before the first of the month.
9. Don't let the dog out of the house!
10. There's a good ballgame this afternoon.

LIST D

1. It's time to go.
2. If you don't want these old magazines, throw them out.
3. Do you want to wash up?
4. It's a real dark night so watch your driving.
5. I'll carry the package for you.
6. Did you forget to shut off the water?
7. Fishing in a mountain stream is my idea of a good time.
8. Fathers spend more time with their children than they used to.
9. Be careful not to break your glasses!
10. I'm sorry.

LIST E

1. You can catch the bus across the street.
2. Call her on the phone and tell her the news.
3. I'll catch up with you later.
4. I'll think it over.
5. I don't want to go to the movies tonight.
6. If your tooth hurts that much you ought to see a dentist.
7. Put that cookie back in the box!
8. Stop fooling around!
9. Time's up.
10. How do you spell your name?

LIST F

1. Music always cheers me up.
2. My brother's in town for a short while on business.
3. We live a few miles from the main road.
4. This suit needs to go to the cleaners.
5. They ate enough green apples to make them sick for a week.
6. Where have you been all this time?
7. Have you been working hard lately?
8. There's not enough room in the kitchen for a new table.
9. Where is he?
10. Look out!

LIST G

1. I'll see you right after lunch.
2. See you later.
3. White shoes are awful to keep clean.
4. Stand there and don't move until I tell you!
5. There's a big piece of cake left over from dinner.
6. Wait for me at the corner in front of the drugstore
7. It's no trouble at all.
8. Hurry up!
9. The morning paper didn't say anything about rain this afternoon or tonight.
10. The phone call's for you.

LIST H

1. Believe me!
2. Let's get a cup of coffee.
3. Let's get out of here before it's too late.
4. I hate driving at night.
5. There was water in the cellar after the heavy rain yesterday.
6. She'll only be gone a few minutes.
7. How do you know?
8. Children like candy.
9. If we don't get rain soon, we'll have no grass.
10. They're not listed in the new phone book.

LIST I

1. Where can I find a place to park?
2. I like those big red apples we always get in the fall.
3. You'll get fat eating candy.
4. The show's over.
5. Why don't they paint their walls some other color?
6. What's new?
7. What are you hiding under your coat?
8. How come I should always be the one to go first?
9. I'll take sugar and cream in my coffee.
10. Wait just a minute!

LIST J

1. Breakfast is ready.
2. I don't know what's wrong with the car, but it won't start.
3. It sure takes a sharp knife to cut this meat.
4. I haven't read a newspaper since we bought a television set.
5. Weeds are spoiling the yard.
6. Call me a little later!
7. Do you have change for a five-dollar bill?
8. How are you?
9. I'd like some ice cream with my pie.
10. I don't think I'll have any dessert.

ATTACHMENT 9
Alpiner-Meline and Aural Rehabilitation (AMAR) Screening Scale

ADMINISTRATION INSTRUCTIONS

INTRODUCTION

The Alpiner-Meline Aural Rehabilitation Screening Scale (AMAR) is designed to identify adults who may need aural rehabilitation. The AMAR allows identification of problems related to hearing loss in three categories: (a) self-assessment, (b) visual aptitude, and (c) auditory aptitude.

APTITUDE

1. The scale should be administered in a quiet room. Items are presented in an interview format.
2. Each subtest is scored independently. Part I, Self-Assessment has nine items rated in terms of five possible responses: ALWAYS, USUALLY, SOMETIMES, RARELY, and NEVER. For all of the items (except number five), ALWAYS refers to maximum negative response possible, that is, a problem exists. For item five, NEVER REFERS TO THE MAXIMUM NEGATIVE RESPONSE.

   A problem is indicated when the response is either ALWAYS, USUALLY, or SOMETIMES. For number five, a problem is counted for either NEVER, RARELY, or SOMETIMES. The possible number of problems for Part 1 can range from 0 to 9. Problems are designated by a minus sign.
3. The five visual aptitude sentences are presented face to face at a distance of three to five feet, with a normal to slow articulatory rate and no voice. Client's oral responses are scored on the basis of whether or not the client identifies the thought or idea of the stimulus sentence. Minus signs are circled for sentences not identified.
4. For auditory aptitude, six CVC or CV items are presented. For each of the six items, the examiner asks the client to circle one of two words. The word is presented live voice in a quiet room at a distance of five feet. A perforated 5×8 card is held three inches from the examiner's mouth so that no visual cues can be received by the client. The minus sign is circled for each incorrect response.
5. AMAR scores are calculated as the total number of problems indicated on the test form.
6. Total time required for administration, scoring, and interpretation is approximately 15 minutes
7. Scoring (according to present norms):
   00–10 PROBLEMS = NO NEED FOR AURAL REHABILITATION
   11–13 PROBLEMS = QUESTIONABLE NEED
   14–20 PROBLEMS = ABSOLUTE NEED

Name: _____

Birthday: _____ Age: _____ SSN: _____

Hearing Aid Status (Circle one):
NONE   ITE   BODY   BONE   EYEGLASS   MONAURAL   BINAURAL

Number of years of hearing aid use: _____

Occupation: _____

Audiologist: _____ Date of Screening: _____

PART I: Self-Assessment of Hearing Handicap

A = Always   U = Usually   S = Sometimes   R = Rarely   N = Never

1. I feel like I am isolated from things because of my hearing loss.	A	U	S	R	N
2. I feel very frustrated when I cannot understand a conversation.	A	U	S	R	N
3. My hearing loss has affected my life.	A	U	S	R	N
4. I tend to avoid people because of my hearing loss.	A	U	S	R	N
5. People in general are tolerant of my hearing loss.	A	U	S	R	N
6. My hearing loss has affected my relationship with my spouse.	A	U	S	R	N
7. I try to hide my hearing loss from my co-workers.	A	U	S	R	N
8. My hearing loss has interfered with job performance.	A	U	S	R	N
9. I feel more pressure at work because of my hearing loss.	A	U	S	R	N

PART I PROBLEMS _____

Source: Alpiner JG, Meline NC, Cotton AD. An aural rehabilitation screening scale: self assessment, auditory aptitude, and visual aptitude. J Acad Aural Rehabil 1991;24:75–83.

PART II: Visual Aptitude

1. Good Morning.   +   −
2. How old are you?   +   −
3. I live in (state of residence).   +   −
4. I only have a dollar.   +   −
5. There is somebody at the door.   +   −

PART II PROBLEMS _____

PART III: Auditory Aptitude

1. FEW   CHEW   +   −
2. FIT   KIT   +   −
3. THIN   FIN   +   −
4. THUMB   SUM   +   −
5. TIE   THIGH   +   −
6. KICK   TICK   +   −

PART III PROBLEMS _____

00–10 Problems: No Need
11–13 Problems: Questionable Need
14–20 Problems: Absolute Need

Mental Status Questionnaire

1. What is the name of this place?

2. Where is it located (address)?

3. What is today's date?

4. What is the month now?

5. What is the year?

6. How old are you?

7. When were you born (month)?

8. When were you born (year)?

9. Who is the president of the United States?

10. Who was the president before him?

Total Correct: _____

Source: Khan R, Goldfarb A, Pollack M, et al. Brief objective measures for the determination of mental status in the aged. Am J Psychiatry 1960;117:326–328.

ATTACHMENT 11 *Speech in Quiet/in Noise Test*

Subject's Name _____

Unaided Test Date: _____   Aided Test Date: _____

PRACTICE ITEMS						
UNAIDED			AIDED			
Item		Item		Item		Item		COMMENTS
1		7		1		7		
2		8		2		8		
3		9		3		9		
4		10		4		10		
5		11		5		11		
6		12		6		12		

SUBJECT'S RESPONSES				
UNAIDED		AIDED		
Item	Quiet Lists 1 & 2	Noise Lists 3 & 4	Quiet Lists 5 & 6	Noise Lists 7 & 8	COMMENTS
1					
2					
3					
4					
5					
6					
7					
8					
9					
10					
11					
12					
13					
14					
15					
16					
17					
18					
19					
20					

* (+) correct responses
(−) incorrect responses

Sentences adapted from Hint Test. Nilsson MJ, Soli SD, Sullivan JA. Development of the Hearing In Noise Test for the measurement of speech thresholds in quiet and in noise. J Acoust Soc Am 1994;95:1085–1099.

ATTACHMENT 12

Hearing Aid Comfort Scale

Check (X) the item that best describes your hearing aid fit and ability to insert the device(s).

Hearing Aid Fit

_____ The hearing aid doesn't fit well—it falls out of my ear and creates a sore.

_____ The hearing aid fits fair—it stays in my ear, but irritates the canal.

_____ The hearing aid fits well—I can wear it several hours before removing it.

_____ The hearing aid fits well—I can wear it all day despite a stuffy feeling.

_____ The hearing aid fits well— I can't tell that it is in my ear.

Hearing Aid Insertion

_____ Insertion is impossible—very difficult—can never insert hearing aid.

_____ Occasionally I can insert the hearing aid.

_____ Insertion is possible only with assistance from another person.

_____ Rarely have problems with insertion of hearing aid.

_____ I am independent with hearing aid insertion—I am always successful.

ATTACHMENT 13

Presence of Feedback Scale

Feedback is the whistling/squealing/squelch "noise" noted from the hearing aid. Check (X) the item which best describes the occurrence of feedback, when using your hearing aids.

I notice feedback . . .

_____ Constantly (100% of the time)

_____ Frequently (50%–100% of the time)

_____ Occasionally (10%–50% of the time)

_____ Seldom (5%–10% of the time)

_____ Never (0% of the time)

_____ Other: _____

ATTACHMENT 14 *Sound Quality Measurement Scale*

Check (X) the item that best describes the quality of sounds (speech, environmental sounds, etc.)

When I am using my hearing aids . . .

_____ Sounds are natural

_____ Sounds are tinny or sharp

_____ Sounds are hollow or like I am "in a barrel"

_____ Other: _____

ATTACHMENT 15   *Cosmetic Assessment Scale*

Check (X) the time which best describes your opinion of how the hearing aids appear/look placed in your ears.

I feel that:

_____ The hearing aids are not seen by others.

_____ The hearing aids are slightly visible to others.

_____ The hearing aids are noticeable to others.

How many hours a day are you wearing your hearing aid(s)?

_____ 0–4 hours   specifically _____ hours

_____ 4.5–8 hours   specifically _____ hours

_____ 8.5–12 hours   specifically _____ hours

_____ 12.5–16 hours   specifically _____ hours

_____ 16 or more hours   specifically _____ hours

ATTACHMENT
16

TINNITUS QUESTIONNAIRE

Date of Onset: _____ Related to Specific Incident: _____

IS TINNITUS: _____ CONSTANT   _____ INTERMITTENT

IS TINNITUS: _____ UNILATERAL   _____ BILATERAL

DESCRIPTION OF TINNITUS: _____ RINGING   _____ BUZZING   _____ HISSING

_____ PULSING   _____ POPPING   _____ WIND   _____ ROARING   _____ INSECTS

_____ CLICKING   _____ OTHER: _____

IS THE TINNITUS:
1. MASKED BY ENVIRONMENTAL SOUNDS?   _____ YES   _____ NO
2. INTERFERING WITH SLEEP?   _____ YES   _____ NO
3. AGGRAVATED BY ANY STIMULI?   _____ YES   _____ NO
       _____ NOISE _____ CAFFEINE _____ ALCOHOL _____ OTHER:_____
4. INTERFERING WITH DAILY ACTIVITIES?   _____ YES   _____ NO
5. HANDICAPPING YOU IN ANY WAY?   _____ YES   _____ NO
6. INTERFERING WITH FAMILY RELATIONSHIPS?   _____ YES   _____ NO

COMMENTS: _____

_____

SUBJECTIVE DEGREE OF PROBLEM

	MILD		MODERATE		SEVERE
PATIENT'S IMPRESSION	1	2	3	4	5
EXAMINER'S IMPRESSION	1	2	3	4	5

_____   _____

DATE   EXAMINER

PATIENT'S NAME: _____ AGE: _____

ATTACHMENT 17   *Profile of Aided Loudness*

Name: _____   Date: _____

Status:_____ unaided _____ previous hearing aids _____ current hearing aids

Instructions:

Please rate the following items by both the level of loudness of the sound and by the appropriateness of that loudness level. For example, you might rate a particular sound as "Very Soft." If "Very Soft" is your preferred level for this sound, then you would rate your loudness satisfaction as "Just Right." If on the other hand, you think the sound should be louder than "Very Soft," then your loudness satisfaction rating might be "Not Too Good" or "Not Good At All." The Loudness Satisfaction rating is not related to how pleasing the sound is to you, but rather, the appropriateness of the loudness. Here is an example:

For example:
The hum of a refrigerator motor:

Loudness Rating

0 do not hear
1 very soft
2 soft
③ comfortable, but slightly soft
4 comfortable
5 comfortable, but slightly loud
6 loud, but OK
7 uncomfortably loud

Satisfaction Rating

⑤ Just right
4. Pretty good
3. Okay
2. Not too good
1. Not good at all

In this example, the hearing aid user rated the loudness level of a refrigerator motor running as "Comfortable, But Slightly Soft" and rated his Loudness Satisfaction for this sound as "Just Right." This satisfaction rating indicates that this person believes that it is appropriate for a refrigerator motor to sound "Comfortable, But Slightly Soft."

Circle the responses that best describe your listening experiences. If you have not experienced one of the sounds listed (or a similar sound), simply leave that question blank.

1. An electric razor:

Loudness Rating

0 do not hear
1 very soft
2 soft
3 comfortable, but slightly soft
4 comfortable
5 comfortable, but slightly loud
6 loud, but OK
7 uncomfortably loud

Satisfaction Rating

5. Just right
4. Pretty good
3. Okay
2. Not too good
1. Not good at all

2. A door slamming:

Loudness Rating

0 do not hear
1 very soft
2 soft
3 comfortable, but slightly soft
4 comfortable
5 comfortable, but slightly loud
6 loud, but OK
7 uncomfortably loud

Satisfaction Rating

5. Just right
4. Pretty good
3. Okay
2. Not too good
1. Not good at all

3. Your own breathing:

Loudness Rating

0 do not hear
1 very soft
2 soft
3 comfortable, but slightly soft
4 comfortable
5 comfortable, but slightly loud
6 loud, but OK
7 uncomfortably loud

Satisfaction Rating

5. Just right
4. Pretty good
3. Okay
2. Not too good
1. Not good at all

4. Water boiling on the stove:

Loudness Rating	**Satisfaction Rating**
0 do not hear	5. Just right
1 very soft	4. Pretty good
2 soft	3. Okay
3 comfortable, but slightly soft	2. Not too good
4 comfortable	1. Not good at all
5 comfortable, but slightly loud	
6 loud, but OK	
7 uncomfortably loud	

5. A car's turn signal:

Loudness Rating	**Satisfaction Rating**
0 do not hear	5. Just right
1 very soft	4. Pretty good
2 soft	3. Okay
3 comfortable, but slightly soft	2. Not too good
4 comfortable	1. Not good at all
5 comfortable, but slightly loud	
6 loud, but OK	
7 uncomfortably loud	

6. The religious leader during the sermon:

Loudness Rating	**Satisfaction Rating**
0 do not hear	5. Just right
1 very soft	4. Pretty good
2 soft	3. Okay
3 comfortable, but slightly soft	2. Not too good
4 comfortable	1. Not good at all
5 comfortable, but slightly loud	
6 loud, but OK	
7 uncomfortably loud	

7. The dryer running:

Loudness Rating	**Satisfaction Rating**
0 do not hear	5. Just right
1 very soft	4. Pretty good
2 soft	3. Okay
3 comfortable, but slightly soft	2. Not too good
4 comfortable	1. Not good at all
5 comfortable, but slightly loud	
6 loud, but OK	
7 uncomfortably loud	

8. You chewing soft food:

Loudness Rating	**Satisfaction Rating**
0 do not hear	5. Just right
1 very soft	4. Pretty good
2 soft	3. Okay
3 comfortable, but slightly soft	2. Not too good
4 comfortable	1. Not good at all
5 comfortable, but slightly loud	
6 loud, but OK	
7 uncomfortably loud	

9. Listening to a marching band:

Loudness Rating	**Satisfaction Rating**
0 do not hear	5. Just right
1 very soft	4. Pretty good
2 soft	3. Okay
3 comfortable, but slightly soft	2. Not too good
4 comfortable	1. Not good at all
5 comfortable, but slightly loud	
6 loud, but OK	
7 uncomfortably loud	

10. A barking dog:

Loudness Rating

0 do not hear
1 very soft
2 soft
3 comfortable, but slightly soft
4 comfortable
5 comfortable, but slightly loud
6 loud, but OK
7 uncomfortably loud

Satisfaction Rating

5. Just right
4. Pretty good
3. Okay
2. Not too good
1. Not good at all

11. A lawn mower:

Loudness Rating

0 do not hear
1 very soft
2 soft
3 comfortable, but slightly soft
4 comfortable
5 comtortable, but slightly loud
6 loud, but OK
7 uncomfortably loud

Satisfaction Rating

5. Just right
4. Pretty good
3. Okay
2. Not too good
1. Not good at all

12. A microwave buzzer sounding:

Loudness Rating

0 do not hear
1 very soft
2 soft
3 comfortable, but slightly soft
4 comfortable
5 comfortable, but slightly loud
6 loud, but OK
7 uncomfortably loud

Satisfaction Rating

5. Just right
4. Pretty good
3. Okay
2. Not too good
1. Not good at all

There are two methods for scoring the PAL. For an individual subject or group of subjects, the clinician may want to take an average score for soft, average, and loud sounds and compare the scores to the average scores of normally hearing individuals. The patient summary sheet is used for this type of scoring. In this manner, the clinician may compare unaided loudness perception to aided loudness perception as well as having a numeric target for the aided condition. Alternatively, the clinician may plot the individual's loudness rating for each item on the plot of ratings from a normally hearing population. The Normative Data for the PAL worksheet is used for this type of scoring. This type of scoring creates a nice counseling tool for the patient because they can see the distribution of loudness ratings provided by normally hearing individuals.

Patient Summary
Profile of Aided Loudness (PAL)

Unaided Performance

Soft Sounds	Q3	Q4	Q5	Q8	Category Average
Loudness	___	___	___	___	___ (target = 2.09)
Satisfaction	___	___	___	___	
Average Sounds	Q1	Q6	Q7	Q12	Category Average
Loudness	___	___	___	___	___ (target = 4.13)
Satisfaction	___	___	___	___	___
Loud Sounds	Q2	Q9	Q10	Q11	Category Average
Loudness	___	___	___	___	___ (target = 5.92)
Satisfaction	___	___	___	___	___

Aided Performance

Soft Sounds	Q3	Q4	Q5	Q8	Category Average
Loudness	___	___	___	___	___ (target = 2.09)
Satisfaction	___	___	___	___	___
Average Sounds	Q1	Q6	Q7	Q12	Category Average
Loudness	___	___	___	___	___ (target = 4.13)
Satisfaction	___	___	___	___	___
Loud Sounds	Q2	Q9	Q10	Q11	Category Average
Loudness	___	___	___	___	___ (target = 5.92)
Satisfaction	___	___	___	___	___

Normative data for PAL

Satisfaction rating scale legend:
1 = very dissatisfied to 5 = very satisfied

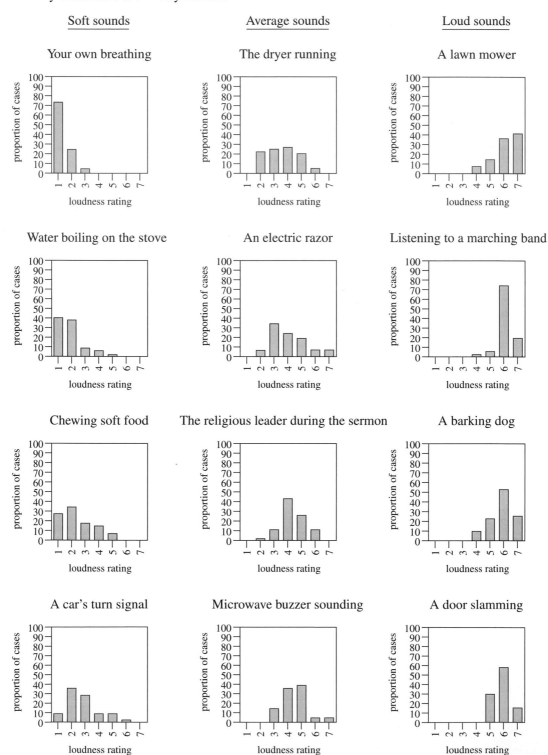

ATTACHMENT 18

The Denver Scale of Communication Function for Senior Citizens Living in Retirement Centers

NAME: _____ DATE OF PRE-TEST: _____

ADDRESS: _____ DATE OF POST-TEST: _____

AGE: _____ EXAMINER: _____

SEX: _____

1. Do you have trouble communicating with your family because of your hearing problem? Yes _____ No _____

   Probe Effect I
   a. Does your family make decisions for you because of your hearing problem? Yes _____ No _____
   b. Does your family leave you out of discussions because of your hearing problem? Yes _____ No _____
   c. Does your family get angry or annoyed with you because of your hearing problem? Yes _____ No _____

   Exploration Effect
   a. Do you have a family? Yes _____ No _____
   b. How often does your family visit you?
   c. How far away does your family live? In a city _____ Other _____
   d. How often do you visit your family?

2. Do you get upset when you cannot hear or understand what is being said? Yes _____ No _____

   Probe Effect I (to be used only if person responds yes)
   a. Do your friends know you get upset? Yes _____ No _____
   b. Does your family know you get upset? Yes _____ No _____
   c. Does the staff know you get upset? Yes _____ No _____

   Probe Effect II (to be used only if person responds no)
   a. Do your friends realize you are not upset? Yes _____ No _____
   b. Does your family realize you are not upset? Yes _____ No _____
   c. Does the staff realize you are not upset? Yes _____ No _____

   Exploration Effect (to be used only if person responds yes)
   a. How does your behavior change when you become upset?

3. Do you think your family, your friends, and the staff understand what it is like to have a hearing problem? Yes _____ No _____

   Probe Effect
   a. Do they avoid you because of your hearing problem? Yes _____ No _____
   b. Do they leave you out of discussions? Yes _____ No _____
   c. Do they hesitate to ask you to socialize with them? Yes _____ No _____

   Exploration Effect
   a. Family   Yes _____ No _____
   b. Friends   Yes _____ No _____
   c. Staff   Yes _____ No _____

4. Do you avoid communicating with other people because of your hearing problem? Yes _____ No _____

Probe Effect

a. Do you communicate with people during meal times? Yes _____ No _____

b. Do you communicate with your roommate(s)? Yes _____ No _____

c. Do you communicate during the social activities in the home? Yes _____ No _____

d. Do you communicate with visiting family or friends? Yes _____ No _____

e. Do you communicate with the staff? Yes _____ No _____

Exploration Effect

a. Is your roommate capable of communication? Yes _____ No _____

b. What are the social activities of the home? _____

c. Which ones do you attend? _____

5. Do you feel that you are a relaxed person? Yes _____ No _____

Probe Effect

a. Do you think you are an irritable person because of your hearing problem? Yes _____ No _____

b. Do you think you are an irritable person because of your age? Yes _____ No _____

c. Do you think you are an irritable person because you live in this home? Yes _____ No _____

Exploration Effect

Do you have to live in this home? Yes _____ No _____

6. Do you feel relaxed in group communicative situations? Yes _____ No _____

Probe Effect

a. Do you get nervous when you have to ask people to repeat what they have said if you have not understood them? Yes _____ No _____

b. Do you feel nervous if you have to tell a person that you have a hearing problem? Yes _____ No _____

Exploration Effect

a. Do you watch facial expression? Yes _____ No _____

b. Do you watch gestures? Yes _____ No _____

c. Do you think you are a good listener? Yes _____ No _____ Why? _____

d. Do you have a hearing aid? Yes _____ No _____

e. Do you wear your aid? Yes _____ No _____

7. Do you think you need help in overcoming your hearing problem? Yes _____ No _____

Exploration Effect I

a. A person can improve his communication ability by using lipreading (or speechreading) which means watching the speaker's lips, facial expressions, and gestures when he's speaking to you.

b. Do you agree with that definition of lipreading?

Probe Effect

a. If lipreading training was available, would you attend? Yes _____ No _____

b. Do you think this home provides adequate activities to make you want to communicate? Yes _____ No _____

Exploration Effect II

a. Is your vision adequate? Yes _____ No _____

b. Are you able to get around unassisted? Yes _____ No _____

Reprinted by permission from Zarnock JM, Alpiner JG. The Denver Scale of Communication Function for Senior Citizens Living in Retirement Centers, unpublished study, 1977.

**THE DENVER SCALE OF COMMUNICATION
FUNCTION FOR SENIOR CITIZENS LIVING
IN RETIREMENT CENTERS**

_____ Initial
Evaluation
_____ Final
Evaluation

by
Janet M. Zarnoch, M. A. and Jerome G. Alpiner, Ph.D.

NAME: _____   DATE OF PRE-TEST: _____

ADDRESS: _____   DATE OF POST-TEST: _____

AGE: _____ SEX: _____   EXAMINER: _____

CATEGORY	MAIN QUESTION	PROBE EFFECTS	EXPLORATION EFFECTS	PROBLEM	NO PROBLEM
Family	1 ☐+ ☐−	a ☐ b ☐ c ☐	a. _____ b. _____ c. _____ d. _____		
Emotional	2 ☐+ ☐−	I a ☐ b ☐ c ☐ II a ☐ b ☐ c ☐	a. _____ _____		
Other Persons	3 ☐+ ☐−	a ☐ b ☐ c ☐	a. _____ _____ b. _____ c. _____		
General Communication	4 ☐+ ☐−	a ☐ b ☐ c ☐ d ☐ e ☐	a. _____ _____ b. _____ _____ c. _____		
Self Concept	5 ☐+ ☐−	a ☐ b ☐ c ☐	a. _____ _____		
Group Situations	6 ☐+ ☐−	a ☐ b ☐ c ☐	a. _____ b. _____ c. _____ d. _____ e. _____		
Rehabilitation	7 ☐+ ☐−	a ☐ b ☐	Ia. _____ b. _____ IIa. _____ b. _____		

Key   + = person responded yes to question
        − = person responded no to question

Additional Client Comments:

1. _____
2. _____
3. _____
4. _____
5. _____
6. _____

ATTACHMENT 19
The Denver Scale of Communication Function—Modified

PRE-THERAPY _____ POST-THERAPY _____

DATE _____

NAME _____ AGE _____ SEX _____

ADDRESS _____

_____

AUDIOGRAM (Examination Date) _____

Pure tone	250	500	1000	2000	4000	8000	Hz
RE	____	____	____	____	____	____	db (re:)
LE	____	____	____	____	____	____	(ANSI)

Speech   Discrimination Score (%)

SRT   Quiet   Noise (S/N =)

RE _____ dB   RE _____   _____

LE _____ dB   LE _____   _____

Hearing Aid Information:

Aided _____ For How Long _____ Aid Type _____

Ear _____ Satisfaction _____

                                                        Examiner _____

INSTRUCTIONS

I am going to say some statements relating to hearing loss. For each statement, I want you to tell me if you: (1) definitely agree, (2) slightly agree, (3) irrelevant, (4) slightly disagree or (5) definitely disagree. If you consider the statement to be irrelevant or unassociated to your communication problem, please tell me.

Scoring

(1) Definitely agree   (2) Slightly agree   (3) Irrelevant   (4) Slightly disagree   (5) Definitely disagree

Attitude Toward Peers

1. The people I live with are annoyed by my loss of hearing. Comments:
   - _____ 1. Definitely agree
   - _____ 2. Slightly agree
   - _____ 3. Irrelevant
   - _____ 4. Slightly disagree
   - _____ 5. Definitely disagree

2. The people I live with sometimes leave me out of conversations or discussions. Comments:
   - _____ 1. Definitely agree
   - _____ 2. Slightly agree
   - _____ 3. Irrelevant
   - _____ 4. Slightly disagree
   - _____ 5. Definitely disagree

3. Sometimes people I live with make decisions for me because I have a hard time following discussions. Comments:
   - _____ 1. Definitely agree
   - _____ 2. Slightly agree
   - _____ 3. Irrelevant
   - _____ 4. Slightly disagree
   - _____ 5. Definitely disagree

4. People I live with become annoyed when I ask them to repeat what was said because I did not hear them. Comments:
   - _____ 1. Definitely agree
   - _____ 2. Slightly agree
   - _____ 3. Irrelevant
   - _____ 4. Slightly disagree
   - _____ 5. Definitely disagree

5. Other people do not realize how frustrated I get when I cannot hear or understand. Comments:
   - _____ 1. Definitely agree
   - _____ 2. Slightly agree
   - _____ 3. Irrelevant
   - _____ 4. Slightly disagree
   - _____ 5. Definitely disagree

6. People sometimes avoid me because of my hearing loss. Comments:

_____ 1. Definitely agree
_____ 2. Slightly agree
_____ 3. Irrelevant
_____ 4. Slightly disagree
_____ 5. Definitely disagree

Socialization

7. I am not an "outgoing" person because I have a hearing loss. Comments:

_____ 1. Definitely agree
_____ 2. Slightly agree
_____ 3. Irrelevant
_____ 4. Slightly disagree
_____ 5. Definitely disagree

8. I now take less of an interest in many things as compared to when I did not have a hearing problem. Comments:

_____ 1. Definitely agree
_____ 2. Slightly agree
_____ 3. Irrelevant
_____ 4. Slightly disagree
_____ 5. Definitely disagree

9. I am not a calm person because of my hearing loss. Comments:

_____ 1. Definitely agree
_____ 2. Slightly agree
_____ 3. Irrelevant
_____ 4. Slightly disagree
_____ 5. Definitely disagree

10. I tend to be negative about life in general because of my hearing loss. Comments:

_____ 1. Definitely agree
_____ 2. Slightly agree
_____ 3. Irrelevant
_____ 4. Slightly disagree
_____ 5. Definitely disagree

11. I do not socialize as much as I did before I began to lose my hearing. Comments:

_____ 1. Definitely agree
_____ 2. Slightly agree
_____ 3. Irrelevant
_____ 4. Slightly disagree
_____ 5. Definitely disagree

12. Since I have trouble hearing, I do not like to participate in activities. Comments:

_____ 1. Definitely agree
2. Slightly agree
_____ 3. Irrelevant
_____ 4. Slightly disagree
5. Definitely disagree

13. Since I have trouble hearing I hesitate to meet new people. Comments:

_____ 1. Definitely agree
_____ 2. Slightly agree
_____ 3. Irrelevant
4. Slightly disagree

_____ 5. Definitely disagree

14. Other people do not understand what it is like to have a hearing loss. Comments:

_____ 1. Definitely agree
_____ 2. Slightly agree
_____ 3. Irrelevant
_____ 4. Slightly disagree
_____ 5. Definitely disagree

15. I do not feel relaxed or comfortable in a communicative situation. Comments:

_____ 1. Definitely agree
_____ 2. Slightly agree
_____ 3. Irrelevant
_____ 4. Slightly disagree
_____ 5. Definitely disagree

Communication

16. Because I have difficulty understanding what is said to me I sometimes answer questions wrong. Comments:

_____ 1. Definitely agree
_____ 2. Slightly agree
_____ 3. Irrelevant
_____ 4. Slightly disagree
_____ 5. Definitely disagree

17. Conversations in a noisy room prevent me from attempting to communicate with others. Comments:

_____ 1. Definitely agree
_____ 2. Slightly agree
_____ 3. Irrelevant
_____ 4. Slightly disagree
_____ 5. Definitely disagree

Reprinted by permission from Kaplan H, Feeley J, Brown J. A modified Denver Scale: test-retest reliability. J Acad Rehab Audiol 1978;11:15–32.

18. I am not comfortable having to communicate in a group situation. Comments:

_____ 1. Definitely agree
_____ 2. Slightly agree
_____ 3. Irrelevant
_____ 4. Slightly disagree
_____ 5. Definitely disagree

19. I seldom watch other people's facial expressions when talking to them. Comments:

_____ 1. Definitely agree
_____ 2. Slightly agree
_____ 3. Irrelevant
_____ 4. Slightly disagree
_____ 5. Definitely disagree

20. Most people do not know how to talk to a hearing-impaired person. Comments:

_____ 1. Definitely agree
_____ 2. Slightly agree
_____ 3. Irrelevant
_____ 4. Slightly disagree
_____ 5. Definitely disagree

21. I hesitate to ask people to repeat if I do not understand them for the first time they speak. Comments:

_____ 1. Definitely agree
_____ 2. Slightly agree
_____ 3. Irrelevant
_____ 4. Slightly disagree
_____ 5. Definitely disagree

22. Because I have difficulty understanding what is said to me, I sometimes make comments that do not fit the conversation. Comments:

_____ 1. Definitely agree
_____ 2. Slightly agree
_____ 3. Irrelevant
_____ 4. Slightly disagree
_____ 5. Definitely disagree

23. I do not like to admit that I have a hearing problem. Comments:

_____ 1. Definitely agree
_____ 2. Slightly agree
_____ 3. Irrelevant
_____ 4. Slightly disagree
_____ 5. Definitely disagree

Specific Difficulty Listening Situations

24. I have trouble hearing the radio or the television unless I turn the volume on very loud. Comments:

_____ 1. Definitely agree
_____ 2. Slightly agree
_____ 3. Irrelevant
_____ 4. Slightly disagree
_____ 5. Definitely disagree

25. If someone calls me when my back is turned, I do not always hear him. Comments:

_____ 1. Definitely agree
_____ 2. Slightly agree
_____ 3. Irrelevant
_____ 4. Slightly disagree
_____ 5. Definitely disagree

26. If someone calls me from another room, I have much trouble hearing. Comments:

_____ 1. Definitely agree
_____ 2. Slightly agree
_____ 3. Irrelevant
_____ 4. Slightly disagree
_____ 5. Definitely disagree

27. When I sit talking with friends in a quite room, I have a great deal of difficulty hearing. Comments:

_____ 1. Definitely agree
_____ 2. Slightly agree
_____ 3. Irrelevant
_____ 4. Slightly disagree
_____ 5. Definitely disagree

28. When I use the phone, I have much difficulty hearing. Comments:

_____ 1. Definitely agree
_____ 2. Slightly agree
_____ 3. Irrelevant
_____ 4. Slightly disagree
_____ 5. Definitely disagree

29. When I play cards, understanding my partner gives me much difficulty. Comments:

_____ 1. Definitely agree
_____ 2. Slightly agree
_____ 3. Irrelevant
_____ 4. Slightly disagree
_____ 5. Definitely disagree

30. At lectures or discussions I have much difficulty hearing the speaker. Comments:

_____ 1. Definitely agree
_____ 2. Slightly agree
_____ 3. Irrelevant
_____ 4. Slightly disagree
_____ 5. Definitely disagree

31. In church, when the minister gives the sermon, I have much difficulty. Comments:

_____ 1. Definitely agree
_____ 2. Slightly agree
_____ 3. Irrelevant
_____ 4. Slightly disagree
_____ 5. Definitely disagree

32. When a movie is shown, I have much difficulty hearing what is said. Comments:

_____ 1. Definitely agree
_____ 2. Slightly agree
_____ 3. Irrelevant
_____ 4. Slightly disagree
_____ 5. Definitely disagree

33. I have difficulty understanding announcements sent through the loudspeaker even when the speaker is in the same room. Comments:

_____ 1. Definitely agree
_____ 2. Slightly agree
_____ 3. Irrelevant
_____ 4. Slightly disagree
_____ 5. Definitely disagree

34. I have trouble understanding messages sent over the intercom. Comments:

_____ 1. Definitely agree
_____ 2. Slightly agree
_____ 3. Irrelevant
_____ 4. Slightly disagree
_____ 5. Definitely disagree

ATTACHMENT 20 Nursing Home Hearing Handicap Index (NHHI): Self Version for Resident

	Very Often				Almost Never
1. When you are with other people do you wish you could hear better?	5	4	3	2	1
2. Do other people feel you have a hearing problem (when they try to talk to you)?	5	4	3	2	1
3. Do you have trouble hearing another person if there is a radio or TV playing (in the same room)?	5	4	3	2	1
4. Do you have trouble hearing the radio or TV?	5	4	3	2	1
5. (How often) do you feel life would be better if you could hear better?	5	4	3	2	1
6. How often are you embarrassed because you don't hear well?	5	4	3	2	1
7. When you are alone do you wish you could hear better?	5	4	3	2	1
8. Do people (tend to) leave you out of conversations because you don't hear well?	5	4	3	2	1
9. (How often) do you withdraw from social activities (in which you ought to participate) because you don't hear well?	5	4	3	2	1
10. Do you say "what" or "pardon me" when people first speak to you?	5	4	3	2	1

Total _____ × 2 = _____

−20

_____ × 1.25 = _____ %

Reprinted by permission from Schow KL, Nerbonne MA. Assessment of hearing handicaps by nursing home residents and staff. J Acad Rehabil Audiol 1977;10:2–12.

Nursing Home Hearing Handicap Index (NHHI): Staff Version

	Very Often				Almost Never
1. When this person is with other people does he/she need to hear better?	5	4	3	2	1
2. Do members of the staff, family and friends make negative comments about this person's hearing problems?	5	4	3	2	1
3. Do they have trouble hearing another person if there is a radio or TV playing in the same room?	5	4	3	2	1
4. When this person is listening to radio or TV do they have trouble hearing?	5	4	3	2	1
5. How often do you feel life would be better for this person if they could hear better?	5	4	3	2	1
6. How often are they embarrassed because they don't hear well?	5	4	3	2	1
7. When they are alone do they need to hear the everyday sounds of life better?	5	4	3	2	1
8. Do people tend to leave them out of conversations because they don't hear well?	5	4	3	2	1
9. How often do they withdraw from social activities in which they ought to participate because they don't hear well?	5	4	3	2	1
10. Do they say "what" or "pardon me" when people first speak to them?	5	4	3	2	1

Total _____ × 2 = _____

−20

_____ × 1.25 = _____ %

Reprinted by permission from Schow KL, Nerbonne MA. Assessment of hearing handicaps by nursing home residents and staff. J Acad Rehabil Audiol 1977;10:2–12.

ATTACHMENT 21 *Communications Assessment Procedure for Seniors (CAPS)*

Name: _____ Date: _____ Birthdate: _____ Sex: _____

Address: _____

Telephone: _____ Pre-Service: _____ Post-Service _____

A. General Communication

1. Do you avoid talking to other people because of your hearing problem?
   Always _____   Never _____
   Sometimes _____   Not applicable _____

2. Do you talk with your roommate?
   Always _____   Never _____
   Sometimes _____   Not applicable _____

3. Do you talk with people during the social activities of this home?
   Always _____   Never _____
   Sometimes _____   Not applicable _____

4. Do you talk with people during your meals?
   Always _____   Never _____
   Sometimes   Not applicable _____

5. Do you talk to the staff here?
   Always _____   Never _____
   Sometimes _____   Not applicable _____

6. Do you have trouble hearing in certain situations? (Example: watching television, listening to the radio, etc.)
   Always _____   Never _____
   Sometimes _____   Not applicable _____

B. Group Situations

1. Do you feel relaxed in group situations?
   Always _____   Never _____
   Sometimes   Not applicable _____

2. Do you ask a person to repeat if you don't understand what he says?
   Always _____   Never _____
   Sometimes _____   Not applicable _____

3. Does it make you nervous to ask a person to repeat what he said?
   Always _____   Never _____
   Sometimes _____   Not applicable _____

4. Does it make you nervous to tell a person you have a hearing problem?
   Always _____   Never _____
   Sometimes _____   Not applicable _____

5. Do you think your hearing problem annoys other people?
   Always _____   Never _____
   Sometimes _____   Not applicable _____

6. Do you get annoyed when people don't speak loudly enough for you to hear?
   Always _____   Never _____
   Sometimes _____   Not applicable _____

7. Do you feel isolated from group discussions because of your hearing loss?
   Always _____   Never _____
   Sometimes _____   Not applicable _____

C. Other Persons: Family, Friends, and Staff

1. Do you think other people understand what it's like to have a hearing problem?
   Always _____   Never _____
   Sometimes _____   Not applicable _____

2. Do others avoid you because of your hearing loss?
   Always _____   Never _____
   Sometimes _____   Not applicable _____

3. Does anyone ever leave you out of conversation because of your hearing problem?
   Always _____   Never _____
   Sometimes _____   Not applicable _____

4. Do you mind telling people that you have a hearing loss?
   Always _____   Never _____
   Sometimes _____   Not applicable _____

5. Do other people understand how frustrated you get when you can't hear them?
Always _____   Never _____
Sometimes _____   Not applicable _____

Comments: Tell me how other people, like your friends, your family, and the staff here, react to your hearing loss.

D. Self-Concept

1. Would you describe yourself as a relaxed person?
Always _____   Never _____
Sometimes _____   Not applicable _____

2. Does your hearing loss make you irritable?
Always _____   Never _____
Sometimes _____   Not applicable _____

3. Do you like living here?
Always _____   Never _____
Sometimes _____   Not applicable _____

4. Are you an interesting person?
Always _____   Never _____
Sometimes _____   Not applicable _____

5. Are you a happy person?
Always _____   Never _____
Sometimes _____   Not applicable _____

6. Do you keep busy with hobbies and other activities?
Always _____   Never _____
Sometimes _____   Not applicable _____

Comments: Is there anything else you'd like to tell me about yourself or about living here?

E. Family

Do you have a family? How much do you see your family? Where do they live? (If the person does not have family, do not use this section.)

1. Does your family get annoyed with you when you can't hear them?
Always _____   Never _____
Sometimes _____   Not applicable _____

2. Do they make decisions for you because of your hearing loss?
Always _____   Never _____
Sometimes _____   Not applicable _____

3. Does your family leave you out of discussions because of your hearing loss?
Always _____   Never _____
Sometimes _____   Not applicable _____

4. Do members of your family speak loudly enough for you to hear them?
Always _____   Never _____
Sometimes _____   Not applicable _____

5. Does your family understand what it's like to have a hearing problem?
Always _____   Never _____
Sometimes _____   Not applicable _____

Comments: How does your family feel about your hearing loss?

F. Rehabilitation

1. Do you think you need help in overcoming your hearing problem?
Always _____   Never _____
Sometimes _____   Not applicable _____

2. Are you a good listener?
Always _____   Never _____
Sometimes _____   Not applicable _____

3. Do you watch facial expressions when someone is speaking to you?
Always _____   Never _____
Sometimes _____   Not applicable _____

4. Do you watch gestures or "body language" when someone is talking to you?
Always _____   Never _____
Sometimes _____   Not applicable _____

5. Do you have a hearing aid? (If person responds yes, proceed.)
Always _____   Never _____
Sometimes _____   Not applicable _____

6. Do you wear your hearing aid?
Always _____   Never _____
Sometimes _____   Not applicable _____

Comments: If lipreading training were available, would you be interested in attending?

Reprinted by permission from Alpiner JG, Baker B. Communication assessment procedures in aural rehabilitation process. Semin Speech Lang Hear 1981;2:189–204.

ATTACHMENT 22
The Hearing Handicap Inventory for the Elderly

Instructions:

The purpose of this scale is to identify the problems your hearing loss may be causing you. Answer YES, SOMETIMES, or NO for each question. *Do not skip a question if you avoid a situation because of your hearing problem.* If you use a hearing aid, please answer the way you hear *without* the aid.

		Yes (4)	Some-times (2)	No (0)
S-1.	Does a hearing problem cause you to use the phone less often than you would like?	____	____	____
E-2.	Does a hearing problem cause you to feel embarrassed when meeting new people?	____	____	____
S-3.	Does a hearing problem cause you to avoid groups of people?	____	____	____
E-4.	Does a hearing problem make you irritable?	____	____	____
E-5.	Does a hearing problem cause you to feel frustrated when talking to members of your family?	____	____	____
S-6.	Does a hearing problem cause you difficulty when attending a party?	____	____	____
E-7.	Does a hearing problem cause you to feel "stupid" or "dumb"?	____	____	____
S-8.	Do you have difficulty hearing when someone speaks in a whisper?	____	____	____
E-9.	Do you feel handicapped by a hearing problem?	____	____	____
S-10.	Does a hearing problem cause you difficulty when visiting friends, relatives, or neighbors?	____	____	____
S-11.	Does a hearing problem cause you to attend religious services less often than you would like?	____	____	____
E-12.	Does a hearing problem cause you to be nervous?	____	____	____
S-13.	Does a hearing problem cause you to visit friends, relatives, or neighbors less often than you would like?	____	____	____
E-14.	Does a hearing problem cause you to have arguments with family members?	____	____	____
S-15.	Does a hearing problem cause you difficulty when listening to TV or radio?	____	____	____
S-16.	Does a hearing problem cause you to go shopping less often than you would like?	____	____	____
E-17.	Does any problem or difficulty with your hearing upset you at all?	____	____	____
E-18.	Does a hearing problem cause you to want to be by yourself?	____	____	____
S-19.	Does a hearing problem cause you to talk to family members less often than you would like?	____	____	____
E-20.	Do you feel that any difficulty with your hearing limits or hampers your personal or social life?	____	____	____
S-21.	Does a hearing problem cause you difficulty when in a restaurant with relatives or friends?	____	____	____
E-22.	Does a hearing problem cause you to feel depressed?	____	____	____
S-23.	Does a hearing problem cause you to listen to TV or radio less often than you would like?	____	____	____
E-24.	Does a hearing problem cause you to feel uncomfortable when talking to friends?	____	____	____
E-25.	Does a hearing problem cause you to feel left out when you are with a group of people?	____	____	____

FOR CLINICIAN'S USE ONLY: Total Score: _____
Subtotal E: _____
Subtotal S: _____

Reprinted by permission from Ventry I, Weinstein B. The Hearing Handicap Inventory for the Elderly: a new tool. Ear Hear 1982;3:128–134.

ATTACHMENT 23 *Hearing Handicap Inventory for the Elderly—Screening Version (HHIE-S)*

Please answer "yes," "no," or "sometimes" to each of the following items. Do not skip a question if you avoid a situation because of a hearing problem. If you use a hearing aid, please answer the way you hear without the aid.

		Yes	No	Some-times
E-1.	Does a hearing problem cause you to feel embarrassed when you meet new people?	____	____	____
E-2.	Does a hearing problem cause you to feel frustrated when talking to members of your family?	____	____	____
S-3.	Do you have difficulty hearing when someone speaks in a whisper?	____	____	____
E-4.	Do you feel handicapped by a hearing problem?	____	____	____
S-5.	Does a hearing problem cause you difficulty when visiting friends, relatives, or neighbors?	____	____	____
S-6.	Does a hearing problem cause you to attend religious services less often than you would like?	____	____	____
E-7.	Does a hearing problem cause you to have arguments with family members?	____	____	____
S-8.	Does a hearing problem cause you difficulty when listening to TV or radio?	____	____	____
E-9.	Do you feel that any difficulty with your hearing limits or hampers your personal or social life?	____	____	____
S-10.	Does a hearing problem cause you difficulty when in a restaurant with relatives or friends?	____	____	____

Reprinted by permission from Ventry I, Weinstein B. Identification of elderly people with hearing problems. Ear Hear 1982;3:128–134.

ATTACHMENT 24 *Abbreviated Profile of Hearing Aid Benefit*

INSTRUCTIONS: Please circle the answers that come closest to your everyday experience. Notice that each choice includes a percentage. You can use this to help you decide on your answer. For example, if a statement is true about 75% of the time, circle C for that item. If you have not experienced the situation we describe, try to think of a similar situation that you have been in and respond for that situation. If you have no idea, leave that item blank.

A Always (99%)
B Almost Always (87%)
C Generally (75%)
D Half-the-time (50%)
E Occasionally (25%)
F Seldom (12%)
G Never (1%)

	Without My Hearing Aid	With My Hearing Aid
1. When I am in a crowded grocery store, talking with the cashier, I can follow the conversation.	A B C D E F G	A B C D E F G
2. I miss a lot of information when I'm listening to a lecture.	A B C D E F G	A B C D E F G
3. Unexpected sounds, like a smoke detector or alarm bell are uncomfortable.	A B C D E F G	A B C D E F G
4. I have difficulty hearing a conversation when I'm with one of my family at home.	A B C D E F G	A B C D E F G
5. I have trouble understanding dialogue in a movie or at the theater.	A B C D E F G	A B C D E F G
6. When I am listening to the news on the car radio, and family members are talking, I have trouble hearing the news.	A B C D E F G	A B C D E F G
7. When I am at the dinner table with several people, and am trying to have a conversation with one person, understanding speech is difficult.	A B C D E F C	A B C D E F G
8. Traffic noises are too loud.	A B C D E F G	A B C D E F G
9. When I am talking with someone across a large empty room, I understand the words.	A B C D E F G	A B C D E F G
10. When I am in a small office, interviewing or answering questions, I have difficulty following the conversation.	A B C D E F G	A B C D E F G
11. When I am in a theater watching a movie or play, and the people around me are whispering and rustling paper wrappers, I can still make out the dialogue.	A B C D E F G	A B C D E F G
12. When I am having a quiet conversation with a friend, I have difficulty understanding.	A B C D E F G	A B C D E F G
13. The sounds of running water, such as a toilet or shower, are uncomfortably loud.	A B C D E F G	A B C D E F G
14. When a speaker is addressing a small group, and everyone is listening quietly, I have to strain to understand.	A B C D E F G	A B C D E F G
15. When I'm in a quiet conversation with my doctor in an examination room, it is hard to follow the conversation.	A B C D E F G	A B C D E F G
16. I can understand conversations even when several people are talking.	A B C D E F G	A B C D E F G
17. The sounds of construction work are uncomfortably loud.	A B C D E F G	A B C D E F G
18. It's hard for me to understand what is being said at lectures or church services.	A B C D E F G	A B C D E F G
19. I can communicate with others when we are in a crowd.	A B C D E F G	A B C D E F G
20. The sound of a fire engine siren close by is so loud that I need to cover my ears.	A B C D E F G	A B C D E F G
21. I can follow the words of a sermon when listening to a religious service.	A B C D E F G	A B C D E F G
22. The sound of screeching tires is uncomfortably loud.	A B C D E F G	A B C D E F G
23. I have to ask people to repeat themselves in one on one conversation in a quiet room.	A B C D E F G	A B C D E F G
24. I have trouble understanding others when an air conditioner or fan is on.	A B C D E F G	A B C D E F G

Reprinted with permission from Cox RM, Alexander GC. The abbreviated profile of hearing aid benefit. Ear Hear 1995;16:176–186.

ATTACHMENT 25

The Hearing Aid Performance Inventory

INSTRUCTIONS

We are interested in knowing the extent to which your hearing aid helps you in your daily life. In this questionnaire you are asked to judge the helpfulness of your hearing aid in a variety of listening situations. You are asked to rate the benefit of your hearing aid in each situation and not the difficulty of the situation itself.

To answer each question, check the phrase that best describes how your hearing aid helps you in that situation.

-Very Helpful
-Helpful
-Very Little Help
-No Help
-Hinders Performance

There are items that appear similar but differ in at least one important detail. Therefore, read each item carefully before checking the appropriate phrase. We know that all people do not talk alike. Some mumble, others talk too fast, and others talk without moving their lips very much. Please answer the questions according to the way most people talk.

If you have never experienced the situation but can predict your hearing aid performance, respond to the item. A "Does Not Apply" response box is also provided. However, use the response "Does Not Apply" only if you do not know how helpful your hearing aid would be in the given situation.

Items

1. You are sitting alone at home watching the news on TV.

2. You are involved in an intimate conversation with your spouse.

3. You are watching TV and there are distracting noises such as others talking.

4. You are at home engaged in some activity and the telephone rings in another room.

5. You are at home in conversation with a member of your family who is in another room.

6. You are at a crowded outdoor auction bidding on an item.

7. You are listening to a speaker who is talking to a large group and you are seated toward the rear of the room. His back is partially turned as he makes notes on a blackboard.

8. You are starting to cross a busy street and a car horn sounds a warning.

9. You are riding on a crowded bus. You are in conversation with a friend seated next to you and you do not want others to overhear your conversation.

10. You are walking in the downtown section of a large city. There are the usual city noises and you are in conversation with a friend.

11. You are in a large office with the usual noise in the background (e.g., typewriters, air conditioners, fans, etc.). A co-worker is telling you the latest gossip from close range in a soft voice.

12. You are riding in the back seat of a taxi. The window is down and the radio is on. The driver strikes up a conversation in a relatively soft voice.

13. You are driving your car and listening to a news broadcast on the radio. You are alone and the windows are closed.

14. You are in a crowded grocery store checkout line and talking with the cashier.

15. You are alone in a small office with the door closed. People are talking quietly outside the door and you want to overhear the conversation.

16. You are at a crowded office picnic talking with a friend.

17. You are at home watching television and the doorbell rings.

18. You are with your family at a noisy amusement park and you are discussing which attraction to go to next.

19. You are taking an evening stroll with a friend through a quiet neighborhood park, there are the usual environmental sounds around (e.g., children playing, dogs barking).

20. You are at home alone listening to your stereo system. (instrumental music).

21. You are listening to an orchestra in a large concert hall.

22. You are in whispered conversation with your spouse at an intimate restaurant.

23. You are in the kitchen in conversation with your spouse during the preparation of an evening meal.

24. You are at home in face to face conversation with member of your family.

25. You are shopping at a large busy department store and talking with a salesclerk.

26. You are at church listening to the sermon and sitting in the front pew.

27. You are listening to a speaker who is talking to a large group and you are seated toward the rear of the room. There is an occasional noise in the room (e.g., whispering, rattling papers, etc.).

28. You are having a conversation in your home with a salesman and there is background noise (e.g., TV, people talking) in the room.

29. You are attending a business meeting where people are seated around a conference table. The boss is talking; everybody is listening quietly.

30. You are at church listening to the sermon and sitting in the back pew.

31. You are talking with a friend outdoors on a windy day.

32. You are driving your car with the windows up and carrying on a conversation with your spouse in the front seat.

33. You are in a small office interviewing for a job.

34. You are ordering food for the family at McDonald's.

35. You are at home reading the paper. Two family members are in another room talking quietly and you want to listen in on their conversation.

36. You are in a courtroom listening to the various speakers (witness, judge, lawyer).

37. You are talking with a teller at the drive-in window bank.

38. You are in a noisy business office talking with a stranger on the telephone.

39. You are in conversation with someone across a large room (such as an auditorium).

40. You are in conversation with a neighbor across the fence.

41. You are in a crowded reception room waiting for your name to be called.

42. You are in your backyard gardening. Your neighbor is using a noisy power lawnmower and yells something to you.

43. You are listening in a small quiet room to someone who speaks softly.

44. You are on an airplane and the stewardess is requiring a meal selection.

45. You are riding in a crowded bus and are in conversation with a stranger seated next to you.

46. You are alone driving your automobile and the cars around you are pulling to the side of the road. You begin to listen for what you anticipate is an emergency vehicle (firetruck, rescue squad, etc.).

47. Someone is trying to tell you something in a small quiet room while you have your back turned.

48. You are driving with your family and are listening to a news broadcast on the car radio. Your window is down and family members are talking.

49. You are driving your car with the windows down and are carrying on a conversation with others riding with you.

50. You are at an exciting sports activity (baseball, football game, etc.) and talk occasionally with those around you.

51. You are in a large business office talking with a clerk. There is the usual office noise (e.g., typing, talking, etc.).

52. You are in a quiet conversation with your family doctor in an examination room.

53. You are talking to a large group and someone from the back of the audience asks a question in a relatively soft voice. Audience is quiet as they listen to the question.

54. You are walking through a large crowded airport and are in conversation with a friend.

55. You are at a large noisy party and are engaged in conversation with one other person.

56. You are alone in the woods listening to the sounds of nature (e.g., birds, insects, small animals, etc.).

57. You are at the dinner table with your whole family and are in conversation with your spouse.

58. You are attending a business meeting where people are seated around a conference table. The discussion is heated as everyone attempts to make a point. The speakers are frequently interrupted.

59. You are one of only a few customers inside your bank and are talking with a teller.

60. You are at a theater watching a movie. There are occasional noises around you (e.g., whispering, wrappers rustling, etc.).

61. You are alone at home talking with a friend on the telephone.

62. You are downtown in a large city requesting directions from a pedestrian.

63. You are riding in a car with friends. The windows of the car are rolled down. You are in the back seat carrying on a conversation with them.

64. You are driving your car with the windows up and radio off and are carrying on a conversation with your spouse who is in the front seat.

ATTACHMENT 26

Hearing Performance Inventory

We are interested in knowing how your hearing problem has affected your daily living. Below you will find a series of questions which describe a variety of everyday listening situations and ask you to judge how much difficulty you would have hearing in these situations. Once we know which situations cause a person difficulty, we can begin to do something about them. Your answers will be confidential.

The questions cover many different listening situations. Some ask you to judge how well you can understand what people are saying when their voices are loud enough. The term <u>understand</u> means hearing the words a person is saying clearly enough to be able to participate in the conversation. Other questions ask whether you can hear enough of a particular sound (doorbell, speech, etc.) to be aware of its presence. Other questions concern occupational, social or personal situations. Still others ask what you <u>do</u> when you miss something that was said.

To answer each question, you are asked to check the phrase that best describes how often you experience the situation being described:

Practically always	(or always)
Frequently	(or about three-quarters of the time)
About half the time	
Occasionally	(about a quarter of the time)
Almost never	(or never)

For example, if you can understand what a person is saying on the telephone about 100% of the time then you should check <u>practically always</u>. On the other hand, if you can understand almost nothing of what a person is saying on the telephone, then you should check <u>almost never</u>. If you can understand what a person is saying on the telephone about 50% of the time, then you should check <u>about half the time</u>.

Your answers to the questions should describe your hearing ability as it is now. If you wear a hearing aid in the situation described, answer the question accordingly. Please check one, and only one, phrase for each question. You should check <u>Does not apply</u> only if you have not experienced a particular situation or one similar to it.

There are also questions that appear identical but differ in at least one important detail. Please read each question carefully before checking the appropriate phrase.

We know that all people do not talk alike. Some mumble, others talk too fast, and others talk without moving their lips very much. Please answer the questions according to the way <u>most</u> people talk to you.

If the question does not specify whether the person speaking is male or female, answer according to which sex you have the most difficulty hearing.

1. You are with a male friend or family member in a fairly quiet room. Can you understand him when his voice is loud enough for you and you can see his face?

2. You are with a female friend or family member in a fairly quiet room. Can you understand her when her voice is loud enough for you and can see her face?

3. You are with a female stranger in a fairly quiet room. Can you understand her when her voice is loud enough for you and you can see her face?

4. You are with a male stranger in a fairly quiet room. Can you understand him when his voice is loud enough for you and you can see his face?

5. You are with a child (6 to 10 years old) in a fairly quiet room. Can you understand the child when his/her voice is loud enough for you and you can see his/her face?

6. You are at a fairly quiet restaurant. Can you understand the waiter/waitress when his/her voice is loud enough for you and you can see his/her face?

7. You are at a restaurant with a friend or family member and the room is fairly quiet. Can you understand the person when his/her voice is loud enough for you and you can see his/her face?

8. You are in a fairly quiet room. Can you carry on a conversation with a man in another room if his voice is loud enough for you?

9. You are in a fairly quiet room. Can you carry on a conversation with a woman in another room if her voice is loud enough for you?

10. You are at a party or gathering of less than ten people and the room is fairly quiet. Can you understand what a friend or family member is saying to you when his/her voice is loud enough for you and you can see his/her face?

11. You are playing cards, monopoly or some similar game with several people and the room is fairly quiet. Can you understand what a friend or family member is saying to you when his/her voice is loud enough for you and you can see his/her face?

12. You are in a fairly quiet room with five or six friends or family members. One person talks at a time. When you are aware of the subject, can you understand what is being said when the speaker's voice is loud enough for you and you can see his/her face?

13. You are in a fairly quiet room talking with five or six strangers. One person talks at a time and the subject of conversation changes from time to time. Can you understand what is being said when the speaker's voice is loud enough for you and you can see his/her face?

14. You are watching your favorite news program on television. Can you understand the news reporter (male) when his voice is loud enough for you?

15. You are watching your favorite news program on television. Can you understand the news reporter (female) when her voice is loud enough for you?

16. You are watching a drama or movie on television. Can you understand what is being said when the speaker's voice is loud enough for you and there is no music in the background?

17. You are watching a drama or movie on television. Can you understand what is being said when the speaker's voice is loud enough for you and there is music in the background?

18. You are in an auditorium listening to a lecturer (male) who is using a microphone. Can you understand what he is saying when his voice is loud enough for you and you can see his face?

19. You are in an auditorium listening to a lecturer (female) who is using a microphone. Can you understand what she is saying when her voice is loud enough for you and you can see her face?

20. When an announcement is given over a public address system in a bus station or airport, can you understand what is being said when the speaker's voice is loud enough for you?

21. Can you understand what a man is saying on the telephone when his voice is loud enough for you?

22. Can you understand what a woman is saying on the telephone when her voice is loud enough for you?

23. You are at a movie. Can you understand what the actors/actresses are saying when their voices are loud enough for you and you can see their faces?

24. You are attending a stage play. Can you understand what the actors/actresses are saying when their voices are loud enough for you and you can see their faces?

25. You are with a male friend or family member and several people are talking nearby. Can you understand him when his voice is loud enough for you and you can see her face?

26. You are with a female friend or family member and several people are talking nearby. Can you understand her when her voice is loud enough for you and you can see her face?

27. You are with a female friend or family member and there is background noise such as traffic, music or a crowd of people. Can you understand her when her voice is loud enough for you and you can see her face?

28. You are with a male stranger and there is background noise such as traffic, music or a crowd of people. Can you understand him when his voice is loud enough for you and you can see his face?

29. You are with a female stranger and there is background noise such as traffic, music or a crowd of people. Can you understand her when her voice is loud enough for you and you can see her face?

30. You are with a child (6 to 10 years old) and several people are talking nearby. Can you understand the child when his/her voice is loud enough for you and you can see his/her face?

31. You are with a child (6 to 10 years old) and there is background noise such as traffic, music or a crowd of people. Can you understand the child when his/her voice is loud enough for you and you can see his/her face?

32. You are at a restaurant and several people are talking nearby. Can you understand the waiter/waitress when his/her voice is loud enough for you and you can see his/her face?

33. You are at a restaurant and there is background noise such as music or a crowd. Can you understand the waiter/waitress when his/her voice is loud enough for you and you can see his/her face?

34. You are at a restaurant with a friend or family member and several people are talking nearby. Can you understand the person when his/her voice is loud enough for you and you can see his/her face?

35. You are at a restaurant with a friend or family member and there is background noise such as music or a crowd of people. Can you understand the person when his/her voice is loud enough for you and you can see his/her face?

36. You are at a party or gathering of less than ten people and several talking nearby. Can you understand what a friend or family member is saying to you when his voice is loud enough for you and you can see his face?

37. You are at a party or gathering of less than ten people and several people are talking nearby. Can you understand what a friend or family member (female) is saying to you when her voice is loud enough for you and you can see her face?

38. You are at a party or gathering of less than ten people and several people are talking nearby. Can you understand what a friend or family member (female) is saying to you when her voice is loud enough for you and you can see her face?

39. You are at a party or gathering of more than twenty people and several people are talking nearby. Can you understand what a friend or family member (male) is saying to you when his voice is loud enough for you and you can see his face?

40. You are at a party or gathering of more than twenty people and there is background noise such as music or a crowd of people. Can you understand what a stranger is saying to you when his/her voice is loud enough for you and you can see his/her face?

41. You are playing cards, monopoly or some similar game with several people and other people are talking nearby. Can you understand what a friend or family member is saying to you when his/her voice is loud enough for you and you can see his/her face?

42. You are playing cards, monopoly or some similar game with several people and there is background noise such as music or a crowd of people. Can you understand what a friend or family member is saying to you when his/her voice is loud enough for you and you can see his/her face?

43. You are with five or six friends or family members at a gathering of more than twenty people and there is a background noise such as music or a crowd of people. One person talks at a time. When you are aware of the subject, can you understand what is being said when the speaker's voice is loud enough for you and you can see his/her face?

44. You are with five or six strangers at a gathering of more than twenty people and there is background noise such as music or a crowd of people. One person talks at a time. When you are aware of the subject, can you understand what is being said when the speaker's voice is loud enough for you and you can see his/her face?

45. You are with five or six friends or family members at a gathering of more than twenty people and several people are talking nearby. One person talks at a time and the subject of conversation changes from time to time. Can you understand what is being said when the speaker's voice is loud enough for you and you can see his/her face?

46. You are with five or six friends or family members at a gathering of more than twenty people and there is background noise such as music or a crowd of people. One person talks at a time and the subject of conversation changes from time to time. Can you understand what is being said when the speaker's voice is loud enough for you and you can see his/her face?

47. You are having dinner with five or six friends or family m embers at home and there is background noise such as music or a crowd of people. Can you understand what is being said when the speaker's voice is loud enough for you and you can see his/her face?

48. You are seated with five or six strangers around a table or in a living room. Often two persons are talking at once and one person frequently interrupts another. Can you understand what is being said when the speaker's voice is loud enough for you and you can see his/her face?

49. You are playing cards, monopoly or some similar game and several people are talking nearby. The subject of conversation changes from time to time. Can you understand what is being said when the speaker's voice is loud enough for you and you can see his/her face?

50. You are riding in an automobile with several friends or family members. The windows are <u>closed</u> and you are sitting in the front seat. Can you understand the driver when his/her voice is loud enough for you and you can see his/her face?

51. You are riding in an automobile with several friends or family members. One or more of the windows are <u>open</u> and you are sitting in the front seat. Can you understand the driver when his/her voice is loud enough for you and you can see his/her face?

52. You are the driver in an automobile with several friends or family members. The windows are closed. Can you understand the passenger behind you when his/her voice is loud enough for you?

53. You are the driver in an automobile with several friends or family members. One or more of the windows are <u>open</u>. Can you understand the passenger behind you when his/her voice is loud enough for you?

54. You are talking to a woman sitting in a ticket or information booth and it is fairly noisy. She is giving directions or information. Can you understand her when her voice is loud enough for you and you can see her face?

55. You are talking to a man sitting in a ticket or information booth and it is fairly noisy. He is giving directions or information. Can you understand him when his voice is loud enough for you and you can see his face?

56. You are in a room with background noise such as music or a crowd of people. Can you carry on a conversation with a person from another room if his/her voice is loud enough for you?

57. Can you hear an airplane in the sky when others around you can hear it?

58. Can you hear birds singing outside when others around you can hear them?

59. Can you hear water running in another room when others around you can hear it?

60. You are reading in a quiet room. Can you hear a person calling you from another room?

61. You are reading in a room with music or noise in the background. Can you hear a person calling you from another room?

62. You are at home reading in a quiet room. Do you hear the telephone ring when it is in another room?

63. You are at home watching television or listening to the radio. Can you hear the telephone ring when is is located in another room?

64. You are at home watching television or listening to the radio. Can you hear the doorbell ring when it is located in the <u>same</u> room?

65. You are at home watching television or listening to the radio. Can you hear the doorbell ring when it is located in <u>another</u> room?

66. When others are listening to speech on the television or radio, is it loud enough for you?

67. If you are riding in a car and you know that others are listening to music on the car radio, do you hear the music?

68. Do you find that children (6 to 10 years old) speak loudly enough for you?

69. When you are in your kitchen, do you hear the refrigerator motor going on and off?

70. You are in a quiet place and the person seated on the side of your better ear whispers to you. Can you hear the whisper?

71. How often do women speak loudly enough for you to hear them?

72. How often do men speak loudly enough for you to hear them?

73. When an announcement is given over a public address system in a bus station or airport, is it loud enough for you to hear?

74. You are in a fairly quiet room and a person is talking to you from a distance of no more than six feet. Would you be aware that he/she is talking if you did not see his/her face?

75. A person is talking to you from a distance of no more than six feet, with music or noise in the background. Would you be aware that he/she is talking if you did not see his/her face?

76. You are at a restaurant. When you miss something important that the waitress/waiter said, do you ask for it to be repeated?

77. You are talking with a close friend. When you miss something important that was said, do you immediately adjust your hearing aid to help you hear better?

78. You are talking with five or six friends. When you miss something important that was said, do you ask the person talking to repeat it?

79. You are talking with a stranger. When you miss something important that was said, do you let him/her know that you have a hearing problem?

80. You are talking with a friend or family member. When you miss something important that was said do you pretend you understood?

81. You are with a friend or family member and you hear only a portion of what was said. Do you repeat that portion before asking him/her for a repetition?

82. You are seated with five or six friends or family members around a table or in a living room. Often two persons are talking at once and one person frequently interrupts another. When you miss something important that was said, do you remind the person talking that you have a hearing problem?

83. You are talking with a friend or family member. When they miss something important that was said, do you ask for it to be repeated?

84. You are having dinner with five or six friends. When you miss something important that was said, do you let the person talking know you have a hearing problem?

85. At the beginning of a conversation, do you let a stranger know that you have a hearing problem?

86. You are seated with five or six strangers around a table or in a living room. Often two persons are talking at once and one person frequently interrupts another. When you miss something important that was said, do you pretend you understood?

87. You are seated with five or six strangers around a table or in a living room. Often two persons are talking at once and one person frequently interrupts another. When you miss something important that was said, do you let the person talking know you have a hearing problem?

88. You are with five or six friends or family members. One person at a time talks to the group. When you miss something important that was said, do you ask the person next to you?

89. You are seated with five or six friends around a table or in a living room. Often two persons are talking at once and one person frequently interrupts another. When you miss something that was said, do you ask the person talking to repeat it?

90. You are at a restaurant and you hear only a portion of something the waitress/waiter said. Do you repeat the portion before asking him/her for a repetition?

91. You are with five or six strangers. One person at a time talks to the group. When you miss something important that was said do you ask the person next to you?

92. You are with five or six strangers and you hear only a portion of what was said. Do you repeat that portion before asking the speaker for a repetition?

93. You are having dinner with five or six friends. When you miss something important that was said, do you ask the person talking to repeat it?

94. You are with five or six friends or family members. One person talks at a time. When you miss something important that was said, do you pretend you understood?

95. You are at a play, movie or listening to a speech. When you miss something important that was said, do you ask the person with you?

96. You are talking with five or six strangers. When you miss something important that was said, do you ask the person talking to repeat it?

97. You are having dinner with five or six friends and you hear only a portion of what was said. Do you repeat that portion before asking the speaker for a repetition?

98. You are talking with a stranger. When you miss something important that was said, do you ask for it to be repeated?

99. You are with five or six friends or family members. One person at a time talks to the group. When you miss something important that was said, do you immediately adjust your hearing aid to help you hear better?

100. You are with five or six friends or family members and you hear only a portion of what was said. Do you repeat that portion before asking the speaker for a repetition?

101. You are talking with five or six strangers. When you miss something important that was said, do you let the person talking know you have a hearing problem?

102. You are at a small social gathering. If you have difficulty hearing what is being said, do you move to a place where you can hear better?

103. When you have difficulty understanding a person with a pipe, toothpick or similar object in his/her mouth, do you ask him/her to remove the object?

104. When you are having difficulty following what someone is saying, do you keep trying until you are able to understand?

105. When you have difficulty understanding a person who speaks quite rapidly, do you ask him/her to speak more slowly?

106. You are at a committee meeting. If you have difficulty hearing what is being said, do you move to a place where you can hear better?

107. When you have difficulty understanding a person because he is holding his hand in front of his mouth, do you ask him to lower his hand?

108. You are at a lecture. If you have difficulty hearing what is being said, do you move to a place where you can hear better?

109. You are with a friend or family member in a fairly quiet room. Can you understand him/her when his/her voice is loud enough for you, but you cannot see his/her face?

110. You are with a stranger in a fairly quiet room. Can you understand him/her when his/her voice is loud enough for you, but you cannot see his/her face?

111. You are with a stranger and there is background noise such as music or a crowd of people. Can you understand the person when his/her voice is loud enough for you, but you cannot see his/her face?

112. You are at a party or gathering of less than ten people and the room is fairly quiet. Can you understand what a friend or family member is saying to you when his/her voice is loud enough for you, but you cannot see his/her face?

113. You are at a party or gathering of less than ten people and there is noise such as music or a crowd of people. Can you understand what a family member is saying to you when his/her voice is loud enough for you, but you cannot see his/her face?

114. You are at a party or gathering of more than twenty people and there noise such as music or a crowd of people. Can you understand what a family member is saying to you when his/her voice is loud enough for you, but you cannot see his/her face?

115. You are at a party or gathering of more than twenty people and there noise such as music or a crowd of people. Can you understand what a stranger is saying to you when his/her voice is loud enough for you, but you cannot see his/her face?

116. You are in a fairly quiet room with five or six friends or family members. One person talks at a time. When you are aware of the subject, can you understand what is being said when the speaker's voice is loud enough for you but you cannot see his/her face?

117. You are with five or six friends or family members and there is background noise such as music or a crowd of people. One person talks at a time. When you are aware of the subject, can you understand what is being said when the speakers voice is loud enough for you, but you cannot see his/her face?

118. You are in a fairly quiet room with five or six strangers. One person talks at a time. When you are aware of the subject, can you understand what is being said when the speaker's voice is loud enough for you, but you can<u>not</u> see his/her face?

119. You are with five or six strangers and there is background noise such as music or a crowd of people. One person talks at a time. When you are aware of the subject, can you understand what is being said when the speaker's voice is loud enough for you, but you cannot see his/her face?

120. You are in a fairly quiet room talking with five or six friends or family members. One person talks at a time. The subject of conversation changes from time to time. Do you understand what is being said when the speaker's voice is loud enough but you cannot see his/her face?

121. You are having dinner with five or six friends or family members at home and there is background noise such as music or a crowd of people. Can you understand what is being said when the speaker's voice is loud enough for you, but you cannot see his/her face?

122. You are playing cards, monopoly or some similar game and the room is fairly quiet. The subject of conversation changes from time to time. Can you understand what is being said when the speaker's voice is loud enough for you, but you cannot see his/her face?

123. You are playing cards, monopoly or some similar game and there is background noise such as music or a crowd of people. The subject of conversation changes from time to time. Can you understand what is being said when the speaker's voice is loud enough for you, but you can<u>not</u> see his/her face?

124. Does your hearing problem discourage you from going to the movies?

125. Does your hearing problem discourage you from attending lectures?

126. Does your hearing problem discourage you from going to concerts?

127. Does your hearing problem discourage you from going to plays?

128. Does your hearing problem lower your self confidence?

129. Does your hearing problem tend to make you nervous and tense?

130. Does your hearing problem tend to make you impatient?

131. Do you feel that others cannot understand what it is to have a hearing problem?

OCCUPATIONAL ITEMS

132. You are with a female co-worker at work in a fairly quiet room. Can you understand her when her voice is loud enough for you and you can see her face?

133. You are with a male co-worker at work in a fairly quiet room. Can you understand him when his voice is loud enough for you and you can see his face?

134. You are with your employer (foreman, supervisor, etc.) at work in a fairly quiet room. Can you understand him when his voice is loud enough for you and you can see his face?

135. You are in a fairly quiet room at work with five or six co-workers. One person talks at a time. When you are aware of the subject, can you understand what is being said when the speaker's voice is loud enough for you and you can see his/her face?

136. You are in a fairly quiet room at work with five or six co-workers. One person talks at a time and the subject of conversation changes from time to time. Can you understand what is being said when the speaker's voice is loud enough for you and you can see his/her face?

137. You are with a female co-worker at work and several people are talking nearby. Can you understand her when her voice is loud enough for you and you can see her face?

138. You are with a female co-worker at work and there is background noise such as traffic, music or a crowd of people. Can you understand her when her voice is loud enough for you and you can see her face?

139. You are with a male co-worker at work and several people are talking nearby. Can you understand him when his voice is loud enough for you and you can see his face?

140. You are with a male co-worker at work and there is background noise such as traffic, music or a crowd of people. Can you understand him when his voice is loud enough for you and you can see his face?

141. You are talking with your employer (foreman, supervisor, etc.) and several people are nearby. Can you understand him/her when his/her voice is loud enough and you can see his/her face?

142. You are with your employer (foreman, supervisor, etc.) and there is background noise such as traffic, music or a crowd of people. Can you understand him/her when his/her voice is loud enough for you and you can see his/her face?

143. You are at work with five or six co-workers and there is background noise such as music or a crowd of people. One person talks at a time and the subject of conversation changes from time to time. Can you understand what is being said when the speaker's voice is loud enough for you and you can see his/her face?

144. You are seated with five or six co-workers around a table at work. Often two persons are talking at once and one person frequently interrupts another. Can you understand what is being said when the speaker's voice is loud enough for you and you can see his/her face?

145. You are with five or six co-workers at work. One person talks at a time. When you miss something important that was said, do you pretend you understood?

146. You are talking with five or six co-workers at work. One person talks at a time. When you miss something important that was said, do you immediately adjust your hearing aid to help you hear better?

147. At the beginning of a conversation do you let your employer (foreman, supervisor, etc.) know that you have a hearing problem?

148. You are with a co-worker at work and you hear only a portion of what was said. Do you repeat that portion before asking the speaker for a repetition?

149. You are talking with your employer (foreman, supervisor, etc.) at work. When you miss something important that was said, do you pretend you understood?

150. At the beginning of a conversation, do you let your co-workers know that you have a hearing problem?

151. You are talking with a co-worker at work. When you miss something important that was said, do you immediately adjust your hearing aid to help you hear better?

152. You are talking with a co-worker at work. When you miss something important that was said, do you pretend you understood.

153. You are with your employer (foreman, supervisor, etc.) at work and you hear only a portion of what was said. Do you repeat that portion before asking the speaker for repetition?

154. You are talking with a co-worker or employer. When you miss something important that was said, do you let him/her know that you have a hearing problem?

155. You are talking with a co-worker at work. When you miss something important that was said, do you ask for it to be repeated?

156. Does your hearing problem interfere with helping or instructing others on the job?

157. Does your hearing problem interfere with your getting a job easily?

158. Does your hearing problem interfere with learning the duties of a new job easily?

ATTACHMENT 27 *Communication Profile for the Hearing Impaired (CPHI)*

The CPHI is a standardized 145-item self-report measure of adjustment to hearing impairment. This comprehensive instrument yields 25 scale scores and 3 importance ratings in 4 general areas. Scores represent mean responses to the items in each scale. The instrument uses a 5-point response scale to represent frequency of occurrence or extent to which respondents agree or disagree with each item. Low scores are indicative of difficulty or areas warranting rehabilitative attention. Most respondents complete the instrument in 30 to 45 minutes. Because of the instrument's length, the CPHI is not included here in its entirety. Copies of the instrument are available at cost from the test developers. The CPHI has been translated into Spanish, Swedish, Portuguese, and Russian. Gender-specific spouse/significant other forms have been developed and are also available at cost, as indicated below. A pass-fail screening measure for hearing disability and handicap has been constructed using CPHI data from more than 1000 individuals with hearing impairment. Computerized scoring programs can generate printed profiles in less than 3 minutes, which includes data entry. Profiles depict mean scores numerically and graphically so the individual's scores can be compared to the normative population.

Communication Performance: The scales in the Communication Performance section assess communication effectiveness in three settings: *Social, Work,* and *Home.* In addition to reporting how frequently effective communication occurs in these situations, respondents are asked to report how important it is to communicate effectively in each of these settings. Responses to these same items are also grouped to yield scores for communication effectiveness in *Average* and *Adverse* listening conditions. A sixth scale in the Communication Performance section is *Problem Awareness.* These items assess the extent to which individuals are aware that communication difficulties related to hearing loss sometimes occur. A low *Problem Awareness* score suggests that the respondent may not be aware of the extent of his or her communication problems or may not admit to these problems. A mid-range score supports the validity of the other Communication Performance scale scores. This can be very helpful to clinicians in ascertaining whether unusually high or low scores are valid or are a function of exaggerated or minimized problems.

Sample Items:

You're at a social gathering with music or other noise in the background. (*Social, Adverse*)
You're at work or a place of business and someone is talking to you from another room. (*Work, Adverse*)
You're at the dinner table with your family. (*Home, Average*)
At social gatherings I sometimes find it hard to follow conversations. (*Problem Awareness*)

Communication Environment: The scales in this section assess the *Need* for communication, the *Physical Characteristics* of listening environments, and the interpersonal environment created by the *Attitudes* and *Behaviors of Others.* A greater need for communication, difficult listening environments, and a poor interpersonal communication environment are likely to contribute to hearing disability and handicap.

Sample Items:

Communicating with others is an important part of my responsibilities. (*Need*)
I have to talk with others when there's a lot of background noise. (*Physical Characteristics*)
Others think I'm ignoring them if I don't answer when they speak to me. (*Attitudes of Others*)
Members of my family talk to me from another room. (*Behaviors of Others*)

Communication Strategies: Three scales comprise the Communication Strategies section of the CPHI. The first, *Maladaptive Strategies,* assesses the extent to which respondents' coping behaviors contribute to ongoing communication difficulties. Examples include ignoring others when they are speaking and pretending to understand. The remaining two scales assess the use of *Verbal* and *Nonverbal Strategies* that can minimize communication problems related to hearing loss. Asking others to repeat or speak up, sitting closer to speakers, and watching the speaker's face are strategies that enhance effective communication. The Communication Strategies scales highlight areas in need of rehabilitative intervention.

Sample Items:

I interrupt others when listening to them is difficult. (*Maladaptive Behaviors*)
I've asked my family to get my attention before speaking to me. (*Verbal Strategies*)
If I'm sitting where I can't hear, I'll move to another seat. (*Nonverbal Strategies*)

Personal Adjustment: The Personal Adjustment items assess several affective components of a person's acceptance of and adjustment to hearing impairment. The scales include attitudes about oneself and the hearing loss, as well as emotional reactions to communication problems. The Personal Adjustment scales include: *Self-Acceptance, Acceptance of Loss, Anger, Displacement of Responsibility, Exaggeration of Responsibility, Discouragement, Stress, Withdrawal,* and *Denial.* Scores in this area help identify those individuals for whom hearing impairment poses emotional distress. As in Communication Performance, one scale in this section, Denial, serves as a validity check for the remaining scales. The *Denial* items describe very common reactions to hearing difficulties and are specifically designed to elicit moderate agreement. Hence, extreme scores for this scale can be indicative of exaggerated or denied emotional responses and alert the clinician to the possibility of malingering or of an unrealistically positive picture of personal adjustment.

Sample Items:

I feel self-conscious because of my hearing loss. (*Self-Acceptance*)
It bothers me to admit that I have a hearing loss. (*Acceptance of Loss*)

I get aggravated when others don't speak up. (*Anger*)
If people want me to understand them, it's up to them to speak more clearly (*Displacement of Responsibility*)
I feel guilty about asking people to repeat for me. (*Exaggeration of Responsibility*)
I get discouraged because of my hearing loss. (*Discouragement*)
Straining to hear upsets me. (*Stress*)
Because of my hearing loss I keep to myself. (*Withdrawal*)
I sometimes feel embarrassed when I can't understand what someone has said. (*Denial*)

BIBLIOGRAPHY

Demorest ME. User's guide to the CPHI database system. Simpsonville, MD: CPHI Services, 1994.
Demorest ME, Erdman SA. Scale composition and item analysis of the Communication Profile for the Hearing Impaired. J Speech Hear Res 1986;29:515–535.
Demorest ME, Erdman SA. Development of the Communication Profile for the Hearing Impaired. J Speech Hear Disord 1987;52:129–143.
Demorest ME, Erdman SA. Retest stability of the Communication Profile for the Hearing Impaired. Ear Hear 1988;9:237–242.
Demorest ME, Erdman SA. Factor structure of the Communication Profile for the Hearing Impaired. J Speech Hear Dis 1989a;54:541–549.
Demorest ME, Erdman SA. Relationships among behavioral, environmental, and affective communication variables: a canonical analysis of the CPHI. J Speech Hear Disord 1989b;54:180–188.
Erdman SA, Demorest ME. CPHI manual: a guide to clinical use. Simpsonville, MD: CPHI Services, 1994.
Erdman SA, Demorest ME. Adjustment to hearing impairment I: description of a heterogeneous clinical population. J Speech Lang Hear Res 1998a;41:107–122.
Erdman SA, Demorest ME. Adjustment to hearing impairment II: audiological and demographic correlates. J Speech Lang Hear Res 1998;b41:123–136.

The following CPHI test forms, database management programs, scoring packages, and test manuals can be obtained at cost from:

Hearing Rehabilitation Laboratory
Department of Psychology
University of Maryland Baltimore County
1000 Hilltop Circle
Baltimore, MD 21250
CPHI
CPHI-H (for husbands or other significant males with hearing impairment)
CPHI-W (for wives or other significant females with hearing impairment)
CPHI Disability and Handicap Screening Test
CPHI-Spanish
CPHI-Portuguese
CPHI-Russian
CPHI Manual: A Guide to Clinical Use (1994)
CPHI Database Management and Scoring System (dBase)
User's Guide to the CPHI Database System (1994)

Windows based scoring programs for the CPHI and the CPHI Disability and Handicap Screening Test are available at cost from:

Computer Programming
School of Audiology and Speech Language Pathology
University of Memphis
Memphis Speech and Hearing Center
807 Jefferson
Memphis, TN 38105

ATTACHMENT 28 — COSI (The NAL Client-Oriented Scale of Improvement)

Name: _____

Audiologist: _____

Date: _____

1. Needs established _____

2. Outcome assessed _____

Degree of Change

"Because of the new hearing instrument, I now hear . . ."

	Worse	No Difference	Slightly Better	Better	Much Better

Final Ability (with hearing instrument)

"I can hear satisfactorily . . ."

	Hardly Ever 10%	Occasion-ally 25%	Half the Time 50%	Most of the Time 75%	Almost Always 95%

ATTACHMENT 29 *Profile of Hearing Aid Benefit (PHAB)*

A Always (99%)   B Almost Always (87%)   C Generally (75%)
D Half-the-time (50%)   E Occasionally (25%)   F Seldom (12%)   G Never (1%)

1. I can understand others in a small group situation if there is no noise.
2. When I am listening to a speaker who is talking to a large group, and I am seated toward the rear of the room, I must make an effort to listen.
3. Women's voices sound "shrill."
4. I find that most people speak too softly.
5. I have trouble comprehending speech when I am in a busy department store talking with the clerk.
6. I can understand my family when they speak softly to me.
7. I can understand a speaker in a small group, even when those around us are speaking softly to each other.
8. I can understand conversations even when several people are talking.
9. When the telephone rings, the sound startles me.
10. I have to ask people to repeat themselves when there is background noise.
11. When I am in a crowded grocery store, talking with the cashier, I can follow the conversation.
12. When I am having a conversation, and people are talking quietly nearby, I have to strain to understand the speaker.
13. If a car horn sounds, it makes me jump.
14. When I am talking to a group, and someone from the back of the room asks a question, I have to ask someone up front to repeat the question.
15. The sounds of construction work are uncomfortably loud.
16. When I am in a crowded reception room waiting to be called, I miss hearing my name.
17. When I am having a quiet conversation with a companion, I have difficulty understanding.
18. When I am listening to the news on the car radio, and family members are talking, I have trouble hearing the news.
19. The sound of screeching tires is uncomfortably loud.
20. I can understand conversation when I am walking with a friend through a quiet park.
21. The sound of a fire engine siren close by is so loud that I need to cover my ears.
22. When I am in conversation with someone across a large empty room (such as an auditorium), I understand the words.
23. When I am on a busy street, asking someone for directions, I have to ask him to repeat them before I really understand.
24. The sounds of running water, such as a toilet or shower, are uncomfortably loud.
25. When a speaker is addressing a small group, and everyone is listening quietly, I have to strain to understand.
26. I have trouble understanding dialogue in a movie or at the theater.
27. When I am in a crowd with a friend who doesn't want others to overhear our conversation, I have trouble hearing as well.
28. When I am at the dinner table with several people, and am trying to have a conversation with one person, understanding speech is difficult.
29. When I'm in a quiet conversation with my doctor in an examination room, it is hard to follow the conversation.
30. I have trouble understanding others when an air conditioner or fan is on.
31. I miss a lot of information when I'm listening to a lecture.
32. I can understand my family when they talk to me in a normal voice.
33. I have to ask people to repeat themselves in one-on-one conversation in a quiet room.
34. I have difficulty hearing a conversation when I'm with one other person at home.
35. When I am riding in the back seat of a car, and the driver talks to me from the front, I have to strain to understand.
36. Music sounds distorted to me.
37. When I'm talking with the teller at the drive-in window of my bank, I understand the speech coming from the loudspeaker.
38. When I am in a small office, interviewing or answering questions, I have difficulty following the conversation.
39. When a lecturer is giving instructions, I can easily follow along.
40. Everyday sounds are too soft for me to hear clearly.
41. I avoid using certain appliances (blender, vacuum cleaner, etc.) because their loudness is uncomfortable.

42. When I am in a busy restaurant and the waitress is taking my order, I can comprehend her questions.

43. I avoid crowds because the noise is uncomfortably loud.

44. When I'm at a large, noisy party, conversation is very confusing.

45. When I am in a theater watching a movie or play, and the people around me are whispering and rustling paper wrappers, I can still make out the dialogue.

46. When I am in a quiet restaurant, I can understand soft conversation.

47. I can't understand the TV news when the volume is set by a normal hearing person.

48. I can understand conversation during a quiet dinner with my family.

49. When I am listening to the news on my car radio, and the car windows are closed, I understand the words.

50. The sound quality of music isn't very good.

51. The ring of a telephone sounds "tinny".

52. I understand the newscaster when I am watching TV news at home alone.

53. I can follow the words of a sermon when listening to a religious service.

54. When I am at home, talking with someone who is in another room, following the conversation is difficult.

55. Unexpected sounds, like a smoke detector or alarm bell are uncomfortable.

56. When I'm talking with a friend outdoors on a windy day, I miss a lot of the conversation.

57. Everyday sounds that don't bother others are too loud for me.

58. It's hard for me to understand what is being said at lectures or church services.

59. When I am in a room with the door closed and I want to overhear a conversation going on outside the door, I have to strain to listen.

60. People's voices sound unnatural.

61. When I am in a face-to-face conversation with one member of my family, I can easily follow along.

62. When I am in a meeting with several other people, I can comprehend speech.

63. Traffic noises are too loud.

64. The sound of glass breaking is uncomfortably loud.

65. I can communicate with others when we are in a crowd.

66. I understand speech when I am talking to a bank teller, and I am one of a few customers at the bank.

Reprinted with permission from Cox RM, Gilmore C, Alexander GC. Comparison of two questionnaires for patient-assessed hearing aid benefit. J Am Acad Audiol 1991;2:134–145.

ATTACHMENT 30

Hearing Handicap Inventory for Adults—Screener

INSTRUCTIONS: The purpose of this questionnaire is to identify the problems your hearing loss may be causing you. Circle Yes, Sometimes, or No, for each question. **DO NOT SKIP A QUESTION IF YOU AVOID A SITUATION BECAUSE OF A HEARING PROBLEM.**

E-1	Does your hearing problem cause you to feel embarrassed when meeting new people?	Yes	Sometimes	No
E-2	Does a hearing problem cause you to feel frustrated when talking to members of your family?	Yes	Sometimes	No
S-1	Does a hearing problem cause you difficulty hearing/understanding co-workers, clients, or customers?	Yes	Sometimes	No
E-3	Do you feel handicapped by a hearing problem?	Yes	Sometimes	No
S-2	Does a hearing problem cause you difficulty when visiting friends, relatives, or neighbors?	Yes	Sometimes	No
S-3	Does a hearing problem cause you difficulty in the movies or theater?	Yes	Sometimes	No
E-4	Does a hearing problem cause you to have arguments with family members?	Yes	Sometimes	No
S-4	Does a hearing problem cause you difficulty when listening to the TV or radio?	Yes	Sometimes	No
E-5	Do you feel that any difficulty with your hearing limits or hampers your personal or social life?	Yes	Sometimes	No
S-5	Does a hearing problem cause you difficulty when in a restaurant with relatives or friends?	Yes	Sometimes	No

Score E:
Score S:
Score T:

ATTACHMENT 31 — *Hearing Aid Needs Assessment (HANA)*

Question	Subscale
1. You are one of only a few customers inside your bank and are talking with a teller.	Quiet
2. You are at home reading the paper. Two family members are in another room talking quietly and you want to listen in on their conversation.	No visual cues
3. You are in a quiet conversation with your family doctor in an examination room.	Quiet
4. You are driving your car with the windows down and are carrying on a conversation with others riding with you.	Noise
5. You are home in face-to-face conversation with one member of your family.	Quiet
6. You are at church listening to a sermon and sitting in the back pew.	No visual cues
7. You are at a large, noisy party and are engaged in conversation with one other person.	Noise
8. You are in your backyard gardening. Your neighbor is using a noisy power lawnmower and yells something to you.	Noise
9. Someone is trying to tell you something in a small quiet room while you have your back turned.	No visual cues
10. You are starting to cross a busy street and a car horn sounds a warning.	Nonspeech
11. You are at home alone listening to your stereo system (instrumental music).	Nonspeech

From Schum D. Perceived hearing aid benefit in relation to perceived needs. J Am Acad Audiol 1999;10:40–45.

Page numbers in parentheses refer to reference list entries.

Page numbers in *italics* denote figures; those followed by a t denote tables.

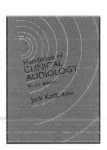
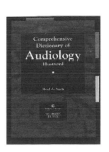
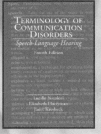
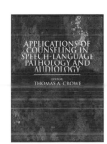